# MEDICAL NEUROSCIENCE

# MEDICAL NEUROSCIENCE

**Stephen E. Nadeau, Tanya S. Ferguson, Edward Valenstein, Charles J. Vierck, Jeffrey C. Petruska, Wolfgang J. Streit, and Louis A. Ritz**

*Departments of Neuroscience and Neurology*
*University of Florida College of Medicine*

*with contributions by:*
Patrick J. Antonelli, Purvis Bedenbaugh, Kevin S. Cahill, Arthur L. Day, John Guy,
N. Scott Howard, Richard D. Johnson, Satya P. Kalra, Robert H. Lenox,
Christina M. Leonard, Michael K. Maraist, David A. Peace, Philip Posner, Paul J. Reier,
Richard P. Schmidt, Jeffrey P. Staab, Dennis A. Steindler, Floyd J. Thompson,
William J. Triggs, Herbert E. Ward, Joseph J. Warner, and Robert T. Watson

*Artwork by George Kelvin*
with contributions by Tanya S. Ferguson, David A. Peace, Edward Valenstein, and Joseph J. Warner

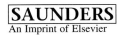
**SAUNDERS**
An Imprint of Elsevier

SAUNDERS

An Imprint of Elsevier

The Curtis Center
Independence Square West
Philadelphia, Pennsylvania 19106

MEDICAL NEUROSCIENCE                                                          ISBN 0-7216-0249-5

**Cover**: The traditional foundation of this text in neuroanatomy and neural systems is symbolized by the
stained sagittal sections of the brain. The sagittal MRI at the center emphasizes the major innovation: the
extensive linking of neuroscientific principles to clinical manifestations in the service of vertical integration of
the neuroscience and neurology curriculum. The strong thematic emphasis of the text on functional principles
coupled with our growing understanding of neural network function in terms of nonlinear dynamic systems is
symbolized by the Lorenz attractor weaving in and out of the brain images. Finally, we wished to capture the
beauty of the nervous system, surely no better exemplified than by the Purkinje cell.

---

**NOTICE**

Medicine is an ever-changing field. Standard safety precautions must be followed, but as new research and
clinical experience broaden our knowledge, changes in treatment and drug therapy may become
necessary or appropriate. Readers are advised to check the most current product information provided by
the manufacturer of each drug to be administered to verify the recommended dose, the method and
duration of administration, and contraindications. It is the responsibility of the licensed prescriber or health
care provider, relying on experience and knowledge of the patient, to determine dosages and the best
treatment for each individual patient. Neither the publisher nor the author assumes any liability for any
injury and/or damage to persons or property arising from this publication.

---

**Library of Congress Cataloging-in-Publication Data**

Medical neuroscience/Stephen E. Nadeau . . . [et al.].—1st ed.
       p. ; cm.
     Includes index.
     ISBN 0-7216-0249-5
     1. Neurophysiology.   I. Nadeau, Stephen E.
     [DNLM:   1. Nervous System Physiology.   2. Neurosciences. WL 102 M489 2004]
     QP361.M39 2004
     612.8—dc22

                                                                            2003066812

Printed in China

Last digit is the print number:   9   8   7   6   5   4   3   2   1

*To Sue Nadeau, Toby A. Ferguson, Candace Valenstein, Cheryl Vierck, Sara Ellen Petruska, Sybil Streit, and Jodi Neely-Ritz, whose unflagging support and patience made all this possible*

# Preface for Educators

The primary goal of this text, and the working principle that guided its writing, was vertical integration: the concept that the teaching of neuroscience through the four years of medical school should be a highly organized, seamless process that assures acquisition of the neurologic skills and knowledge demanded of today's medical generalist. The process of vertical integration requires from the beginning a clear understanding of the clinical capabilities that will be needed. From these clinical capabilities can be inferred the basic scientific principles necessary to understand them. A vertically integrated neuroscientific curriculum confers a number of benefits. It defines what subset of the vast realm of neuroscientific knowledge should be presented to medical students. To the extent that basic and clinical science are linked throughout the teaching process, there is a measure of redundancy that helps students retain knowledge. Medical students, unsurprisingly, are particularly intrigued by clinical material, and case vignettes in a basic science text can thus serve to enhance their interest. The time-tested rule of basic science graduate education—that students should be introduced to the laboratory as soon as possible—applies equally to medical students, with the qualification that their laboratory is the clinic. Case vignettes provide for them a halfway step into the clinical domain, in the same way that the discussion of how discoveries were made provides an equivalent halfway step for the graduate student.

Vertical integration carries some potential risks, which we have strived to avoid. In the extreme, it can lead to a sort of medical apprenticeship, in which students focus exclusively on a set of case scenarios, and the basic science becomes so limited and fragmented that students never really have the opportunity to develop the most essential skill of all: the ability to think creatively and scientifically in dealing with the ever varying and perplexing problems posed by patients. In this extreme, there is also the risk that all courses, in effect, teach clinical medicine. This text avoids these problems in several ways. It is organized around the basic science. Case vignettes serve exclusively to illustrate or elaborate basic scientific principles, not to teach clinical medicine. The text is heavily focused on concepts, problem solving, and thinking skills, the fundamental tools medical students will need at the bedside, but it eschews clinical detail. Although learning neuroscience inevitably involves the acquisition of a rather substantial vocabulary, we have attempted to get away, to the extent possible, from teaching facts. Fact knowledge is required only to the extent that it is needed to understand concepts.

Vertical integration, narrowly construed, risks exposing students only to the narrow channels of knowledge absolutely necessary to understand targeted clinical skills. It therefore risks depriving students of the wonder and beauty of the vast landscape of neuroscience as we know it today. We have taken a broad view of vertical integration and have not hesitated to delve into many topics in some depth. In the process, we have risked overwhelming students with far more information than even the most brilliant could effectively master in a medical school course. In fact, we encourage students to use the text as a reference two years later, during their neurology clerkship, and the text is sophisticated enough to serve usefully as a neuroscience primer for neurology residents. To keep our neuroscience course from becoming overwhelming, we teach strictly to the objectives and the problem sets in the text. We also explicitly introduce the concept of graded knowledge, that students must acquire knowledge of differing degrees of detail, some precise and highly detailed, some at the level of only a rough sense of very broad relationships. For many students, this type of knowledge acquisition, although it reflects the reality of clinical medicine, will be a novel experience, and quite stressful, accustomed as they are to learning the precise facts that will appear on the final examination and none other.

*Medical Neuroscience* is not intended to be comprehensive. For material to be included in the text, it had to be (1) of direct clinical import for the medical generalist; (2) crucial to understanding a key neuroanatomic or physiologic principle; or (3) sufficiently exciting or dramatic to merit inclusion even in the absence of direct or indirect clinical relevance. During our writing of the text, these three criteria repeatedly guided the resolution of controversies regarding inclusion or exclusion of selected topics. More generally, our annual trials of the text with students served to repeatedly remind us that in a very real sense, a medical neuroscience course is a zero sum game: all but the very best students tend to be overwhelmed by the amount of material presented, mandating that detail added in one area be balanced by detail deleted in another. In our emphasis on concepts, functions, and problem solving approaches, and our strict adherence to the three major inclusion criteria, we have excluded or attenuated the treatment of a number of traditional topics. Developmental neurobiology has not been included except in passing. In our focus on the principles of clinicoanatomic correlation in the brainstem and thalamus, we have included fewer histologic sections and made greater use of diagrams and other drawn illustrations than is traditional. Ascending auditory pathways, and the details of thalamic, cerebellar, and hypothalamic connections have not been described at all because these topics did not meet our

inclusion criteria. We are satisfied that *Medical Neuroscience* uniquely meets the needs of our students as a neuroanatomic atlas and a neuroscience text. However, all students will benefit from supplementation of the text with laboratory exposure to gross and histologic material and from access to more comprehensive atlases, more advanced texts (e.g., Kandel, Schwartz, and Jessell, *Principles of Neural Science;* and Zigmond, Bloom, Landis, Roberts, and Squire, *Fundamental Neuroscience*), and the many useful Web sites and other computer-based material that are now available.

This text is testimony to the capacity of clinicians and basic scientists to work together in developing the details of a basic science course in a way that meets the goals and requirements of all, and helps assure that the material included is accurate and up to date. The process has also included three first- and second-year medical students, Kevin Cahill, Scott Howard, and Michael Maraist, who helped us better understand the perspective of students in the course and were instrumental in detecting areas of weakness or lack of clarity. Though often arduous, writing this text has for many of us been one of the most positive experiences of our academic careers.

# Preface for Medical Students

This introductory neuroscience text is written specifically for medical students. It focuses on the basic neuroscientific knowledge base that the physician generalist needs in order to deal intelligently and flexibly with the clinical problems she or he will face.

Chapter 1 introduces some basic anatomy and a considerable amount of vocabulary. Thereafter, anatomy and function are discussed together in an integrated fashion, and many clinical case discussions appear in the text. The goal is to enable you to understand the basic science, including anatomy and physiology, in a clinical context. We hope that this will prepare you better for your future work with patients and help you remember basic neuroscience when you work with patients. This approach to medical education is often referred to as vertical integration. The idea is that basic science faculty and clinical science faculty collaborate to assemble a comprehensive educational program, all parts of which are melded together in a seamless whole. The ultimate goals of this program are to assure the clinical competencies that you will need to have by the time you graduate. The requisite clinical competencies determine the requisite basic science competencies. Any medical student could bypass the basic sciences and do an apprenticeship on clinic services. He or she would become reasonably adept at handling the actual clinical problems encountered during that apprenticeship. However, most patients do not fit any exact mold, and it requires creative, scientifically based thinking to figure out what they really have and what to do about it. This is why basic science knowledge and the ability to use it creatively to solve clinical problems are so important. Medical education must fuse basic and clinical science throughout. In early courses, such as this one, the logical emphasis is on the basic science, but its relationship to clinical science, and the ultimate importance of problem solving (rather than simple fact learning) cannot be forgotten. This text provides this basic science–clinical science fusion and strongly emphasizes thinking skills and problem solving over learning facts.

This text contains far more material than anyone, however brilliant, could possibly master in any one medical school neuroscience course. It was written in this way for several reasons. We hope to give you a vivid glimpse of the marvels of the human nervous system, something that cannot be done with an exclusive focus on what you absolutely need to know. We intend this text to be a useful reference later in medical school, and perhaps later in your career. We are also introducing what may be, for many of you, a novel responsibility— a responsibility for acquiring varying depths of knowledge, some absolute and precise, some at the level of general concepts, some at the level of awareness or "gut feeling." In many of your courses so far, you have been able to divide knowledge into what you absolutely needed to know and what you absolutely did not need to know. Good physicians cannot do this. Rather, they must maintain precise and comprehensive knowledge and skills in their immediate area of expertise, general knowledge about their overall field (e.g., medicine, surgery), and a sense of what is happening across the entire breadth of medicine. This "graded" knowledge base is critical to good clinical judgment. This course is an explicit exercise in the acquisition of a graded knowledge base.

How can you know what we expect you to know and what you will be held responsible for on tests? The text provides many explicit guides. At the beginning of each section is a set of objectives. At the end of most sections, there are some problems. Throughout the text, selected terms and fundamental principles are set in italic type. If you can provide answers that satisfy the objectives, you can solve the problems, and if you know the key terms and principles, then you have learned what we intended and you will do well in the course. As you read the text the first time and as you review for tests, use the objectives, problems sets, and italicized text to guide your studies. All material in smaller font, whether within the body of the text or in footnotes, is optional and is included for your interest only.

A note of caution: Some of you will view this as a basic science course and conclude that the clinical cases throughout the text are "window dressing." To the contrary, much of this course is taught through the cases. Many of the cases are somewhat complicated (as real life cases are), but if you understand the essential neuroscientific point being made by every case, you will have made a great deal of progress toward learning what you need to know and achieving the nec-essary thinking and problem-solving skills. If you accomplish the objectives of this course, you will have made a remarkable achievement, about which you can be quite proud, even as you are aware of the vast amount of neuroscience you do not yet know or understand.

# Acknowledgments

Many other people contributed to the creation of this book. We gratefully acknowledge the assistance of M. Tariq Bhatti, Pushpa S. Kalra, Katherine A. Karpinia, Pamela J. LaFrentz, Albert L. Rhoton, Gerard P.J. Shaw, Ryusui Tanaka, Natalie K. Thomas, and Greg Weslye. The leadership provided by Robert T. Watson, Senior Associate Dean for Educational Affairs, and Lynn J. Romrell, Associate Dean for Education, University of Florida College of Medicine, has been instrumental in creating the fertile environment that makes innovative medical education projects like this one possible. We wish to thank Jason Malley and Inta Ozols, our editors at Elsevier Science, and Joan Sinclair and Karen O'Keefe Owens, also of Elsevier Science; they have enthusiastically supported us from our first contacts with them, have been of inestimable assistance, and have made our working relationship with Elsevier a great pleasure. Finally, we thank Lee Jackson, our copy editor, and we are tremendously indebted to Peggy M. Gordon, who did a magnificent job of bringing together all the threads of the complex publication process.

# Contents

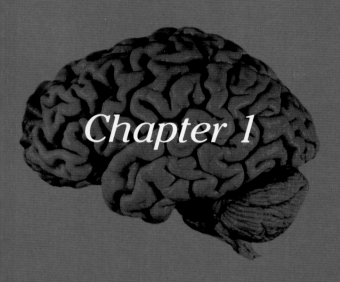

*Chapter 1*

# MAJOR DIVISIONS OF THE CENTRAL NERVOUS SYSTEM

## An Introduction and Overview

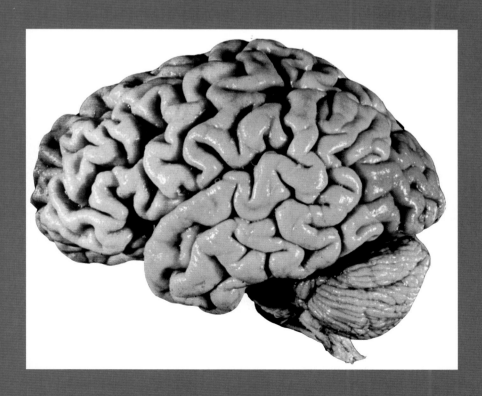

# Chapter 1

# MAJOR DIVISIONS OF THE CENTRAL NERVOUS SYSTEM
## An Introduction and Overview

# Introduction

We study the brain at many levels, from specific molecules to complex systems. At each of these levels, we are exposed to a bewildering body of details. If we are to fit these details into a broad view of nervous system structure and function, we must begin with a broad picture of the basic three-dimensional brain anatomy. The goal of this chapter is to create a three-dimensional perspective that will remain clear, even if memory of the details begins to fade.

In this chapter, we will encounter the brain in three increasing levels of detail. First (Cycle 1-1), we will learn some of the general terms that are used for describing locations and structures in the brain. Second (Cycles 1-2 and 1-3), we will identify the major divisions of the brain and spinal cord and will see how these divisions relate to the fluid-filled cavities within the brain—the ventricular system. Third, in Cycle 1-4, we will review the membranous coverings of the brain and the structures that anchor the brain within the skull.

In Cycles 1-5 through 1-11, we will consider each of these major divisions in some detail, looking at basic anatomic structure with some reference to function. In the final cycle (1-12), we will review the membranous coverings of the spinal cord. At the end of each cycle throughout the book there is a list of terms that you should know, and there may be one or more problems that test your understanding of the material in the cycle. Feedback on these problems is located at the end of each chapter.

This chapter is intended to be used as a laboratory manual, in conjunction with actual brain material, both intact and partially dissected. Brain models will be useful at times, particularly in understanding the spatial relationships of some of the deep structures. Two atlases will be useful in identifying specific brain structures, particularly in cross section:

1. DeArmond SJ, Fusco MM, Dewey MM. Structure of the Human Brain, 3rd ed. New York, Oxford, 1989.

2. Nolte J, Angevine JB. The Human Brain, 2nd ed. St. Louis, Mosby, 2000.

The following Web sites may be useful:

http://www.neurophys.wisc.edu/

One of the world's largest collections of well-preserved, sectioned, and stained brains of mammals, this site offers over 100 different species (including humans) representing 17 mammalian orders, includes a discussion of evolution, and gives links to many other Web sites.

http://www9.biostr.washington.edu/da.html

http://www.anatomy.wisc.edu

These interactive atlases of the human brain include gross views, histologic sections, drawings, computer-aided reconstructions, and movies that show complex structural relationships.

http://www.med.Harvard.edu/AANLIB/cases/caseM/case.html

This magnetic resonance image (MRI) atlas of the human brain offers a choice of labeled or unlabeled slices. It includes MRIs of normal human brains and of brains of patients with a variety of pathologic conditions, correlated with single photon emission computed tomographic (SPECT) images.

http://www.neuropat.dote.hu/

The Web site of neuroscience/neuropathology.

http://www.meddean.luc.edu/lumen/MedEd/Neuro/Neuro.html

Major Divisions of the Central Nervous System

This particularly well done atlas of brainstem, thalamus, basal ganglia and immediately adjacent structures pairs unadorned histologic sections with color demarcated sections demonstrating the location and extent of various structures and pathways. It also contains a tutorial on vasculature.

At the end of this chapter, Table 1-8 summarizes the organization of many of the structures and pathways discussed within the chapter into functional systems. You may find it helpful to refer to this table as you proceed through the chapter.

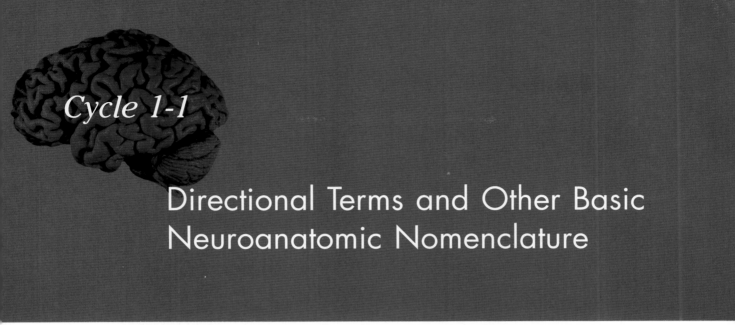

# Cycle 1-1

# Directional Terms and Other Basic Neuroanatomic Nomenclature

## Objective

Learn the terminology that is used for describing locations and structures in the brain.

Neuroanatomists use a standard set of terms to refer to specific directions in the brain (Fig. 1-1). This terminology is generally consistent with that used in gross anatomy. There is, however, a minor complication introduced by the fact that much of our knowledge of neuroanatomy comes from the study of quadrupedal animals (e.g., rats and cats), in which the long axis of the brain lies in a straight line with the brainstem and spinal cord. In a quadruped, we use *rostral* to indicate forward (i.e., toward the rostrum, or "beak") and *caudal* to indicate rear (i.e., toward the caudum, or "tail"). The back of a quadruped is continuous along a straight line with the top of the head, so *dorsal* consistently indicates toward the animal's back, and *ventral* consistently indicates toward the belly surface. *Medial* is toward the midline, and *lateral* is toward the side (away from the midline).

The human nervous system, in contrast, is flexed such that the long axis of the brain is at approximately a right angle with the axis of the brainstem and spinal cord. We use the same directional terms as in quadrupeds, but the orientation of the dorsal-to-ventral axis in humans differs between brain and spinal cord.

That is, the *dorsal* surface consists of the back of the spinal cord and the top surface of the brain. Also, in the human, we use the terms *anterior* to indicate front and *posterior* to indicate rear, and the terms *superior* and *inferior*, in the brain, correspond to dorsal and ventral, respectively. These terms are summarized below and in Figure 1-1.

*In human brain:*
rostral = anterior = forward
caudal = posterior = back
dorsal  = superior = toward the top of the skull
ventral = inferior = away from the top of the skull
medial = toward the midline
lateral  = toward the side

*In human brainstem and spinal cord:*
rostral  = toward the brain
caudal  = toward the tail end of the spinal cord
dorsal  = posterior = back
ventral = anterior = forward
medial  = toward the midline
lateral  = toward the side

We study the brain by cutting it into slices oriented in standard planes. These planes are represented in Figure 1-2. A *coronal* section through the brain is oriented parallel to the coronal suture of the skull, roughly parallel to the face. Coronal sections are left/right symmetrical, and one can refer to dorsal, ventral, medial, and lateral directions within each section. A horizontal or *axial* section of the brain is oriented horizontally (i.e.,

**Major Divisions of the Central Nervous System**

5

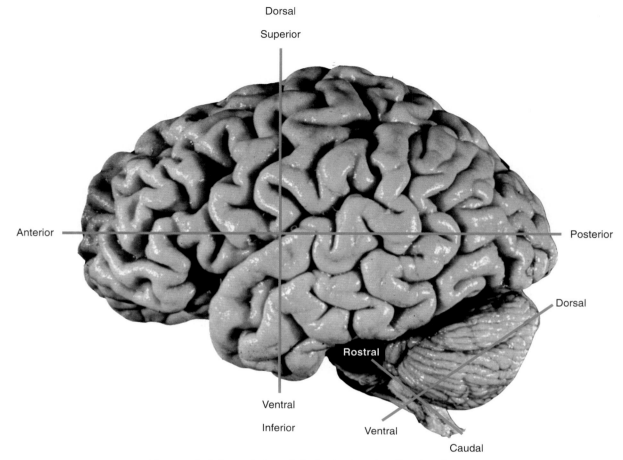

**Figure 1-1** Lateral view of the brain showing directional terms.

parallel to the floor) in an upright human. An axial section is also left/right symmetrical, and one can refer to anterior (rostral), posterior (caudal), medial, and lateral directions within the section. The term *transverse* is most often used to refer to horizontal sections of the brainstem and spinal cord. A *sagittal* section is oriented parallel to the midline, i.e., parallel to the sagittal suture of the skull. Sagittal sections are not front/back symmetrical. One can refer to anterior (rostral), posterior (caudal), dorsal (superior), and ventral (inferior) directions.

It is convenient at this point to introduce some of the general terms that are used for naming anatomic structures in the brain. The *central nervous system (CNS)* is the brain plus the spinal cord. A simple definition of the *peripheral nervous system (PNS)* is all the neural tissue outside the CNS. Regions of nerve cell bodies in the PNS are referred to as *ganglia*, whereas

in the CNS they are *nuclei*. Bundles of nerve fibers in the PNS are nerves, whereas they are referred to as *tracts* or pathways in the CNS.

Some CNS tracts that carry information in one direction are named for their origin and termination, in that order. For example, the spinothalamic tract carries information from the spinal cord to the thalamus, not from thalamus to spinal cord. Some tracts have other descriptive names, like *fasciculus* (a bundle), funiculus (a cord), or a *lemniscus* (a ribbon). Tracts that terminate on the same side of the nervous system as their origin are said to terminate *ipsilaterally*, whereas those that terminate on the opposite side terminate *contralaterally*. The point at which a tract crosses the midline of the CNS is known as its *decussation*. Some tracts branch to terminate on both sides of the midline—these terminate *bilaterally*.

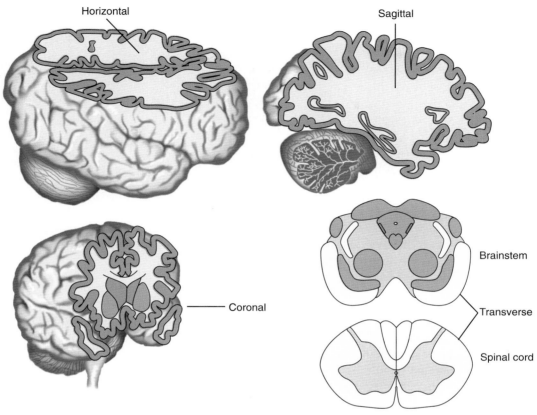

Horizontal

Sagittal

Coronal

Brainstem

Transverse

Spinal cord

**Figure 1-2** Standard planes of a section.

Nerves and tracts often are named according to whether they carry information toward or away from the periphery. Fibers that bring input to a given neural structure are known as *afferents*, whereas those that carry the output from a structure are *efferents*. Thus, sensory nerves are afferents and motor nerves are efferents.

In examining unstained cut brain specimens, you will notice that some areas have a shiny white appearance, whereas other areas are darker. The white areas, *white matter*, owe their color to the presence of large numbers of myelinated nerve fibers. *Myelin* is a fatty substance that surrounds some nerve fibers and results in an increase in the rate of nerve conduction. The darker areas, *the gray matter*, are made up of nerve cell bodies and are relatively devoid of myelin. Some of the brain sections illustrated in this chapter were stained for myelin. In these illustrations, areas that contain myelin appear dark, and myelin-free areas appear light.

## PRACTICE 1-1

**A.** Make sure you know the meaning of the following in both the cerebrum and the brainstem/spinal cord:

| | |
|---|---|
| dorsal | anterior |
| ventral | posterior |
| medial | coronal |
| lateral | axial |
| rostral | transverse |
| caudal | sagittal |

**B.** Make sure you know the meaning of the following:

| | |
|---|---|
| CNS | myelin |
| PNS | ganglia |
| decussation | nuclei |
| afferents | nerves |
| efferents | tracts |
| white matter | fasciculus |
| gray matter | lemniscus |

**Major Divisions of the Central Nervous System**

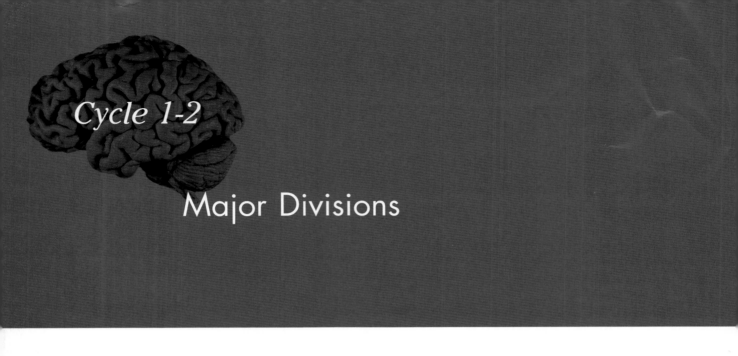

Cycle 1-2

# Major Divisions

### Objective

To identify in human brain material the major subdivisions of the brain and spinal cord.

The best way to become familiar with gross brain anatomy is to don rubber gloves and examine actual brain material. In this cycle, we will begin by identifying the major divisions of the brain and spinal cord in the intact and hemisected brain and in the isolated brainstem and cerebellum.

The brain is illustrated in lateral view in Figure 1-3. Any view of the intact brain is dominated by the two hemispheres of the highly convoluted *cerebral cortex*. This is the region of the brain that is most conspicuously developed in humans relative to other animals and to which we attribute our highest sensory, motor, and cognitive abilities. The folded appearance of the cerebral cortex reflects the large cortical surface area that is packed into a skull of limited volume. The outward ridges of the folds are known as *gyri*, and the inward grooves are *sulci*.

Posterior and ventral to the cerebral hemispheres is the *cerebellum* ("little brain") (Table 1-1). The cerebellum integrates the activity of the cerebral cortex with that of brainstem and spinal motor systems to coordinate movement. The light-colored structure that emerges from under the cerebral hemispheres and cerebellum is a portion of the *brainstem*. Caudally, the brainstem is continuous with the *spinal cord*, which has been cut off most of the specimens of whole brains.

On the cerebral hemispheres, one can identify four major lobes of the cerebral cortex. Named for the

**TABLE 1-1 Structures of the Brain and Their Functions**

| Structure | Function |
|---|---|
| Corpus callosum | Interconnects cerebral hemispheres |
| Septum pellucidum | Separates the lateral ventricles |
| Thalamus | Relays information from brainstem to cortex and between cortical regions |
| Hypothalamus | Regulates appetite, thirst, sexual drive; neuroendocrine; autonomic |
| Cerebral peduncles | Carry motor information from cerebrum to brainstem and spinal cord |
| Pyramids | Carry motor information from brainstem to spinal cord |
| Cerebellum | Coordinates movement of the body |
| Cerebellar peduncles | Carry information to and from the cerebellum |
| Superior colliculus | Visual system component |
| Inferior colliculus | Auditory system component |

*8*

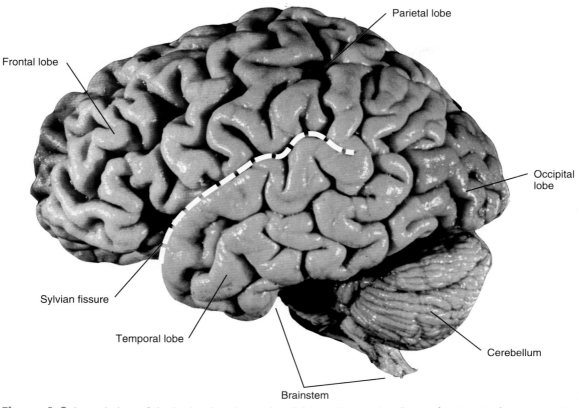

**Figure 1-3** Lateral view of the brain, showing major divisions. The sylvian fissure (*dashed line*) separates the frontal and parietal lobes from the temporal lobe.

skull bones that overlie them, they are the *frontal*, *parietal*, *occipital*, and *temporal lobes*. These lobes contain, among other things, the motor (frontal lobe), somatosensory (parietal lobe), visual (occipital lobe), and auditory (temporal lobe) cortical areas. We will distinguish these areas more precisely in Cycle 1-5. The lateral or *sylvian* fissure separates the frontal and parietal lobes from the temporal lobe.

The medial aspect of a cerebral hemisphere can be examined on a hemisected brain (Fig. 1-4). One can see the cut surface of a large white matter structure, the *corpus callosum*. This structure is an enormous bundle of fibers that interconnect the two cerebral hemispheres. In the hemisected brain, one sees the cut ends of the fibers. Beneath the corpus callosum is the *lateral ventricle*, a fluid-filled space within the cerebral hemisphere. Depending on exactly where the brain was hemisected, one might have a clear view into the ventricle, or the ventricle might be closed by a membranous midline *septum pellucidum*. The lateral ventricles (one in each hemisphere) are part of a series of fluid-

filled spaces within the brain that will be discussed more fully in the next cycle.

In the center of the medial view of the hemisphere, ventral to the corpus callosum, is an area of gray matter known as the *thalamus*. The thalamus lies on either side of the midline and, in some brains, extends across the midline at a restricted area known as the massa intermedia. The thalamus relays information from subcortical areas to the cerebral cortex and from one portion of the cortex to another. The ventral-most portion of the central area of gray matter is the *hypothalamus*. The hypothalamus is involved in aspects of appetitive ("motivated") behavior and neuroendocrine function, and it is the "head nucleus" of the autonomic nervous system. If the cerebellum is in place, one can see, on the cut surface, the gray cerebellar cortex and the underlying cerebellar white matter.

Next, examine a brainstem specimen from which the cerebral hemispheres and cerebellum have been cut away. The brainstem contains three major divisions: the *midbrain*, the *pons*, and the *medulla*. These three

**Major Divisions of the Central Nervous System**

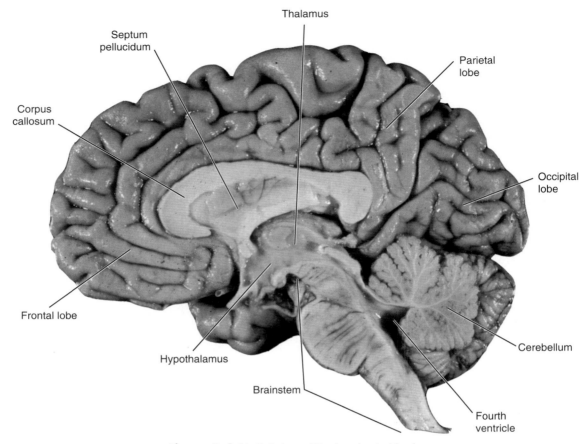

**Figure 1-4** Medial view of the hemisected brain.

divisions are clearly visible on the ventral surface (Fig. 1-5). The midbrain is identified by the paired *cerebral peduncles*. These bundles of longitudinal fibers carry largely motor information from the cerebral cortex to the brainstem and spinal cord. Caudal to the cerebral peduncles is the pons. The medulla is marked by the *pyramids*, which are longitudinal fiber bundles on the ventral surface that are in continuity with many of the fibers of the cerebral peduncles. Many of these fibers continue caudally to the spinal cord.

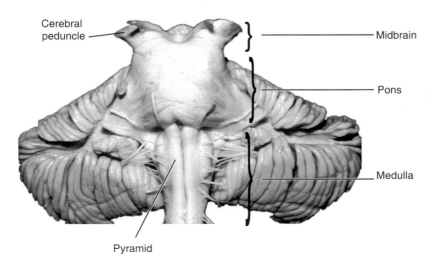

**Figure 1-5** Ventral view of the brainstem.

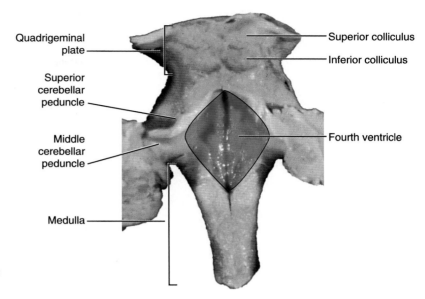

Quadrigeminal plate
Superior cerebellar peduncle
Middle cerebellar peduncle
Medulla
Superior colliculus
Inferior colliculus
Fourth ventricle

**Figure 1-6** Dorsal view of the brainstem with the cerebellum removed.

On the dorsal surface of the brainstem (Fig. 1-6) are four small bumps, which form the *tectum* ("roof") of the midbrain. The rostral bump on each side of the brainstem is the *superior colliculus* ("little hill"), which is a component of the visual system, and the caudal bump is the *inferior colliculus*, which is a component of the auditory system. The four colliculi form the *quadrigeminal plate*. At the level of the pons are the *cerebellar peduncles*, bundles of fibers that carry information to or from the cerebellum. These fibers have been cut to remove the cerebellum. Try to fit a cerebellum specimen on top of the pons to see the position of the cerebellum on the brainstem. Between the cerebellar peduncles is a space, the *fourth ventricle*. The dorsal surface of the brainstem forms the floor of the fourth ventricle, and the cerebellum forms most of the roof. The medulla begins caudal to the pons and tapers caudally toward the spinal cord. The spinal cord has been cut away; we will examine it in a later cycle.

## PRACTICE 1-2

Make sure you know the meaning and location of the following:

| | |
|---|---|
| sulci | medulla |
| gyri | spinal cord |
| cerebral cortex | tectum |
| frontal lobe | quadrigeminal plate |
| parietal lobe | superior colliculus |
| temporal lobe | inferior colliculus |
| occipital lobe | lateral ventricle |
| sylvian fissure | septum pellucidum |
| thalamus | fourth ventricle |
| hypothalamus | corpus callosum |
| brainstem | cerebral peduncles |
| midbrain | cerebellar peduncles |
| pons | pyramids |
| cerebellum | |

Major Divisions of the Central Nervous System

# The Ventricular System

## Objective

To learn the anatomy of the ventricular system and its relationship to the major CNS structures that surround it.

Deep within all the structures of the CNS is a series of fluid-filled cavities, which form the ventricular system. *Cerebrospinal fluid* is produced by a specialized tissue, the *choroid plexus*, lying within the ventricles. This fluid passes through several foramina into the subarachnoid space surrounding the brain. The brain literally floats in cerebrospinal fluid. We will have more to say later about cerebrospinal fluid circulation, but at this point, we will review the ventricular system as a useful set of landmarks or points of reference for other brain structures.

Figures 1-7 and 1-8 depict lateral and dorsal views of the ventricular system, respectively, and Figure 1-9 depicts the relationship of the parts of this system to the CNS structures surrounding them. For the insets at the tops of Figure 1-9A to F the brain has been sliced down the middle into two hemispheres and we are looking at the medial surface of one hemisphere. The line drawn on this inset figure shows the level of the coronal slice through the brain and brainstem. These coronal slices are depicted immediately below. At the bottom is a lateral view of the ventricular system showing the relationship of these coronal slices to the ventricles.

In Figure 1-9A, the slice cuts through the *frontal (anterior) horns* of the lateral ventricles. The lateral ventricles are delimited above by the *corpus callosum*, the enormous bundle of fibers connecting the two cerebral hemispheres. The frontal horns are separated by a thin membrane, the *septum pellucidum*. Directly lateral to the frontal horns are masses of *deep cerebral white matter* carrying connections between anterior and posterior parts of each hemisphere and between the frontal lobes (anterior to this section) and the brainstem. Ventrolateral to the frontal horns are large masses of gray matter, the *basal ganglia* (Table 1-2). These ganglia are divided by another important white matter tract, the *internal capsule* (barely visible in Fig. 1-9A, better seen in Fig. 1-9B), into a medial portion immediately adjacent to the ventricles, the *caudate nucleus*, involved in frontal lobe function, and a lateral portion, the *putamen*, involved in motor function.

Slice B also cuts through the frontal horns of the lateral ventricles but a little more posteriorly, so that it passes through the anterior-most part of the *third ventricle*. The passages from the lateral ventricles to the third ventricle are the *foramina of Monro*. The gray matter in the walls of this anterior portion of the third ventricle comprises the *hypothalamus*, which is involved in autonomic and neuroendocrine function. The caudate and putamen are again visible, still separated by the internal capsule. The putamen has been joined medially by another gray matter structure, intimately connected with it, the *globus pallidus*. Just lateral to the putamen is the *insular cortex*, a phyloge-

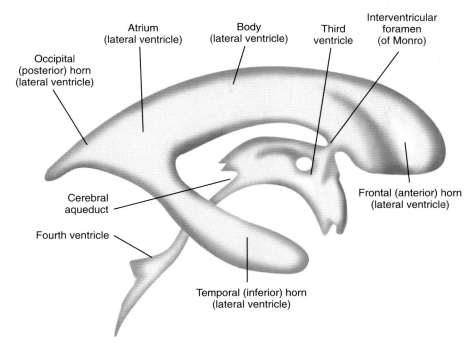

**Figure 1-7** Lateral view of ventricular system. (Modified from Warner JJ. Atlas of Neuroanatomy. Boston, Butterworth Heinemann, 2001.)

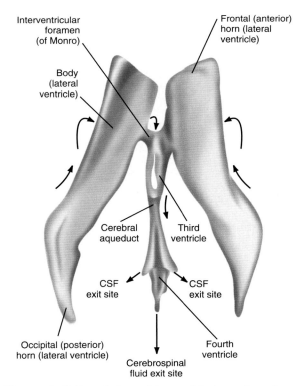

**Figure 1-8** Dorsal view of the ventricular system. Arrows indicate flow patterns of cerebrospinal fluid (CSF). (Modified from Warner JJ. Atlas of Neuroanatomy. Boston, Butterworth Heinemann, 2001.)

netically ancient cortex that has been overgrown by the frontal and temporal lobes, which here overlie it even more laterally. The cerebrospinal fluid space lying over the insula is the circular sulcus. The *circular sulcus* lies immediately beneath the sylvian fissure separating the frontal and parietal from the temporal lobes, on the lateral surface of the brain. Ventral to (below) the putamen and globus pallidus is another large gray matter structure, the *amygdala*, located in the medial temporal lobe. The amygdala is involved in emotional function. Just posterior to the ventrolateral margin of the amygdala is the *temporal horn* of the lateral ventricle. The amygdala lies immediately beneath the surface of a prominence on the anteromedial surface of the temporal lobe known as the *uncus*.

Slice *C* cuts through the body of the lateral ventricles and posterior regions of the third ventricle. Structures already familiar to you include the corpus callosum, septum pellucidum, deep cerebral white matter, putamen, and insula. The lateral walls of the third ventricle are now formed by the *thalamus*, a giant relay station within the brain. The thalamus is separated from the putamen by the internal capsule. Immediately below the putamen, the amygdala has been supplanted by the *hippocampus*, a structure that plays a crucial role in memory. Like the amygdala, the hippocampus lies adjacent to the temporal horn of the lateral ventricle.

*Text continued on p. 20*

**Major Divisions of the Central Nervous System**

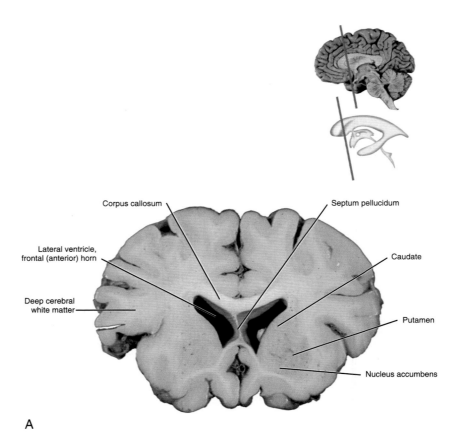

**Figure 1-9** The relationship of major CNS structures to the ventricular system. *A* through *C* show coronal sections; *D* through *F* show transverse sections stained for myelin; see insets.

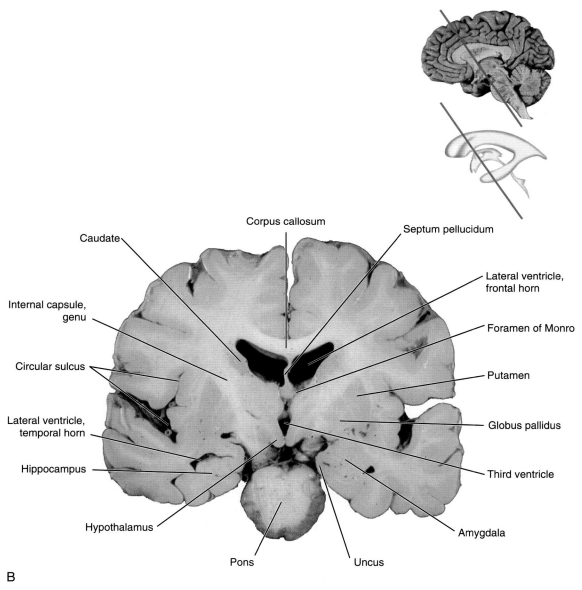

Figure labels:
Corpus callosum
Caudate
Septum pellucidum
Internal capsule, genu
Lateral ventricle, frontal horn
Circular sulcus
Foramen of Monro
Lateral ventricle, temporal horn
Putamen
Hippocampus
Globus pallidus
Hypothalamus
Third ventricle
Pons
Uncus
Amygdala

B

**Figure 1-9**, cont'd

*Figure continued*

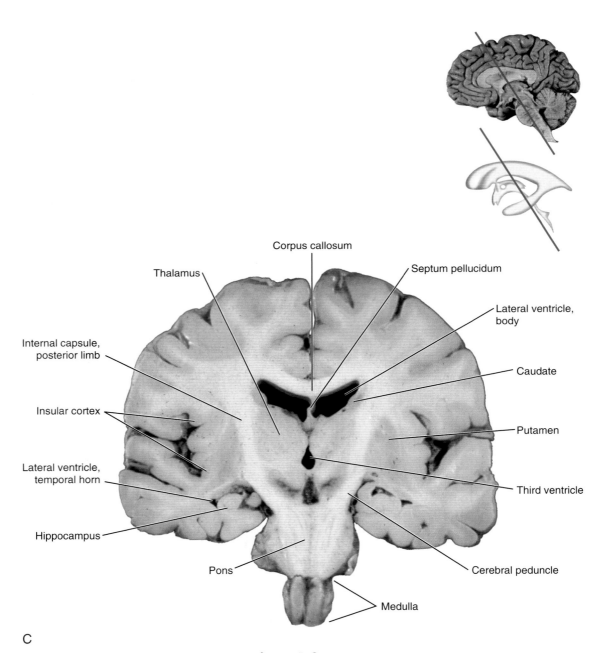

C

**Figure 1-9**, cont'd

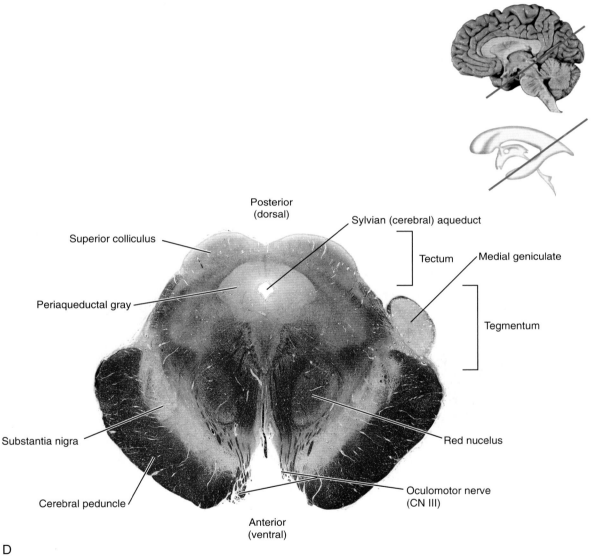

D

**Figure 1-9**, cont'd

*Figure continued*

**Major Divisions of the Central Nervous System**

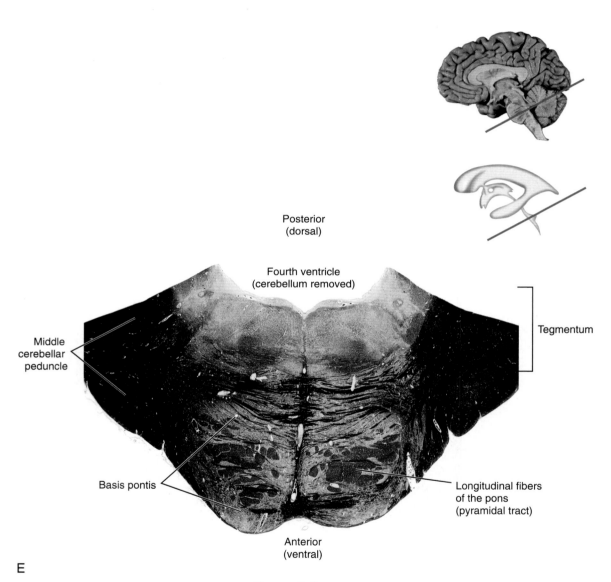

Posterior
(dorsal)

Fourth ventricle
(cerebellum removed)

Tegmentum

Middle
cerebellar
peduncle

Basis pontis

Longitudinal fibers
of the pons
(pyramidal tract)

Anterior
(ventral)

E

**Figure 1-9**, cont'd

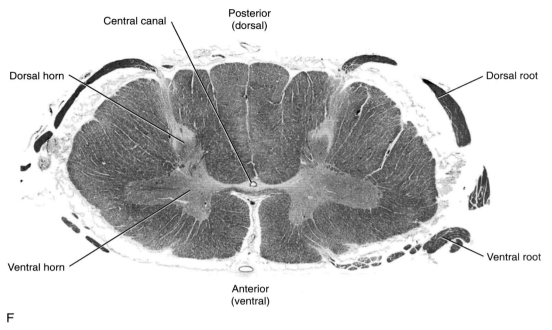

Central canal

Posterior
(dorsal)

Dorsal horn

Dorsal root

Ventral horn

Ventral root

Anterior
(ventral)

F

**Figure 1-9**, cont'd

| TABLE 1-2 Structures and Their Function | |
|---|---|
| **Structure** | **Function** |
| Basal ganglia | |
|   Caudate | Frontal lobe related |
|   Putamen | Motoric |
|   Globus pallidus | Output structure of basal ganglia |
| Internal capsule | Connections between cerebral cortex and subcortical/brainstem structures, especially cerebral cortex and cerebral peduncles |
| Foramina of Monro | Connect lateral and third ventricles |
| Sylvian aqueduct (midbrain) | Connects third and fourth ventricles |
| Central canal | Continuation of ventricular system in the spinal cord |
| Circular sulcus | CSF space between insula and overlying opercular cortex |
| Insula | Emotions/autonomic |
| Amygdala | Emotions/autonomic |
| Hippocampus | Memory |
| Periaqueductal gray | Pain experience/modulation |
| Middle cerebellar peduncles | Inflow pathway from cerebrum, via pons, to cerebellum |
| Superior cerebellar peduncles | Outflow pathway from cerebellum |

Major Divisions of the Central Nervous System

Slice *D* is an axial (transverse) cut through a rostral portion of the brainstem, the *midbrain*. Because the brainstem is more or less at right angles to the long axis of the cerebrum, slice *D* also comprises an axial cut through the cerebrum. This is the most common cut displayed in computed tomographic (CT) scans and magnetic resonance images (MRI) obtained for diagnostic purposes in patients. Slice *D* cuts through the slender cerebrospinal fluid connection between the third and fourth ventricles, the *sylvian (cerebral) aqueduct*. Surrounding the aqueduct is the *periaqueductal gray* substance, a structure important in pain sensation and modulation. The tissue dorsal to the aqueduct is referred to as the midbrain *tectum* (roof), at this level comprising the *superior colliculi*, which are important in vision. The tissue ventral to the aqueduct here and at lower levels (i.e., more caudally) is referred to as the *tegmentum* (floor). The massive white matter structures forming the lower margins of this section are the *cerebral peduncles*, the caudal continuation of the internal capsule.

Slice *E* is an axial cut through the fourth ventricle. The inset in Figure 1-9*E* shows that the structures visualized are dwarfed dorsally by the *cerebellum*, a motor structure. The dorsolateral walls of the fourth ventricle here are composed of the *superior cerebellar peduncles*, the major outflow pathway of the cerebellum. The entire mottled structure beneath the fourth ventricle is the *pons*. The pontine tissue just below the fourth ventricle is the *pontine tegmentum*. Below this, marked by transverse bands of white matter, is the *basis pontis*. The pons is framed on either side by massive white matter structures, the *middle cerebellar peduncles*, which are the inflow pathways from the cerebrum to the cerebellum.

Slice *F* is an axial cut through the spinal cord. Notice that the gray matter–white matter distribution exhibited in the cerebrum is reversed here: the core of the spinal cord is gray matter and all the surrounding tissue is white matter. In the middle of the cord, in the gray matter bridge between the two halves, lies a small hole. This opening is the *central canal*, the caudal continuation of the fourth ventricle. Although the central canal is a structural extension of the ventricular system, it is irregularly interrupted and does not support the flow of cerebrospinal fluid.

## PRACTICE 1-3

Make sure you know the meaning and location of the following:

| | |
|---|---|
| lateral ventricles | basal ganglia |
| body, atrium, frontal horn, temporal horn, occipital horn of lateral ventricles | caudate nucleus |
| | putamen |
| | globus pallidus |
| septum pellucidum | thalamus |
| third ventricle | hypothalamus |
| foramina of Monro | amygdala |
| fourth ventricle | uncus |
| sylvian aqueduct | hippocampus |
| central canal | insular cortex |
| choroid plexus | circular sulcus |
| cerebrospinal fluid | |
| corpus callosum | midbrain |
| deep cerebral white matter | periaqueductal gray |
| | pons |
| internal capsule | cerebellum |
| cerebral peduncles | tectum |
| superior cerebellar peduncles | tegmentum |
| middle cerebellar peduncles | basis pontis |
| | superior colliculi |
| | inferior colliculi |

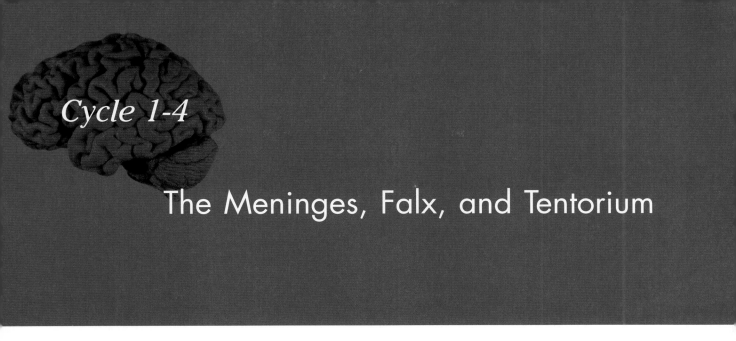

# Cycle 1-4

# The Meninges, Falx, and Tentorium

## Objectives

1. To learn the membranous coverings of the brain, the structures (falx and tentorium) that stabilize the brain within the skull, the venous sinus system within these structures, and the cerebrospinal fluid pathways outside the brain.

2. To learn the principle of herniation within the skull and the major types of herniation that may occur.

The membranous coverings of the brain, referred to as the *meninges*, consist of three fibrous layers: the *dura*, *arachnoid*, and *pia*.

## THE DURA

The outermost, thickest, and toughest layer, the dura, is closely adherent to the inner surface of the skull. The dura is composed of two portions—an outer periosteal layer that forms the periosteum of the inner surface of the skull (often referred to as the inner table), and an inner fibrous layer. For the most part, these two layers are closely adherent to one another, but there are areas of separation that form the *venous sinus system* (superior sagittal sinus, inferior sagittal sinus, straight sinus, confluence of sinuses, and the lateral and sigmoid sinuses) (Fig. 1-10). We will discuss these at greater length later when we review the blood supply to the brain (Chapter 2). Large extensions of the inner fibrous layer of the dura form the *falx* and the *tentorium* (Figs. 1-10 and 1-11). The falx forms a partition between the two cerebral hemispheres. Its inferior margin lies just above the corpus callosum. The caudal, infratentorial portion of the falx forms a partition between the two cerebellar hemispheres. The tentorium, a tent-shaped structure, forms a roof over the cerebellum and provides a partition between the cerebrum and the cerebellum. The occipital and the posterior portions of the temporal lobes of the cerebrum lie above the tentorium. A hole in the tentorium, the *incisura* (also referred to as the tentorial notch) accommodates the brainstem. The midbrain is centered within the incisura. The junction between the falx and the tentorium forms another venous structure, the straight sinus.

The falx and the tentorium help to stabilize the brain within the skull. Because of the great weight of the brain (on average 1.5 kg), it has considerable inertia. Consequently, there is inevitably some delay in the transmission of skull movements to the brain. This results in, at times, considerable movement of the brain within the skull. Such movement has the capacity for damaging the brain, particularly when the movement is rotational. The falx and the tentorium help to reduce the amplitude of these movements. Case 1-1 illustrates, however, that during extreme skull decelerations, as in motor vehicle accidents, the stabilizing effects of the falx and tentorium cannot prevent the occurrence of severe injury to the brain.

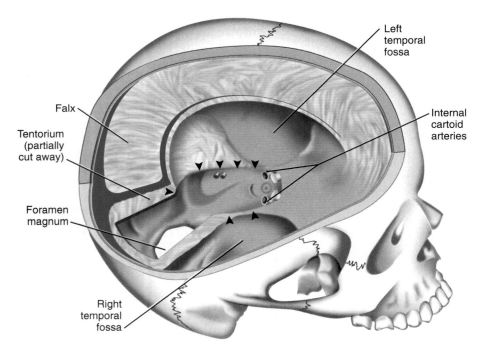

Left
temporal
fossa

Falx

Tentorium
(partially
cut away)

Foramen
magnum

Right
temporal
fossa

Internal
cartoid
arteries

**Figure 1-10** Diagram of the falx and tentorium in relation to the skull. The tentorium divides the middle cranial fossa from the posterior cranial fossa. The incisura (*arrowheads*) is the opening in the tentorium that accommodates the midbrain.

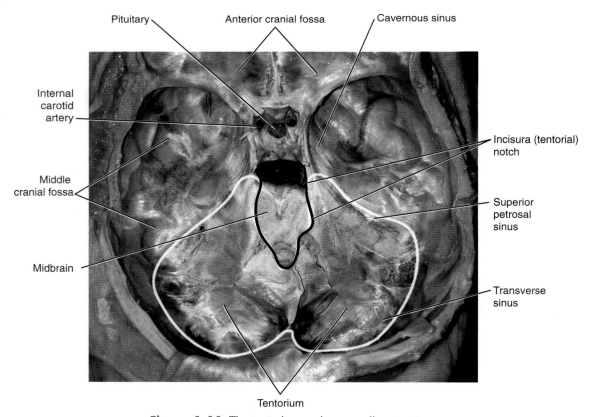

Pituitary

Anterior cranial fossa

Cavernous sinus

Internal
carotid
artery

Middle
cranial fossa

Midbrain

Incisura (tentorial)
notch

Superior
petrosal
sinus

Transverse
sinus

Tentorium

**Figure 1-11** The tentorium and surrounding structures.

## Case 1-1

**Head Trauma**
*A 17-year-old high school student is involved in a high-speed collision on the way back from a graduation party. He is not wearing a seat belt and his head strikes the windshield. He arrives at the nearest hospital comatose. He has a fractured femur but no skull fracture. However, over the next 24 hours, massive brain swelling occurs to the degree that intracranial pressure exceeds arterial pressure and his brain dies for lack of a blood supply. A postmortem examination reveals extensive evidence of shearing of neural pathways within the brain, brainstem, and cerebellum.*

**Comment:** *The great disparity between brain velocity and skull velocity at the moment of impact has literally torn the brain, notwithstanding the stabilizing influence of the falx and the tentorium.*

## INTRACRANIAL COMPARTMENTS AND HERNIATION SYNDROMES

The falx and the tentorium divide the cranial vault into two major compartments. The space above the tentorium is referred to as the *supratentorial* compartment and that below the tentorium as the *infratentorial* compartment (often referred to as the *posterior fossa*). The supratentorial compartment is divided into left and right halves by the falx. Because the falx and the tentorium are extremely stiff and resistant fibrous structures, they strictly limit the volume of the various compartments within the closed vault of the skull. When pathologic processes involving the brain increase the volume of brain beyond the capacity of a compartment, the brain expands from that compartment into adjacent compartments (*herniates*), with very serious consequences (Case 1-2).

An analogous process can occur in the presence of a mass (blood, tumor, tissue damaged by stroke) in the infratentorial compartment. In such a situation, the contents of the infratentorial compartment squeeze upward through the incisura and downward through the *foramen magnum* (the hole at the bottom of the skull through which the medulla and spinal cord pass). The *cerebellar tonsils* (lima bean–shaped structures at the medial caudal aspect of the cerebellum) are

## Case 1-2

**Head Trauma**
*The driver of the car involved in the accident described in Case 1-1 was wearing a seatbelt but still was very seriously injured. He also arrives at the hospital comatose. However, a CT scan reveals a large collection of blood over the left hemisphere between the brain and the dura (an acute subdural hematoma). The combined mass of the hematoma and the left hemisphere exceeds the volume of the left half of the supratentorial compartment. As a result, portions of the left hemisphere squeeze beneath the falx (subfalcine herniation). The large excess of mass in the left supratentorial compartment and the somewhat more modest excess in mass in the right supratentorial compartment (as a result of the subfalcine herniation) together push the brainstem to the right and downward through the incisura and squeeze the medial portions of the temporal lobes against the thalamus and midbrain. The downward thrust of the midbrain is referred to as central herniation. The squeezing of the medial temporal lobes against the thalamus and midbrain and into the incisura is referred to as uncal herniation (actually both the uncus, overlying the amygdala, and the more posterior hippocampus are deformed by the edge of the tentorium as the downward force pushes them through the incisura).*

**Comment:** *The compression of the midbrain and thalamus causes coma by interfering with the function of the core system underlying wakefulness (the midbrain reticular activating system). The lateral shift of the midbrain compresses the cerebral peduncle against the edge of the tentorium, causing paralysis on the opposite side of the body. The oblique downward movement of the brainstem produces traction on some cranial nerves, damaging them (a topic to which we will return later). If the subdural hematoma is drained sufficiently quickly, this process, which may become terminal in less than an hour, can be arrested and the patient's life saved.*

squeezed against the medulla as they are pushed downward, resulting in potentially fatal compression of medullary cardiorespiratory centers (*tonsillar herniation*). Table 1-3 summarizes the herniation syndromes.

**Major Divisions of the Central Nervous System**

**TABLE 1-3** Herniation Syndromes

| Type | Description |
|------|-------------|
| Subfalcine | Shift of midline cerebrum to one side, beneath the falx, because of excess mass (tumor, blood, edema) in one hemicranial compartment |
| Central | Downward shift of the brainstem through the tentorial notch (incisura) because of excess mass in the supratentorial compartment |
| Uncal | Medial shift of one uncus against the midbrain (because of ipsilateral mass effect), causing contralateral shift of the midbrain, and sometimes, compression of the midbrain against the opposite margin of the tentorium |
| Tonsilar | Downward shift of the medulla and cerebellar tonsils through the foramen magnum, with compression of the medulla, as a result of excess mass in the posterior fossa, either because of posterior fossa pathology, or because of severe central herniation |

## THE ARACHNOID AND PIA

The middle meningeal layer, the *arachnoid*, is much thinner than the dura. It is adherent to the brain (as opposed to the skull as in the case of the dura), but it does not follow the contours (gyri and sulci) of the brain. Rather, it forms a weblike membrane that bridges over the sulci. In the parasagittal region of the dorsal surface of the cerebrum (adjacent to the interhemispheric fissure), the arachnoid tissue forms tufted projections, the *arachnoid granulations*, that extend upward into the superior sagittal venous sinus (Figs. 1-12 and 1-13). Recall that cerebrospinal fluid flows through the ventricular system and exits at several foramina at the caudal aspect of the fourth ventricle into the *subarachnoid space*, beneath the arachnoid. It flows through the subarachnoid space over the convexities of the brain into the arachnoid granulations and into the superior sagittal sinus.

The deepest, thinnest layer of the meninges, the *pia* (Fig. 1-13), is entirely adherent to the surface of the brain and follows the contours of the gyri and sulci. The space between the arachnoid and the pia constitutes the subarachnoid space.

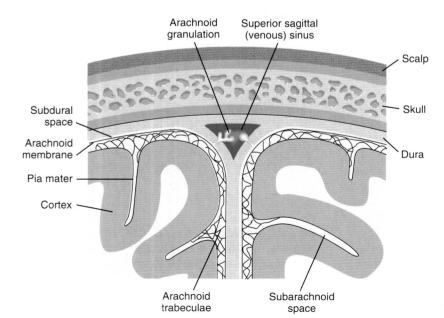

**Figure 1-12** Anteroposterior view of the arachnoid granulations. (Modified from Warner JJ. Atlas of Neuroanatomy. Boston, Butterworth Heinemann, 2001.)

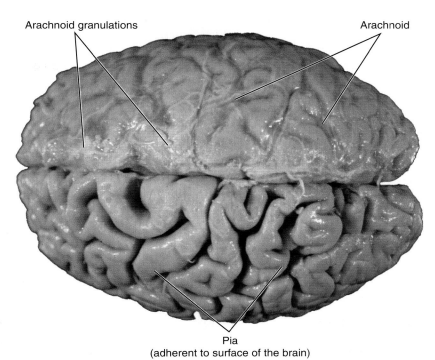

Arachnoid granulations

Arachnoid

Pia
(adherent to surface of the brain)

**Figure 1-13** View of the top of the brain showing the arachnoid granulations.

## PRACTICE 1-4

**A.** Make sure you know the meaning and location of the following:

| | |
|---|---|
| meninges | incisura |
| dura | foramen magnum |
| arachnoid | venous sinus system |
| subarachnoid space | supratentorial compartment |
| pia | infratentorial compartment |
| arachnoid granulations | posterior fossa |
| | subfalcine herniation |
| | uncal herniation |
| falx | central herniation |
| tentorium | tonsillar herniation |

**B.** A 25-year-old man presents with a very large mass centered in his right temporal lobe and basal ganglia. He is nearly comatose. An MRI shows that he has severe subfalcine, uncal, and central herniation (see Fig. 1-14). Uncal herniation is compressing the midbrain and driving it against the margin of the tentorium on the left side. The right lateral ventricle is compressed to a thin slit, and the left lateral ventricle is dilated because the subfalcine herniation has occluded the left foramen of Monro. The central herniation has used up all extra space in the posterior fossa and compressed the fourth ventricle. Tonsillar herniation has begun. A member of the medical team wants to perform a lumbar puncture (a spinal tap) in order to analyze the cerebrospinal fluid. This analysis would help to rule out an abscess—a pocket of pus within the brain. Would you agree with this decision?

In answering this question, consider the following: nearly all the cerebrospinal fluid normally passes over the surface of the brain into the arachnoid granulations. However, because of all the pressure in the supratentorial compartment, this flow is interrupted and an unusually large proportion of the fluid flows down through the foramen magnum into the spinal canal. From there it passes against great resistance along the exiting nerve roots into the soft tissues surrounding the spinal cord. Considering the great resistance to fluid flow out of the spinal canal, what do you think the fluid pressure will be in the spinal canal? What effect will this pressure have on the impending descent of the cerebellar tonsils through the foramen magnum? During a lumbar puncture (the insertion of a needle into the spinal canal in the lumbar region) not very much fluid is removed. However, the puncture produces a leak in the arachnoid and the dura through which a great deal of fluid can pass before the leak eventually seals. Given this persistent leak, what is going to happen to the cerebrospinal fluid pressure in the spinal canal? What consequences will this have for the cerebellar tonsils? How will that affect the medulla and the patient? Do you think a lumbar puncture is a good idea? (See Cycle 1-4 Feedback at end of chapter.)

Major Divisions of the Central Nervous System

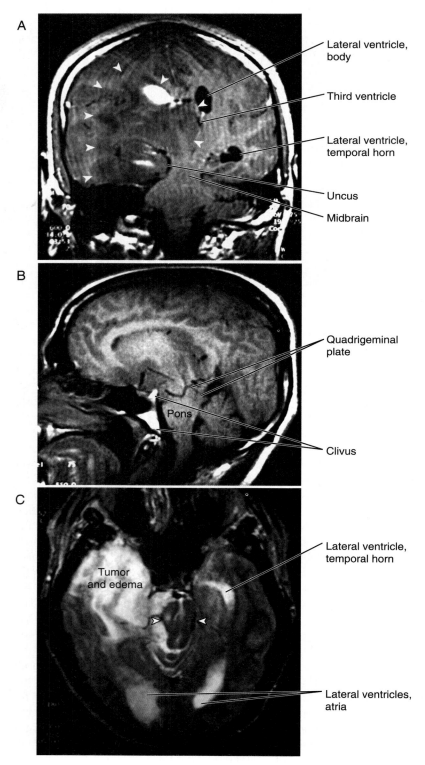

A

Lateral ventricle, body

Third ventricle

Lateral ventricle, temporal horn

Uncus

Midbrain

B

Quadrigeminal plate

Pons

Clivus

C

Lateral ventricle, temporal horn

Tumor and edema

Lateral ventricles, atria

**Figure 1-14** (Practice B) Magnetic resonance image of brain demonstrating a very large right hemispheric mass with herniation. *A,* This coronal section shows the dilated body and temporal horn of the left lateral ventricle (*black oval spaces*). Note how far to the left of midline the third ventricle has been driven. Most of the tumor appears as a gray mass (outlined by the *white arrowheads*). The tumor is not much different in color than surrounding brain except for an area roughly where you would normally expect the body of the right lateral ventricle, which is white, reflecting a hemorrhage. Notice the uncus of the right temporal lobe pressed up against the midbrain, pushing it toward the left. *B,* From a sagittal view, one can see the entire brainstem has been driven downward (central herniation) such that the midbrain, instead of being centered posterior to the upper tip of the clivus (white because of fat in the bone marrow), is now well below the tip of clivus. The midbrain appears to be very thick (you can see the quadrigeminal plate situated far more posteriorly than normal) because it is being squashed by the descending thalamus. The excessive pressure within the posterior fossa (due to central herniation) is apparent in the flattening of the anterior aspect of the pons against the clivus. *C,* Note from this horizontal or axial section the extent of the tumor and tumor-related edema, which appear as white or nearly white tissue in this image sequence. You can also appreciate how much the midbrain (*arrowheads*) has been compressed and pushed over to the left by the uncal herniation.

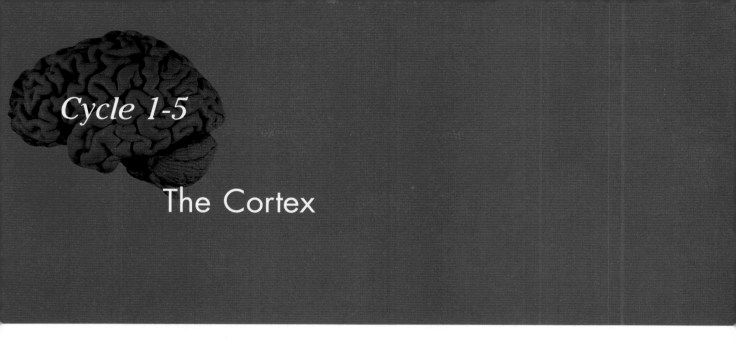

# Cycle 1-5

# The Cortex

**Objective**

Learn the major divisions of the cortex (frontal, temporal, parietal, and occipital lobes; parahippocampal and limbic cortices) and their general functions.

One of the central tenets of neuroscience is that particular aspects of perception and behavior can be identified with specific areas of the neocortex. This belief derives from perceptual and behavioral deficits that are known to result from restricted cortical lesions, from results of electrophysiologic recording and stimulation experiments in humans and experimental animals, and from imaging studies (e.g., functional magnetic resonance imaging [fMRI], positron emission tomography [PET], and single photon emission computed tomography [SPECT]) of brain function. We use as cortical landmarks the fissures, sulci, and gyri that are readily visible in gross brain material. These landmarks generally are reliable at the level at which they will be considered in this chapter, although they can differ in detail between individual specimens.

We will identify four lobes of the *neocortex* in the whole or hemisected brain material. A cerebral hemisphere is shown in lateral and medial views in Figures 1-15 and 1-16, respectively. The two most important landmarks for demarcating the cortical lobes are the

*central sulcus* and the *sylvian fissure*. The *central sulcus* forms the dividing line between the frontal and parietal lobes. It crosses the dorsolateral surface of the hemisphere obliquely. Dorsally, the central sulcus curves over the dorsal medial aspect of the hemisphere to enter the *median longitudinal fissure*, which is the large fissure on the midline of the brain that divides the two hemispheres. The central sulcus travels ventrally and somewhat anteriorly to end near the sylvian fissure. The central sulcus can be distinguished from other sulci by the presence of paired *pre-* and *postcentral gyri*, which lie anterior and posterior to the central sulcus. The sylvian fissure separates the frontal and parietal lobes from the temporal lobe.

Recall from Cycle 1-3 that each lobe of the cerebral cortex is associated with a particular division of the lateral ventricle. The frontal lobe overlies the frontal (anterior) horn of the lateral ventricle. It extends from the central sulcus anteriorly to the frontal pole of the hemisphere (i.e., to the most anterior point on the hemisphere). Posterior to the central sulcus is the parietal lobe, which overlies the *body* and part of the *atrium* of the lateral ventricle. The parietal lobe extends posteriorly to the *parieto-occipital fissure*. The parieto-occipital fissure is prominent on a medial view of the hemisphere, but it extends only a short distance onto the lateral aspect of the hemisphere. The parietal lobe is bounded ventrally on the hemispheric surface by a line extending straight posteriorly from the sylvian fissure to the parieto-occipital fissure. The occipital lobe overlies the posterior horn of the lateral ventricle.

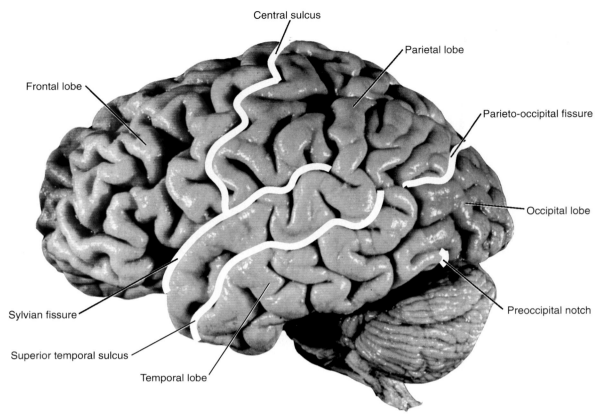

Central sulcus

Parietal lobe

Frontal lobe

Parieto-occipital fissure

Occipital lobe

Sylvian fissure

Preoccipital notch

Superior temporal sulcus

Temporal lobe

**Figure 1-15** Lateral view of the left cerebral hemisphere.

The occipital lobe is most visible in a medial view: only a small portion extends onto the posterolateral surface of the hemisphere. The occipital lobe lies posterior to the parieto-occipital fissure. On the lateral surface of the hemisphere, the occipital lobe is bounded by a line drawn from the dorsal end of the parieto-occipital fissure to the preoccipital notch, located ventrally. The temporal lobe, which overlies the inferior horn of the lateral ventricle, lies ventral to the sylvian fissure. The insula is folded within the sylvian fissure and can be seen by gently pulling the temporal lobe laterally (Fig. 1-17).

We now can identify specific functional areas on the cortical lobes. Cortical areas have been distinguished at the microscopic level on the basis of the sizes and packing densities of cell bodies (the cytoarchitecture) and on the distribution of myelinated fibers (the myeloarchitecture). One of the most influential cytoarchitectonic classifications of the neocortex was published in 1909 by the German anatomist, Korbinian Brodmann. We often will refer to specific cortical areas

by their numbers in Brodmann's scheme. The areas that we will consider are shown, as designated by Brodmann, in Figures 1-18 and 1-19 (see also Table 1-4).

## THE FRONTAL LOBES

The frontal lobe contains several areas that are involved in initiation of movements. The *primary motor cortex* (Brodmann's area 4) is located on the *precentral gyrus*, immediately anterior to the central sulcus. Anterior to the primary motor cortex are the *premotor* and *supplementary motor areas* (area 6). Further anterior, in Brodmann's area 8, are the *frontal eye fields*, which are involved in initiating rapid eye movements and directing attention. In the ventral frontal lobe, bordering the lateral fissure, are areas 44 and 45. In the dominant hemisphere (usually the left), this area is known as *Broca's area*. Observations dating back to Paul Broca, a French anatomist who published his work in the 1860s, suggest that this area is important for language

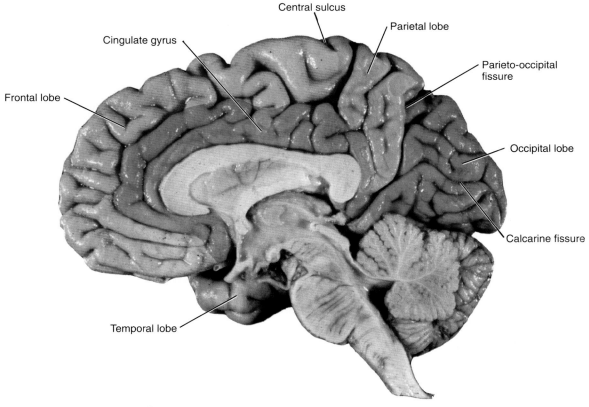

**Figure 1-16** Medial view of the right cerebral hemisphere.

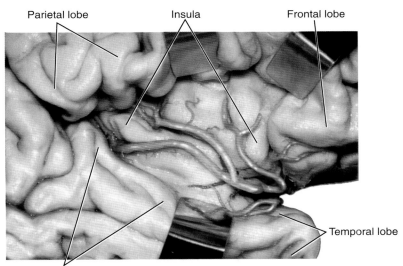

**Figure 1-17** Lateral view of the left hemisphere with the temporal lobe retracted to show the insula.

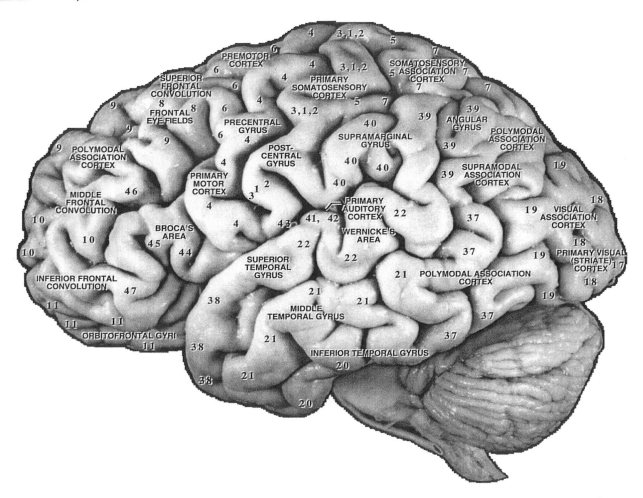

**Figure 1-18** Lateral view of the left hemisphere, showing cortical areas, numbered according to Brodmann. (From Warner JJ. Atlas of Neuroanatomy. Boston, Butterworth Heinemann, 2001.)

production. The remainder of the frontal lobe, anterior to the frontal eye fields and premotor cortex, is known as the *prefrontal cortex*, which contains the *frontal association areas*. Prefrontal cortex is involved in developing goals and plans for action and carrying them out.

## THE PARIETAL LOBE

The parietal lobe contains the areas for somatic sensation, for example, the sense of touch on the body and face. The *primary somatosensory cortex* lies on the *postcentral gyrus* (areas 3, 1, and 2), which is immediately posterior to the central sulcus. Most of the remainder of the parietal lobe is occupied by *somatosensory*

and *visual association areas* and area 7 (parasagittal parietal lobe in humans). One major function of area 7, to align our body-centered coordinate frame within the environmentally centered coordinate frame, subsumes both somatosensory and visual modalities. Ventral in the posterior association areas are the *supramarginal* and *angular* gyri, so-called "supramodal" association cortices, most of whose function is complex and unrelated to any specific sensory modality. Parts of the dominant (left) angular gyrus and posterior and ventral parts of the supramarginal gyrus are involved in language function. The supramarginal gyrus wraps around the dorsoposterior tip of the sylvian fissure, whereas the angular gyrus has a similar relation to the dorsoposterior tip of the *superior temporal sulcus* (Fig. 1-18).

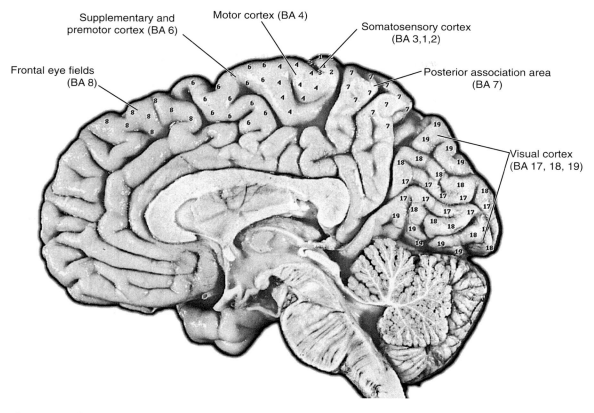

**Figure 1-19** Medial view of the right hemisphere, showing cortical areas, numbered according to Brodmann. (Modified from Warner JJ. Atlas of Neuroanatomy. Boston, Butterworth Heinemann, 2001.)

## THE OCCIPITAL LOBE

Much of the occipital lobe is buried within the hemisphere, folded around the *calcarine* fissure; the calcarine fissure is visible on the medial aspect of the hemisphere (Fig. 1-16). The occipital lobe is the site of the visual cortex (Fig. 1-19). The *primary visual cortex* (area 17) is largely hidden from view, but portions can be seen on the dorsal and ventral lips of the calcarine fissure. The primary visual cortex receives the major projection of fibers carrying visual input from the thalamus. The primary visual cortex goes by many names: it is called *V1*, because it is the first site of visual cortical processing; *calcarine cortex*, because of its location around the calcarine fissure; or *striate cortex*, because it contains a prominent white stripe (stria) within its gray matter. Area 17 sends fibers to the adjacent *areas 18 and 19* for higher-level visual processing.

## THE TEMPORAL LOBE

The temporal lobe has important auditory and visual functions. One can view the superior surface of the temporal lobe by removing the structures (frontal and parietal lobes) above the lateral fissure (Fig. 1-17). The *primary auditory cortex* (areas 41 and 42) is located on the transverse temporal gyrus of Heschl. Auditory association cortex posterior to Heschl's gyrus is referred to as the *planum temporale*. The planum temporale, together with adjacent regions of the superior temporal gyrus, is Brodmann's area 22. In the hemisphere that is dominant for language (usually the left), this region is called Wernicke's area. Lesions in *Wernicke's area* produce deficits in both the comprehension and production of language. Consistent with its involvement in language function, the planum temporale is significantly larger in the left hemisphere than in the right in

**TABLE 1-4** Summary of Brodmann's Areas of the Cerebral Cortex

| Location | Brodmann's Area | Function |
| --- | --- | --- |
| **Frontal Lobe** | | |
| Precentral gyrus | 4 | Primary motor cortex |
| Anterior to precentral gyrus | 6 | Premotor area |
| Anterior to area 6 on middle and superior frontal gyri | 8 | Frontal eye fields |
| Perisylvian frontal cortex | 44, 45 | Broca's area—language (dominant hemisphere) |
| Prefrontal cortex | | Frontal association areas |
| **Parietal Lobe** | | |
| Postcentral gyrus | 3, 1, 2 | Primary somatosensory cortex |
| Parietal convexity posterior to postcentral gyrus | 5, 7 | Visual and somatosensory association areas |
| Parasagittal parietal lobe | 7 | Bimodal (visual and somatosensory) association area |
| **Occipital Lobe** | | |
| Calcarine (striate) cortex | 17 | Primary visual cortex (VI) |
| Para- and peri-striate cortex | 18, 19 | Higher level visual cortex |
| **Temporal Lobe** | | |
| Heschl's gyri | 41, 42 | Auditory cortex |
| Planum temporale and posterior superior temporal gyrus | 22 | Wernicke's area—language cortex (in the dominant hemisphere) |
| Middle and inferior temporal gyri, undersurface of temporal lobe | | Visual association areas |
| **Limbic Cortex** | | |
| Temporal pole, insula, orbitofrontal cortex, cingulate gyrus | | Emotional and motivational function |

most human brains. Ventral to the superior temporal gyrus, in the middle and inferior temporal gyri, as well as the entire inferior surface of the temporal lobe, are the *temporal visual association areas* (Fig. 1-20), which are involved in higher level visual processing. The most anterior aspect of the temporal lobe, the *temporal pole*, is polymodal cortex (linked to two sensory modalities, auditory and visual) and supramodal cortex (not directly associated with any given sensory modality). This supramodal cortex is linked functionally to the amygdala and subserves emotional and motivational functions.

## THE PARAHIPPOCAMPAL AND LIMBIC CORTEX

On the inferior aspect of the temporal lobe, we can follow the transition in the medial portions of the lobe from neocortex to a more primitive three-layered cortex (Fig. 1-20). The *parahippocampal gyrus*, the lateral border of which is formed anteriorly by the rhinal fissure and posteriorly by the collateral sulcus, represents a transition between six-layered cortex laterally and three-layered cortex more medially. Continuous with the parahippocampal gyrus and folded within it is the three-layered *hippocampus*, which we will discuss in a later cycle. On the anteromedial aspect of the parahippocampal gyrus is the uncus (Latin for "hook"). The *uncus*, which is composed of transitional cortex (six to three layers), overlies the *amygdala*, a spherical nucleus that lies just anterior to the temporal horn of the lateral ventricle. This ventral view of the brain also provides a view of the *orbitofrontal* cortex, which is part of the prefrontal cortex.

The major remaining structure on the medial surface of the hemisphere is the cingulate gyrus, lying both dorsal and rostral to the corpus callosum

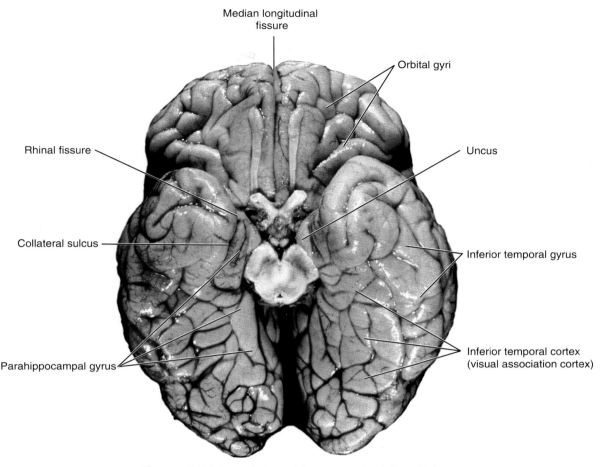

**Figure 1-20** Ventral view of the temporal and frontal lobes.

(Fig. 1-16). The *cingulate gyrus*, the temporal pole, the posteromedial orbitofrontal cortex, the insula, the amygdala, the hypothalamus (Cycle 1-3), and the lateral septal nuclei (buried in the most posterior portions of the frontal cortex on the medial surface of the hemisphere, just anterior to the hypothalamus) compose the *limbic system*. This system is involved in motivation and emotional function. The hippocampus and the parahippocampal gyrus traditionally have been included in the limbic system but this designation no longer seems appropriate, because they are clearly structures involved in encoding new memories.

The *insula* is an area of transitional cortex that is folded within the sylvian fissure. It can be seen by retracting the temporal lobe (Fig. 1-17). The "lips" of neocortex that overlie the insula are the frontal, parietal, and temporal *opercula*.

## PRACTICE 1-5

Make sure you know the meaning and location of the following:

median longitudinal fissure
sylvian fissure
central sulcus
precentral gyrus
primary motor cortex (area 4)
premotor cortex (area 6)
supplementary motor cortex (part of area 6)

frontal eye fields (area 8)
frontal association areas
prefrontal cortex
Broca's area (dominant 44, 45)
orbitofrontal cortex
postcentral gyrus
primary somatosensory cortex (areas 3, 1, 2)

**Major Divisions of the Central Nervous System**

parieto-occipital
  fissure
somatosensory
  association cortex
supramarginal gyrus
angular gyrus
area 7

calcarine fissure

primary visual cortex
  (V1, calcarine
  cortex, area 17,
  striate cortex)
areas 18, 19

primary auditory
  cortex (areas 41, 42)
Wernicke's area
  (area 22)

temporal visual
  association areas
temporal pole
superior temporal
  sulcus
parahippocampal
  gyrus
hippocampus

limbic system
  (including its major
  cortices)
amygdala
uncus
cingulate gyrus
insula
operculum

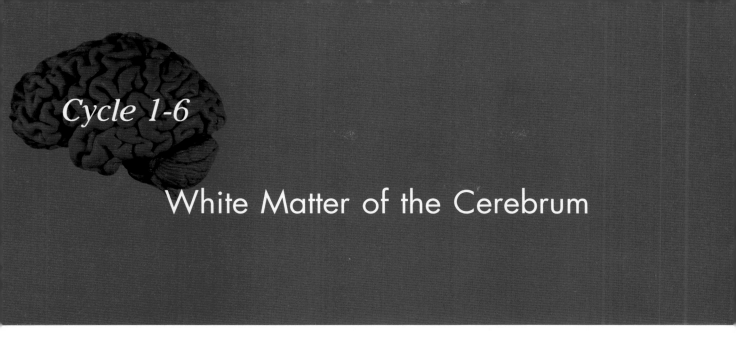

# Cycle 1-6

# White Matter of the Cerebrum

### Objective

To learn the major components of the cerebral white matter.

In any cross section through the cerebral hemisphere, one can see that the cerebral cortex consists of a relatively thin layer of gray matter, about 1.3 to 4.5 mm thick, deep to which is a large mass of white matter. The white matter is called the *centrum semiovale*, and it contains all the fibers that provide input to and output from the cortical gray matter (Fig. 1-21). These fibers include *projection fibers*, which interconnect the cortex with subcortical structures, commissural fibers, which connect one cerebral hemisphere with the other, and *association fibers*, which interconnect one cortical area with another in the same hemisphere.

*Projection fibers* carry ascending input from subcortical nuclei to the cortical gray matter and descending output from the cortex to various sites in the basal ganglia, thalamus, brainstem, and spinal cord. Particular tracts can be named according to their origins and terminations. For example, the frontopontine tract transmits activity in the frontal eye fields, motor and premotor cortex to the pons. Other tracts have more function-related names, such as the acoustic radiations, which carry auditory input to the cortex. Most projection fibers connecting to the brainstem and spinal cord

pass through a major fiber bundle called the *internal capsule* (Fig. 1-22). In the horizontal view, the internal capsule exhibits a V shape. One can identify three regions of this V: (1) the *anterior limb*, (2) the *genu* (the "knee"), and (3) the *posterior limb*. For now, just learn to identify these three divisions. Later, we will learn the location of specific fiber bundles within the internal

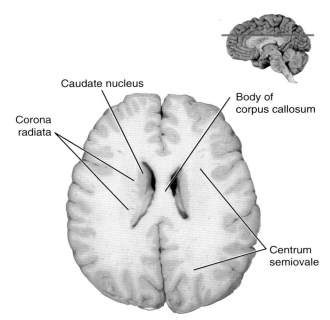

**Figure 1-21** Horizontal section through the cerebrum demonstrating the centrum semiovale.

*35*

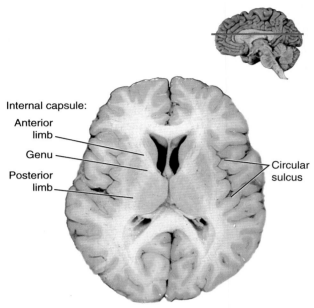

Internal capsule:
Anterior limb
Genu
Posterior limb
Circular sulcus

**Figure 1-22** Horizontal section through the cerebrum several centimeters ventral to section in Figure 1-21, demonstrating the internal capsule.

capsule. The white matter immediately dorsal to the internal capsule, lying adjacent to the bodies of the lateral ventricles (Fig. 1-21), which contains the continuation of fibers in the internal capsule, is referred to as the *corona radiata* ("radiant crown").

Association fibers carry information from one cortical area to another in the same hemisphere. The majority of these fibers travel only a short distance and are unnamed; this type of fiber is called a U fiber

because it descends into the subcortical white matter, travels a short distance, then reenters the cortical gray matter. Later, we also will encounter several well-defined bundles of association fibers connecting distant cortices that are named.

Commissural fibers travel from one cerebral hemisphere to the other. In a midsagittal section of the brain (Fig. 1-23), one sees the cut ends of these fibers. The most conspicuous commissural bundle is the corpus callosum. We name four regions of the corpus callosum: the *splenium* at the posterior end, the *body*, the *genu*, and the tapering, anteroventral *rostrum*. The *anterior commissure* interconnects the olfactory cortices and the association cortices of the temporal lobes. The *posterior commissure* interconnects structures in the two halves of the rostral brainstem, principally those involved in eye movement control and pupillary responses.

## PRACTICE 1-6

Make sure you know the meaning and location of the following:

centrum semiovale
corona radiata
association fibers
projection fibers
anterior commissure
posterior commissure
internal capsule
   anterior limb
   posterior limb
   genu

corpus callosum
rostrum
genu
body
splenium

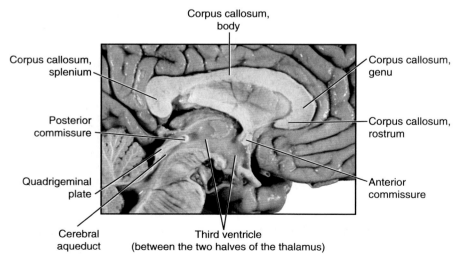

Corpus callosum, body

Corpus callosum, splenium

Posterior commissure

Quadrigeminal plate

Cerebral aqueduct

Third ventricle (between the two halves of the thalamus)

Corpus callosum, genu

Corpus callosum, rostrum

Anterior commissure

**Figure 1-23** Midsagittal section through the cerebrum demonstrating the major commissures.

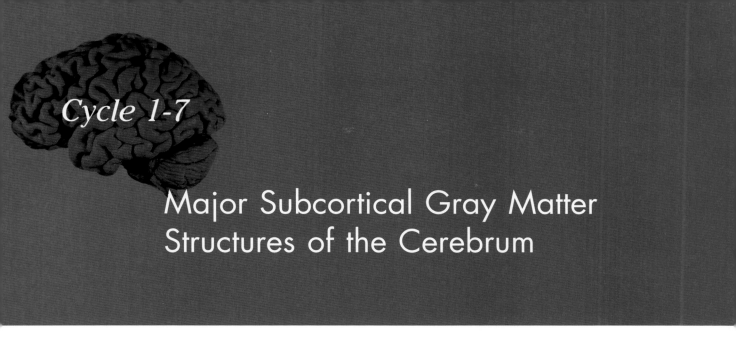

## Cycle 1-7

# Major Subcortical Gray Matter Structures of the Cerebrum

### Objective

Be able to identify the major subcortical gray matter structures within the cerebral hemispheres.

Deep within the cerebral hemispheres, one finds more or less homogeneous deep nuclei as well as structures that are cortical in organization. We will consider the *basal ganglia*, the *hippocampal formation*, the *amygdala*, and the *basal forebrain*.

## THE BASAL GANGLIA

The *basal ganglia* modulate the functions of the frontal cortex. They have three major components: the *caudate nucleus*, *putamen*, and *globus pallidus* (often referred to collectively as the striatum). The caudate nucleus has an elongated, tapered shape (caudate is from the Latin for "tail") (Fig. 1-24). Its large anterior *head* lies on the lateral wall of the frontal (anterior) horn of the lateral ventricle. The *body* curves posteriorly and ventrally, along the dorsolateral aspect of the thalamus. The *tail* curves down and finally anteriorly as it follows the temporal (inferior) horn of the lateral ventricle into the temporal lobe. The head and body of the caudate lie medial to the anterior limb of the internal capsule. All portions of the caudate lie on the lateral wall of the lateral ventricle. Because of its arched shape,

one often can find two pieces of the caudate in a single coronal section from a hemisphere: one fairly substantial piece, from the head or body, and a thin piece, from the tail.

The lenticular nucleus, so-named because it is shaped like a lens, consists of the *putamen* and the *globus pallidus* (Figs. 1-24 and 1-25). The lenticular nucleus lies deep in the white matter of the hemisphere, separated from the caudate by the anterior limb of the internal capsule (Fig. 1-24). A vertically oriented sheet of fibers, the external medullary lamina, divides the lenticular nucleus into a lateral *putamen* and a medial *globus pallidus* (a pallid, or pale, globe). The fibers of the internal medullary lamina of the globus pallidus further divide it into internal and external parts. At the most ventral levels, below the fibers of the anterior limb of the internal capsule, the caudate and the putamen join each other as the *nucleus accumbens* (an adjunct to the limbic system) (see Fig. 1-30A).

The V shape of the internal capsule in horizontal section defines three compartments: anterior, lateral, and posterior (Fig. 1-24). The anterior compartment of the V is occupied by the head of the caudate. The body and tail of the caudate arch posteriorly and dorsally, out of the plane of the horizontal section, then the tail arches ventrally back into the section. The lateral compartment is occupied by the lenticular nucleus. Passing through the lateral compartment from medial to lateral, one can locate the genu of the internal capsule, the globus pallidus, the putamen, and ultimately, the gray matter of the insular cortex. The posterior compartment

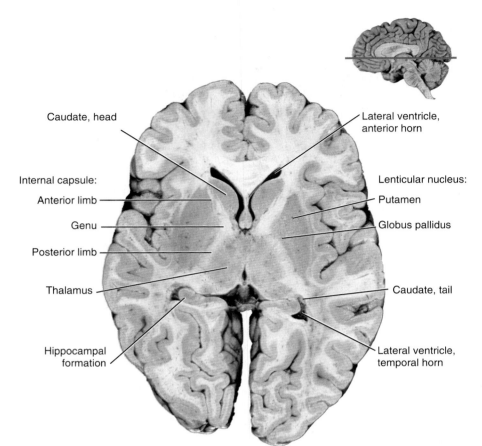

**Figure 1-24** Horizontal section through the cerebral hemispheres.

of the V is occupied by the thalamus. Try to predict the arrangement of the basal ganglia structures and the thalamus in coronal sections through the anterior limb, genu, and posterior limb of the internal capsule, then check your prediction by referring to an atlas.

## THE HIPPOCAMPAL FORMATION

The *hippocampal formation* is located within the temporal lobe, folded within the parahippocampal gyrus (Figs. 1-26 and 1-27). The hippocampus is the core of the system responsible for formation of new memories. It is continuous medially with the cortex of the parahippocampal gyrus. Dorsolateral to the hippocampus is the temporal horn of the lateral ventricle.

The hippocampus has two major input-output structures. The most important is the parahippocampal gyrus, which has extensive afferent and efferent connections with the cerebral cortex. A second system can be seen as fibers coalescing on the dorsal surface of the

hippocampus to form the fimbria (Fig. 1-28). At the posterior end of the hippocampus, the fimbria on the two sides close to form the cylindrical bundles of the *fornix*, which arch up, anteriorly, and ultimately down again as the *columns of the fornix*. As the columns of the fornix meet the anterior commissure, they split into the precommissural (in front of) and postcommissural (in back of) fornix. The precommissural fornix terminates in the medial septal nuclei of the basal forebrain (see below), and the postcommissural fornix terminates in the *mammillary bodies* of the hypothalamus. The arched shape of the fornix, like that of the caudate nucleus, implies that one will often encounter two pieces of the fornix in a single coronal or horizontal section.

## THE AMYGDALA

Immediately anterior to the hippocampus and inferior to the lenticular nucleus lies a complex nucleus, the

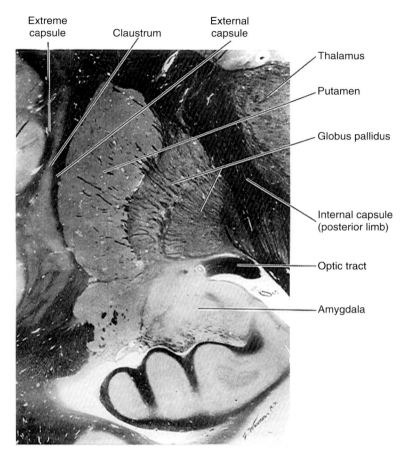

**Figure 1-25** Coronal section through the left cerebral hemisphere, stained for myelin, showing the lenticular nucleus. Lateral is left. (Modified from Warner JJ. Atlas of Neuroanatomy. Boston, Butterworth Heinemann, 2001, with permission from Elsevier Science.)

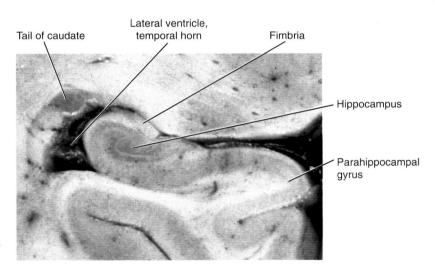

**Figure 1-26** Coronal section through the hippocampal formation. Lateral is left.

**Major Divisions of the Central Nervous System**

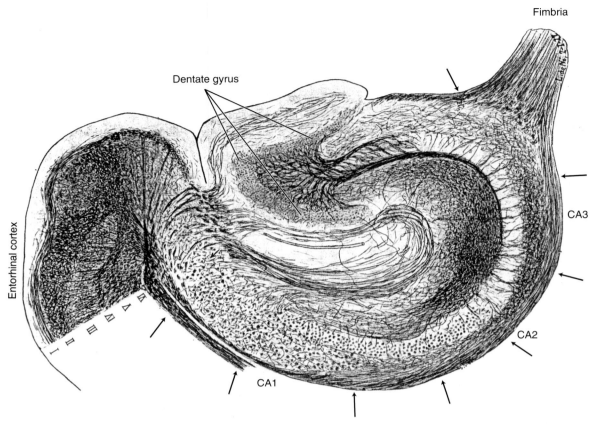

**Figure 1-27** Drawing from a silver stain of a horizontal section through the hippocampal formation of an adult mouse demonstrating the complex, but precisely organized neural fiber structure. Arrows delineate the actual hippocampus. The fimbria has a different spatial relationship to the hippocampus in the mouse. (Modified from R. Lorente de Nó. Studies on the structure of the cerebral cortex. II. Continuation of the study of the Ammonic system. J Psychol Neurol 1934;46:113-177.)

*amygdala*, which is involved in defining the motivation for behavior and in emotional function (Figs. 1-25 and 1-29*A*, *B*). The most important inputs to the amygdala are from the frontal and temporal lobes, and its most important outputs are to the hypothalamus and the cerebral cortex, directly and via the nucleus accumbens and ventral caudate.

## THE BASAL FOREBRAIN

The *basal forebrain* refers to a group of midline structures ventromedial to the frontal horns of the lateral ventricles bordering the anterior hypothalamus and lying in the general vicinity of the anterior commissure

(Fig. 1-30*A*, *B*). Despite their peculiar location at the edge of the ventricles and between other much larger gray matter structures such as the basal ganglia, the nuclei of the basal forebrain have profound import for complex behavior. Most dorsally, along the inferior margin of the septum pellucidum, lie the *septal nuclei*. The *medial septal nuclei* are linked via the fornix to the hippocampus (remember medial for memory). The *lateral septal nuclei* are part of the limbic system (remember lateral for limbic), involved, like the amygdala, in motivation and emotional function. Ventrolateral to the septal nuclei lies the *nucleus accumbens*. This structure is part of the basal ganglia and forms a gray matter bridge between the ventral head of the caudate and the putamen (which are no longer

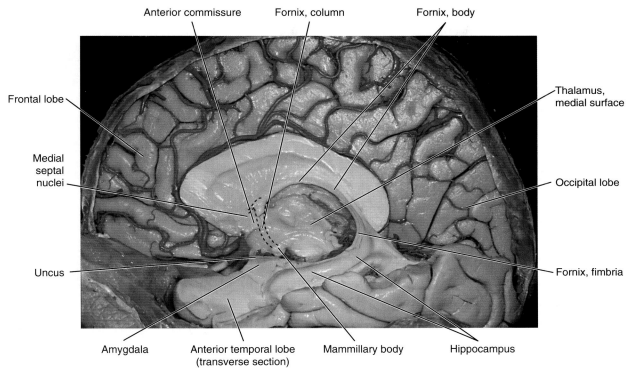

**Figure 1-28** The hippocampus and fornix. All of the left hemisphere has been dissected away except for the inferior temporal and occipital lobes, exposing the hippocampus and the amygdala. The column of the left fornix (the continuation of the fornix to the mammillary body) and the continuation of the left fornix in front of the anterior commissure to the medial septal nucleus were lost in the dissection. These pathways are therefore delineated by dashed lines. (Dissection by Riusui Tanaka.)

separated by the anterior limb of the internal capsule at this level). The nucleus accumbens is also a limbic structure. Just posterior to the nucleus accumbens and immediately below the globus pallidus lies the *nucleus basalis of Meynert*, a cluster of neurons that project widely to the cerebral cortex. The nucleus basalis is primarily involved in the formation of memory, both for facts and for skills; it helps to define what cortical neural activity is of sufficient importance to contribute to memory formation. It is particularly affected in patients with Alzheimer's disease.

## SUMMARY

The locations of several of the deep telencephalic structures are easiest to learn relative to the lateral ventricle. Just remember that the caudate, head, body, or tail, is always found lateral to the lateral ventricle, whereas structures related to the hippocampus, including the hippocampus itself, the fimbria, the fornix, and the septal nuclei, are found on the floor of or medial to the lateral ventricle. In the temporal lobe, both the tails of the caudate and the hippocampus end at the anterior end of the inferior horn of the lateral ventricle. The amygdala is found in the temporal lobe mostly anterior to the inferior horn; its caudal end lies dorsal to the tip of the inferior horn. Thus, in the temporal lobe region of a coronal section, if there is no inferior horn, an area of gray matter will be the amygdala. If the inferior horn is present, a small spot of gray matter lateral to the ventricle would be the tail of the caudate and a laminated structure medial to the ventricle would be the hippocampus. The amygdala and the inferior horn can be seen in the same coronal section only at the most anterior end of the inferior horn and most posterior end of the amygdala.

Major Divisions of the Central Nervous System

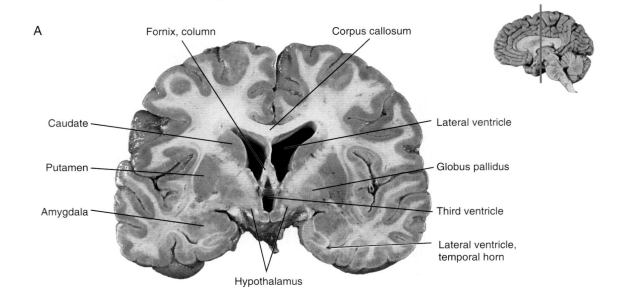

A

Fornix, column
Corpus callosum
Caudate
Lateral ventricle
Putamen
Globus pallidus
Amygdala
Third ventricle
Lateral ventricle, temporal horn
Hypothalamus

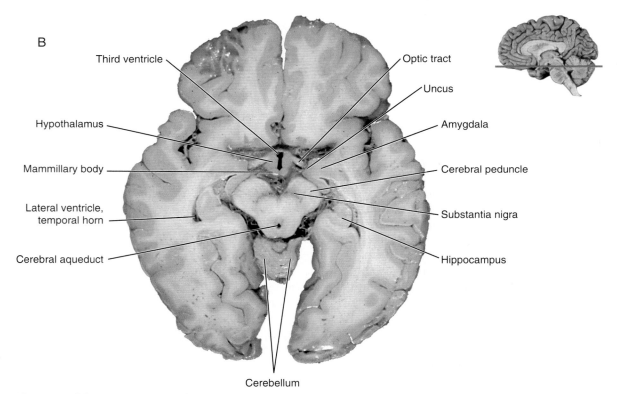

B

Third ventricle
Optic tract
Uncus
Hypothalamus
Amygdala
Mammillary body
Cerebral peduncle
Lateral ventricle, temporal horn
Substantia nigra
Cerebral aqueduct
Hippocampus
Cerebellum

**Figure 1-29** *A*, Coronal section through the amygdala showing the relationship of the amygdala, hypothalamus, and the temporal horn. *B*, Axial section through the amygdala showing relationship to the hippocampus, uncus, and temporal horn.

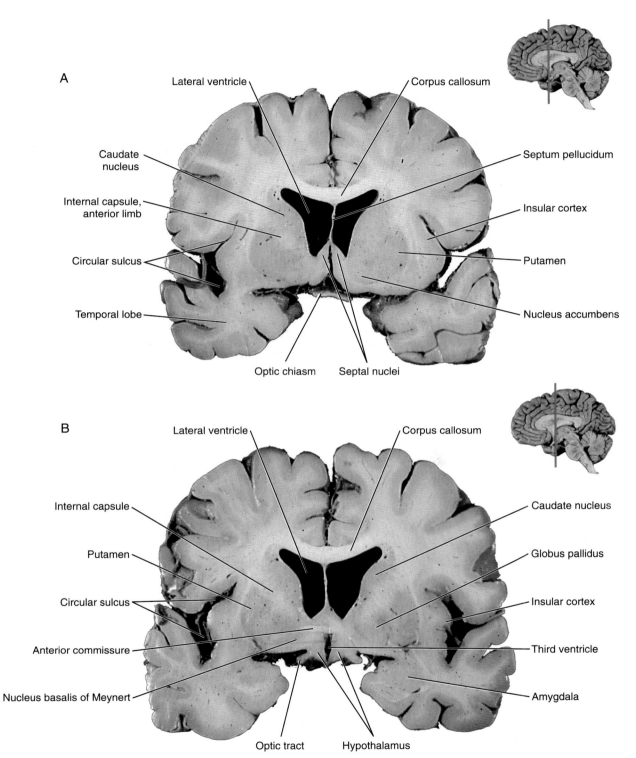

**Figure 1-30** *A*, Coronal section, showing the anterior basal forebrain. *B*, Coronal section, approximately 8 mm posterior to the section in *A*, showing posterior regions of the basal forebrain.

Major Divisions of the Central Nervous System

## PRACTICE 1-7

Make sure you know the meaning and location of the following structures:

basal ganglia
caudate nucleus (head, body, tail)
putamen
globus pallidus

internal capsule

hippocampal formation
parahippocampal gyrus

fornix (and columns of the fornix)
mammillary bodies

amygdala
basal forebrain
septal nuclei
nucleus basalis of Meynert
nucleus accumbens

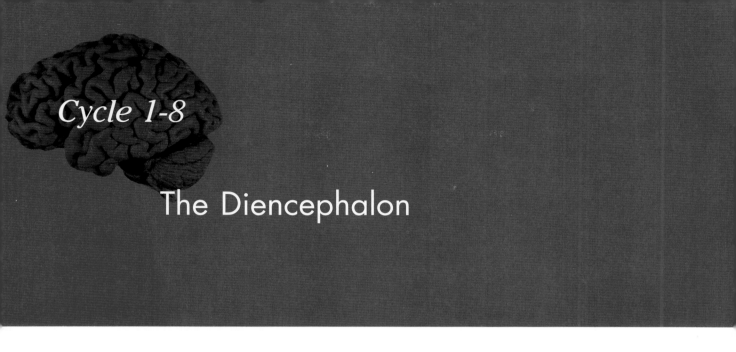

# The Diencephalon

## Objective

To learn the major divisions of the diencephalon.

The diencephalon comprises the *thalamus*, the *epi-thalamus*, the *subthalamus*, and the *hypothalamus* (Table 1-5). It is buried deep within the cerebral hemispheres. The total volume of tissue is small compared to the cerebral cortex, but the functions of the diencephalon are no less important. For example, virtually all sensory projections ascending to the cortex synapse first in portions of the thalamus, and the hypothalamus is the principal regulator of the autonomic (visceral) nervous system and the endocrine system.

The diencephalon forms the lateral walls of the third ventricle (see Fig. 1-9C and 1-31). It is bounded rostrally and laterally by the genu and posterior limb, respectively, of the internal capsule. Dorsomedially, it is bounded by a cerebrospinal fluid space (the cistern of the velum interpositum). Dorsolaterally, the diencephalon is bounded by deep cerebral white matter. Caudally, it runs into the midbrain as the third ventricle funnels down into the cerebral aqueduct, and one can expect to see a number of midbrain structures in coronal sections through the diencephalon. A midsagittal view of the brain (Fig. 1-31) offers a good view of the major divisions of the diencephalon: the hypothalamus, located ventral to the hypothalamic sulcus;

the subthalamus, not visible in this medial view; the thalamus, dorsal to the hypothalamic sulcus; and the epithalamus, the posterodorsal portion of the diencephalon (comprising the pineal gland and the posterior commissure).

## THE HYPOTHALAMUS

The hypothalamus interacts closely with the limbic system and is regarded as the "head ganglion" of the autonomic nervous system. It exerts neuronal and hormonal control over systems involved in maintaining homeostasis. Small tumors or infarcts involving the various nuclei of the hypothalamus can have devastating effects on water balance, energy regulation, temperature regulation, cardiovascular function, sleep, sexual development or behavior, and emotional behavior. These functions will be discussed in more detail in subsequent chapters.

The ventral surface of the hypothalamus is formed by three structures (Fig. 1-32). From rostral to caudal, these are (1) the *optic chiasm*, the site at which many of the fibers of the optic nerve cross the midline on their way to the thalamus; (2) the midline *infundibulum*, which is the *pituitary stalk*, the pathway via which the hypothalamus regulates pituitary function; and (3) the paired *mammillary bodies*, which receive a major input from the hippocampus via the postcommissural fornix. A well-defined bundle of fibers, the *mammillothalamic tract*, passes from the mammillary bodies to the

**TABLE 1-5** Structures and Their Functions

| Structure | Function |
|---|---|
| Hypothalamus | Autonomic, emotional, and neuroendocrine function |
| Subthalamus | |
|   Subthalamic white matter | Various, e.g., arousal and attention, motor, oculomotor control |
|   Subthalamic nucleus | Motor (linked to globus pallidus) |
| Thalamus | |
|   Relay nuclei | |
|     Medial geniculate | Auditory (brainstem to auditory cortex) |
|     Lateral geniculate | Visual (retinas, via optic nerves, chiasm and tracts, to the calcarine cortex) |
|     Ventral posterior (VPL, VPM) | Somatosensory (brainstem to sensory cortex) |
|     Ventral anterior, Ventral lateral | Motor (basal ganglia and cerebellum to motor and premotor cortex) |
|     Associative (e.g., pulvinar, dorsomedial, anterior) | Linkage of association cortices with each other and some subcortical structures |
|   Nucleus reticularis | Regulation of thalamic transmission |
| Epithalamus | |
|   Pineal | Radiologic landmark |
|   Posterior commissure | Fibers important in eye movement and control of pupillary size |

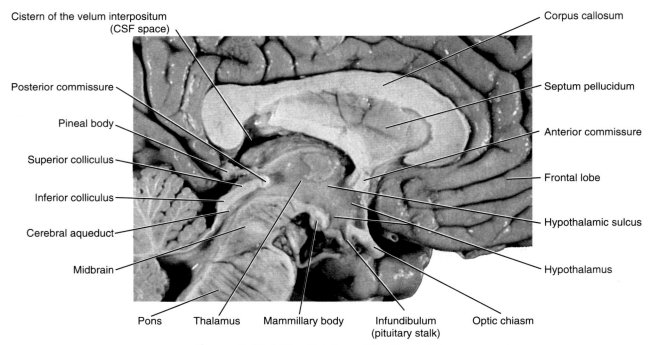

**Figure 1-31** Midsagittal view of the diencephalon.

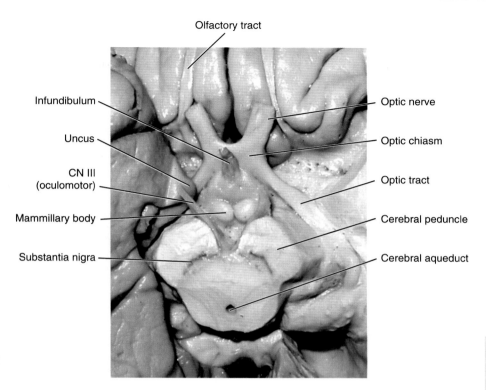

Olfactory tract

Infundibulum

Uncus

CN III
(oculomotor)

Mammillary body

Substantia nigra

Optic nerve

Optic chiasm

Optic tract

Cerebral peduncle

Cerebral aqueduct

**Figure 1-32** Ventral view of the hypothalamus.

anterior nucleus of the thalamus; this can be seen best in coronal section (Fig. 1-33).

## THE SUBTHALAMUS

The *subthalamus* is located ventral to the thalamus and posterior and lateral to the hypothalamus (Fig. 1-34). The subthalamus consists largely of a dense tangle of white matter pathways involved in a large spectrum of functions ranging from arousal and attention to movement to oculomotor control. Within this white matter lies the lens-shaped *subthalamic nucleus*, a structure closely linked with globus pallidus (part of the basal ganglia) and involved in motor function. Lesions of this tiny nucleus produce a very dramatic movement disorder (hemiballismus), which we will discuss in a later chapter.

## THE THALAMUS

The thalamus is the largest division of the diencephalon. It functions as a precisely controllable relay station between the brainstem and the cerebral cortex and between various parts of the cerebral cortex. Each of its subdivisions (nuclei) has a *precise topographic*

*relationship to its afferent and efferent systems*. The caudal inferior portion of the thalamus is composed of three nuclei that relay afferent sensory input to the cerebral cortex (Fig. 1-35): (1) the *medial geniculate nucleus* (MGN), which relays transmission from ascending auditory pathways in the brainstem to Heschl's gyrus (primary auditory cortex, Brodmann's areas 41 and 42) on the superior surface of the temporal lobe deep within the sylvian fissure; (2) the *lateral geniculate nucleus* (LGN), which receives visual transmission from the retina via the optic tract and transmits it to the banks of the calcarine fissure in the medial occipital lobe via the optic radiations; and (3) the *ventral posterior nucleus* (divided into ventral posterolateral [VPL] and ventral posteromedial [VPM] nuclei), which relay transmission from ascending somatosensory pathways within the brainstem to the postcentral gyrus (the primary somatosensory cortex). The information relayed by other thalamic nuclei is more difficult to characterize, but the topographic relationship to afferent and efferent systems is maintained throughout:

Immediately anterior to VPL and VPM is the ventral lateral nucleus; posterior portions of this nucleus relay projections from the cerebellum to the motor and premotor cortices, and anterior portions relay projections coming

*Major Divisions of the Central Nervous System*

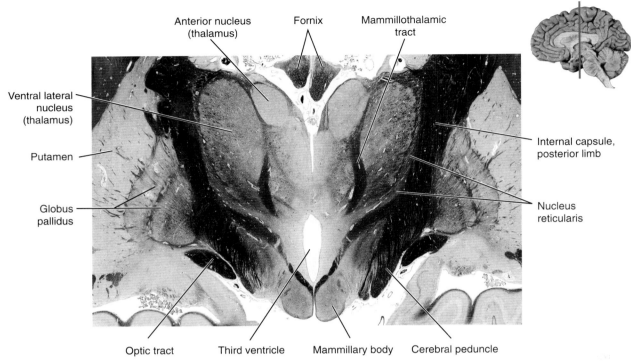

**Figure 1-33** Coronal section of the thalamus at the level of the mammillothalamic tract. (Modified from Warner JJ. Atlas of Neuroanatomy. Boston, Butterworth Heinemann, 2001, with permission from Elsevier Science.)

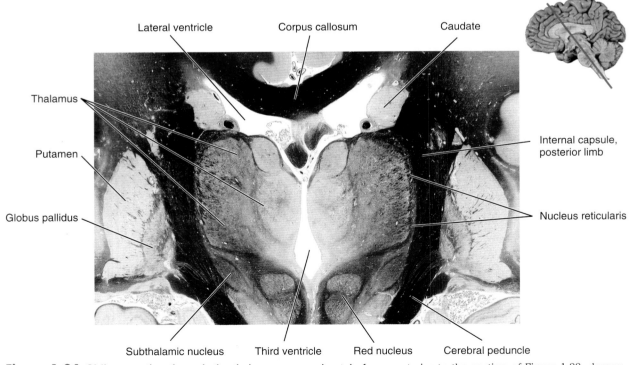

**Figure 1-34** Oblique section through the thalamus, approximately 1 cm posterior to the section of Figure 1-33, demonstrating the subthalamus. (Modified from Warner JJ. Atlas of Neuroanatomy. Boston, Butterworth Heinemann, 2001, with permission from Elsevier Science.)

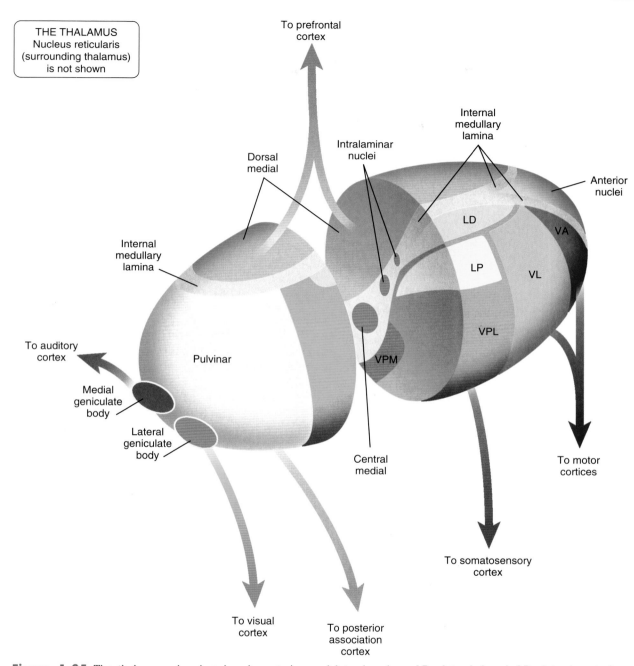

THE THALAMUS
Nucleus reticularis
(surrounding thalamus)
is not shown

To prefrontal
cortex

Dorsal
medial

Intralaminar
nuclei

Internal
medullary
lamina

Anterior
nuclei

LD

VA

Internal
medullary
lamina

LP

VL

To auditory
cortex

Pulvinar

VPL

VPM

Medial
geniculate
body

Central
medial

Lateral
geniculate
body

To motor
cortices

To somatosensory
cortex

To visual
cortex

To posterior
association
cortex

**Figure 1-35** The thalamus, showing dorsal, posterior, and lateral regions. LD = lateral dorsal; LP = lateral posterior; VA = ventral anterior; VL = ventral lateral; VPL = ventral posterolateral; VPM = ventral posteromedial.

from the putamen via the globus pallidus to motor and premotor cortices. At the anterior pole of the thalamus, the ventral anterior nucleus relays projections coming from the caudate via the globus pallidus to the prefrontal cortex. Dorsomedial to a fibrous partition within the thalamus (the internal medullary lamina), lies the dorsomedial nucleus (DM). The major afferent and efferent connec-

tions of DM are with prefrontal cortex. Immediately ventral to DM are the midline nuclei, which have extensive limbic connections. At the caudal pole of the thalamus is the pulvinar, the major connections of which are with overlying temporal and parietal cortex. At the superior anterior pole of the thalamus, between the sheaves of the internal medullary lamina, is the anterior nuclear group. These

Major Divisions of the Central Nervous System

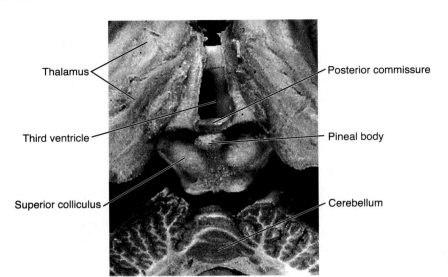

Thalamus

Posterior commissure

Third ventricle

Pineal body

Superior colliculus

Cerebellum

**Figure 1-36** Dorsal view of the epithalamus. (Dissection by JJ Warner.)

nuclei are connected by the mammillothalamic tract to the mammillary bodies, which are in turn connected to the hippocampus by the fornix. Predictably, the anterior nuclear group is involved in memory function.

The exquisite *topographic organization of the thalamus* and its links to every major cortical and brainstem system provide the basis for thalamic regulation of neural transmission throughout the brain. The thalamus is wrapped in another fiber layer, the external medullary lamina. Immediately outside this lamina, enveloping the entire thalamus except the anterior nuclear group, is a paper-thin sheet of neurons, the thalamic reticular nucleus (or *nucleus reticularis*) (Figs. 1-33 and 1-34), which projects to the various nuclei within the thalamus and not to the cortex. Nucleus reticularis has the capability for enabling or blocking transmission from the thalamus to the cortex: it is the switch on the thalamic relay. This switch is regulated by overlying temporoparietal cortex and the frontal lobes, which enable selective transmission to the cortex, and by connections from the midbrain reticular formation and ascending biogenic amine systems (norepinephrine and serotonin), which enable the general release of thalamic transmission to cortex. This switching device transforms the thalamus from a simple relay station into a mechanism for regulating the flow of information throughout the brain.

## THE EPITHALAMUS

The *epithalamus* (Fig. 1-36) is situated immediately posterior to the thalamus. The two most important structures here are the pineal gland and the posterior commissure. The *pineal gland* is a small pine cone–shaped structure thought to influence biologic responses to the light/dark cycle (circadian rhythms) by releasing the hormone melatonin. It is also thought to inhibit gonadal function in children. In practice, its chief importance is as a radiologic landmark. The *posterior commissure* marks the boundary between the midbrain and the thalamus. It crosses the midline dorsal to the cerebral aqueduct at the point where the aqueduct opens into the third ventricle. The posterior commissure contains fibers important to eye movement control and pupillary light responses.

## PRACTICE 1-8

Make sure you know the meaning and location of the following structures:

hypothalamus
optic chiasm
infundibulum (pituitary stalk)
mammillary bodies
mammillothalamic tract
subthalamus
subthalamic nucleus
thalamus
medial geniculate nucleus
lateral geniculate nucleus

ventral posterior nuclei (VPL and VPM)
ventral anterior/ventral lateral (VA/VL)
nucleus reticularis
principle of topographic organization of thalamus
epithalamus
pineal gland
posterior commissure

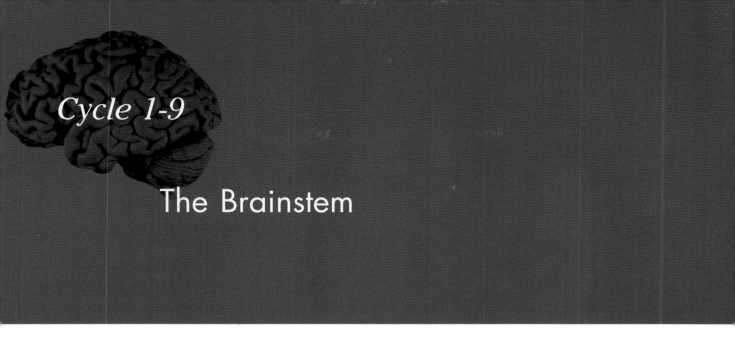

## Cycle 1-9

# The Brainstem

*Objective*

To learn the major divisions of the brainstem and the locations of the cranial nerves.

At this point, we will concentrate on surface features and a few deep structures that can be seen in unstained sections. We will save the internal details for Chapter 8 (Cranial Nerves).

The brainstem consists of the midbrain, the pons, and the medulla. Within a small volume, it contains all the ascending and descending pathways between the cerebral cortex and the spinal cord as well as all but two of the 12 cranial nerves (CNs). Inasmuch as a small brainstem lesion can have profound consequences for a patient's well-being and survival, an understanding of brainstem anatomy is of great clinical importance.

## THE MIDBRAIN

The *midbrain* contains the cerebral aqueduct, or aqueduct of Sylvius. The midbrain is identified on the dorsal surface of the brainstem by four colliculi that form the *quadrigeminal plate* ("fourfold") (Fig. 1-37). The two superior hills are the *superior colliculi* (Fig. 1-38). The superior colliculus, often referred to as the optic tectum, is involved in the direction of attention and in the reflexive orienting movements of the eyes and head necessary to direct sensory organs to the focus of attention. The inferior hills are the *inferior colliculi* (Fig. 1-39). The inferior colliculus is an obligatory relay in the ascending auditory pathway. The colliculi and all other tissue dorsal to the cerebral aqueduct are referred to collectively as the *tectum* of the midbrain. The cerebral peduncles identify the midbrain on the ventral surface of the brainstem. The cerebral peduncles, forming the "basement" of the midbrain, are the caudal continuation of the internal capsule. All the tissue ventral to the cerebral aqueduct, except for the cerebral peduncles, is the *tegmentum* ("floor"). Figure 1-38 also shows two prominent structures of the tegmentum, the *red nuclei* and the *substantia nigra*, both of which are parts of the motor system. The tissue surrounding the aqueduct comprises the *periaqueductal gray*, a structure important in the modulation of pain sensation that also serves as an adjunct to the limbic system. On either side of the periaqueductal gray is *midbrain reticular formation*, which is the major structure regulating our level of arousal or alertness.

Approximately 1 cm caudal to the brainstem slice we have been reviewing, we see the caudal continuation of many of the structures already discussed (Fig. 1-39). The superior colliculi have now been replaced by the inferior colliculi. In the very center of the section we see a new white matter tract, the *decussation (crossing) of the brachium conjunctivum* (another name for superior cerebellar peduncles, the major outflow tract from the cerebellum to the cerebrum).

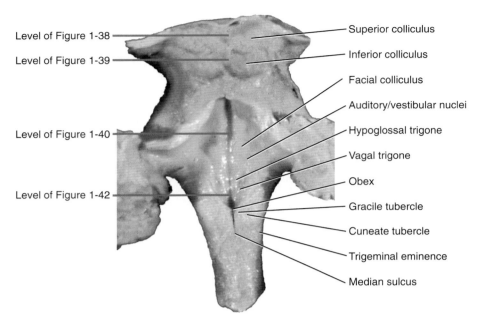

Level of Figure 1-38 — Superior colliculus
Level of Figure 1-39 — Inferior colliculus
Facial colliculus
Auditory/vestibular nuclei
Hypoglossal trigone
Level of Figure 1-40 — Vagal trigone
Obex
Level of Figure 1-42 — Gracile tubercle
Cuneate tubercle
Trigeminal eminence
Median sulcus

**Figure 1-37** Dorsal view of the brainstem.

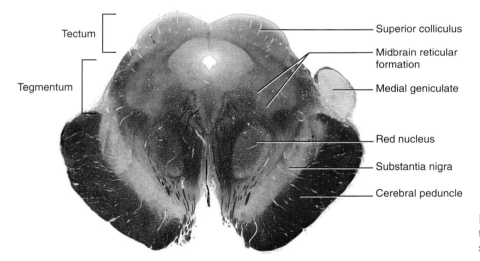

Tectum
Superior colliculus
Midbrain reticular formation
Tegmentum
Medial geniculate
Red nucleus
Substantia nigra
Cerebral peduncle

**Figure 1-38** Transverse section through the rostral midbrain, stained for myelin.

## THE PONS

The *pons* is identified on the ventral surface of the brainstem by the transverse fibers of the pons, which continue up the lateral surface of the pons as the middle cerebellar peduncles (Figs. 1-40 and 1-41). The dorsal surface of the pons forms the rostral half of the floor of the fourth ventricle. In a cross section of the pons we see the fourth ventricle dorsally and the transverse fibers streaming across through the entire ventral half (the *basis pontis*) (Fig. 1-40). Within the basis pontis we see some islands of tissue, which are actually the caudal extension of the cerebral peduncles we identified in the midbrain and of the internal capsule. The two sides of the pons are framed by the *middle cerebellar peduncles*, the inflow tract to the cerebellum from the cerebrum. The dorsolateral aspects of the fourth ventricle are framed by the *superior cerebellar peduncles*, the major outflow tracts of the cerebellum. More rostrally, these cross within the caudal midbrain (the decussation of the brachium conjunctivum). All

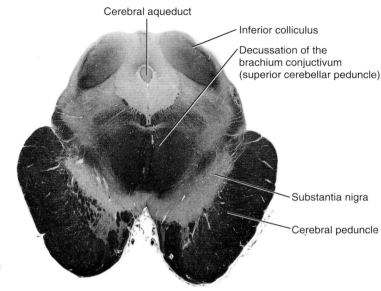

**Figure 1-39** Transverse section through the caudal midbrain, stained for myelin.

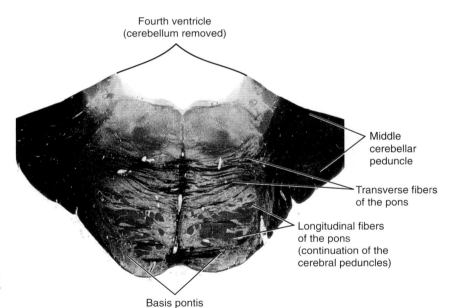

**Figure 1-40** Transverse section through the mid-pons, stained for myelin.

the structures that we have identified in the pons are involved in motor function.

## THE MEDULLA

The *medulla* is identified on the ventral surface of the brainstem by the *pyramids*, which contain the caudal continuation of some of the fibers of the cerebral peduncles (Fig. 1-41). Dorsolateral to the pyramids are the *inferior olives*, which function as an adjunct to the cerebellum. On cross section (Fig. 1-42), the inferior olives are the two striking, serpiginous structures composing most of the ventral quadrants. The most ventral aspect of the medulla is composed of the medullary pyramids—the caudal continuation of the internal capsule, cerebral peduncles, and descending motor pathways of the basis pontis. Immediately dorsal to the pyramids, lying between the olives, is a major ascending sensory pathway, the *medial lemniscus*, ultimately

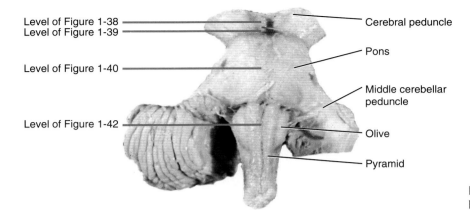

Level of Figure 1-38
Level of Figure 1-39
Level of Figure 1-40
Level of Figure 1-42

Cerebral peduncle
Pons
Middle cerebellar peduncle
Olive
Pyramid

**Figure 1-41** Ventral view of the brainstem.

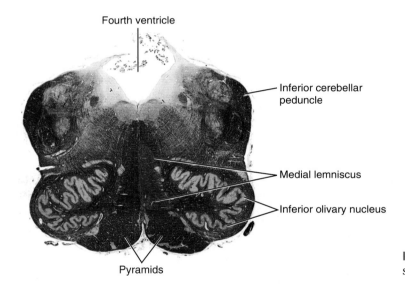

Fourth ventricle

Inferior cerebellar peduncle

Medial lemniscus

Inferior olivary nucleus

Pyramids

**Figure 1-42** Transverse section of the medulla, stained for myelin.

destined for the thalamus. The dorsal surface of the medulla forms the caudal floor of the fourth ventricle. The roof of the fourth ventricle at this level is formed by the cerebellum. At the dorsolateral margins of the medulla are the *inferior cerebellar peduncles*, the inflow pathway from the spinal cord and the inferior olives to the cerebellum.

One can identify landmarks on the dorsal surface of the medulla that correspond to underlying sensory and motor nuclei (Fig. 1-37). The groove that runs along the midline of the dorsal surface is the median sulcus. Caudal to the *obex* (the caudal recess of the fourth ventricle), beginning at the median sulcus and passing laterally, one can see three elevations: the gracile tubercle, the cuneate tubercle, and the trigeminal eminence, overlying the *gracile nucleus*, the

*cuneate nucleus*, and the *spinal nucleus of the trigeminal nerve*, respectively. These nuclei are involved in the sense of touch and proprioception on the lower and upper body, and pain and temperature sensation on the face, respectively. Rostral to the obex, beginning at the median sulcus, one can identify the hypoglossal trigone and the vagal trigone, which overlie the motor nuclei for the tongue (CN XII) and the vagus nerve (CN X), respectively. Further rostral is the *facial colliculus* (a caudal pontine structure), formed by motor fibers from the facial nucleus as they loop over the nucleus of the abducens nerve (one of the nerves controlling movement of the eyes). Laterally, one can see the nuclei of the cochlear and vestibular nerves, which convey the senses of hearing and balance, respectively.

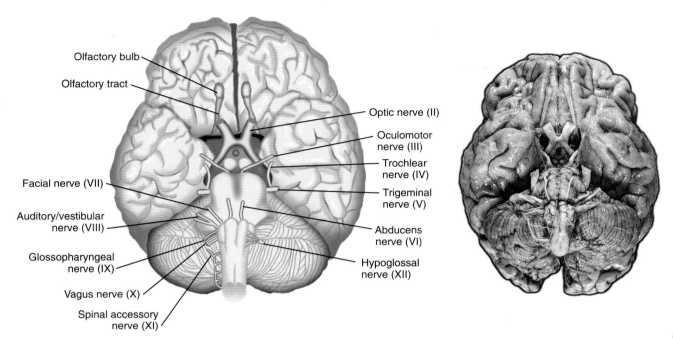

**Figure 1-43** Ventral view of the brain, showing the cranial nerves. (Dissection by JJ Warner.)

## THE CRANIAL NERVES

The 12 pairs of *cranial nerves* exit from the forebrain and brainstem (Fig. 1-43, Tables 1-6 and 1-7). They provide sensory and motor function for the head, convey the "special senses" (sight, smell, hearing, balance, and taste), and participate in control of the viscera. Cranial nerves can be purely sensory, purely motor, or mixed. They can also contain efferent or afferent autonomic fibers. In some cases, one pair of cranial nerves can provide input to or output from several cranial nerve nuclei. In this cycle, we will locate the cranial nerves and learn their functions in only a most general sense. The details will follow in Chapter 8.

Students throughout the years have invented mnemonic phrases to help remember the names of the cranial nerves. One of the few that is suitable for print is: "<u>O</u>n <u>O</u>ld <u>O</u>lympus's <u>T</u>owering <u>T</u>op, <u>A</u> <u>F</u>at <u>A</u>rmed <u>G</u>orilla <u>V</u>ends <u>S</u>nowy <u>H</u>ops." Table 1-7 lists the full names, the general functions of the nerves, and whether they carry sensory (S), motor (M), or parasympathetic autonomic (P) information.

All but one of the cranial nerves exit the brain tissue from the ventral or lateral surface and are visible in a ventral view (Fig. 1-43). Two of the nerves are found in the forebrain. The *olfactory nerves* (CN I) are tiny nerves that pass from the olfactory mucosa in the nose, through the cribriform plate, to terminate in the *olfactory bulb*. Neurons in the olfactory bulb project to frontal and temporal lobe structures. The olfactory tract, visible on the ventral aspect of the frontal lobe, carries the output of the olfactory bulb. The *optic nerve* (CN II) carries visual input from the retina of the eye toward the *lateral geniculate nucleus* (LGN) of the thalamus. Optic "nerve" refers to the fibers that pass from the retina to the *optic chiasm*. At the optic chiasm, half of the fibers from each retina cross the midline. The fibers from the chiasm to the LGN are called the *optic tract*. The fibers from the LGN to the calcarine cortex are called the *optic radiations*.

**TABLE 1-6 Summary of Points of Entry/Exit of the Cranial Nerves**

| Region | Cranial Nerves |
|---|---|
| Temporal lobe (uncus) and posterior inferior frontal lobes | I (olfactory tract) |
| Thalamus (lateral geniculate nucleus) | II |
| Midbrain | III, IV |
| Pons | V |
| Pontomedullary junction | VI, VII, VIII |
| Medulla | IX, X, XII |
| Cervicomedullary junction | XI |

**Major Divisions of the Central Nervous System**

**TABLE 1-7 The Cranial Nerves**

| | Nerve | Type* | Function |
|---|---|---|---|
| I | Olfactory | S | Sense of smell |
| II | Optic | S | Vision |
| III | Oculomotor | M, P | Control of four of the six extraocular muscles |
| | | | Pupillary constriction |
| IV | Trochlear | M | Control of the superior oblique extraocular muscle |
| V | Trigeminal | S, M | Sensation on the face, in the mouth, and in the anterior and middle cranial fossae |
| | | | Control of the muscles of mastication |
| VI | Abducens | M | Control of the lateral rectus extraocular muscle |
| VII | Facial | S, M, P | Sense of taste in the anterior $2/3$ of the tongue |
| | | | Control of muscles of facial expression |
| | | | Control of the lacrimal glands (tears) |
| VIII | Auditory/vestibular | S | Hearing/balance |
| IX | Glossopharyngeal | S, M, P | Sense of taste in the posterior $1/3$ of the tongue |
| | | | Control of the stylopharyngeus muscle |
| | | | Control of the parotid salivary gland |
| X | Vagus | S, M, P | Control of pharyngeal musculature (swallowing, the larynx) |
| | | | Visceral autonomic sensation and control |
| XI | Accessory | M | Control of the sternocleidomastoid and trapezius muscles |
| XII | Hypoglossal | M | Control of the tongue |

*S = sensory; M = motor; P = parasympathetic autonomic.

Two cranial nerves have their cell bodies in the mesencephalon: the *oculomotor nerve* (CN III) and the *trochlear nerve* (CN IV). The oculomotor nerve has its cell bodies at the level of the superior colliculus, and the nerve emerges ventrally, near the midline, from between the cerebral peduncles. The trochlear nerve has its cell bodies at the level of the inferior colliculus. The trochlear nerve emerges caudal to the inferior colliculi and is the only nerve to emerge from the dorsal surface of the brainstem. It is visible in a ventral view as it wraps around the lateral aspect of the cerebellar peduncle. The *trigeminal nerve* (CN V) penetrates the middle cerebellar peduncle at mid-pons. Three pairs of nerves emerge at the junction of pons and medulla. The *abducens nerve* (CN VI) emerges near the midline. Further lateral is the *facial nerve* (CN VII). The most lateral is CN VIII, consisting of the *auditory* and *vestibular* nerves. The remainder of the cranial nerves can be located with reference to the inferior olive of the medulla (Fig. 1-41). Small rootlets of the *glossopharyngeal* (CN IX), *vagus* (CN X), and *spinal accessory* (CN XI) nerves emerge in a rostral-to-caudal line along a sulcus dorsal to the olive. The rootlets of the *hypoglossal nerve* (CN XII) emerge along a sulcus ventral to the olive.

## PRACTICE 1-9

Make sure you know the meaning and location of the following structures:

tectum
tegmentum
midbrain
quadrigeminal plate
superior colliculus
inferior colliculus
red nuclei
substantia nigra
cerebral peduncle
periaqueductal gray
   substance
midbrain reticular
   formation (site of
   midbrain reticular
   activating system)
decussation of
   brachium
   conjunctivum
   (superior cerebellar
   peduncles)

pons
basis pontis
superior cerebellar
   peduncle
middle cerebellar
   peduncle
inferior cerebellar
   peduncle
facial colliculus

medulla
inferior olives
gracile nucleus
cuneate nucleus
spinal nucleus of the
   trigeminal nerve
medial lemniscus

cranial nerves I to XII

olfactory bulb

optic tract
optic chiasm
optic radiations

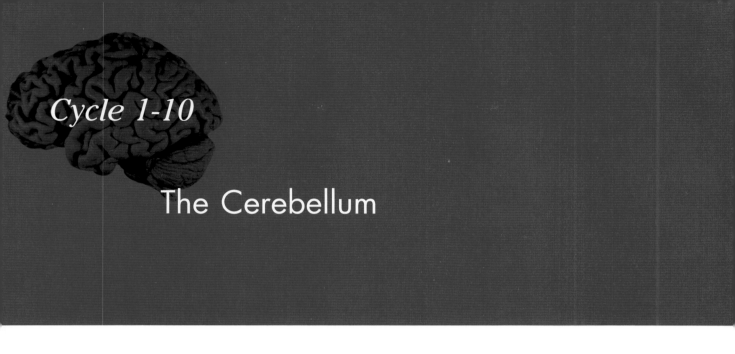

# Cycle 1-10

# The Cerebellum

## Objective

To learn the major functional divisions of the cerebellum.

The cerebellum acts with the motor system to formulate movements. It forms most of the roof of the fourth ventricle. Although there are many named anatomic subdivisions in the cerebellum, we will learn only those few that are functionally most relevant.

Most of the volume of the cerebellum is occupied by the laminated cerebellar cortex and its accompanying white matter (Fig. 1-44). The gyri of the cerebellar cortex are called *folia*. In the mediolateral dimension, the cerebellum is divided into the midline *vermis* ("worm") and the lateral *cerebellar hemispheres*. The

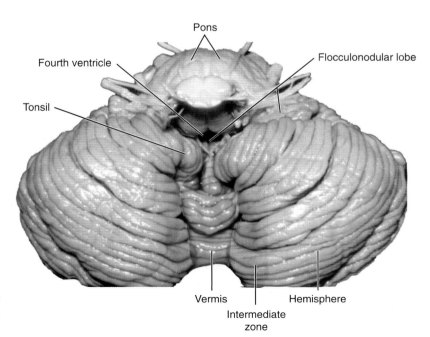

**Figure 1-44** Lobes of the cerebellar cortex, caudal-rostral view. Note, the nodulus cannot be seen in this view.

Major Divisions of the Central Nervous System

57

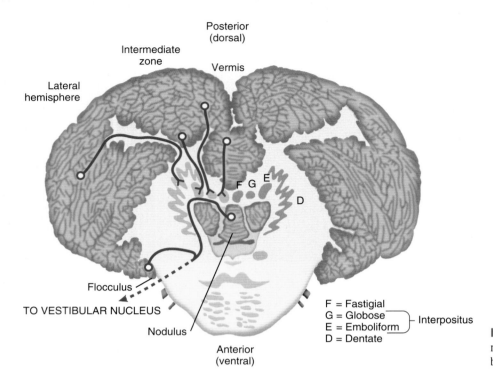

**Figure 1-45** Deep cerebellar nuclei. (Modification of drawing by JJ Warner.)

vermis extends from near the brainstem at its superior end, wrapping most of the way around the cerebellum in the sagittal plane, to end near the brainstem at its inferior end. The cerebellar hemispheres are involved in coordination of the most lateral body parts (arms and hands), whereas the vermis is involved in coordination of the body midline (gait and balance). The caudal-most aspect of the cerebellum forms the *flocculonodular lobe*. The flocculonodular node includes the nodule, which is the most anterior folium at the inferior end of the vermis, and its two lateral appendages, which form the flocculi. The flocculonodular lobe is involved in the coordination of eye movements.

Deep to the cerebellar cortex, within the white matter, are the deep cerebellar nuclei (Fig. 1-45). Inputs to the cerebellum from everywhere but the inferior olives send a branch to one of the deep nuclei before proceeding to the cerebellar cortex, and the entire output of the cerebellar cortex terminates in the deep nuclei. The four pairs of nuclei, from medial to lateral, are the *fastigial*, globus, emboliform, and *dentate*. We normally will refer to the globus and emboliform together as the *nucleus interpositus* (the interposed nuclei). Each of these nuclei has a strict topographic

relationship with overlying cerebellar cortex, the dentate with the cerebellar hemispheres, the nucleus interpositus with intermediate zone, and the fastigial nucleus with the vermis.

We have seen in cross sections of the brainstem the three major fiber bundles connecting the cerebellum with the brainstem. The *superior cerebellar peduncle* carries most of the output of the cerebellar hemisphere. The *middle cerebellar peduncle* carries input that is relayed from the cerebral cortex to the cerebellum via the gray matter of the pons. The *inferior cerebellar peduncle* carries connections of the cerebellum to and from the medulla and spinal cord.

## PRACTICE 1-10

Make sure you know the meaning and location of the following structures:

| | |
|---|---|
| vermis | superior cerebellar |
| cerebellar hemispheres | peduncle |
| flocculonodular lobe | middle cerebellar |
| fastigial nucleus | peduncle |
| nucleus interpositus | inferior cerebellar |
| dentate nucleus | peduncle |

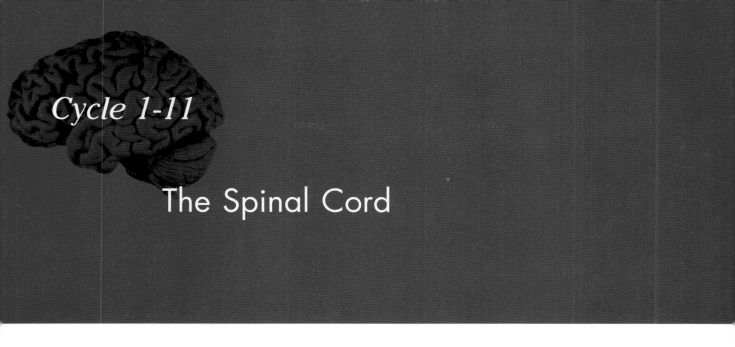

# Cycle 1-11

# The Spinal Cord

## Objective

To learn the cross-sectional and segmental organization of the spinal cord.

The core of the spinal cord, which is gray matter, carries out integrative functions similar to those carried out in the brain and, in fact, many of the early advances in CNS physiology were made in the spinal cord. The spinal cord presents an example of *topographic organization* in which locations on the body surface and muscles map onto locations within the cord. Because of the vulnerability of the spinal cord to traumatic injury, the clinician often must deal with this topography rather directly.

A transverse section through the spinal cord (Fig. 1-46) reveals a portion of the ventricular system found in the spinal cord, the central canal, which typically is not patent in the adult. The central canal is surrounded by a region of gray matter, the *central gray*. The gray matter has the general shape of a letter H; the exact shape of the H varies according to the rostrocaudal level of the spinal cord. The dorsal arms of the H are called the *dorsal horns*; in humans, the dorsal horns often are called the *posterior horns*. They are *sensory* in function. The ventral arms of the H are called the *ventral*, or *anterior*, *horns*. They are *motoric* in function.

The intermediolateral column is a spike-like lateral extension of the gray matter, intermediate between the dorsal and ventral horns (Fig. 1-47). It is found only at cord levels T1 to L2. The intermediolateral column is the lateral extension of the *intermediate zone* of the spinal cord, the band of gray matter between the dorsal and ventral horns that contains preganglionic autonomic neurons, sympathetic from T1 through L2, parasympathetic from S2 through S4.

Projections from the ventral horns and the intermediate zone to the periphery exit the spinal cord in the *ventral roots* to terminate on muscles and autonomic ganglia, respectively. *Dorsal root fibers* (the cell bodies of which lie in the *dorsal root ganglia*) (Figs. 1-53 and 1-54) enter the spinal cord at the edges of the dorsal horn. These fibers carry sensory information into the spinal cord. Some dorsal root fibers form synapses within the dorsal horn immediately upon entry into the spinal cord, whereas others ascend or descend some distance in the white matter before synapsing. Peripherally, the dorsal and ventral roots from each segment of the spinal cord coalesce to form a spinal nerve. There are a total of 31 spinal cord segments: 8 *cervical*, 12 *thoracic*, 5 *lumbar*, 5 *sacral*, and 1 *coccygeal*. The area of the body served by a single dorsal root is called a *dermatome*. Sensory fibers from the dorsal roots coalesce more peripherally in various ways to form peripheral sensory nerves. Figure 1-48 shows the distribution of dermatomes and sensory nerves on the body surface. Neurologists maintain a pretty precise mental image of the dermatomes but can routinely recall only the peripheral sensory nerves most commonly affected by disease. You need learn only the general organization of the dermatomes.

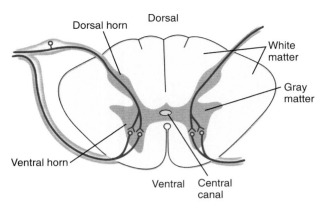

**Figure 1-46** Transverse section of the spinal cord.

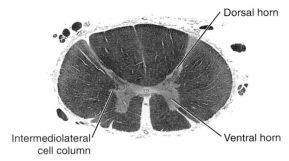

**Figure 1-47** Transverse section through the spinal cord, T6 level, stained for myelin.

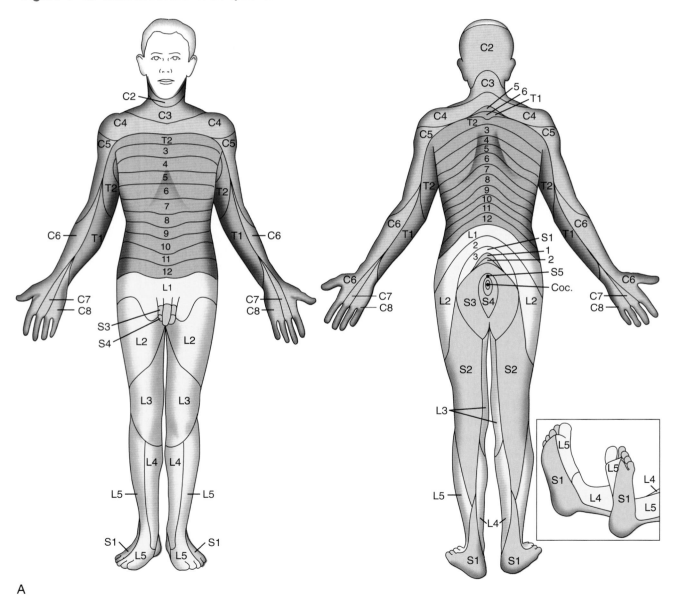

A

**Figure 1-48** Distribution of the dermatomes and body surface supplied by the peripheral sensory nerves. (Modified from W. Haymaker, B. Woodhall. Peripheral Nerve Injuries, Principles of Diagnosis, 2nd ed. Philadelphia, WB Saunders, 1953.)

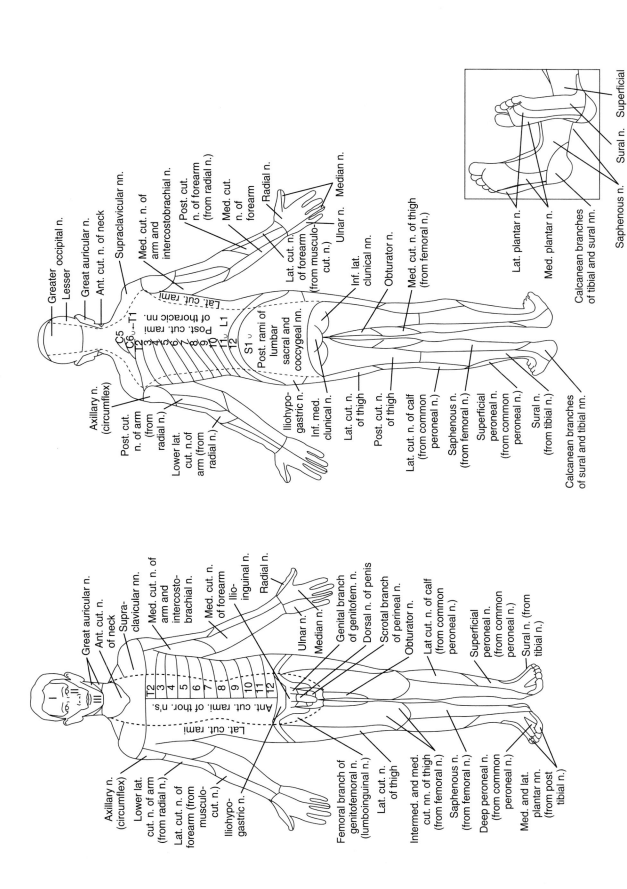

**Figure 1-48**, cont'd      **Major Divisions of the Central Nervous System**

B

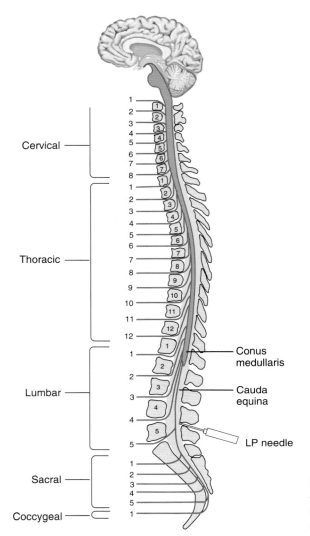

Cervical

Thoracic

Lumbar

Sacral

Coccygeal

Conus medullaris

Cauda equina

LP needle

**Figure 1-49** Location of the spinal cord within the bony spinal canal. Note that the site at which lumbar puncture (LP) is routinely done, at the L4-L5 level, is well below the terminus of the spinal cord.

In development, up to about the third month of fetal life, the spinal cord segments are aligned with the corresponding vertebrae, and spinal roots exit the vertebral column at the nearest intervertebral space. At later developmental stages, however, the vertebral column grows faster than the spinal cord, and a spinal root can become greatly elongated as it spans the distance from a given cord segment to what was once the adjacent intervertebral space. In the adult, the caudal end of the spinal cord (the *conus medullaris*) is aligned

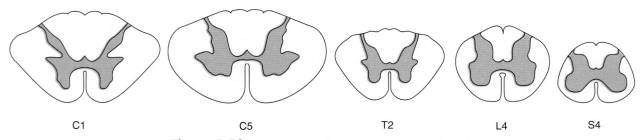

C1    C5    T2    L4    S4

**Figure 1-50** Transverse sections through the spinal cord.

with the first lumbar vertebra (Fig. 1-49). The spinal roots that extend caudal to the caudal end of the spinal cord form what is called the *cauda equina* ("horse's tail").

The shape and relative size of gray matter and white matter areas vary between different regions of the spinal cord. Figure 1-50 shows transverse sections through the cord at various levels. Two general principles apply:

1. The gray matter, particularly in the ventral horns, is enlarged at cord segments that supply the extremities. The *brachial (cervical) enlargement*, which supplies the arms (i.e., the brachial plexus), extends from C5 to T1. The *lumbosacral enlargement*, which supplies the legs, extends from L1 to S3.

2. The total thickness of white matter increases from caudal to rostral. This is because the white matter of the coccygeal segment contains only the axons that serve that segment, whereas the white matter

of, say, C1 contains the ascending and descending axons that serve C1 plus all segments located further caudally.

## PRACTICE 1-11

Make sure you know the meaning and location of the following:

central gray
posterior (dorsal) horn
anterior (ventral) horn
dorsal root ganglion
dorsal root fibers
ventral root fibers
dermatome
conus medullaris
cauda equina
brachial (cervical)
    enlargement

lumbosacral
    enlargement
intermediate zone
topographic
    organization of
    the spinal cord
spinal cord regions
    (cervical, thoracic,
    lumbar, sacral,
    coccygeal)

**Major Divisions of the Central Nervous System**

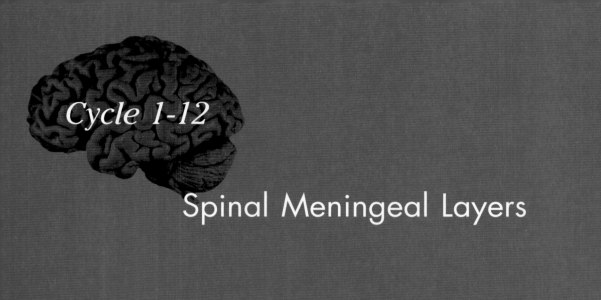

# Spinal Meningeal Layers

Learn the relationship of the meningeal layers to the spinal cord and nerve roots.

The three meningeal layers investing the brain, the outer *dura*, intermediate *arachnoid*, and inner *pia*, which we discussed in Cycle 1-4, continue down the bony spinal canal. However, there are important differences in their architecture within the spinal canal. The dura is not closely adherent to the vertebral bones because the inner vertebral surface has its own periosteal layer (unlike within the cranial vault, where the outer layer of the dura forms the inner periosteum of the skull). A layer of fat and a network of veins are interposed between the periosteum and the spinal dura. It is the puncture of these veins that is most often responsible for a "traumatic" (bloody) lumbar puncture.

The dura is separated from the arachnoid by a potential space. The arachnoid is a thin membrane and its extent parallels that of the dura. The two membranes form a sac-like space that is continuous with the cranial meninges at the foramen magnum and ends as a closed sac at the level of the second sacral vertebral body.

The pia is a filamentous structure that is adherent to the spinal cord and separated from the arachnoid by a subarachnoid space, which contains cerebrospinal fluid. Therefore, this site is targeted for lumbar punctures (spinal taps) and for introducing contrast material for myelography. Spinal taps are usually performed at the L4-L5 or L5-S1 interspaces and always below the second lumbar vertebral body to avoid the risk of penetrating the spinal cord with the needle (Fig. 1-49).

The pia of the spinal cord has a series of lateral projections (which appear as scalloped or tooth-like structures) called denticulate ligaments. These ligaments penetrate the arachnoid layer and attach to the inner aspect of the dura, providing a lateral stabilizing force on the spinal cord within the spinal canal. The spinal pia is also specialized at the caudal termination of the cord. Below L1, the pia continues as a threadlike extension from the terminal spinal cord, the *filum terminale*, which is anchored to the coccygeal vertebral surface (Figs. 1-51 to 1-53).

An investment of meninges is carried with spinal nerve rootlets for a short distance peripheral to the cord. The dura actually continues beyond the dorsal root ganglia, which lie within the bony intervertebral foramina, whereas the arachnoid terminates proximal to the ganglion. The same arrangement is found with the cranial nerves.

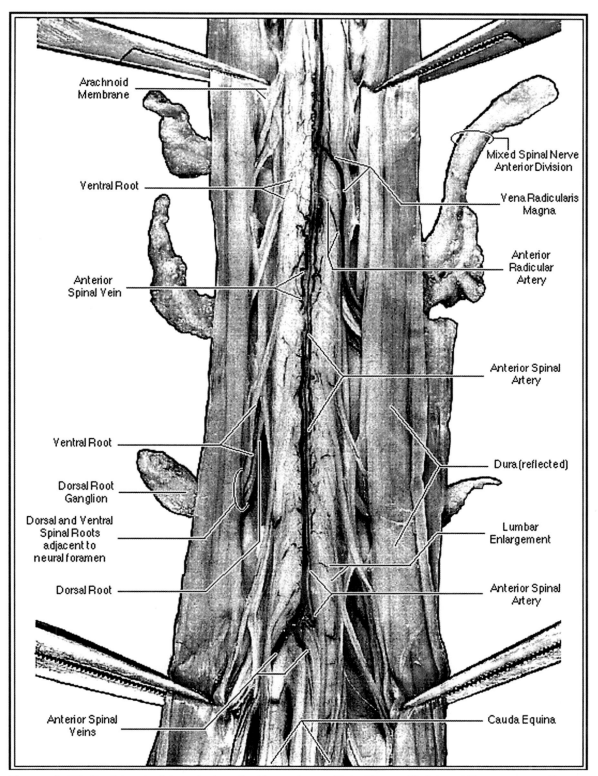

Arachnoid Membrane

Ventral Root

Anterior Spinal Vein

Ventral Root

Dorsal Root Ganglion

Dorsal and Ventral Spinal Roots adjacent to neural foramen

Dorsal Root

Anterior Spinal Veins

Mixed Spinal Nerve Anterior Division

Vena Radicularis Magna

Anterior Radicular Artery

Anterior Spinal Artery

Dura (reflected)

Lumbar Enlargement

Anterior Spinal Artery

Cauda Equina

**Major Divisions of the Central Nervous System**

**Figure 1-51** Caudal end of the spinal cord with meninges. (From Warner JJ. Atlas of Neuroanatomy. Boston, Butterworth Heinemann, 2001, with permission from Elsevier Science.)

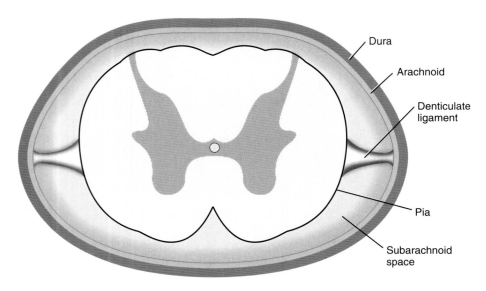

**Figure 1-52** Cross section of the spinal cord with meninges.

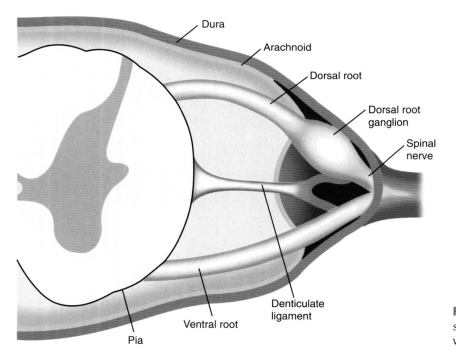

**Figure 1-53** Cross section of the spinal cord with meninges, dorsal and ventral roots.

## Case 1-3

### Herniated Intervertebral Disk with Nerve Root Compression

*A 45-year-old man presents to the neurology clinic with a 3-day history of excruciating, sharp pain radiating from his left hip down his left leg, sometimes all the way to the foot. The pain is sharp and stabbing in quality but it is often associated with a tingling or burning sensation over the lateral aspect of his leg. He can obtain some relief by sitting on his right buttock and holding the left leg flexed and adducted. Coughing, sneezing, or the Valsalva maneuver (forcibly exhaling against a closed glottis) precipitate unbearable stabs of pain in the leg. He has hardly slept since the pain started. One year ago he slipped on some ice and landed on his buttocks. He experienced some low back pain at the time, but it resolved over a week or so. On examination, straightening the leg beyond about 30 degrees markedly aggravates the pain. If the leg is straightened and lifted to about 20 degrees, he experiences no pain; however, forceful dorsiflexion of the ankle with the leg in this position elicits a stab of pain.*

**Comment:** *This patient has a herniated lumbar disk (Fig. 1-54), most likely the L5-S1 disk, both because it is the one most commonly affected and because the episodic tingling of the left lateral calf suggests involvement of the L5 nerve root, which exits between L5 and S1. Intervertebral disks are composed of a fibrous ring containing a semigelatinous core. Herniation occurs because of fracture of the fibrous ring, in which case it may protrude, most often posterolaterally, where it is least likely to be contained by the long paraspinous ligaments. The protruding fragment may then entrap the exiting nerve root, along with its meningeal investment, as it passes into the bony intervertebral foramen. Raising the straightened leg or dorsiflexing the ankle with the leg held immobile both pull on the sciatic nerve running up the back of the leg, and thus, indirectly, pull on the affected nerve root. It is the traction on the meningeal investment that causes the stabbing pain. An L5-S1 disk herniation is shown in the MRI depicted in Figure 1-54.*

## PRACTICE 1-12

**A.** Make sure you know the meaning and location of the following:

| | |
|---|---|
| spinal dura | spinal arachnoid |
| spinal pia | filum terminale |

**B.** (Optional) The spinal column is encased and stabilized by a number of major ligaments: the anterior longitudinal ligament, running along the anterior margin of the vertebral bodies; the posterior longitudinal ligament, running along the posterior margins of the vertebral bodies; the ligamentum flavum, running along the posterior aspect of the spinal canal; and the interspinous ligaments, linking the spinous processes of the vertebral bodies.

In patients such as the one depicted in Case 1-3, gravitational force tends to compress the ruptured intervertebral disk, forcing the herniated segment to protrude further. By contrast, the tension of the posterior longitudinal ligament tends to resist the protrusion and press the herniated tissue back into place. Based on this knowledge, what kind of treatment (short of surgery) would you recommend for this patient? What physical maneuvers or activities would you counsel him to avoid? (See Cycle 1-12 Feedback at end of chapter.)

**C.** (Optional) Ruptured cervical disks can be surgically removed through the anterolateral aspect of the neck (between the trachea and larynx medially and the sternocleidomastoid muscle laterally), in which case the evacuated disk is often replaced with a chip of bone from the iliac crest. Ultimately, this graft matures into a fusion of the two vertebral bodies. An alternative surgical approach is to enter posteriorly, removing the spinous process and the bony ring forming the posterior margin of the spinal canal, thus relieving the pressure on the spinal cord. Bone chips are placed laterally, on both sides, over the facet joints and lateral vertebral processes, and eventually form a fusion mass. Which surgical approach would logically be preferable? (See Cycle 1-12 Feedback.)

Major Divisions of the Central Nervous System

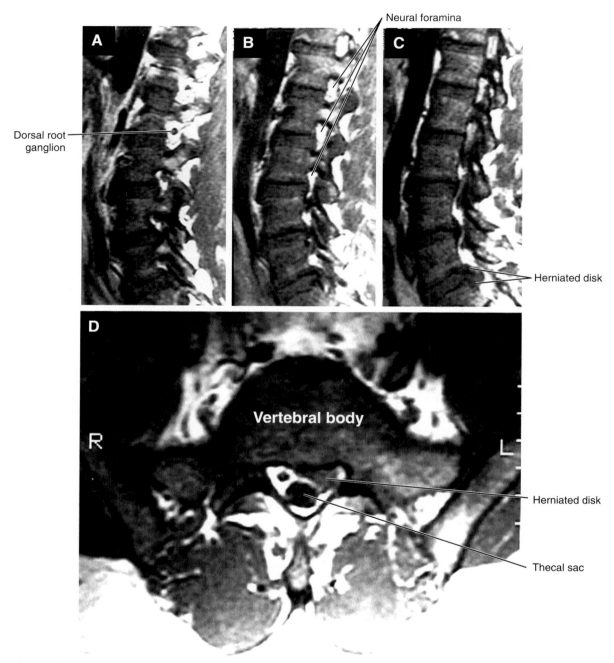

**Figure 1-54** Magnetic resonance image (MRI) of the lumbar spine demonstrating herniation of the L5-S1 disk on the left side (Case 1-3). *A, B,* and *C* depict sagittal sections of the lumbar spine, progressing from far lateral (*A*) medially. Even the most medial image (*C*) is lateral to the spinal canal. The most superior vertebral body is T12 and the most inferior is S1. *D* shows an axial section through the caudal portion of L5, which cuts through the herniated disk within the spinal canal.

**TABLE 1-8** Functional Groups

| System | Components |
|---|---|
| Motor, "pyramidal" | Premotor cortex (area 6) $\Rightarrow$ <u>precentral gyrus (motor cortex, area 4)</u> $\Rightarrow$ <u>corona radiata</u> $\Rightarrow$ <u>internal capsule, anterior limb</u> $\Rightarrow$ <u>cerebral peduncles</u> $\Rightarrow$ brainstem motor nuclei<br><u>Internal capsule (posterior limb)</u> $\Rightarrow$ <u>cerebral peduncles</u> $\Rightarrow$ <u>descending fibers in basis pontis</u> $\Rightarrow$ <u>medullary pyramids</u> $\Rightarrow$ <u>ventral horns of spinal cord</u> $\Rightarrow$ <u>ventral roots</u> $\Rightarrow$ <u>peripheral motor nerves</u> $\Rightarrow$ muscles |
| Motor, "extrapyramidal" | Premotor and motor cortex $\Rightarrow$ putamen $\Rightarrow$ globus pallidus $\Rightarrow$ thalamus $\Rightarrow$ supplementary motor area (part of area 6) |
| Somatosensory | Parietal association cortex (area 5) $\Leftarrow$ postcentral gyrus (primary somatosensory cortex, areas 3, 1, 2) $\Leftarrow$ <u>corona radiata</u> $\Leftarrow$ <u>VPL</u> $\Leftarrow$ <u>medial lemniscus</u> $\Leftarrow$ <u>gracile (leg) and cuneate (arm) nuclei</u> $\Leftarrow$ dorsal horns of spinal cord $\Leftarrow$ <u>dorsal root ganglia</u> $\Leftarrow$ <u>dorsal roots (dermatomal distributions)</u> $\Leftarrow$ <u>peripheral (sensory) nerves</u><br>Parietal association cortex (area 5) $\Leftarrow$ postcentral gyrus $\Leftarrow$ VPM $\Leftarrow$ spinal nucleus of CN V |
| Cerebellar motor | <u>Premotor and motor cortex (areas 6 and 4)</u> $\Rightarrow$ <u>internal capsule (anterior limb)</u> $\Rightarrow$ <u>cerebral peduncles</u> $\Rightarrow$ <u>basis pontis gray matter</u> $\Rightarrow$ <u>middle cerebellar peduncles</u> $\Rightarrow$ cerebellar cortex $\Rightarrow$ <u>dentate and interpositus nuclei</u> $\Rightarrow$ <u>superior cerebellar peduncles</u> $\Rightarrow$ <u>decussation of brachium conjunctivum</u> $\Rightarrow$ red nuclei, thalamus $\Rightarrow$ premotor and motor cortex<br>Spinal cord $\Rightarrow$ inferior cerebellar peduncles $\Rightarrow$ cerebellar cortex and interpositus nuclei |
| Oculomotor | Frontal eye fields (area 8) $\Rightarrow\Rightarrow$ CN III, IV, VI<br>Flocculonodular lobe and fastigial nuclei of cerebellum |
| Visual | <u>Retina</u> $\Rightarrow$ <u>optic nerves</u> $\Rightarrow$ <u>optic chiasm</u> $\Rightarrow$ <u>optic tracts</u> $\Rightarrow$ <u>lateral geniculate nucleus</u> $\Rightarrow$ <u>optic radiations</u> $\Rightarrow$ primary visual cortex (medial occipital, calcarine, striate cortex, area 17, VI) $\Rightarrow$ visual association cortex $\Rightarrow$ superior colliculus |
| Auditory | CN VIII (auditory branch) $\Rightarrow$ inferior colliculus $\Rightarrow$ medial geniculate nucleus $\Rightarrow$ Heschl's gyrus (areas 41 and 42, superior temporal lobe) |
| Memory | Parahippocampal gyrus/hippocampus/fimbria/fornix/medial septal nuclei/mammillary bodies/mammillothalamic tract/anterior nuclear group of thalamus/cingulate gyrus |
| Limbic system | Temporal pole, insula, cingulate gyrus, amygdala, lateral septal nuclei, nucleus accumbens, midline thalamic nuclei, periaqueductal gray, hypothalamus ($\Rightarrow$ intermediolateral column of spinal cord, CN X) |
| Arousal/attention | Midbrain reticular formation, intralaminar nuclei of thalamus, nucleus reticularis of thalamus |

*Note*: Some may find that organizing structures into functional groupings, as opposed to relative anatomic locations, is helpful in learning them. This table provides such a functional grouping. Most pathways in the cerebrum and some in the brainstem and spinal cord are bidirectional; the arrows in this table indicate the direction of neural transmission that best captures the functionality of the systems indicated. Underlined sequences define continuous tracts together with the neuronal pools that give rise to them. All these systems will be considered in greater detail in later chapters.

**Major Divisions of the Central Nervous System**

## CYCLE 1-4 FEEDBACK

**B.** Lumbar puncture, though often frightening to patients, is under most circumstances an extraordinarily safe procedure. However, this situation is one of the few circumstances in which it absolutely should not be done. The resultant sudden drop in cerebrospinal fluid pressure within the spinal canal could markedly potentiate the herniation process, leading to medullary compression and cardiorespiratory arrest. This patient turned out to have a malignant brain tumor. Aggressive surgery combined with radiation therapy will give him a life expectancy of approximately a year.

## CYCLE 1-12 FEEDBACK

**B.** Several days of complete bed rest will remove the compressive force of gravity, allowing the posterior longitudinal ligament to push the herniated fragment back where it can scar down in a position that will not produce symptoms. This "conservative" approach is successful in about 80 percent of cases. Jumping, lifting, bending, or twisting at the waist should be strongly proscribed because these movements will transmit a compressive shock to the herniated disk. Patients should be very cautious when going down stairs, as some tend to strike the heels fairly forcibly when going down. It may be worth while having them go down stairs backward for a few weeks.

**C.** The anterior approach is strongly favored because it minimally disrupts any of the stabilizing ligamentous structures. Unfortunately, some patients have a very narrow cervical spinal canal, marked thickening and kinking of the ligamentum flavum, and spinal cord compression at multiple levels, necessitating a multilevel posterior decompression. This removes the interspinal ligaments, a particularly important anteroposterior stabilizing force because the interspinous ligaments exert their action on a long lever of bone against the fulcrum located at the intervertebral disk.

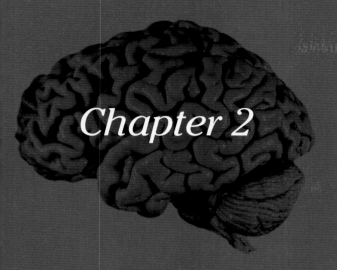

*Chapter 2*

# CENTRAL NERVOUS SYSTEM VASCULATURE, BLOOD FLOW, AND METABOLISM

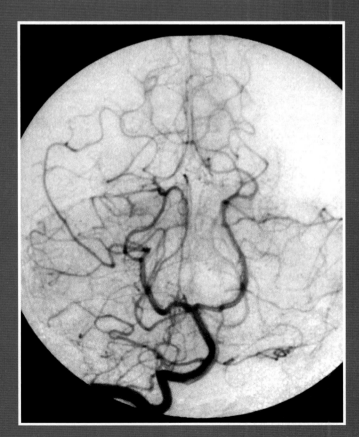

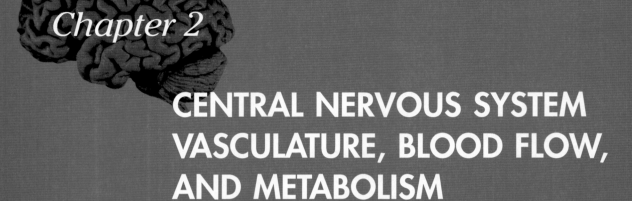

# Chapter 2

# CENTRAL NERVOUS SYSTEM VASCULATURE, BLOOD FLOW, AND METABOLISM

# Introduction

Physicians must deal with the blood flow to the brain from two major perspectives. From the generalist's perspective, the brain is like any other organ in its dependence on systemic oxygen delivery. The delivery of oxygen to the brain is a function of systemic blood pressure, cardiac output, degree of oxygen saturation of the blood, and the oxygen-carrying capacity of the blood (related to hemoglobin concentration). The brain is similar to the heart and the kidneys in its relative intolerance of low blood flow and reduced oxygen delivery. It is unique in that reductions in brain oxygenation beyond a critical minimum are immediately manifested in dramatic behavioral alterations, the first being lethargy, which is quickly followed by stupor and coma. Any physician dealing with the systems responsible for maintaining systemic oxygenation must have an understanding of the constraints imposed by brain oxygen requirements.

From the neurologist's perspective, the brain, because of its intricate structure, is unique in its susceptibility to the consequences of vascular occlusion.

Even more than the heart, the brain is distinctive for the devastating consequences of focal infarction. Each year 750,000 Americans experience stroke, and about 500,000 of them are left with significant disability. Stroke is the third leading cause of death in the United States. Until very recently, the principal focus of physicians' efforts in caring for patients with stroke was to prevent stroke recurrence. We are now entering an exciting new era in which we are developing the capability for limiting the extent of stroke.

The first major division of this chapter, Central Nervous System Vasculature, focuses on a principle central to the prevention of stroke recurrence: by precisely defining the neuroanatomic localization of a stroke, we can infer the blood vessels involved and the likely pathophysiology and, thereby, initiate the correct treatment. Division II, Cerebral Blood Flow and Metabolism, will deal with the relationship of brain function to systemic oxygen delivery and will touch on the opportunities for mitigating stroke damage.

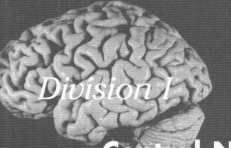

# Division I

# Central Nervous System Vasculature

# The Cervicocranial Arteries: Origin of the Blood Supply to the Brain

## Objective

Be able to describe the organization and territories of supply of the major cervical arteries to the brain.

The entire brain receives its blood supply from two sets of paired arteries, the right and left *internal carotid arteries* (ICAs) and the right and left *vertebral arteries* (Fig. 2-1). These vessels all derive indirectly from the *aortic arch*. On the right side, the brachiocephalic trunk bifurcates to form the right subclavian artery and the right common carotid artery. On the left side, the common carotid artery branches directly from the aortic arch. Both common carotid arteries bifurcate at the level of the superior border of the thyroid cartilage to form the internal and external carotid arteries. The internal carotid arteries ascend in the neurovascular bundle medial to the sternocleidomastoid muscle to supply the cerebrum and the eye. The external carotid arteries supply nearly all the meninges, the skull, and the extracranial and facial soft tissues. The vertebral arteries branch from the subclavian arteries on both sides. They ascend in the foramina transversaria in the transverse processes of the cervical vertebral bodies to supply the cervical spinal cord, the medulla, parts of the cerebellum, and some of the meninges in the posterior fossa. Just after entering the foramen magnum at the base of the skull, the vertebral arteries merge on the ventral aspect of the brainstem to form the *basilar artery*. The basilar artery supplies the remainder of the brainstem and cerebellum, and posterior parts of the cerebrum.

## PRACTICE 2-1

You should be able to identify all the vascular structures labeled in Figure 2-1.

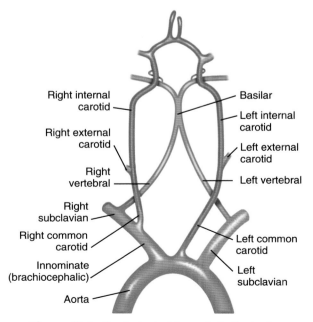

**Figure 2-1** Cervical arterial supply to the brain.

# Internal Carotid and Vertebral Artery Relationships to the Base of the Brain and the Circle of Willis

Be able to describe the organization of arteries at the base of the brain.

Each internal carotid artery ascends from the carotid bifurcation through the petrous bone at the base of the skull to emerge at the posterior medial edge of the middle cranial fossa just lateral to the sella turcica (Fig. 2-2). It then travels anteriorly along one side of the *sella turcica*, within a blood-filled dural venous space, the *cavernous sinus* (Fig. 2-3). It shares the cavernous sinus with two branches of cranial nerve V (V₁ and V₂), as well as cranial nerves III, IV, and VI (Fig. 2-4). Each internal carotid artery then curls up to penetrate the roof of the cavernous sinus just behind and medial to the anterior clinoid process of the sella turcica, continuing posteriorly and then superiorly as the supraclinoid segment of the internal carotid artery. The nearly S-shaped segment of the internal carotid artery, beginning at its entrance into the cavernous sinus and ending as the supraclinoid carotid artery wends its way superiorly, is often referred to as the carotid siphon. The supraclinoid carotid artery ends as it bifurcates to form the *anterior* and *middle cerebral arteries* at a point

referred to, for obvious reasons, as the *carotid T-junction* (Fig. 2-5).

The vertebral arteries enter the foramen magnum and merge to form the basilar artery just caudal to the junction of the pons and the medulla (Fig. 2-6). The basilar artery ascends along the anterior pons and ultimately terminates within the interpeduncular fossa of the midbrain (formed by the cerebral peduncles on either side) to form the *two posterior cerebral arteries*.

The *circle of Willis* consists of an anastomotic connection of the carotid and vertebrobasilar systems (Fig. 2-7). A branch of the supraclinoid carotid artery, the *posterior communicating artery*, links the internal carotid artery to the *posterior cerebral artery*. The *anterior cerebral arteries* wend their way anterior, superior, and medial from their points of origin at the carotid T-junctions; at the point where they come together in the cerebral midline, they are joined together by the *anterior communicating artery*. The circle thus formed lies immediately above the sella turcica, occupying the lateral reaches of the suprasellar cistern, and surrounds the pituitary stalk (the infundibulum) and the optic chiasm (Fig. 2-7).

The circle of Willis provides the major source of collateral blood supply to intracranial arteries in the event of cervical arterial occlusion. The importance of this vascular structure is illustrated in Case 2-1.

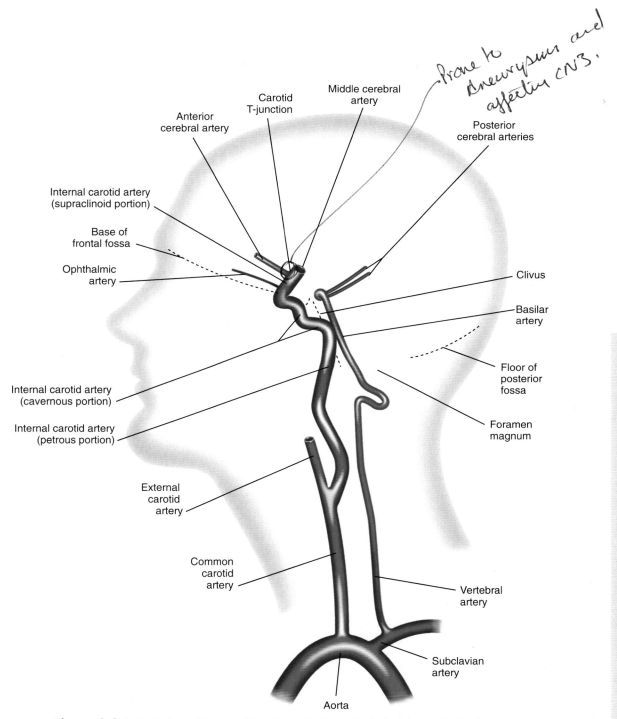

**Figure 2-2** Lateral view of the carotid and vertebral arteries in their ascent to the brain.

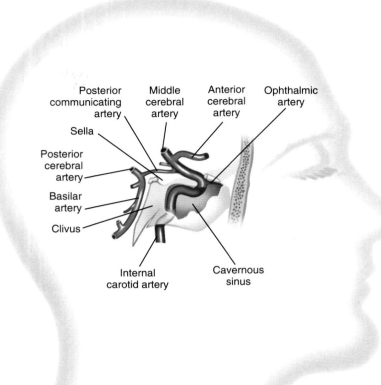

**Figure 2-3** Lateral view of the cavernous portion of the intracranial internal carotid artery in relation to the cavernous sinus and the sella turcica.

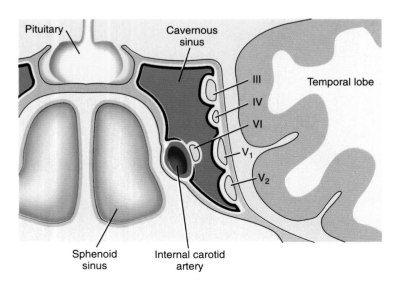

**Figure 2-4** Anterior-posterior view of the internal carotid artery and cranial nerves (see Roman numerals) within the cavernous sinus.

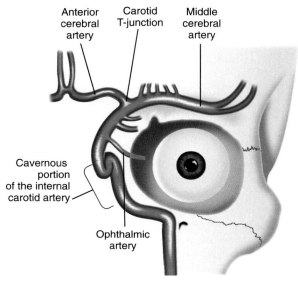

**Figure 2-5** Anteroposterior view of the proximal intracranial internal carotid artery depicting its termination at the carotid T-junction.

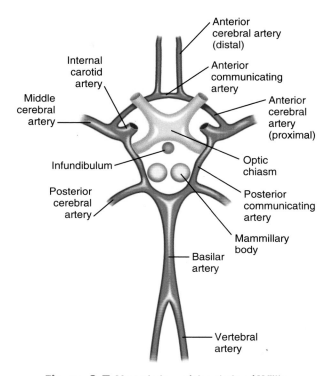

**Figure 2-7** Ventral view of the circle of Willis.

VENTRAL SURFACE OF BRAINSTEM

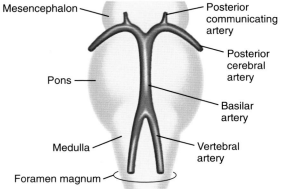

**Figure 2-6** The posterior circulation: the basilar and vertebral arteries in their relationship to the ventral surface of the brainstem.

Central Nervous System Vasculature, Blood Flow, and Metabolism

## Case 2-1

### Asymptomatic Carotid Stenosis

*A physician performing a routine physical examination on a 65-year-old man discovers a right carotid bruit (a blowing sound synchronous with the heartbeat, possibly signaling the presence of internal carotid artery stenosis). He recommends the performance of a carotid duplex study of the cervical carotid bifurcation, the most common site of carotid stenosis due to atheromatous plaque. This examination combines two modalities: a carotid Doppler study in which sound waves are bounced off passing red blood cells, and a carotid "B-mode" ultrasound, in which sound waves are bounced off the wall of the carotid artery. The Doppler study provides a measure of the velocity of blood flow (manifested as the Doppler shift), which becomes quite high when blood must pass through a narrowed segment. The B-mode ultrasound provides information on the structure of the arterial wall. In this patient, the duplex study suggests the presence of 90 percent stenosis of the right internal carotid artery. The physician becomes quite alarmed and tells the patient that he must immediately undergo surgery to remove the atheroma that is stenosing the artery, because if the artery becomes completely occluded, the patient will experience a massive right hemisphere stroke. Is this good advice?*

**Comment:** *No. Even if the internal carotid artery becomes completely occluded, the anastomotic network provided by the circle of Willis assures that, with only occasional exceptions, the right brain will get adequate blood. In fact, to perform a carotid endarterectomy (remove the atheroma), surgeons temporarily clamp the internal carotid artery. The real danger of the carotid bifurcation atheroma is that it will break down, leading to the formation of blood clot, which can then propagate or embolize to the intracranial arteries beyond the circle of Willis, where vascular anastomoses are far more limited, as we shall see. The pros and cons of performing a carotid endarterectomy on an asymptomatic patient, as in this case, are hotly debated, and there has not yet been a definitive clinical trial of carotid endarterectomy under these circumstances.*

## PRACTICE 2-2

**A.** If you cannot describe the carotid and vertebral arteries in their relationship to the base of the skull and the brain, and their anastomotic relationships, review this section.

**B.** Studies performed on cadavers suggest that 1 in 3 people, when they rotate their head as far as they can to one side, occlude one vertebral artery. Why don't we see neurologic symptoms of brainstem ischemia under such circumstances? What are the alternative sources of blood to the brainstem?

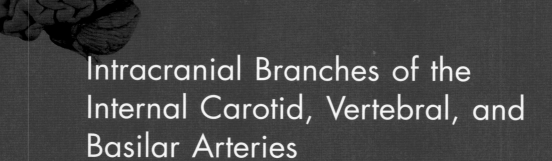

# Intracranial Branches of the Internal Carotid, Vertebral, and Basilar Arteries

## Objectives

1. Be able to describe the courses and the regions of supply of the anterior, middle, and posterior cerebral arteries.

2. Be able to describe the approximate course and territories supplied by the posterior inferior cerebellar artery (PICA).

3. Be able to describe the anatomic principles of vascular supply to the brainstem.

## CEREBRAL HEMISPHERES

In the last section, we noted that the supraclinoid carotid artery ascends to bifurcate at the T-junction to form the anterior and middle cerebral arteries. Before its bifurcation, it has two important branches: (1) the *ophthalmic artery*, which supplies the eyeball, emerges from the anterior aspect of the proximal supraclinoid carotid artery just above the anterior clinoid process of the sella turcica; and (2) the *posterior communicating artery*, which originates from the posterior aspect of the supraclinoid carotid artery somewhat distal to the ophthalmic artery take-off and proceeds posteriorly to terminate at the posterior cerebral artery.

The *anterior cerebral arteries* proceed anteriorly and medially until they approach each other, at which point they are linked by the anterior communicating artery. From this point they proceed in tandem upward and then posteriorly over the rostrum, genu, and body of the corpus callosum (Figs. 2-8, 2-9). They supply the entire medial surface of the hemispheres, generally to about the splenium of the corpus callosum (Fig. 2-10).

The *middle cerebral arteries* proceed laterally from the carotid T-junction through the depths of the sylvian fissure. They subsequently form multiple branches that course over the surface of the insula and then curl around the frontal, temporal, and parietal operculae to emerge from the sylvian fissure on the lateral surface of the hemisphere. These branches then course over the surface of the frontal, temporal, and parietal lobes to supply most of the lateral surface of the hemisphere (Figs. 2-11, 2-12).

The *basilar artery* ends within the interpeduncular fossa of the midbrain to form the *posterior cerebral arteries*, which wrap around the midbrain and then proceed posteriorly, sending branches over the inferior surfaces of the temporal lobes all the way to the occipital pole. Some branches extend medially to supply the medial surface of the posterior portion of the hemisphere, including the calcarine (visual) cortex. Other branches curl onto the ventrolateral surface of the hemisphere to supply posterior portions of the inferior temporal gyrus (Figs. 2-13, 2-14, 2-15).

The distributions of the three major cerebral arteries vary somewhat from brain to brain. The portion of the medial surface of the hemisphere supplied by the posterior cerebral artery often extends more anteriorly, sometimes as far as the midbody of the corpus callosum. The posterior cerebral artery may supply no cortex on the lateral surface of the hemisphere or it may extend quite superiorly to supply posterior portions of

Central Nervous System Vasculature, Blood Flow, and Metabolism

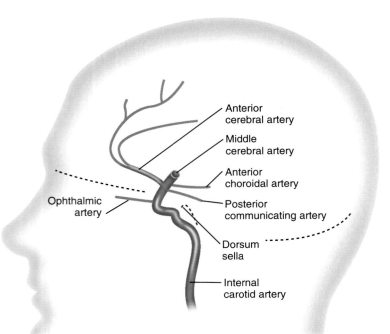

**Figure 2-8** Lateral view of the intracranial carotid artery circulation illustrating the course of the anterior cerebral artery.

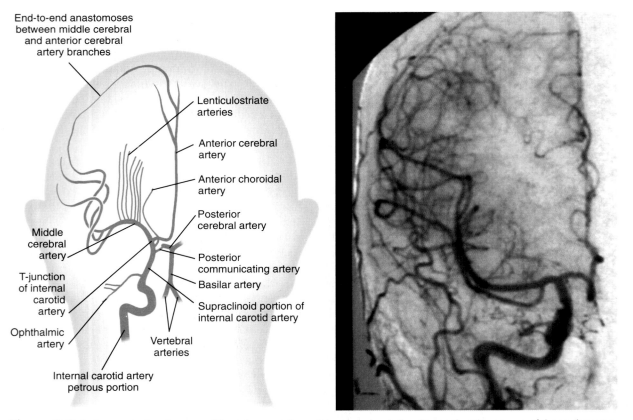

**Figure 2-9** Anteroposterior diagram of the intracranial carotid artery circulation illustrating the course of the major cerebral vessels (*left*) and a comparable view of a cerebral angiogram (*right*). The common carotid artery was injected in this study, so both internal and external carotid artery branches are seen.

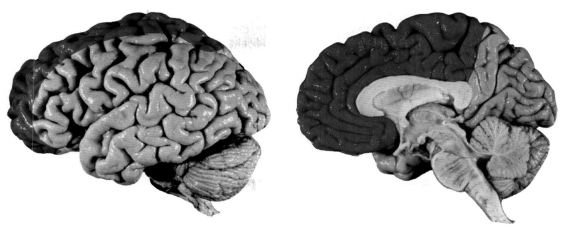

**Figure 2-10** Lateral and medial views of the regions of the brain supplied by the anterior cerebral artery (*shaded areas*).

the lateral surface of the inferior temporal gyri. However, the *middle cerebral artery always supplies the perisylvian cortex*. This fact is of clinical importance in that, in the dominant hemisphere, language networks supporting the processes necessary to repeat words and phrases are always located in the perisylvian region. Therefore, if a patient with a stroke has difficulty repeating, we know that he has a dominant perisylvian lesion, hence a middle cerebral artery event. This finding in turn tells us that the clot causing the stroke had to originate in the internal carotid artery or travel through the internal carotid artery from the heart or from an atheromatous lesion in the aorta.

## BRAINSTEM, CEREBELLUM, AND SPINAL CORD

The blood supply to the brainstem and the cerebellum is provided by branches of the vertebral and basilar arteries. *The blood supply to the brainstem is organized like slices of a pie* (Fig. 2-16, Table 2-1). For example, midline branches from the basilar artery (pontine arteries) penetrate the ventral pons and supply the median portions of the pons. The arteries on the two sides generally respect the midline. Short circumferential arterial branches of the basilar artery course for a short distance laterally before penetrating the ventral pontine surface to supply the paramedian pons. Long circumferential arteries, variably named (anterior inferior cerebellar artery [AICA], superior cerebellar artery [SCA]), originate at the basilar artery and follow

a long course around the pons or midbrain, send branched twigs into the lateral brainstem, and then proceed laterally to supply parts of the cerebellar hemispheres.

The posterior cerebral arteries, which we have already discussed, also constitute long circumferential branches of the basilar artery. Their relationship to the brainstem (the midbrain and thalamus) is comparable to that of the other long circumferential arteries, and proximal occlusions of the posterior cerebral arteries may cause ischemic damage to the most rostral portions of the brainstem, including the thalamus and the junction of the internal capsule and the cerebral peduncles.

Caudally, branches from each of the two vertebral arteries course medially where they join to form the rostral end of the *anterior spinal artery*, which courses in the midline for the entire length of the spinal cord (Fig. 2-17). Twigs from the rostral-most anterior spinal artery supply the paramedian slices of the medulla, in a fashion analogous to the basilar artery twigs supplying the pons. Long circumferential arteries originating at the distal vertebral arteries, the *posterior inferior cerebellar arteries (PICAs)*, wrap around the medulla, send branched twigs to supply the dorsolateral quadrants of the medulla, and then proceed laterally, like the superior cerebellar arteries, to supply the inferior cerebellum (Fig. 2-18). At this point, it is most important that you remember the organization of the vascular supply to posterior fossa structures, and that you remember the posterior inferior cerebellar and anterior spinal arteries, for reasons that will soon be made clear.

*Text continued on p. 88*

Central Nervous System Vasculature, Blood Flow, and Metabolism

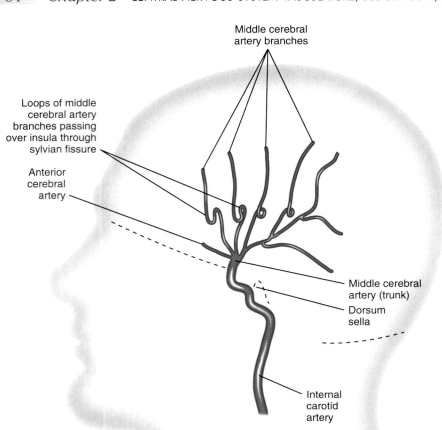

Middle cerebral
artery branches

Loops of middle
cerebral artery
branches passing
over insula through
sylvian fissure

Anterior
cerebral
artery

Middle cerebral
artery (trunk)

Dorsum
sella

Internal
carotid
artery

**Figure 2-11** Lateral view of the intracranial carotid artery circulation illustrating the course of the middle cerebral artery.

**TABLE 2-1** Vascular Supply of the Brainstem

| Arterial Territory | Midbrain | Pons | Medulla |
|---|---|---|---|
| Median | Midline branches from basilar artery | Midline branches from basilar artery | Midline branches from anterior spinal artery |
| Paramedian | Short circumferential branches from basilar artery | Short circumferential branches from basilar artery | Short circumferential branches from anterior spinal artery |
| Dorsolateral/ cerebellum | Posterior cerebral artery; superior cerebellar artery | Anterior inferior cerebellar artery (AICA) | Posterior inferior cerebellar artery (PICA) |

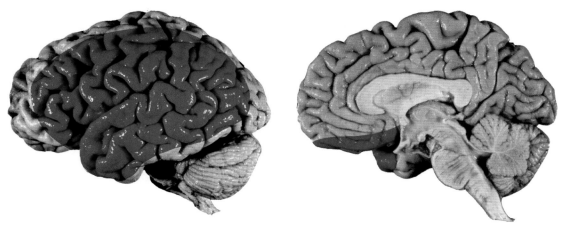

**Figure 2-12** Lateral (*left*) and medial (*right*) views of the regions of the brain supplied by the middle cerebral artery (*shaded areas*).

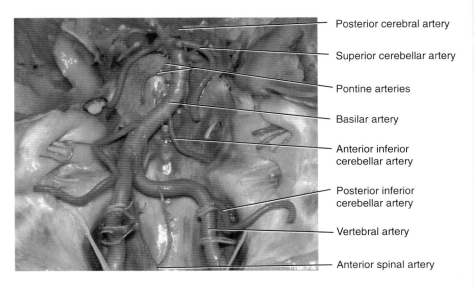

**Figure 2-13** Anteroventral view of the vertebrobasilar arterial system.

Posterior cerebral artery

Superior cerebellar artery

Pontine arteries

Basilar artery

Anterior inferior cerebellar artery

Posterior inferior cerebellar artery

Vertebral artery

Anterior spinal artery

**Central Nervous System Vasculature, Blood Flow, and Metabolism**

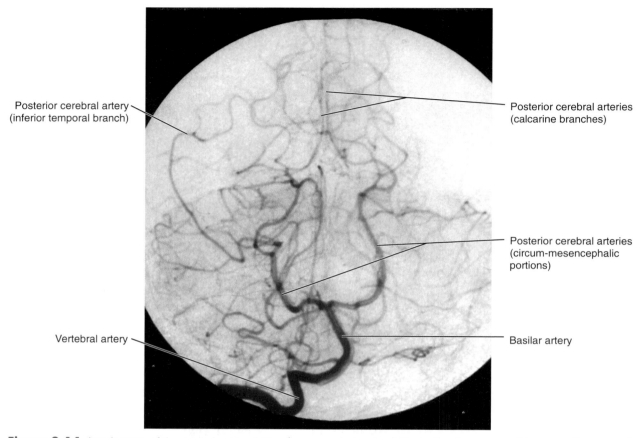

Posterior cerebral artery
(inferior temporal branch)

Posterior cerebral arteries
(calcarine branches)

Posterior cerebral arteries
(circum-mesencephalic
portions)

Vertebral artery

Basilar artery

**Figure 2-14** Arteriogram of the posterior circulation (anteroposterior view) illustrating the course of the posterior cerebral arteries.

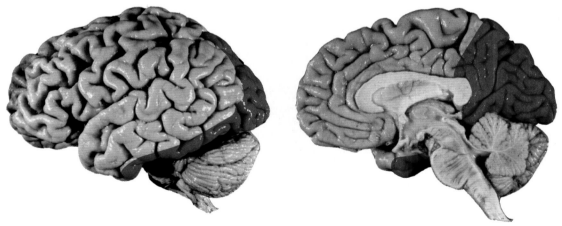

**Figure 2-15** Lateral (*left*) and medial (*right*) views of the regions of the brain supplied by the posterior cerebral arteries (*shaded areas*).

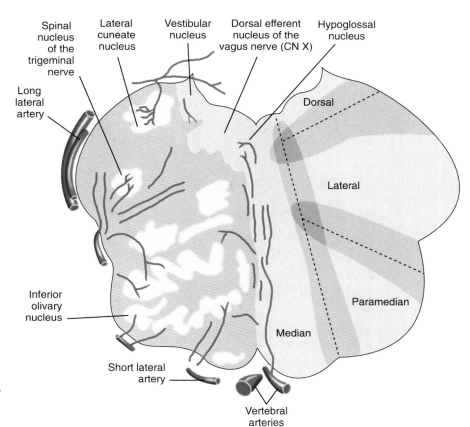

**Figure    2-16** Axial section through the medulla illustrating the organization of the blood supply to the brainstem. (Modified from Gillilan LA. The correlation of the blood supply to the human brain stem with clinical brainstem lesions. J Neuropathol Exp Neurol 23:73–108, 1964. Reproduced with permission from the *Journal of Neuropathology and Experimental Neurology.*)

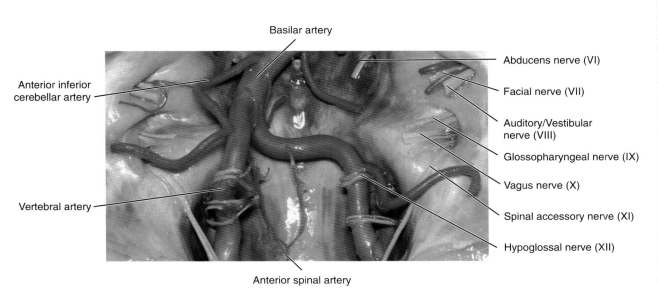

**Figure 2-17** The formation of the anterior spinal artery from branches of the vertebral arteries, and the course of the anterior spinal artery down the ventral (anterior) aspect of the spinal cord.

Central Nervous System Vasculature, Blood Flow, and Metabolism

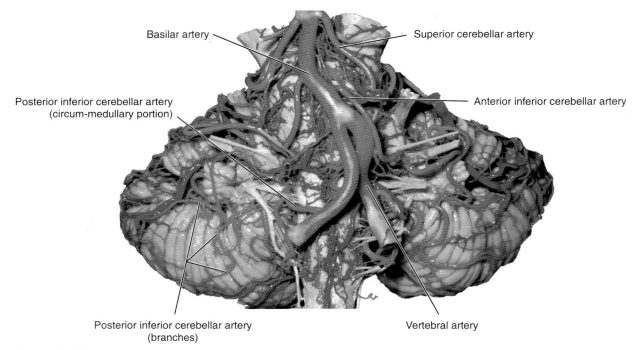

Basilar artery

Superior cerebellar artery

Posterior inferior cerebellar artery
(circum-medullary portion)

Anterior inferior cerebellar artery

Posterior inferior cerebellar artery
(branches)

Vertebral artery

**Figure 2-18** The course of the posterior inferior cerebellar artery (PICA) and branches from their origin at the rostral vertebral arteries, around the medulla, ultimately to terminate over the inferior surface of the cerebellum.

## PRACTICE 2-3

**A.** If you cannot describe the intracranial courses and regions of the brain supplied by the anterior, middle, and posterior cerebral arteries, review this section.

**B.** A 70-year-old man with a long history of hypertension and heavy smoking has extensive atheromatous disease of the basilar artery, demonstrated on a magnetic resonance angiogram obtained last year when he was evaluated following a minor carotid artery distribution stroke. An atheromatous plaque on the dorsal inner surface of the basilar artery occludes the orifice of a small median artery, causing a right hemiparesis. Draw an outline of the pons and sketch the distribution of the resulting infarct.

**C.** A 35-year-old mother suddenly brakes her car to avoid striking a driver who failed to yield right of way. She immediately turns to check on her 2-year-old, who is strapped into a car seat. As she does so, she experiences a stab of pain in the posterior right side of her neck that persists. Two weeks later, she suddenly develops nausea, vomiting, dizziness, difficulty swallowing, incoordination of her right arm, and a tendency to fall to her right side. A magnetic resonance angiogram demonstrates occlusion of the right vertebral artery as a result of thrombosis complicating a vascular dissection (a separation of the inner layer [intima] and middle layer [media] of the artery by blood that has dissected into the tissue from a tear in the intima). The thrombosis occludes the orifice of the posterior inferior cerebellar artery. Draw an outline of the medulla and sketch the distribution of the infarct.

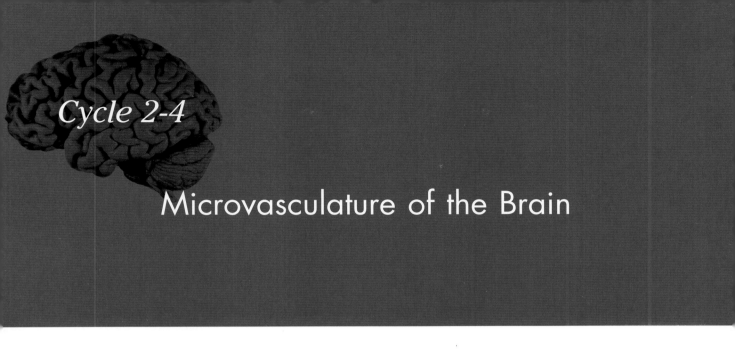

# Cycle 2-4

# Microvasculature of the Brain

Be able to describe the major sources of blood supply to the basal ganglia, thalamus, deep cerebral white matter, and brainstem.

The deep gray matter structures of the cerebral hemispheres are supplied by small penetrating branches of the anterior, middle, and posterior cerebral arteries and the supraclinoid internal carotid artery. The branches of the anterior and middle cerebral arteries, which supply the basal ganglia, are referred to as the *lenticulostriate arteries* (Fig. 2-19). The thalamus is supplied by a number of small arteries that emerge from the tip of the basilar artery, the proximal posterior cerebral arteries, and the posterior communicating arteries, which can simply be referred to as *thalamoperforators*.

The deep cerebral white matter receives its blood supply jointly from the lenticulostriate and thalamoperforating vessels and from small penetrating arteries that emerge from cortical branches of the anterior, middle, and posterior cerebral arteries as they course over the surface of the brain (Fig. 2-20).

The microvasculature of the brainstem (see Cycle 2-3) consists of the small penetrating arteries emerging from the basilar and anterior spinal arteries medially, from short circumferential branches from the basilar and vertebral arteries ventrolaterally, and from long circumferential branches of the basilar and vertebral arteries dorsolaterally.

Central Nervous System Vasculature, Blood Flow, and Metabolism

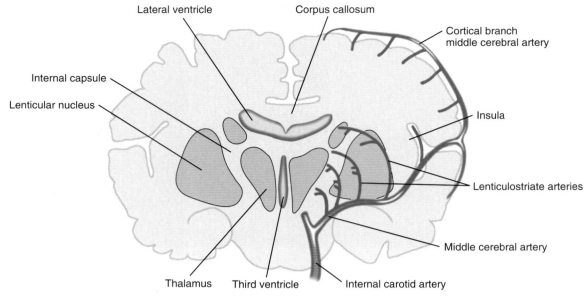

**Figure 2-19** Anteroposterior view of the lenticulostriate arteries on one side of the brain.

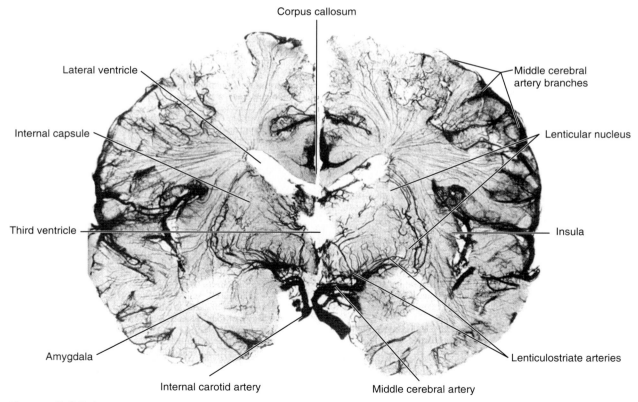

**Figure 2-20** Coronal section of the brain illustrating the normal organization of the microvasculature. This slice is anterior to the drawing in Figure 2-19, so the thalamus is not included. (Modified from Román GC. Senile dementia of the Binswanger type: A vascular form of dementia in the elderly. JAMA 258:1782–1788, 1987. Copyrighted 1987, American Medical Association.)

# Cycle 2-5

# Principles of Function of the Cerebral Vasculature

## Objectives

1. Be able to list the major loci of thrombus formation that lead to stroke.

2. Be able to describe where emboli usually land and explain why emboli to the brain stop moving.

3. Be able to describe what influences the path that emboli take at arterial bifurcations. Be able to explain the implications of this phenomenon for the pathogenesis of microvascular strokes.

4. Be able to explain how probabilistic principles governing the trajectories and functional impact of emboli support the following statements:

   a) Cardiogenic embolism is a concern in every stroke patient.
   b) Cardiogenic embolism is unlikely in the patient with repeated events in a single vascular territory.
   c) Artery-to-artery thromboembolism is unlikely in the patient with strokes in multiple vascular territories.
   d) Large vessel embolism is less likely and microvascular thrombosis, migraine, or seizures

are more likely in the case of multiple stereotyped events.

5. Be able to explain why infarction in the lenticulostriate end zone is a common sequel of anterior circulation large vessel occlusive events.

6. Be able to describe and explain the pattern of infarction in a patient with major anomalies of the circle of Willis producing an isolated intracranial carotid circulation when cervical carotid artery occlusion occurs.

7. Be able to explain why "silent" infarcts occur, why right hemisphere infarcts are more likely to be silent than left hemisphere infarcts, and why lacunar infarcts are more likely to be silent than large vessel infarcts.

8. Be able to explain how an arterial aneurysm could cause neurologic manifestations without rupturing.

9. Be able to explain why a patient with a brain tumor causing a cerebral herniation syndrome is at risk for a posterior cerebral artery territory infarction.

In the introduction to this chapter, we defined a crucial clinical scientific principle: by precisely defining the neuroanatomic localization of a stroke, we can infer the blood vessels involved and the likely pathophysiology, and thereby, initiate the correct treatment. Computed tomographic (CT) scans can enable us to distinguish hemorrhage from infarction. CT and magnetic resonance image (MRI) scans often help with neuroanatomic localization of infarcts, although frequently they are unrevealing, particularly early in the course of stroke when the initiation of correct treatment may be crucial. In such cases, we must rely on the neu-

*91*

**TABLE 2-2** Summary of Principles of Function of Brain Vasculature

| Feature | Effect |
|---|---|
| Major sites of clot formation | Heart, aorta, proximal cervical internal carotid arteries, distal (intracranial) vertebral arteries, proximal and middle basilar artery, perforating microvessels of the cerebrum, and brainstem are major sites. |
| Movement of emboli | Emboli wedge at points of vascular narrowing, usually bifurcations; at bifurcations, they enter a vessel that is larger and branches at a lesser angle. |
| Probabilistic phenomena affecting brain infarction | Systemic embolism is most likely to manifest as stroke because embolization of organs other than the brain is likely to be clinically silent. |
| | Recurrent emboli to a single cerebral vessel are likely to reflect local atheromatous disease because of the low probability of multiple recurrent emboli from the heart to a single vessel. |
| | Emboli to multiple cerebrovascular territories are likely to reflect cardiogenic embolism because of the low probability of multiple concurrent sites of arterial thrombosis. |
| | Recurrent transient ischemic attacks (TIAs) reflecting large vessel thromboembolism are likely to vary in their manifestations because of variability in clot size and trajectory. |
| | Recurrent, highly similar events are more likely to reflect microvascular TIAs, migraine, or seizures, because these processes tend to be intrinsically stereotyped. |
| Extent and distribution of stroke | These features are defined by locus of thromboembolism and availability and pattern of collateral blood supply. |
| Clinical manifestations of stroke | These manifestations reflect the functional significance of the infarcted territory. |
| | May be absent when stroke does not affect somatosensory, visual, motor or conspicuous higher neural functions (e.g., language). |
| Neurologic manifestations related to subarachnoid course of arteries | Aneurysms may cause neurologic manifestations through compression of adjacent neural structures. |
| | Cerebral herniation syndromes may cause (1) posterior cerebral artery distribution stroke by compressing the posterior cerebral artery against the margin of the tentorium; (2) CN III palsies by pulling the posterior cerebral artery down onto CN III. |

rologic examination, particularly the examination of higher neural functions. Even when we have accurately localized a stroke, it is necessary to have an understanding of principles of cerebrovascular function to define pathogenic mechanisms, hence the best treatment. Now that you have a basic understanding of cerebrovascular anatomy, we can consider cerebrovascular function. The major principles discussed in this section are summarized in Table 2-2.

## A. THE ROLE OF THROMBOSIS IN PATHOGENESIS OF STROKE

Although the details of stroke pathogenesis will be found in future courses, it is important at this point to understand that the way in which the cerebral vasculature functions as a system is most clearly reflected in those situations in which it has to deal with vascular occlusion by thrombus (blood clot). Thrombus tends to develop at a very limited number of locations:

- within the heart

and at sites of atheromatous disease in

- the aorta
- the most proximal, extracranial portions of the internal carotid arteries (just distal to the common carotid artery bifurcations in the neck)
- the distal-most, intracranial portions of the vertebral arteries, just before they come together to form the basilar artery
- the proximal half of the basilar artery
- the perforating microvessels of the cerebrum and brainstem

Clot may occlude a blood vessel at the location at which it forms, but often, particularly in the case of blood clot originating in the heart, aorta, or internal carotid or vertebral arteries, clot may break off and travel as an embolus, ultimately to wedge in and occlude a more distal vessel.

# B. THE COURSE TRAVELED BY EMBOLI

Emboli continue to move with the blood flow until they wedge in a blood vessel too small to allow further passage. Typically this occurs at bifurcation points. For example, blood clots originating in the heart or at atheromatous lesions at the carotid bifurcation in the neck may be large enough to wedge in the supraclinoid internal carotid artery but more often wedge at the carotid T-junction, the point at which the internal carotid artery bifurcates to form the anterior and middle cerebral arteries. Clots traversing the vertebrobasilar system often travel until they wedge at the basilar artery tip or the proximal-most portion of one of the posterior cerebral arteries. Carotid T-junction occlusions and tip of the basilar artery occlusions account for the vast majority of large vessel cerebral strokes.

When a clot is capable of entering either branch at a bifurcation point, it tends to enter the artery that is both the largest and emerges at the least angle from the parent artery. The best example of this is that smaller clots coming to the carotid T-junction almost invariably pass into the middle cerebral artery, rarely into the anterior cerebral artery, because the anterior cerebral artery is the smaller of the two branches and because it tends to emerge from the internal carotid artery at a sharper angle. This simple hemodynamic principle provides the basis for a very important clinical principle: strokes due to occlusion of cerebral penetrating vessels must be due to intrinsic (atheromatous) disease of these vessels and not due to embolism from the cervicocranial vessels or the heart, because penetrating arteries take off at right angles from the parent vessel and are much smaller. The application of this principle is illustrated in Case 2-2.

## Case 2-2

### Lacunar Stroke

*A 75-year-old right-handed man with a history of high blood pressure, diabetes, and smoking awakes one morning with severe weakness of his right arm and, to a lesser extent, his right leg. His language and other higher cerebral functions are completely normal and he has no impairment of vision. Auscultation of the neck reveals a loud bruit (sound of high velocity blood flow) over the left carotid artery. Should carotid endarterectomy be considered, assuming cerebral angiography does demonstrate high-grade stenosis of the left internal carotid artery?*

**Comment:** *Because language capacity is localized to the left brain in 99.5 percent of right-handed individuals, we can be quite confident that this man's weakness did not result from middle cerebral artery occlusion. In fact, the absence of any abnormalities in cerebral cortical function clearly indicates that his paralysis is due to the occlusion of a small penetrating artery supplying motor pathways at one of the points at which they become highly focused, for example, the posterior limb of the internal capsule (Fig. 2-21). The posterior limb of the internal capsule is supplied by tiny branches of the anterior choroidal artery, a minor branch of the supraclinoid internal carotid artery. The anterior choroidal artery, like other small branch arteries supplying penetrating vessels to the brain, including the lenticulostriate vessels and the thalamoperforators, emerges at a relatively sharp angle from a vastly larger parent vessel. Therefore, there is an extremely low probability that an embolus would enter it, rather than traveling with the mainstream blood flow in the supraclinoid carotid artery. Thus, we conclude that this man's stroke was caused by local microvascular disease, not by embolism from clot at an atheroma at the carotid bifurcation (or for that matter, clot from the heart). Thus, we do not have to subject him to the risks of cerebral angiography or unnecessary carotid endarterectomy. Instead, we would treat him with drugs that inhibit thrombus formation (e.g., aspirin, dipyridamole) and drugs that inhibit atheroma formation (e.g., hepatic HMG-CoA reductase inhibitors such as pravastatin, which reduce cholesterol levels, and angiotensin-converting enzyme inhibitors).*

# C. THE ROLE OF PROBABILITY IN CEREBROVASCULAR EVENTS

We have already introduced concepts of variability and probability in our discussion of stroke pathogenesis. Thus, variability in the size of emboli determines whether they will wedge in large or small vessels. Hemodynamic principles reduce the probability of an embolus traveling out a smaller branch artery emerging from the parent vessel at an acute angle. At this point we introduce some further probabilistic aspects of stroke pathogenesis, and show how they can be

Central Nervous System Vasculature, Blood Flow, and Metabolism

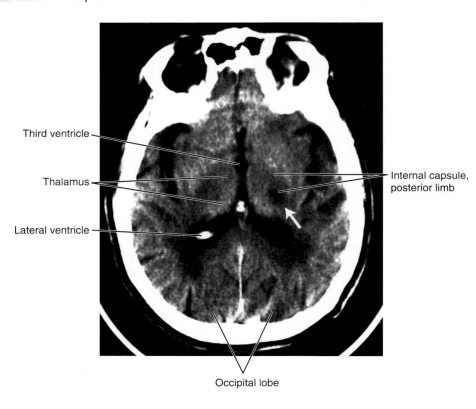

Third ventricle

Thalamus

Lateral ventricle

Internal capsule, posterior limb

Occipital lobe

**Figure 2-21** Axial computed tomographic (CT) scan of the brain illustrating a lacunar infarction of the posterior limb of the left internal capsule (*white arrow*).

turned to our advantage to determine stroke pathogenesis and thus, optimal treatment.

The brain receives approximately 20 percent of cardiac output. However, approximately 80 percent of emboli from the heart appear to involve the brain. Does this mean that the cervicocranial vessels vacuum emboli from the aortic blood stream? Obviously not: it means that most systemic emboli but few cerebral emboli are clinically silent. For these reasons, the possibility of cardiogenic embolism is very carefully considered in every stroke patient.

Most emboli from the heart to the brain enter the carotid arteries, because they provide 90 percent of the blood flow to the brain. A single internal carotid artery provides 45 percent. What is the likelihood that two successive cardiac emboli would go to the same carotid artery? It is $(.45)^2$, or 21.25 percent. Because this is a substantial probability, if a patient presented with two left internal carotid artery distribution events, we would still have to consider the possibility of cardiogenic embolism. What if a patient experienced two vertebrobasilar artery events? The likelihood of two cardiogenic emboli traveling to the posterior circulation is $(0.1)^2$, or 1 percent. Thus, in such a patient, we would

deem cardiogenic embolism to be highly unlikely and search for an arterial source of clot.

The likelihood that one patient would have more than one arterial source of clot formation is low because atheromas only occasionally develop the hemorrhage and necrosis that makes them at risk for thromboembolism, and the period for which such unstable atheromas pose this risk is relatively short. If we saw a CT scan showing multiple large vessel distribution strokes in different vascular territories (e.g., a middle cerebral artery territory stroke on both the left and right sides and a posterior cerebral artery distribution stroke), we would conclude that the clots must be coming from the heart.

Serial clots traveling in large vessels are likely to vary in size, and therefore wedge at different points in cerebral vessels. Serial clots of nearly equal size traveling out the middle cerebral artery are likely to end up in different middle cerebral arterial branches. Thus, each one of several serial internal carotid artery territory thrombi is likely to affect a different portion of the terminal vascular territory, and the volume of brain affected by these emboli is going to be quite variable. On the other hand, clots involving a single small penetrating vessel are going to produce exactly the same manifestations every time, corresponding to dysfunction of all the neural structures supplied by that tiny vessel. These simple probabilistic principles provide the basis for some very powerful clinical principles. Thus, if a patient experiences multiple events that sound like strokes but are transient (transient ischemic attacks [TIAs]), and these events are both highly stereotyped (clinical manifestations nearly identical every time) and do not involve cerebral cortical dysfunction, we would infer that the TIAs were due to atheromatous disease with thrombosis in a small penetrating vessel. Therefore, we would not worry about carotid or heart disease. If a patient experienced multiple, variable TIAs, some involving language impairment (aphasia), we would conclude that the combination of variability and cortical arterial involvement indicated large vessel clots, possibly of internal carotid atheromatous origin or cardiac origin, something very serious and calling for aggressive diagnostic evaluation and treatment. If a patient experienced multiple, absolutely stereotyped, TIA-like events affecting the cortex, we would reason that they could not be microvascular in origin because they affect the cortex, and that they are unlikely to be embolic in origin because they are stereotyped. We would therefore suspect some other pathophysiologic basis for the patient's events, most likely migraines, possibly seizures, both capable of producing this clinical picture.

## D. THE EXTENT AND DISTRIBUTION OF STROKE ARE DEFINED BY THE AVAILABILITY OF COLLATERAL BLOOD SUPPLY

We noted earlier in this chapter that occlusion of an internal carotid or vertebral artery in the neck is unlikely to produce a stroke, as long as it does not result in embolism or distal propagation of clot, because the circle of Willis almost always provides alternative channels of blood flow to the regions of the brain distal to the occlusion. The danger of blood clots that travel to or extend into the circle of Willis is that they interfere with this usually robust source of collateral flow, making regions of the brain distal to the occluded artery dependent on sources of collateral flow that are often tenuous and may be completely inadequate.

Consider what we have identified as the most common large vessel occlusive event: occlusion of the distal internal carotid artery at the T-junction, either

because an embolus from the heart or an internal carotid artery atheromatous lesion in the neck has become trapped there, or because clot has formed at a cervical internal carotid artery atheroma and propagated all the way up the internal carotid artery into the T-junction. Clot at the T-junction now occludes the proximal middle and anterior cerebral arteries. What happens to the brain distal to these arteries? If an anterior communicating artery exists (usually the case), blood can flow from the opposite internal carotid artery territory to the proximally occluded anterior cerebral artery, preventing infarction in the territory of this vessel. Furthermore, Figure 2-9 reveals that blood flowing into the anterior cerebral artery can also flow through end-to-end anastomoses between branches of the anterior and middle cerebral arteries, thereby saving some of the middle cerebral artery territory. The same thing can happen via end-to-end anastomoses between posterior cerebral artery and middle cerebral artery branches. If all these anastomoses are large, most of the middle cerebral artery territory will be spared ischemic damage and a potentially devastating stroke can be averted. The great importance of these collateral vessels is illustrated in Figure 2-22.

In most patients, one region is nearly always at serious risk, even under the best of circumstances: the *lenticulostriate end zone*. Note that in the case of a proximal middle cerebral artery occlusion, for blood to get to this territory, it must travel via the anterior and posterior cerebral arteries into distal middle cerebral branches, flow backward along these branches all the way into the main trunk of the middle cerebral artery, and finally, the length of the lenticulostriate vessels. Often, because the various cortical anastomoses are not large enough, the blood supply essentially runs out before the distal lenticulostriate territory is adequately supplied, much like the Colorado and Yangtze rivers often end before reaching the ocean because of all the water diverted for municipal and agricultural use along the way. In this way, proximal middle cerebral artery occlusion often results in infarction (stroke) in the lenticulostriate end zone (Fig. 2-22*D*). The lenticulostriate end zone lies in the deep hemispheric white matter just lateral and superior to the body of the lateral ventricle. When this type of infarct involves the posterior third of the periventricular white matter, it causes hemiparesis and sensory loss due to damage to motor and sensory fibers in the corona radiata.

A considerably less common situation may arise in patients who have major anomalies of the circle of Willis. Modest anomalies of the circle of Willis are the

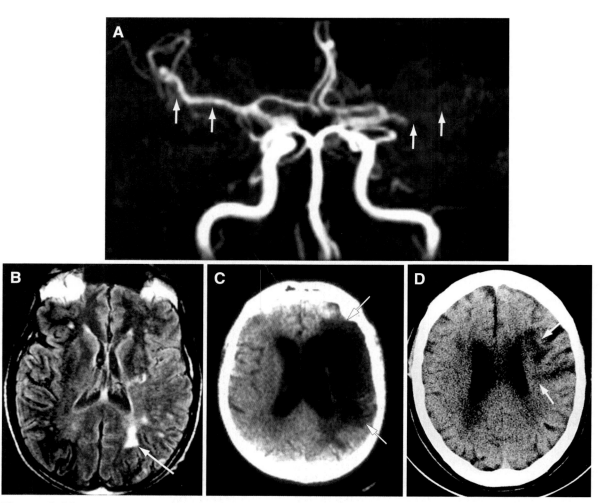

**Figure 2-22** *A,* A magnetic resonance angiogram (MRA) demonstrating complete occlusion of the proximal left middle cerebral artery by an embolus. The only clinical evidence of this was mild confusion. *B,* An MR image (MRI) of this patient, revealing minimal infarction in the parietal lobe. This patient's middle cerebral artery territory was almost completely spared by the presence of large cortical arterial anastomoses. *C,* A CT scan of a patient with a similar proximal middle cerebral occlusion but with poor anastomatic connections, illustrating nearly complete infarction of the entire middle cerebral artery territory. *D,* An axial CT scan of the brain illustrating a lenticulostriate end zone infarction.

rule rather than the exception. However, consider the rare patient with more extensive anomalies, for example, (1) the anterior communicating artery is absent; (2) the left posterior cerebral artery originates at the left supraclinoid carotid artery (in lieu of the posterior communicating artery); and (3) the portion of the proximal posterior cerebral artery originating from the basilar artery is vestigial or absent. This patient has an "isolated" intracranial carotid circulation. What will happen to this patient if the left internal carotid artery undergoes thrombotic occlusion? To the extent that there is a vestigial proximal posterior cerebral artery

emerging from the basilar tip, this artery will provide some blood to the isolated portion of the circle of Willis on the side of the occlusion. In addition, the internal and the external carotid arteries anastomose with each other via the ophthalmic artery. Thus, in this situation, blood can flow from the external carotid artery, backward through the ophthalmic artery, into the supraclinoid carotid artery on the side of the proximal internal carotid artery occlusion. We now have two admittedly inadequate sources of blood supply to the proximal anterior, middle, and posterior cerebral arteries on the side of the occlusion. The region of maximal ischemia will now be over the cerebral convexity in the end zones of these three arteries, territory that is often referred to as the "watershed" zone. Brain supplied by more proximal portions of the three major hemispheric arteries will tend to be spared to the extent that the two anastomotic sources we have noted prove adequate to supply them.

Finally, we will consider the very common situation that occurs when a small atheroma within a cerebral penetrating vessel forms a clot that occludes that vessel. These small penetrating vessels may have very tenuous anastomoses via terminal capillary networks with other deep penetrating vessels. The result is that proximal occlusion of these penetrating vessels, whether it occurs in the cerebrum or the brainstem, typically results in infarction of most of the territory supplied by the vessel. These infarcts are typically small (<1 cm in diameter), and are commonly referred to as *lacunar infarcts* (Fig. 2-21).

## E. THE MANIFESTATIONS OF STROKES REFLECT THE FUNCTIONAL SIGNIFICANCE OF THE INFARCTED TERRITORY

This statement seems fairly obvious, but the full ramifications are not always considered. For example, when patients with TIAs were first systematically evaluated with CT and MRI scans, it came as quite a surprise that many of them had evidence of both old and new cerebral infarctions. It had been assumed that a TIA, defined as a cerebrovascular event resulting in neurologic deficits lasting less than 24 hours, was not associated with permanent damage to the brain. These imaging studies demonstrated that many TIAs produced actual "silent" infarcts. This effect had not been appreciated because the infarcts commonly occurred in regions of the brain having to do exclusively with higher neural functions that were either too subtle or too widely distributed through the brain for the effects of a single, limited stroke to be recognized. The evidence of old strokes in these imaging studies further emphasized this point: these strokes had occurred without producing any symptoms recognizable by the patient or his/her family. In fact, it is only when strokes affect somatosensory, visual, motor, or language systems that they are reliably recognized.

Large vessel distribution strokes commonly produce these types of symptoms because they so often occlude the proximal middle cerebral artery, less often the proximal posterior cerebral artery, and cortical anastomoses are seldom adequate to assure essential perfusion to cortical systems subserving somatosensory, visual, motor, or language function in the dominant hemisphere. Because events affecting the nondominant hemisphere rarely produce obvious language dysfunction, and because patients with nondominant hemisphere lesions often have anosognosia (denial of illness), something we will discuss later in the course, "silent" cortical infarctions are far more likely to occur in the nondominant hemisphere.

Strokes produced by occlusion of small, penetrating vessels (lacunar infarcts, Figs. 2-21, 2-23) commonly affect regions of the brain in which small lesions will be inapparent (e.g., the putamen, or white matter pathways subserving highly distributed higher neural functions). They produce symptoms only when they happen to be located in regions where pathways subserving somatosensory, visual, motor, or language function are concentrated. By far the most common exemplars are motor pathways in the corona radiata (the lenticulostriate end zone), the posterior limb of the internal capsule, and the basis pontis. Far less common are sensory pathways in the ventral posterior nucleus of the thalamus. Lacunar infarctions affecting vision (via infarction of the lateral geniculate nucleus) or language function (via infarction of other portions of the thalamus) are rare. Because lacunar infarctions affecting any other portions of the vast extent of the deep cerebral gray and white matter are unlikely to affect somatosensory, visual, motor, or language functions, most lacunar infarctions are silent, and we commonly see evidence of such silent infarcts on imaging studies.

## F. NEUROLOGIC EVENTS RELATED TO THE SUBARACHNOID COURSE OF ARTERIES

Up to this point, we have considered the dynamics of events produced by clots within arteries. However, some relatively unusual events occur in relation to the routes that arteries take over the surface of the brain.

One class of events occurs when an artery becomes unusually enlarged, that is, forms a spherical outpouching or aneurysm, usually at arterial junctions such as the point where the anterior cerebral arteries are joined together by the anterior communicating artery, or the point at which the posterior communicating artery emerges from the supraclinoid carotid artery. Most commonly, the symptoms of aneurysms

Central Nervous System Vasculature, Blood Flow, and Metabolism

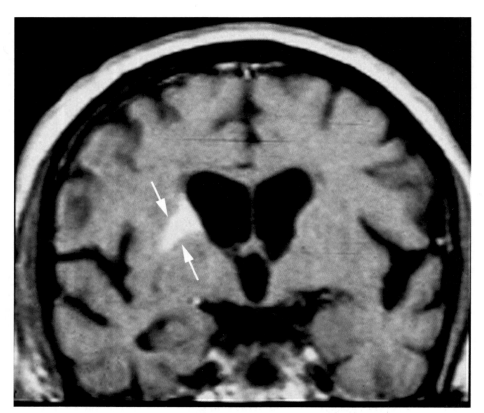

**Figure 2-23** Coronal magnetic resonance image (MRI) demonstrating a lacunar infarct involving the entire territory of a lenticulostriate vessel (*arrows*). This image was obtained after administration of a contrast agent, gadolinium, which flows across a blood-brain barrier rendered leaky by ischemic injury, into the surrounding tissue: hence the increased MR signal in the territory of the infarct.

## Case 2-3

### Cranial Nerve III Compression by an Arterial Aneurysm

*A 55-year-old woman suddenly develops headache and diplopia (double vision). On examination, her left pupil is widely dilated and there is some impairment in her ability to look up, down, or medially with the left eye. These findings indicate damage to left cranial nerve (CN) III. The absence of any other abnormalities on examination suggests that the area of damage is outside the brainstem. Furthermore, because brain lesions do not produce pain, the presence of headache also suggests that the lesion is outside the brainstem and involves the meninges or blood vessels. Because the CN III fibers subserving pupillary function travel on the medial upper surface of the nerve, the disproportionate involvement of pupillary function in this case suggests pressure on the nerve from above and medially.*

**Comment:** *This picture is the characteristic clinical signature of an aneurysm originating at the junction of the posterior communicating artery and the supraclinoid carotid artery (see Fig. 8-20). These aneurysms characteristically protrude downward from the carotid artery such that the dome of the aneurysm compresses CN III as the nerve enters the roof of the cavernous sinus, a point at which the nerve is firmly anchored and thus cannot slide out of the way of the aneurysm. It is absolutely critical for physicians to recognize the significance of this clinical presentation because this aneurysm can be clipped readily, thus saving the patient from the consequences of outright rupture of the aneurysm, which would have an approximately 50 percent likelihood of being fatal.*

reflect aneurysmal rupture, in which case arterial blood floods into the subarachnoid space (almost always a catastrophic event). However, these aneurysms, when they become sufficiently large, may produce symptoms by compressing nearby neural structures. Cases 2-3 and 2-4 illustrate this situation.

## Case 2-4

### Giant Aneurysm Compromising Frontal Lobe Function

*Over the course of a year a 70-year-old man becomes progressively more apathetic and inactive. Once a very colorful character with a dozen stories for every occasion, warm and jovial in his interactions with everyone, he is now uncharacteristically quiet. He tends to sit around all day doing nothing. He speaks only when spoken to and then usually responds with a single word answer. An imaging study demonstrates a 2.5-cm diameter midline spherical mass beneath the rostrum of the corpus callosum (Fig. 2-24). Subsequent arteriography confirms a giant aneurysm originating at the anterior communicating artery.*

**Comment:** *This aneurysm has grown slowly and ultimately compressed white matter pathways connecting the prefrontal cortex with other deep systems in the thalamus and brainstem. The result is profound impairment in all prefrontal functions, marked by loss of goal-oriented activity and akinesia affecting both language and motor function. In theory, a spring-loaded titanium clip can be placed across the neck of this aneurysm, thus isolating it from its arterial source and allowing decompression of the brain around it. In practice, this surgery is technically quite demanding and a favorable outcome is not always assured.*

The other major circumstance in which the routes that arteries take is important to the clinical picture is in patients who have large intracranial masses producing herniation (see Chapter 1, Case 1-2 and Practice Case 1-4B). The patient described in this case would be at risk for two other serious consequences that we did not mention at the time because we had not yet introduced the vascular anatomy necessary to understand them. First, herniation of the medial temporal lobe through the hole in the tentorium through which the brainstem passes (the incisura) may compress the posterior cerebral artery against the margin of the tentorium sufficiently forcefully to occlude it, resulting in a

stroke in the distribution of this artery. Second, central herniation, coupled with uncal herniation, pushes the entire brainstem downward and to the contralateral side, pulling the basilar artery with it because the basilar artery is tethered to the pons by the penetrating vessels it supplies to the pons. CN III, after it emerges from the interpeduncular fossa of the midbrain, passes between the superior cerebellar artery inferiorly and the posterior cerebral artery superiorly on its way to the cavernous sinus. The basilar artery pulls the posterior cerebral artery on the side of the intracranial mass down on the superior surface of the nerve, buckling the nerve and compressing its fibers (see Fig. 8-22). As in the case of the internal carotid artery–posterior communicating artery aneurysm, the fibers most immediately affected are those supplying the pupil. Thus, one particularly alarming sign of cerebral transtentorial herniation is a dilated or "blown" pupil, because it indicates that central/uncal herniation is quite advanced and that the patient's death is imminent unless the mass causing the herniation is immediately decompressed.

## PRACTICE 2-5

**A.** List the major sites where clots responsible for strokes most commonly form.

**B.** Bacterial meningitis (bacterial infection with secondary inflammation of the meninges) is often complicated by stroke. Explain the likely mechanism. (Hint: Where do the major arteries to the brain and brainstem travel with respect to the brain and the meninges?)

**C.** Which stroke is more likely to reflect cardiogenic embolism—a tip of the basilar artery stroke (e.g., a posterior cerebral artery occlusion resulting in loss of vision in one-half field) or a distal vertebral artery occlusion resulting in a lateral medullary (Wallenberg) infarction? Explain why.

**D.** A 75-year-old woman with a history of myocardial infarction suddenly develops severe right-sided sensory loss. Neurologic examination confirms the sensory loss and in addition reveals subtle loss of vision in the right half field. An MRI scan reveals a small infarction in the portion of the thalamus receiving sensory projections from the brainstem (ventral posterior nucleus). An echocardiogram (a test in which sound waves bounced off the heart enable us to define heart chamber size and motion) shows an enlarged left ventricle with an area

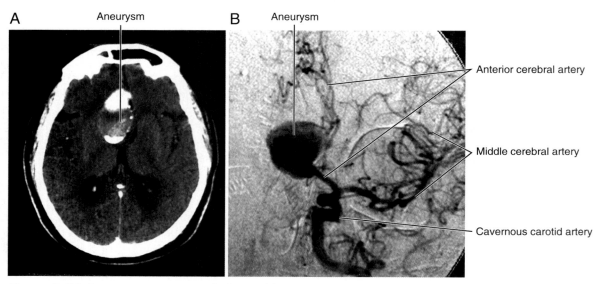

**Figure 2-24** Computed tomographic (CT) scan (*A*) and arteriogram (*B*) showing a giant aneurysm of the anterior communicating artery. The white material seen within the aneurysm on the CT scan is clotted blood.

of protrusion (ventricular aneurysm) lined with clot (mural thrombus). Does this patient have a microvascular infarct (due to thrombosis of a thalamoperforator), in which case she should receive antiplatelet therapy (e.g., aspirin and dipyridamole), or is she more likely to have had embolism from the heart causing her stroke, in which case she should be anticoagulated with warfarin. Explain why. (Hint: think about all the neurologic manifestations in this patient and about the common sites of atheromatous disease.)

**E.** A 60-year-old man with a history of hypertension, diabetes, and heavy smoking, suddenly notices a terrible smell while he is watching television. He discovers to his horror that it is the smell of the index and third fingers of his left hand being burned by the cigarette he is holding—something he cannot feel. An MRI scan reveals extensive infarction limited to the right postcentral gyrus (primary somatosensory cortex). What does the extent of this infarct tell you about the state of collateral circulation in this man's right hemisphere? Be specific.

**F.** A 50-year-old man with coronary artery disease experiences a myocardial infarction. Shortly after arriving at the hospital, he has a cardiorespiratory arrest, dropping his blood pressure to zero. After 10 minutes of cardiopulmonary resuscitation, a pulse is reestab-

lished and his blood pressure rises to 90/50 mm Hg. He is comatose for 24 hours but then rapidly recovers. However, he is left with significant, permanent neurologic deficits. Based on your knowledge of the territories supplied by the major cerebral arteries, predict the location of his lesion(s).

**G.** In Practice Case 2-3C, you mapped out the distribution of the brainstem stroke resulting from occlusion of the posterior inferior cerebellar artery—the lateral medullary or Wallenberg infarction. The posterior inferior cerebellar artery supplies the entire inferior surface of the cerebellar hemisphere and yet, in Wallenberg infarcts, there is often minimal, if any, cerebellar infarction. Explain why this might be so. (Hint: apply your knowledge about arterial anastomoses in the cerebrum.)

**H.** Binswanger's disease, the most common vascular cause of dementia, is caused by the accumulation of very large numbers of cerebral microinfarctions which eventually, in aggregate, cause extensive damage to the deep cerebral white matter. Prefrontal and memory functions are most severely affected because these are the systems most dependent on long, white matter connections. Patients become forgetful and akinetic. Typically, the dementia is insidiously progressive and patients do not relate a history of multiple strokes. How can this be?

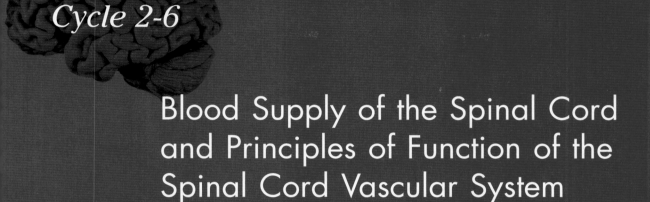

# Blood Supply of the Spinal Cord and Principles of Function of the Spinal Cord Vascular System

1. Be able to describe the vascular anatomy of the spinal cord.
2. Be able to explain the pattern of spinal cord infarction that occurs with occlusion of the artery of Adamkiewicz.

## A. ANATOMY

The spinal cord is supplied by the *anterior spinal artery*, which continues as a single vessel along the entire ventral aspect of the cord, and the posterior spinal arteries, which are discontinuous and form the most conspicuous vessels of a plexus along the dorsal aspect of the cord (Fig. 2-25). At their rostral end, both the anterior and the posterior spinal arteries begin as branches of the vertebral arteries (see Figs. 2-13, 2-17). As they descend along the spinal cord, they are supplied from radicular branches of lateral spinal arteries, which in the neck derive from the vertebral arteries, and below the neck, derive from the intercostal arteries. In the neck, there are two lateral spinal arteries at every level, but thoracic, lumbar, and sacral portions of the cord are supplied by a far more limited number of lateral spinal arteries, sometimes as few as two or three, typically clustered along lumbosacral portions of the cord. One of these, a particularly large vessel often referred to as

the *artery of Adamkiewicz*, usually enters from the left side from as high as the ninth thoracic or as low as the fourth lumbar level.

Branches from the anterior spinal artery supply the ventromedial portion of the cord (Fig. 2-25). They also penetrate the cord deeply and branch to supply the dorsal and ventral horns and the lateral corticospinal tracts immediately lateral to the spinal cord gray matter. The posterior spinal artery plexus supplies the margins of the entire cord with the exception of the ventromedial portions immediately adjacent to the anterior spinal artery.

## B. FUNCTION

Because the cervical spinal cord has such a redundant blood supply, it is very rarely affected by ischemic events. However, if one or more of the lateral spinal arteries in the lumbosacral region are occluded, particularly the artery of Adamkiewicz, either by atheromatous disease or by surgery (e.g., during abdominal aortic aneurysectomy), the blood supply to the spinal cord may be seriously compromised. Because the thoracic region of the cord receives the least number of spinal arteries, it is the region typically affected by vascular occlusions at the lumbosacral level. Thus, the thoracic cord is often referred to as a "watershed" region, although "terminal drought" region would be more appropriate.

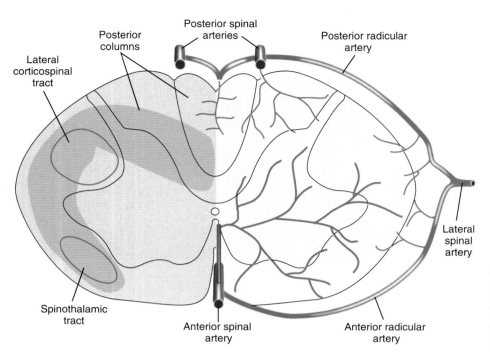

**Figure 2-25** Cross section of the spinal cord illustrating the vascular supply. In the left half of the figure, the distribution of the watershed territory is depicted in darker gray.

The peculiarities of the cross-sectional blood supply to the spinal cord define the pattern of cord infarction produced by occlusion of lumbosacral lateral spinal arteries. Loss of perfusion by, for example, occlusion of the artery of Adamkiewicz, leads to infarction in the end zone (the "watershed distribution") of anterior and posterior spinal artery perforators (Fig. 2-25). The most severely affected structures are the lateral corticospinal tracts (the spinal cord extension of the medullary pyramids) and the lateral spinothalamic tracts more ventrally, below the level of the lesion (the midthoracic level). The resultant symptom complex is often referred to as the "anterior spinal artery syndrome," which is illustrated in Case 2-5.

## Case 2-5

### Spinal Cord Infarction
*A 72-year-old man with a long history of hypertension, hyperlipidemia, and heavy smoking awakes one day to find his legs paralyzed. Examination reveals flaccid paralysis of both legs. His bladder is distended. The touch of a hand to his legs feels normal and he is also able to perceive vibratory stimulation to his feet with normal sensitivity. However, he cannot differentiate hot from cold below the*

## Case 2-5—cont'd

*midthoracic level and the prick of a sharp stick caudal to this level is perceived as dull.*

**Comment:** *The lateral corticospinal tracts, the spinal cord extension of the medullary pyramids (see Chapter 1), provide the basis for movement. Fibers helping to control urinary function are located in the general vicinity of the corticospinal tracts. The lateral spinothalamic tracts are located in the ventrolateral portions of the cord and carry sensory fibers predominantly subserving pain and temperature sensation. Sensory pathways subserving vibratory sensation (the dorsal/posterior columns) are located in the dorsal midline portion of the cord, which is usually adequately supplied by penetrating vessels deriving from the posterior spinal artery plexus.*

## PRACTICE 2-6

Most people are able to undergo repair of abdominal aortic aneurysms (with attendant risk of compromise to lateral spinal arteries) without experiencing neurologic deficits. What does this tell you about the typical vascular supply to the spinal cord?

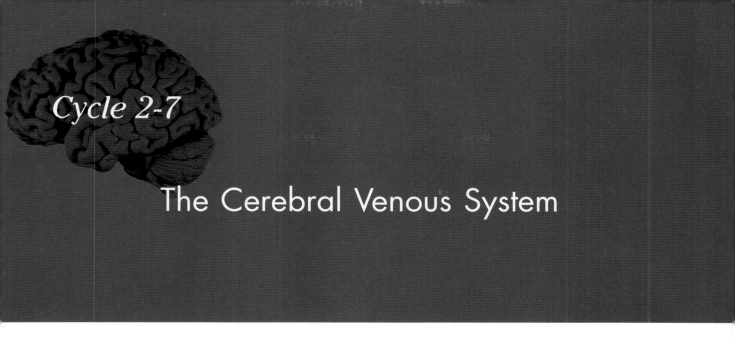

# Cycle 2-7

## The Cerebral Venous System

### Objectives

1. Be able to explain why a patient with elevated central venous pressure due to congestive heart failure has high cerebrospinal fluid pressure.

2. Be able to explain why cerebral sinus thrombosis may cause elevated intracranial pressure and pseudotumor cerebri.

3. Be able to explain how sinus thrombosis can sometimes cause cerebral infarction.

4. Be able to explain the implications of patterns of cranial venous flow for central facial infections.

Because the cerebral venous system is uncommonly implicated in disease processes, we will confine the discussion in this section to an anatomic overview and a focus on some essential principles of the venous system that often have implications for clinical phenomena.

Figure 2-26 demonstrates the major structures in the cerebral venous system. The "trunks" of the system are the dural sinuses, venous channels enclosed within the leaves of the dura. The superior sagittal sinus, located at the junction of the falx and the dura covering the inner table of the skull, drains backward into the confluens of sinuses. The inferior sagittal sinus, forming the inferior margin of the falx, drains backward into the straight sinus, a channel within the intersection of the falx and the tentorium, which in turn drains backward into the confluens. Blood from the confluens then drains laterally into the transverse sinuses, formed at the junction of the tentorium and the inner table of the skull, then into the sigmoid sinuses, and ultimately, into the internal jugular veins. The surface of the brain is drained by cortical veins, which terminate in one of the venous sinuses. Deep structures of the brain drain backward into the straight sinus. The cavernous sinuses, on either side of the sella turcica, are linked to the transverse and sigmoid sinuses by the superior and inferior petrosal sinuses. Veins from the periorbital and paranasal regions of the face drain backward into the cavernous sinuses.

We will review four important principles governing the venous system:

1. Central venous pressure is communicated through the arachnoid granulations to the cerebrospinal fluid compartment (Case 2-6).

2. Obstruction of cerebral venous flow due to sinus thrombosis leads to elevation of cerebrospinal fluid pressure. A variety of circumstances may lead to thrombosis of one or more of the venous sinuses. The most common cause of this infrequent event is a generally enhanced tendency to form blood clots, as is seen with a variety of inherited and acquired abnormalities of coagulation mechanisms. Often this is potentiated by drugs (oral contraceptives) or cigarette smoking. This situation is illustrated by Case 2-7.

Central Nervous System Vasculature, Blood Flow, and Metabolism

## Case 2-6

### Elevated Central Venous Pressure and Cerebrospinal Fluid Pressure[1]

*A 35-year-old woman born with a single cardiac ventricle is admitted to the hospital in severe heart failure. Her central venous pressure is 25 mm Hg. Because she is confused and has a low-grade fever, a lumbar puncture is performed. The opening pressure is 450 mm $H_2O$ (approximately 40 mm Hg). A normal opening pressure is less than 200 mm $H_2O$. Should one be alarmed by this extremely high pressure?*

**Comment:** *No. The central venous pressure is transmitted directly through the arachnoid granulations to the cerebrospinal fluid compartment. Because the pressure is transmitted evenly throughout the intracranial compartment, there is no danger of shifts of intracranial contents (herniation) as there would be if the high pressure were due to a large tumor pressing on the arachnoid granulations and interfering with the normal egress of cerebrospinal fluid. If this patient's severe congestive heart failure and elevated venous pressure were not treated, the persistent elevation of venous pressure could lead, in theory, to transudation of plasma into the CNS tissue in the same manner as in the lungs, liver, and lower extremities in such cases. In practice, these patients keep themselves in a semiupright position to minimize venous distention in the lungs (thus making it possible for them to breathe) and they thereby reduce the cerebral venous pressure simply by the force of gravity.*

## Case 2-7

### Superior Sagittal Sinus Thrombosis

*A 25-year-old woman presents with a 2-month history of unrelenting headache. Her examination is normal but for the presence of bilateral papilledema (swelling of the optic nerve heads or "disks," visible on funduscopic examination). An MRI scan of the head fails to reveal any abnormalities, most particularly a tumor. A lumbar puncture reveals an opening pressure of 350 mm $H_2O$. A magnetic resonance angiogram reveals little blood flow in the superior sagittal sinus and in the larger of the two transverse sinuses. She takes oral contraceptives and smokes one pack of cigarettes per day. Studies of her coagulation system reveal that she has the Leiden allelic variant of factor V, which renders the prothrombin activator complex (factors V and X and phospholipid) relatively resistant to degradation.*

**Comment:** *This patient has three factors that increase her risk for pathologic thrombosis (smoking, oral contraceptive use, factor $V_{Leiden}$). As a result, she has developed thrombosis of the cerebral venous sinus system. This in turn has obstructed the egress of cerebrospinal fluid through the arachnoid granulations, hence the very high intracranial pressure. This pressure is sufficiently high (and sufficiently persistent, unlike the situation in Case 2-6) to interfere with normal flow of cytoplasmic constituents along the axons of retinal ganglion cells (axoplasmic flow) as they pass through the optic nerves, ultimately to terminate at the lateral geniculate nuclei. As a result, there is swelling of the optic nerve heads. If this swelling is not addressed soon, she will develop progressive loss of peripheral vision. This situation of increased intracranial pressure in the absence of a mass, caused by obstruction to the outflow of cerebrospinal fluid, is called pseudotumor cerebri. It may occur for a variety of reasons, sinus thrombosis being a common one. Headache is a common accompaniment, possibly because cerebral edema leads to traction of pain-sensitive structures, such as the meninges, against the skull. This patient will probably respond favorably to cessation of smoking, discontinuation of oral contraceptives, and chronic anticoagulation. However, it may be necessary to decompress her optic nerves to save her vision and provide an alternative pathway for egress of cerebrospinal fluid with a procedure called optic nerve sheath fenestration, or simply to reduce the elevated intracranial pressure with a lumbar-peritoneal cerebrospinal fluid shunt.*

---

[1]Central venous pressure can be measured by inserting a catheter (a thin, hollow tube) connected to a pressure transducer into either the external jugular vein in the neck or the subclavian vein (just beneath the clavicle) and threading it in until the tip is in the superior vena cava. A normal pressure would be 5 mm Hg. Cerebrospinal fluid (CSF) pressure is measured by connecting a calibrated plastic tube (a manometer) to a lumbar puncture needle. The CSF will rise in the manometer until the height of the fluid column equals the CSF pressure in millimeters of water.

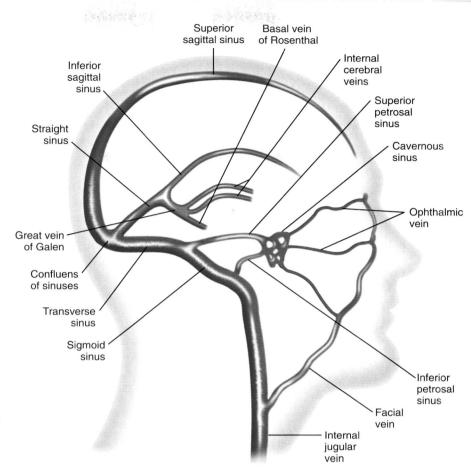

**Figure 2-26** Lateral view of the intracranial venous system demonstrating the major venous sinuses.

3. Sinus thrombosis associated with venous thrombosis may cause stroke.

From time to time, for poorly understood reasons, sinus thrombosis is associated with thrombosis of cortical veins. When thrombosis is limited to the sinuses, the network of cerebral veins provides alternative routes (collaterals) that enable blood to drain, even if venous pressure is on average increased. However, when thrombosis extends to within the veins, collaterals no longer can serve their purpose, all local venous drainage and hence the perfusion of local portions of the brain stop, and the tissue is infarcted. Because sinus thrombosis most commonly occurs in the superior sagittal sinus, the tissue most commonly affected by this venous infarction is in the parasagittal region of the brain. This portion of the motor cortex (precentral gyrus) subserves leg movement. Thus, these patients often present with difficulty in walking and leg weakness.

4. Venous drainage from ocular and paranasal tissues into the cavernous sinuses carries the risk of transmitting facial infections to within the cranial vault. Case 2-8 illustrates the potential consequences.

## Case 2-8

### Midline Facial Infection

*A 45-year-old man develops a minor infection around an ingrown hair just below his nose. Three days later, his wife notes that he is spending more and more time in bed and at times is hard to arouse. On arrival at the hospital, he is by turns lethargic and combative. It requires four security guards to hold him still during a lumbar puncture. Later that day he becomes deeply comatose. The following morning, a neurology resident, suspecting an infectious cause of the patient's coma, initiates an oxacillin infusion as he*

*Continued*

## Case 2-8—cont'd

*takes the patient for a CT scan. The scan is normal. When it comes time to load the patient back on his gurney to return to the intensive care unit, he suddenly sits up and asks where he is.*

**Comment:** *Staphylococcal infections such as this one are commonly associated with alterations of mental status, whether because of bacterial products or cytokines induced by the infection. In this case, blood from the infection was draining back into the cavernous sinuses and associated venous systems. The precise mechanisms by which this affects the brain are unclear, but as this case demonstrates, termination of the sustained bacteremia with appropriate antibiotics can have very rapid and dramatic effects. Failure to treat this infection in a timely fashion would lead to staphylococcal meningitis and death.*

## PRACTICE 2-7

A lumbar puncture is obtained in a 25-year-old woman in an attempt to clarify the diagnosis of multiple sclerosis (an autoimmune disease causing areas of demyelination within the central nervous system). The medical student performing the lumbar puncture records an opening pressure of $350\,mm\,H_2O$ and becomes quite alarmed. The resident instructs the patient to partially straighten her body (lumbar punctures are performed with patients curled into the fetal position to maximally spread the spaces between the vertebral spinous processes) and to relax. She assures the patient that everything is going smoothly, that the medical student did a fine job, and that the procedure is nearly complete. The cerebrospinal fluid pressure drops to $140\,mm\,H_2O$. Explain why.

# Division II

# Cerebral Blood Flow and Metabolism

## Cycle 2-8

# Cerebral Blood Flow and Metabolism

### Objectives

1. Be able to list the major principles governing cerebral energy metabolism.

2. Be able to explain what is meant by cerebral vascular autoregulation and the role of arterial $CO_2$ in influencing cerebral flood flow, and give an clinical example of how these phenomena can prove useful in clinical care.

3. Be able to provide approximate ranges for normal cerebral blood flow rates, blood flow rates associated with neuronal silence without infarction, and blood flow rates that, when sustained, lead to infarction. Be able explain the relevance of this information to cardiac surgery and mitigating the size of strokes.

4. Be able to explain why reduction of blood pressure in patients with acute stroke may be catastrophic.

Intermediate metabolism in the brain is not fundamentally different than in other organ systems. However, to fully understand the brain's function in normal and pathologic states, one needs to recognize that neurons and glia also have several unusual metabolic attributes:

1. For practical purposes, glucose is the only metabolic substrate for the brain.

2. Central nervous system glucose uptake depends upon an ATP-linked active transport mechanism but does not require insulin.

3. The brain is reliant almost exclusively on aerobic metabolism.

4. The brain has no facility for oxygen storage (e.g., like myoglobin in muscles) and its capacity for glucose storage is minimal and limited to glia.

5. For most neural tissue, intermediate metabolism accounts for less than half of all energy consumption. The rest is spent on maintenance of ion gradients that are constantly being dissipated in the course of repeated neuronal firing (up to 1000 Hz) and the energy costs of synthesis, transport, packaging, release, and reuptake or catabolism of neurotransmitters (see Chapters 4 and 5). This enormous energy requirement is indirectly reflected in the extremely high blood flow to cerebral tissue, 50 to 60 mL/100 g/min (Table 2-3), and in that fact that the brain, constituting 1.5 to 2 percent of body mass, receives 20 percent of resting cardiac output.

An adequate supply of glucose and oxygen must constantly be provided to neural tissue despite variability in both the metabolic demands of that tissue and variability in the parameters affecting the delivery of these metabolic substrates. The brain has evolved two fundamental means to deal with this double variability:

**TABLE 2-3** Normal Values of Variables Relevant to Cerebral Oxygen Delivery

| Variable | Normal Values |
| --- | --- |
| Cerebral blood flow | 50-60 mL/100 g/min |
| Hemoglobin | 13-14 g/dL |
| Arterial $P_{CO_2}$ | 90-95 mm Hg |
| Arterial oxygen saturation | 100% |
| Arterial $P_{CO_2}$ | 35 mm Hg |
| Systemic blood pressure | 120/70 mm Hg |
| Systemic pulse pressure | 85 mm Hg |

(1) a capacity for autoregulation of its blood flow; and (2) a high tolerance for substantial reductions in metabolic substrate. We will consider each of these mechanisms in further detail.

## AUTOREGULATION

Cerebral resistance vessels (arterioles) respond to a variety of substances that enable increases in local blood flow in response to increased metabolic demand, two of the most important being interstitial potassium and $CO_2$. The response to potassium is almost instantaneous. Thus, it provides a mechanism by which increased activity at neural synapses (the most energy intensive focus of neural systems), associated with outflow of potassium from within the neural cytosol into the extracellular space, triggers instant local vasodilatation in anticipation of increased metabolic demand. Carbon dioxide is also a potent central nervous system vasodilator. Although vascular responses to $CO_2$ are not sufficiently rapid to entrain local fluctuations in synaptic activity, they are homeostatic in that they help to increase blood flow when and where metabolism is high. The role of $CO_2$ is particularly important because of the large fluctuations in arterial $CO_2$ that occur in relation to breathing rates and systemic acid-base balance. Neurosurgeons are able to take great advantage of this mechanism, as Case 2-9 illustrates.

Cerebral blood flow is also responsive to arterial oxygen concentrations, although to a considerably lesser extent than to blood $CO_2$ concentrations.

### Case 2-9

**Temporary Treatment of Cerebral Herniation with Hyperventilation**

*A 50-year-old man notices one morning that he is having some difficulty walking, tending to drag his left leg. By the time he arrives at the hospital 6 hours later, he has a left hemiparesis. A CT scan reveals a massive right frontal lobe tumor producing incipient herniation (see Cycle 1-4, Practice B). By nightfall, the patient is stuporous. Operative decompression is being arranged but the neurosurgeon needs several hours to prepare for surgery and carry out the craniotomy. He promptly intubates the patient and hyperventilates him, bringing his arterial $P_{CO_2}$ down from 35 mm Hg to 25 mm Hg. The patient becomes more easily arousable and surgery is successfully carried out before herniation can take place.*

**Comment:** *The patient became stuporous because the combination of brain, tumor mass, and cerebrospinal fluid blocked in an obstructed ventricular system had exceeded the volume of the closed vault provided by the skull, particularly the supratentorial compartment. This increased volume led to an incipient herniation process. The marked reduction in $P_{CO_2}$ produced by hyperventilation induced constriction of cerebral resistance vessels, thereby markedly reducing the amount of blood in the downstream venules and veins (the cerebral capacitance system). This reduced the total mass of the brain by enough to arrest and partially reverse the herniation process until the bulk of the tumor could be removed.*

Central Nervous System Vasculature, Blood Flow, and Metabolism

Cerebral autoregulatory capacity not only enables the brain to match the demands of local increases in synaptic activity with appropriate increases in blood flow, but it also enables the maintenance of nearly constant cerebral blood flow despite wide fluctuations in blood pressure. In fact, blood flow is well maintained until cerebral blood pressure drops below 60 mm Hg. Below this point of maximal vasodilatation and minimal cerebrovascular resistance, blood flow becomes proportional to perfusion pressure.

## TOLERANCE FOR REDUCTIONS IN BLOOD FLOW

Normal cerebral blood flow is in the range of 50 to 60 mL/100 g/min, somewhat higher in women, most likely because of higher neuronal density in smaller brains. This blood flow can be reduced to as low as 23 mL/100 g/min without any alteration in cerebral function. In other words, the brain has a metabolic reserve of nearly two thirds. Between 18 and 23 mL/100 g/min, neural activity essentially ceases, but there is enough energy substrate to sustain intermediate metabolism (though not protein synthesis, which ceases promptly with greater than 50 percent reductions in blood flow). Only when blood flow drops below 18 mL/100 g/min do irreversible neuronal changes start. The extent of these changes depends upon how far below 18 mL/100 g/min blood flow falls and how long it remains there. Thus, levels of 17 mL/100 g/min might be tolerated for a number of hours, whereas levels of less than 10 mL/100 g/min, or the zero flow associated with cardiac arrest, will induce irreversible changes within minutes. The tolerance of the brainstem for ischemia may be even greater as this ancient structure long ago evolved to function under conditions of extremely low oxygen availability.

The remarkable cerebral tolerance for even relatively severe reductions in blood flow has two very important practical implications: (1) it makes feasible cardiac surgery, in which patients are maintained on the cardiopulmonary bypass pump at blood pressures of 40 to 50 mm Hg; and (2) it provides enormous opportunity for the acute treatment of stroke.

The reduction of systemic blood pressure to 40 to 50 mm Hg at first seems like a guarantee of massive cerebral anoxic injury. However, from the data we have reviewed, you can appreciate that this pressure is enough to maintain cerebral blood flow well over the 18 mL/100 g/min minimum. However, it is also important to keep in mind that the crucial variable here is oxygen delivery, and two major factors other than blood flow affect oxygen delivery: hemoglobin concentration and arterial oxygen saturation. Drops in hemoglobin concentration from average normal levels of 13 to 14 g/dL to approximately 12 g/dL actually slightly increase oxygen delivery by reducing blood viscosity. However, further drops reduce oxygen delivery. Thus, performing cardiac surgery on a patient with a hemoglobin concentration of 8 g/dL would be quite risky because this 33 percent further drop in oxygen-carrying capacity would seriously risk the equivalent of dropping cerebral blood flow to less than 18 mL/100 g/min.[2] Arterial oxygen saturation is also a factor, but a less important one, because of the shape of the hemoglobin-oxygen desaturation curve. Thus, even dropping arterial oxygen pressure from 95 mm Hg to 60 mm Hg results in a reduction in blood oxygen concentration of only 10 percent.

In earlier cycles of this chapter, we described how extensive anastomoses in the cerebral arterial network effectively maintain at least some blood flow to nearly all the tissue downstream to the point of vascular occlusion. Regions in which blood flow is severely reduced quite promptly undergo extensive infarction. However, with nearly every arterial occlusion, there is a volume of tissue, referred to as the ischemic penumbra, in which the blood flow is in the range of 15 to 23 mL/100 g/min. All the neurons in this region will be silent, and some of them will be in serious jeopardy but potentially salvageable if the right measures are taken quickly enough. In practical terms, the period of opportunity appears to be limited to about 3 hours. Measures that might be taken to salvage the ischemic penumbra ("hyperacute" stroke care) range from accelerating clot lysis, a therapeutic approach first introduced in 1996, to inhibiting any one of the numerous biochemical mechanisms that eventuate in neuronal death. Two of the most important mechanisms are glutamate-mediated cytotoxic effects (which we will discuss in Chapter 4) and damage caused by free radicals.

Although the existence of ischemic penumbra provides a great opportunity for mitigating stroke size, it

---

[2]Brain damage is relatively common in cardiac operations, but it is primarily due to the effects of hundreds or even thousands of cerebral emboli that may occur in the course of aortic clamping and unclamping.

also carries with it a serious danger. In the penumbra region, because of brain blood flow autoregulation, resistance vessels are maximally dilated. Under these circumstances, cerebral blood flow becomes a linear function of perfusion pressure, and reductions in systemic blood pressure can increase the size of the infarction, as illustrated in Case 2-10.

## Case 2-10

**Worsening of Stroke by Aggressive Treatment of High Blood Pressure**
*A 65-year-old man acutely develops mild difficulty speaking and clumsiness of his right hand. His blood pressure is 190/110 mm Hg. The admitting team administers antihypertensive agents and brings the blood pressure down to 120/70 mm Hg. One hour later, a nurse reports that the patient cannot speak, cannot understand spoken commands, and cannot move his right side.*

**Comment:** *This patient had a carotid T-junction embolic occlusion from thrombosis at a proximal internal carotid artery atheroma. Like most acute stroke patients, he developed compensatory hypertension, which maintained sufficient perfusion to*

## Case 2-10—cont'd

*an exceptionally large ischemic penumbra to keep it not only alive but substantially functional (i.e., cerebral blood flow >23 mL/100 g/min). However, the over 30 percent reduction in systemic pulse pressure dropped blood flow well below that necessary to maintain function and perhaps to levels likely to produce infarction. The sequence of events in this unfortunate gentleman illustrates why treatment of blood pressures of less than 200/120 mm Hg in patients with acute stroke is not recommended.*

## PRACTICE 2-8

**A.** Electroencephalograms (EEGs) are most commonly employed to detect and characterize potentially epileptiform activity. However, they also provide an accurate, online measure of the function of cortical neurons. Explain how an EEG could prove useful to a neurosurgeon cross-clamping an internal carotid artery in the course of performing a carotid endarterectomy. Consider the circle of Willis and the impact of various levels of cerebral blood flow in your answer.

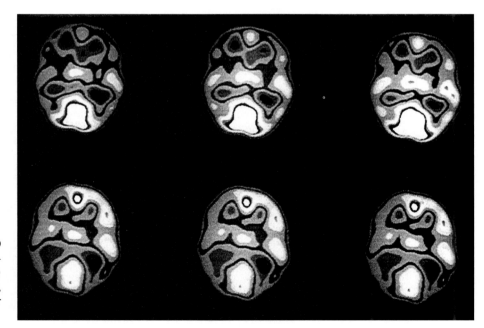

**Figure 2-27** [$^{99m}$Tc]-HMPAO single photon emission computed tomographic (SPECT) scans of three subjects. See text, Practice Problem 2-8B for explanation.

**B.** The tomographic scans (Fig. 2-27) were made with a radiolabeled ligand [$^{99m}$Tc]-HMPAO that binds to vascular endothelium in proportion to the magnitude of blood flow. The scans in the bottom row were made while the subjects had their eyes closed. Those in the top row were made while the subjects had their eyes open and were looking at a rapidly oscillating checkerboard pattern on a television screen. High signal in the medial occipital (calcarine) cortex is readily evident in these scans, reflecting the high synaptic activity in this area during the high intensity, rapidly changing visual input. Explain why it is possible to use a radioligand that tracks blood flow to image neural (actually synaptic) activity.

## CYCLE 2-2

**B.** Blood can still flow to the basilar artery territory via the other vertebral artery and both posterior communicating arteries.

## CYCLE 2-3

**B.** In your further encounters with cases like this one, later in the course, you will eventually be able to explain all the various neurologic manifestations. At this point, from your review of anatomy in Chapter 1, you can appreciate that the infarct damages descending corticospinal pathways in the basis pontis, hence the contralateral hemiparesis (Fig. 2-28).

**C.** This particular, fairly common infarct is referred to as a lateral medullary or Wallenberg infarct. We will reconsider this type of infarct at several points later in this course. The clinical manifestations described reflect damage to vestibular and cerebellar structures and a small nucleus adjacent to the inferior olive that innervates musculature involved in swallowing (Fig. 2-29).

## CYCLE 2-5

**A.** See Cycle 2-5, Table 2-2. (page 92)

**B.** The arteries and veins travel in the subarachnoid space, which in a patient with bacterial meningitis is full of inflammatory cells (pus). The arteries and veins are caught up in the inflammation and may thrombose. In the text, we discussed the most common sites of clot formation, those related to cardiac or atheromatous disease. Uncommon pathology (e.g., meningitis) can lead to thrombosis at other loci.

**C.** Because embolic clots tend to lodge at bifurcation points, and because we know that the distal vertebral arteries are sites of thrombogenic atheromatous disease (Cycle 2-5A), a tip-of-the-basilar-artery stroke is more likely to be due to cardiogenic embolism. This type of clinical reasoning is employed routinely in trying to decide stroke pathogenesis and, thus, the best therapy for patients with stroke.

**D.** This case nicely illustrates the reasoning that goes into choice of therapy for patients with stroke. Normally, we would think that a small stroke of the thala-

*Central Nervous System Vasculature, Blood Flow, and Metabolism*

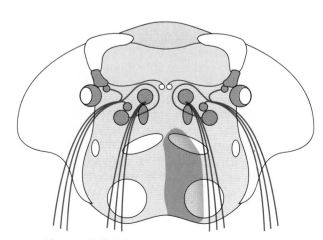

**Figure 2-28** See text for Cycle Feedback 2-3B.

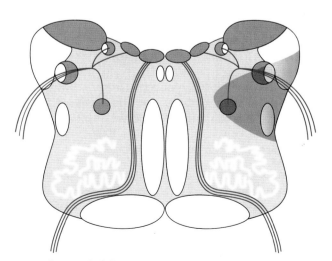

**Figure 2-29** See text for Cycle Feedback 2-3C.

mus was due to microvascular disease. However, this patient also has a visual field cut, indicating an infarction of the calcarine cortex and providing clear evidence that this was a large vessel event. It could conceivably be due to thrombosis at the site of atheromatous disease in the proximal left posterior cerebral artery, occluding both this artery and the thalamoperforator in the process, but this is an extraordinary location for such disease. Thus, even though emboli usually lodge at branch points, we are inclined to think that this was indeed a case of cardiogenic embolism. Thus, we would anticoagulate with warfarin. To arrive at the correct therapeutic decision, we have considered the neurologic examination, the types of lesions one could see with microvascular and large vessel events, sites of atheromatous disease, the course traveled by emboli, and the relative probabilities of various scenarios.

**E.** This stroke clearly involves a large vessel distribution. Whether it reflects clot wedged at the carotid T-junction or in the proximal portions of the middle cerebral artery branch supplying the postcentral gyrus, it indicates that the end-to-end anastomosis between this middle cerebral artery branch and the corresponding anterior cerebral artery branch is small or nonexistent, and thus is inadequate to save the postcentral gyrus. This case emphasizes the role of collateral blood supply in defining the distribution of infarction.

**F.** This situation demonstrates the classic cause of "watershed" infarction. If you answered the cortical zones between the anterior, middle, and posterior cerebral arteries, you are correct. Often, the worst damage is in the "triple" watershed zone in the medial parietal lobes that falls at the margin of the territories of all three vessels. Because this part of the brain is important in enabling us to visually relate the environmental coordinate system to our personal, head- and body-centered coordinate system, these patients are often very inaccurate in pointing to things, and have great difficulty voluntarily directing their eyes to a target, major components of what is known as Balint's syndrome (to be discussed further in Chapter 12).

**G.** Just as the branches of the major cerebral arteries anastomose with each other over the cerebral hemispheres, the branches of the long circumferential brainstem arteries supplying the cerebellar hemispheres have anastomotic connections with each other that in most cases serve to prevent large cerebellar infarctions.

**H.** The infarcts are small and occur in "silent" areas of the brain. Thus, only their cumulative impact becomes evident. This case is yet one more illustration that the manifestations of strokes reflect the functional significance of the infarcted territory.

# CYCLE 2-6

It indicates that most people have sufficient lumbar and thoracic lateral spinal arteries that loss of one or more does not sufficiently compromise the blood supply to the cord to cause infarction.

# CYCLE 2-7

Because the patient was tense and curled in the fetal position, she was straining and thus elevating her intrathoracic pressure. This was elevating her central venous pressure, which, transferred through the cerebral venous sinus system to the arachnoid granulations, elevated the cerebrospinal fluid pressure.

# CYCLE 2-8

**A.** Although the circle of Willis usually provides adequate collateral blood supply when an internal carotid artery is occluded, we have seen that there can be major anomalies, most important, those that result in an isolated intracranial carotid circulation. The uncommon patient with such an anomalous circulation could experience extensive hemispheric infarction when the internal carotid artery is cross-clamped. Fortunately, there is a margin for error in that cerebral blood flows in the range of 18 to 23 mL/100 g/min lead to neuronal dysfunction without infarction. The sudden appearance of slowing on the electroencephalogram when the carotid artery is clamped—indicative of widespread neuronal dysfunction—serves as a warning that hemispheric blood flow has fallen into this critical region, if not below. The neurosurgeon can then employ a shunt from the proximal to the distal cervical internal carotid artery to help perfuse the hemisphere while the atheromatous lesion is being resected.

**B.** The capacity for vascular autoregulation within the central nervous system enables the brain to focally increase blood flow to areas of high metabolic need in which neurons are consuming a great deal of energy in order to maintain their ion gradients and process neurotransmitter substances in the course of rapid firing. Other functional imaging modalities, such as $H_2^{15}O$ positron emission tomography (PET) and functional magnetic resonance imaging (fMRI) make use of the same autoregulatory principle. Functional imaging is used widely in research efforts to decipher human brain function.

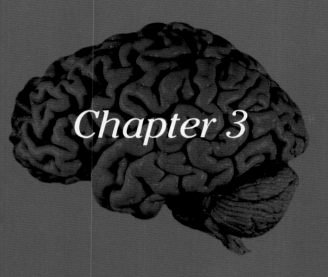

# Chapter 3

# NEUROHISTOLOGY

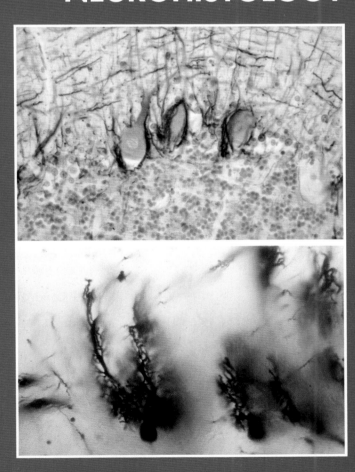

## Chapter 3

# NEUROHISTOLOGY

# Introduction

Neural networks, composed of hundreds, thousands, or even millions of highly interconnected neurons, form the essential units of function in the nervous system. We will touch on various attributes of neural network function in succeeding chapters of this book. In this chapter, we focus on the neurons that make up these networks.

Neurons are extraordinarily active, highly specialized and messy machines. For these reasons, they rely heavily on the presence of a variety of support cells, the glia, particularly astrocytes and oligodendrocytes (and their peripheral nervous system analog, Schwann cells). Astrocytes provide the structural matrix in which neurons reside, and they are instrumental in maintaining a stable ionic and molecular environment for neurons. Oligodendrocytes and Schwann cells produce the myelin or insulation surrounding neuronal processes. They thereby markedly potentiate the speed of neural transmission from one locus to another. Although much of the nervous system is encased in bone and relatively insulated from the periphery by the blood-brain barrier, the central nervous system (CNS) is not impervious to traumatic, vascular, infectious, immunologic, toxic, or metabolic injury. It is in dealing with the neural consequences of these hazards that a third class of glia, the microglia (actually the CNS form of the monocyte) becomes important.

Until quite recently, it was thought that we entered life with all the neurons we would ever have, and that neurons were incapable of dividing except in the case of certain brain tumors of neural origin. We now know that within the nervous system there reside precursor cells that are capable of division and maturation into neurons of any type, as well as into glial cells. These cells are activated by brain injury, thus providing a potential endogenous source for replacement of dead neurons. One of the most exciting areas of neuroscientific investigation today concerns the study of neuronal precursor cells with the aim of learning how to manipulate them to the end of treating brain injury, whether acquired or due to degenerative diseases such as Parkinson's disease, Alzheimer's disease or amyotrophic lateral sclerosis. It now also appears likely that neural precursor cells play a role in normal brain function, for example, providing a steady supply of new neurons to the hippocampus, which may be necessary to sustain a capacity for acquisition of certain types of memories throughout life.

# Division I

## Cellular Classes Within the Nervous System

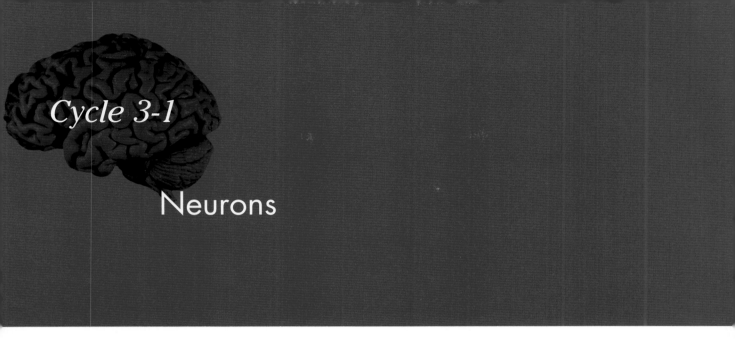

# Neurons

## Objectives

1. Be able to describe the major morphologic features of neurons.

2. Be able to summarize the metabolic demands that are unique to neurons.

3. Be able to define the major elements of the cytoskeleton—microtubules, neurofilaments, and microfilaments—and summarize their function.

4. Be able to describe axoplasmic transport and provide some examples of phenomena that reflect normal and disrupted axoplasmic transport.

5. Be able to describe a chemical synapse.

## GENERAL STRUCTURE

There are approximately 100 billion neurons in the human CNS. Neurons come in a great variety of sizes and shapes, reflecting their various specializations of function (Fig. 3-1). However, all neurons share common structural elements (Fig. 3-2). The dendrites provide a vast expansion of the geographic and membrane area available for contact by other neurons. The membrane available for contact is typically even further expanded by the presence of large numbers of *dendritic spines*—small hairlike or bulbous excrescences of dendritic neural membrane. The output of the neuron is conveyed to other neurons, or to muscle and other effector cells, via the axon, which typically has many terminal branches. The proximal-most portion of the axon, the *initial segment*, is the region at which neural impulse (action potential) formation occurs. The initial segment arises from a slight outpouching of the neuronal cell body known as the *axon hillock*. In most circumstances, the axons (and sometimes dendrites) are encased in a multilayered lipid-laden envelope of myelin, which by virtue of its insulating properties vastly increases axonal conduction velocity (see Chapter 5). Axons terminate in *boutons*, buttonlike enlargements that form the proximal component of neural *synapses*. Synapses provide the major means by which a neuron elicits responses, through the release of chemical neurotransmitters, in target cells (see Chapter 4). In Figure 3-2, the target happens to be a muscle cell, the synapse is referred to as a neuromuscular junction, and the distal component of the synapse is referred to as the *motor end plate*.

## INTERNAL STRUCTURE

Most of the internal organelles of neurons are no different from those of cells throughout the body. Thus, neurons have nuclei (with prominent nucleoli), rough and smooth endoplasmic reticulum (ER), free ribosomes, Golgi apparatus, lysosomes, and mitochondria (Fig. 3-3). However, neurons also have some unique attributes that relate to their peculiar structure and the

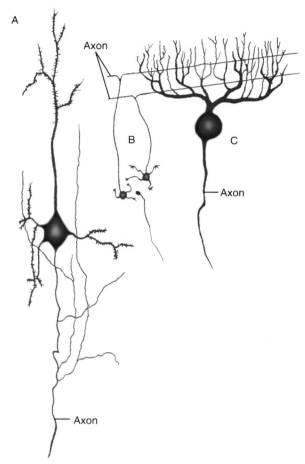

**Figure 3-1** Drawings of various types of neurons. *A,* Cortical pyramidal neuron. *B,* Cerebellar granule cells. *C,* Cerebellar Purkinje cell.

synthesized. The requirements for protein synthesis are reflected in an exceptional amount of free ribosomes and rough ER. These components stain prominently with certain basophilic dyes, an observation first made by Franz Nissl, hence the commonly used term "Nissl substance" to refer to this material.

In order to define and maintain their structure, cells throughout the body rely on a *cytoskeleton* composed of microtubules, intermediate filaments, and microfilaments. Because of the complex and highly extended structure of neurons, these cytoskeletal elements are particularly numerous. There is evidence from studies of the very large axons found in squids that axonal structure (and considerable function) can be maintained by the cytoskeleton even when the cell membrane is stripped off.

Microtubules are composed of 13 thick linear protofilaments aligned side by side to form a 25-nm diameter cylindrical structure. Neurofilaments, the special class of intermediate filaments found in the nervous system, comprise 24 thin protein filaments of the cytokeratin family that coil in a complex way to form a 10-nm diameter solid fibril. Neurofilaments characteristically have many short side arms. Microfilaments are 7-nm diameter fibers composed of two actin filaments twisted in a helix. Each of these three cytoskeletal elements comes in a variety of forms.

The cytoskeleton serves a number of purposes, including the definition and maintenance of gross neural morphology; the positioning of membrane proteins such as receptors and ion channels and the protein structures responsible for inserting them in the cell membrane and subsequently replacing them; the positioning of the protein structures involved in release of neurotransmitters; and the distribution of membrane-bound organelles within the cytoplasm. The cytoskeleton also provides the scaffold along which molecular motors transport protein and membrane bound vesicles within axons and dendrites. Microtubules are the structural correlate of the mitotic spindle and the functional core of cilia and flagella. All cytoskeletal elements are particularly crucial during maturational neural growth and neural repair after injury. Several human disorders have now been linked to dysfunctional cytoskeletal elements. Neurofibromatosis type 2, a disease characterized by the relentless formation of tumors of Schwann cell origin (the myelinating cells of nerves and nerve roots) within the cranial vault and spinal column, is caused by a mutation in a protein that regulates microfilament length and anchors microfilaments to other structures. Duchenne

very high levels of protein synthesis that they must maintain. A neuron 30 μm in diameter may support an axon up to a meter in length. If a neuronal cell body were the size of a house or apartment, its axon would be 200 km long. Axons contain as much as 10,000 times the cytoplasmic volume of the cell body. Thus, in a very real sense, the functional component of a neuron consists of its axonal and dendritic processes. The cell body merely serves as the factory needed to keep these extended neural processes in perfect structural and functional condition. Intermediate metabolism must be sustained at a brisk rate throughout the apparatus. Vast quantities of proteins must be synthesized constantly to maintain turnover of membrane proteins and maintenance of intracellular organelles. In many cases, large amounts of protein neurotransmitter must be

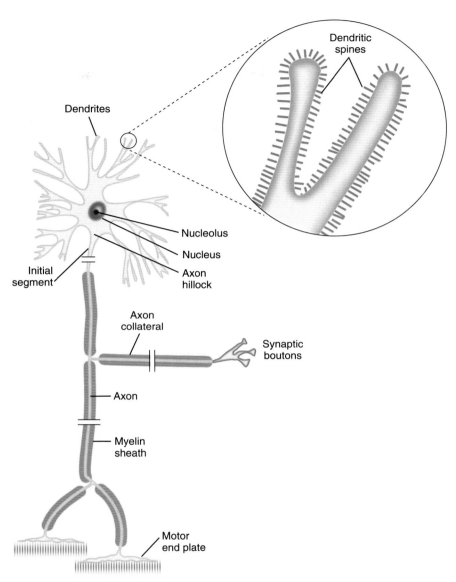

**Figure 3-2** Diagram of a generic neuron.

muscular dystrophy, an X-linked disease of muscles that is typically fatal within the second decade of life, is caused by a mutation in the gene for dystrophin, which appears to be critical for microfilament-mediated clustering of receptors in muscle. Disorders that may be related to impaired axoplasmic transport as a result of cytoskeletal dysfunction are discussed next.

## AXOPLASMIC TRANSPORT

*Axoplasmic transport*, the process of moving proteins and organelles along axons, is both anterograde (from

the cell body distally) and retrograde. Axoplasmic transport requires energy and depends on a local supply of adenosine triphosphate (ATP).

## Anterograde Axoplasmic Transport

There are two major types of anterograde axoplasmic transport: fast and slow. Fast transport occurs at rates of 50 to 500 mm per day. It primarily subserves the movement of membrane-bound intracellular organelles (e.g., synaptic vesicles, lysosomes, mitochondria).

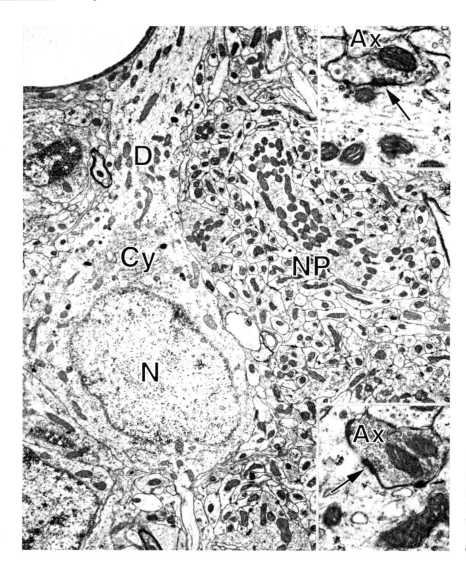

**Figure 3-3** Electron micrograph of a neuron. N = nucleus, Cy = cytoplasm, D = dendrite, NP = neuropil (axonal, dendritic, and glial) processes; *insets,* Ax = axon terminals (synaptic densities indicated by *arrows*).

Movement is achieved by repeated binding and release of these organelles to successive points along microtubules via a molecular motor composed of proteins of the kinesin class. Slow axoplasmic transport achieves movement rates of 0.1 to 10 mm per day. It primarily subserves the movement of proteins (including cytoskeletal proteins). The regrowth of axons after injury occurs at a rate of approximately 1 mm per day, suggesting that it is limited by slow axoplasmic transport. Slow axoplasmic transport is severely disrupted by drugs such as vinca alkaloids (vincristine, vinblastin), which are toxic to microtubules, as illustrated in Case 3-1.

There is circumstantial evidence that suggests the enormous demands made upon neurons to maintain the structural and functional integrity of axons and

### Case 3-1

**Vincristine Neurotoxicity**
*A 35-year-old woman with Hodgkin's disease (a cancer involving lymphocytes) receives a multidrug chemotherapy regimen that includes vincristine. Her cancer goes into remission, but she subsequently notes loss of feeling in her feet.*

**Comment:** *Selective damage to large axons, as a result of disruption of microtubule-facilitated axonal transport, has permanently damaged peripheral nerves, including those supporting sensation. Because the requirements for axonal transport are greatest in the longest axons, the most distal portions of the body (the feet and distal legs) are most severely affected.*

## Case 3-2

### Alzheimer's Disease

*A 70-year-old woman experiences progressive impairment in her ability to remember new things, difficulty expressing herself, loss of motor skills (once a gifted cook, she now cannot be allowed to work in the kitchen because of her hazardous misuse of utensils), and a tendency to get lost. On examination, 3 minutes after being given the names of three objects to remember, she can recall none. Her language is lacking in detail and substance. When asked why she is in the clinic, she responds "Well, I have been having a lot of trouble with things. I can't seem to get it. We go there and then, I can't. All these things. My daughter says that's what it is." She makes major errors in copying simple drawings. However, she exhibits a warm and engaging personality. The remainder of her neurologic examination is normal.*

**Comment:** *This picture presents the classic profile of cognitive impairment in Alzheimer's disease, and it reflects the function of both those portions of the cerebral cortex that are damaged most severely, and those that are relatively spared by this disease. Although much has been made of certain histologic features of Alzheimer's disease (e.g., neuritic plaques, neurofibrillary tangles), the cognitive impairment associated with this disease results predominantly from the loss of axonal and dendritic processes. A normal cortical neuron might be likened to a live oak tree, the cell body corresponding to the short trunk, and the dendritic arborization corresponding to the huge canopy of branches. Using this analogy, in Alzheimer's disease, a cortical neuron may be likened to a live oak after an overzealous municipal electrical utility worker has finished trimming it to free power lines. Axonal and dendritic arborizations are often reduced to jagged stumps. The precise mechanism of this selective destruction of axons and dendrites has not yet been determined. It could reflect a specific defect in axoplasmic transport. Tau, which is one of the proteins that prevents the depolymerization of microtubules, is heavily and pathologically phosphorylated in Alzheimer's disease. Many neurons are filled with polymerized tau aggregates known as neurofibrillary tangles (Fig. 3-4). There is a group of rare, inherited, dementing disorders that occur as a result of single point polymorphisms involving tau protein, the gene for which is located on chromosome 17. The selective destruction of axons and dendrites could also reflect the inability of a diseased neuron to maintain adequate protein synthesis to support the entire extended axodendritic array (see Case 3-3).*

dendrites through protein synthesis and axoplasmic transport may exceed neuronal capacity in the face of disease. Cases 3-2 and 3-3 are exemplary.

The complete dependence of axons in both the CNS and the peripheral nervous system (PNS) on a constant supply of proteins and organelles from the neural cell body is perhaps best illustrated by *Wallerian degeneration*, named after Augustus Wall, who first described the phenomenon in the middle of the 19th century. Wallerian degeneration refers to the process an axon undergoes after it has been severed at some point from the cell body (axotomy). In the distal segment, immediate cessation of transmission is followed by gradual degradation of the axon and its enveloping myelin sheath, and ultimately, removal of all remnants by phagocytic cells (microglia in the CNS, macrophages and Schwann cells in the PNS) (Fig. 3-5).

Axotomy also has an impact on the affected neuron, most likely because it results in loss of retrograde axoplasmic transport of trophic factors. With

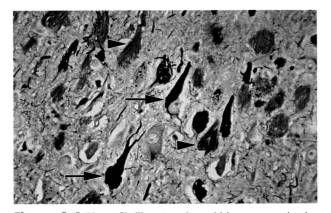

**Figure 3-4** Neurofibrillary tangles within neurons in the cortex of a patient with Alzheimer's disease. In neurons slightly out of the plane of section, the cytoplasm is completely opacified by dark-staining neurofibrillary material (*arrows*). In neurons that have actually been sectioned, individual spicular tangles can be discerned (*arrowheads*). (Ubiquitin, ×250)

Neurohistology

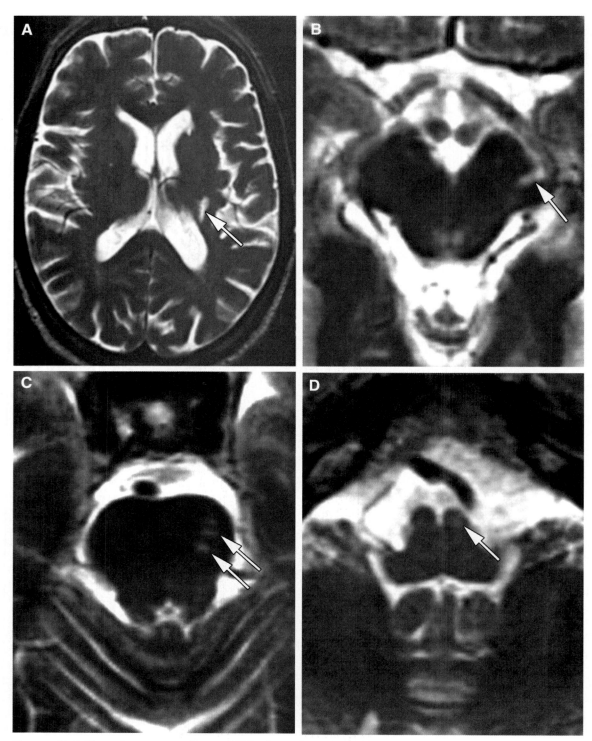

**Figure 3-5** Magnetic resonance image (MRI) of a patient who has experienced a lacunar infarction involving axons of cortical neurons projecting to the brainstem and spinal cord as they pass through the corona radiata and the posterior limb of the internal capsule (*A*). The arrows show where ischemic damage to these axons has resulted in Wallerian degeneration that is visible in the cerebral peduncle (*B*), the basis pontis (*C*), and very subtly, in the medullary pyramid (*D*).

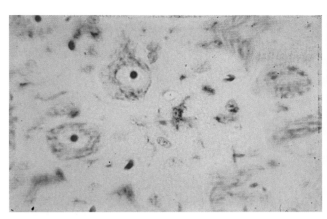 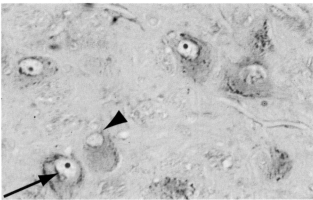

**Figure 3-6** Normal neurons (*left*) and chromatolytic neurons (*right*). Note rearrangement of Nissl substance (*arrow*) and swelling of the cell body with displacement of the nucleus (*arrowhead*) in chromatolytic neurons. (Nissl, ×250)

### Case 3-3

**Late Progression of Poliomyelitis**

*A 55-year-old man experienced poliomyelitis as a child. He was left with substantial weakness of his legs but was able to ambulate quite well with the aid of crutches. He now complains of progressive weakness and cramping in his legs and he fears he soon will no longer be able to walk.*

**Comment:** *In genetically susceptible individuals, poliovirus binds to, infects, and ultimately destroys anterior horn cells in the spinal cord. These cells are the large neurons in the ventral horn of the cord that innervate muscles. As some anterior horn cells die, surviving anterior horn cells sprout new branches that grow and reinnervate denervated muscle fibers. This regrowth provides the basis for recovery of function after poliovirus infection. However, it also results in the remaining anterior horn cells having an unusually large number of axonal branches. Consequently, unusually high demands are made upon these neurons. We currently believe that, with aging, progressively more of these neurons are no longer able to meet this demand, resulting in death of the neurons or loss of axonal processes, further denervation of muscle, and progressive weakness.*

axotomy, most neurons exhibit a chromatolytic reaction: the cell body swells, the nucleus moves to an eccentric location, and the rough endoplasmic reticulum (Nissl substance) fragments (Fig. 3-6). Later, the neuron may shrink somewhat, and the nucleus and cytoplasm may stain more intensely with hematoxylin and eosin. Some neurons will die after axotomy.

### Retrograde Axoplasmic Transport

A retrograde transport mechanism mediates the transfer of substances providing trophic support for the neuron (e.g., nerve growth factors) from the axon terminal to the cell body. Retrograde transport also subserves the routine processes of cell maintenance by returning proteins and lipids to the cell body for reuse or degradation, and transporting endosomes and mitochondria back to the cell body. Unfortunately, the retrograde transport mechanism also proves the means by which herpes, polio, and rabies viruses and tetanus toxin are carried from the periphery into the CNS.[1]

## NEURAL SYNAPSES

Neurons communicate with each other through two types of synapses: electrical and chemical. Electrical synapses are plentiful in invertebrates, but their role in mammals, to the extent that we understand it, appears

[1]The existence of a retrograde transport mechanism has been an enormous boon to neuroscientists studying neural connectivity. When horseradish peroxidase or any of a number of other proteins is injected into a particular locus within the CNS, it is taken up by axonal endings and transported retrogradely to the cell bodies. With appropriate histochemical staining, the entire pathway from cell body to axonal termination can then be delineated.

Neurohistology

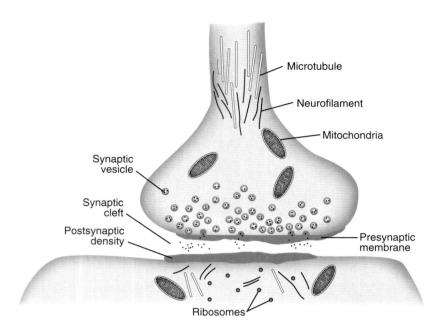

Figure 3-7 A neural synapse.

to be relatively limited.[2] Our focus will therefore be on chemical synapses. At a chemical synapse, neurotransmitter is released at the presynaptic terminal and binds to the postsynaptic terminal where it elicits a response in the postsynaptic neuron or effector cell (e.g., a muscle cell).

A chemical synapse is defined by pre- and postsynaptic regions of thickening of the synaptic membrane that define a distinct intercellular synaptic cleft 20 to 40 nm wide (Fig. 3-7). The thickening of the presynaptic membrane reflects its specialization for neurotransmitter release, whereas the thickening of the postsynaptic membrane reflects the insertion in the membrane of large numbers of neurotransmitter receptor molecules. On the presynaptic side, large numbers of synaptic vesicles can be seen, as well as mitochondria, reflecting the energy intensive process of neurotransmitter release and, in some synapses, neurotransmitter uptake or synthesis.

Synapses are predominantly between the terminal boutons of axons and dendritic spines (axo-dendritic), but they may be axo-somatic, axo-axonic, or even dendro-dendritic. We will have considerably more to say about chemical synapses in Chapter 4.

---

[2]There is good evidence that the function of neurons in the locus ceruleus is critically dependent on electrical synapses. This pigmented nucleus is located in the lateral pontine tegmentum and is the source of norepinephrine for nearly the entire brain.

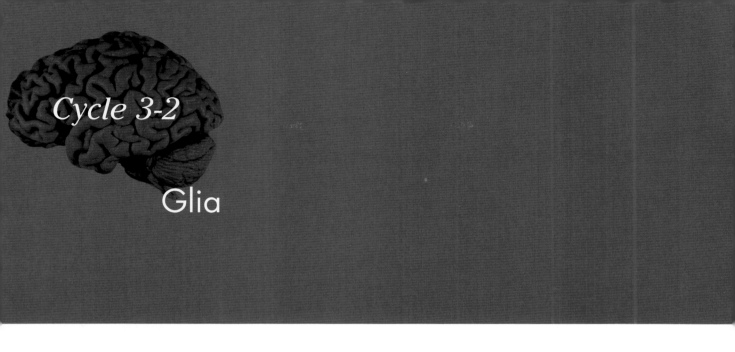

# Cycle 3-2

## Glia

### Objective

Be able to briefly describe the major functions of astrocytes, oligodendrocytes, Schwann cells, ependymal cells, and microglia.

Glia constitute at least 90 percent of all cells in the CNS (Fig. 3-8). Macroglia, which include *astrocytes*, *oligodendrocytes*, and *ependymal cells*, are of ectodermal origin. *Microglia*, the macrophages of the CNS, are of mesodermal origin. Glial cells differ from neurons in that (1) they do not form synapses; (2) they have only one type of process; (3) they retain the ability to divide throughout their life span; and (4) they are electrically inexcitable.

## ASTROCYTES

Astrocytes perform two major functions within the CNS. They provide the structural matrix in which neurons reside, and they play a major homeostatic role in maintaining the environment of neurons.

Neurons in the cerebral cortex are heavily admixed with astrocytes (Fig. 3-9). The astrocytes and their processes, in conjunction with neuropil—axons and dendrites—compose the sea in which the neuronal cell bodies reside. Terminal enlargements of the processes of some astrocytes—foot processes—abut

blood vessels and thereby form a component of the *blood-brain barrier* (Figs. 3-10, 3-11) (see also Division II). The other components include the vascular basement membrane and vascular endothelial cells, which in the CNS uniquely form tight junctions with each other. Astrocytes are responsible for inducing and maintaining these tight endothelial junctions. Astrocytic foot processes also form a continuous sheet beneath the pia known as the glia limitans.

Astrocytes also play a major homeostatic role in maintaining the ionic and molecular environment of neurons. They regulate the extracellular potassium concentration. They are involved in the reuptake of certain neurotransmitters, most notably peptide neurotransmitters and glutamate. Glutamate may be neurotoxic if allowed to accumulate in excessive concentrations. They produce a large number of neurotrophic substances known as growth factors. These factors play a major role in the proliferation, migration, and differentiation of neurons and the guidance of axonal and dendritic growth in early life. They may be vital to the survival of injured neurons, the proliferation of new neurons, and for the general capacity for adaptive responses to injury (neural plasticity) later in life. Astrocytes may to some degree insulate electrically active elements such as axons and synapses, thereby preventing cross talk. They also act to insulate neurons from pathologic processes.

Almost any insult to the CNS will elicit astrogliosis—astrocytic hypertrophy and proliferation of astrocytic processes. One of the most extreme forms of

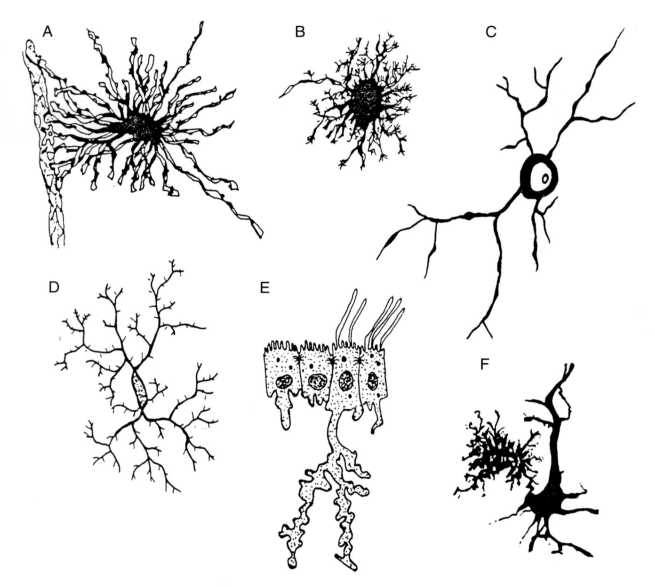

**Figure 3-8** Drawings of various types of glial cells. *A*, Fibrous astrocyte. *B*, Protoplasmic astrocyte. *C*, Oligodendrocyte. *D*, Microglial cell. *E*, Ependymal cells. *F*, A fibrous astrocyte (*left*) next to a neuron.

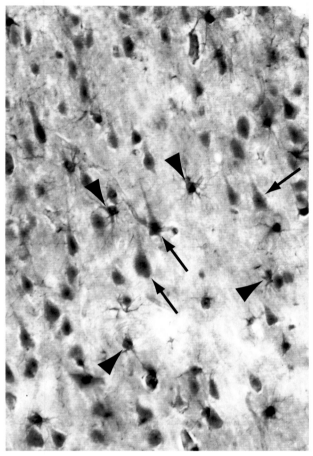

**Figure 3-9** Cerebral cortex. Note neurons (*arrows*), and astrocytes (*arrowheads*). (Rio-Ortega silver stain, ×320)

nerve roots and peripheral nerves. These cells wrap axons and some large dendrites in concentric layers of cell membrane (Figs. 3-12, 3-13). Besides the phospholipids of the closely opposed cell membranes, myelin contains cholesterol and other complex lipids (cerebrosides), as well as a number of proteins, the most clinically important being myelin basic protein.

Myelination is segmental: long continuous stretches of myelin are interrupted by narrow gaps or *nodes of Ranvier*, where the axon is relatively bare. Myelin facilitates axonal conduction; nodes of Ranvier play a particularly important role in this process (see Chapter 5). A single oligodendrocyte may contribute to the myelination of 50 or more adjacent nerve processes. Unlike oligodendrocytes, Schwann cells also appear to share most of the capacities of astrocytes, they are responsible for secretion of the extracellular matrix in dorsal root ganglia and peripheral nerves, and under conditions of inflammation or injury, they can become phagocytes.

## EPENDYMAL CELLS

Ependymal cells line the ventricles of the brain and the central canal of the spinal cord (Fig. 3-14). The ventricular surface is covered with cilia, which are involved in the circulation of cerebrospinal fluid. Specialized ependymal cells form the choroid plexus of the lateral, third, and fourth ventricles. The choroid plexus manufactures cerebrospinal fluid.

## MICROGLIA

Microglia populate the developing nervous system during embryonic and fetal development. They arise from primitive precursor cells called fetal macrophages. In the adult CNS, microglial cells are distributed throughout all brain regions and are quite numerous: there are about as many microglia as there are neurons. Following injury to neural tissue, microglia migrate to and multiply at the site of injury, where they may become brain macrophages if neural cell death occurs (Fig. 3-15). Thus, microglia are the primary source of endogenous brain macrophages responsible for clearing out debris after injury. Microglia, like peripheral macrophages, also mediate immunologic responses
*Text continued on page 135*

astrogliosis is seen in the dramatic astrocytic reaction to parenchymal bacterial infection, in which astrogliosis serves to effectively form a wall around the cerebral abscess. Unfortunately, this phenomenon can also be detrimental. Astrogliosis at a site of injury may impede the regrowth of axons through the site. This appears to be a major factor in limiting axonal regeneration after CNS injury.

## MYELIN-FORMING CELLS: OLIGODENDROCYTES AND SCHWANN CELLS

Oligodendrocytes form and maintain myelin in the CNS. *Schwann cells* perform the same function for

Neurohistology

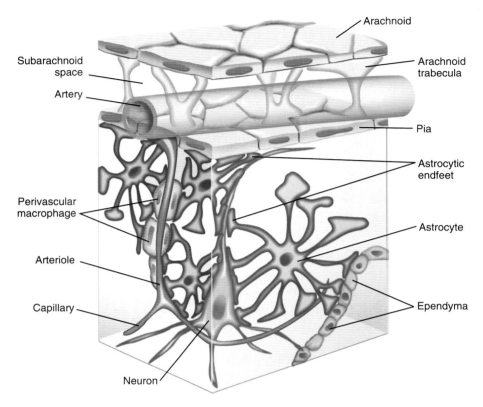

Arachnoid

Subarachnoid space

Artery

Arachnoid trabecula

Pia

Astrocytic endfeet

Perivascular macrophage

Astrocyte

Arteriole

Capillary

Ependyma

Neuron

**Figure 3-10** Illustration of the relationships of glia to surfaces of the CNS and to vascular and neuronal elements. Note the coating of the pial surface, blood vessels, ependyma, and neurons by astrocytic foot processes.

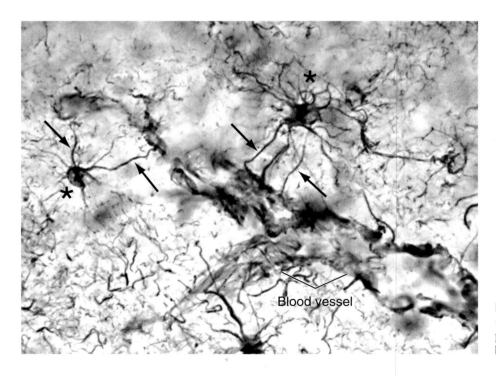

Blood vessel

**Figure 3-11** Astrocytes (*asterisks*) extending multiple processes (*arrows*) to abut a blood vessel. (GFAP, ×700)

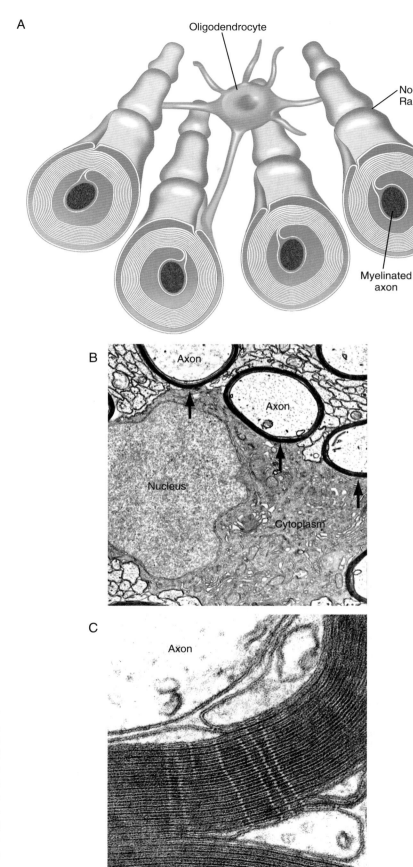

A, Oligodendrocyte; Node of Ranvier; Myelinated axon; Myelin sheath

B, Axon; Axon; Nucleus; Cytoplasm

C, Axon

**Figure 3-12** *A,* Oligodendrocyte wrapping axons in myelin. Several nodes of Ranvier are evident. *B,* Electron micrograph of a cross section through myelinated axons demonstrating the many dark-staining myelin lamellae (*arrows*) as well as an adjacent oligodendrocyte (nucleus and cytoplasm); *C,* Higher magnification view of myelin lamellae around an axon.

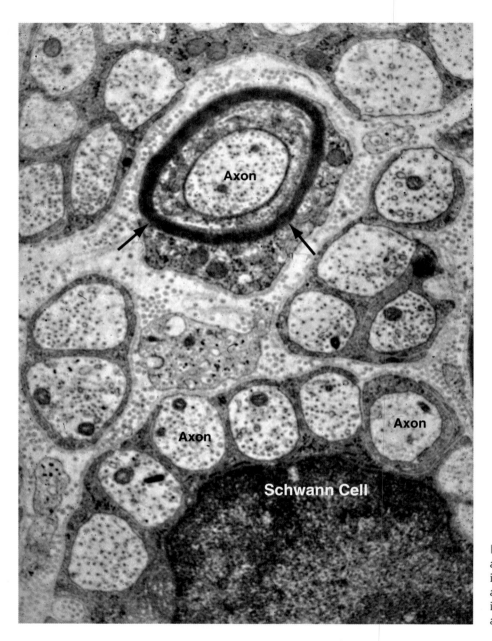

**Figure 3-13** Cross section of a peripheral nerve demonstrating myelinated axons (*arrows*) and a Schwann cell enveloping a number of unmyelinated axons.

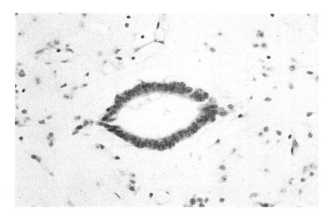

**Figure 3-14** Ependymal cells surrounding a portion of the ventricular system. (Nissl, ×220)

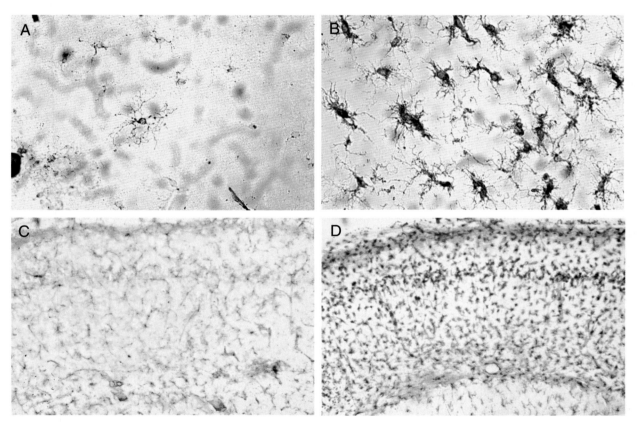

**Figure 3-15** *A,* Quiescent microglia. *B,* Activated microglia. *C,* Microglia in normal cerebral cortex. *D,* Microglia in cortex 4 days after a period of ischemia (an early infarct). (*A, B,* LN-3, ×200; *C, D,* GS-1 B4 isolectin, ×50)

to injury or infection, and like macrophages, they are capable of antigen presentation. They have been referred to as the brain's immune system. In some pathologic conditions, microglial cells become targets themselves; for example, the human immunodeficiency virus (HIV), which infects lymphocytes peripherally, also infects microglia in the CNS, rendering these cells dysfunctional.

**Neurohistology**

# Cycle 3-3

## Stem Cells

### Objectives

1. Be able to list the major loci of stem cells in the adult CNS.
2. Be able to describe two normal brain functions that appear to rely on a continuous supply of new neurons.
3. Be able to describe the impact of brain injury or degeneration on neural precursor cells and briefly summarize the mechanisms involved.

Until recently, it was accepted dogma that the adult mammalian brain did not contain any cells capable of dividing and generating new neurons. It is now known, however, that neuronal precursor cells do exist in the subependymal zone of the ventricular system throughout its extent, from the lateral ventricles of the telencephalon to the caudal reaches of the central canal in the spinal cord, in the dentate gyrus of the hippocampal formation, and likely in scattered clusters throughout the neural parenchyma. The subependymal zone of the telencephalon is the region in which, during embryogenesis, all cortical neurons originate and differentiate. It appears that at least some of the cells in the adult subependymal zone are indeed pluripotent stem cells, capable of differentiating into any cell type within the body. Clearly they are capable of differentiating into neurons, astrocytes, and oligodendrocytes, and furthermore, cells that have a neuronal fate can

further differentiate, depending upon the specific environment, into neural types specific to any particular region of the CNS.

During embryogenesis, and likely in the adult brain, the proliferation, differentiation, migration, and morphologic development of cellular precursors in general and neuronal precursors in particular is dependent upon a temporally evolving interaction between endogenous cellular processes and exogenous time- and location-dependent molecular signals. Exogenous molecular signals include a host of growth factors, signaling molecules, hormones, and extracellular matrix adhesion molecules. At any one time in the state of maturation, proliferation, differentiation, and migration of a precursor cell, it is susceptible to the influence of a specific set of exogenous signals. If these signals are present, generally in one of a variety of complex combinations, then the precursor will respond with a specific measure of proliferation, differentiation, movement, or morphologic alteration. As these changes occur, the precursor will become unresponsive to certain exogenous signals, responsive to new ones, and some opportunities for proliferation, differentiation, migration, and morphologic change will be lost, seemingly permanently. Thus, both the state and the future possibilities of a precursor cell evolve over time, and the manner in which they evolve depends upon the location of the precursor cell within the nervous system. The term "stem cell" is usually reserved for undifferentiated cells that have the capacity for asymmetric division resulting in two daughters, one identical and one more differentiated. It may be pluripotent, that is, capable of giving rise to any cell type in the body, or its parenting possibilities may be more limited. Although pluripotent stem cells have been identified in the adult CNS, it is more precise to refer to cells in the brain capable of division and further differentiation as precursor cells.

At present in this very rapidly advancing field, it appears that neural precursor cells in the adult CNS are involved in two separate processes: one occurs in normal brain, and one evolves only in response to injury. Precursor cells in the subependymal zone of the lateral ventricles migrate to the olfactory bulb, where they apparently contribute to the routine turnover of granule cells as part of the normal process of olfactory function. Neural precursors in the dentate gyrus of the hippocampal formation apparently contribute in an essential way, by virtue of the connections that their progeny form, to the ongoing process of encoding new fact memories.

Injury to the brain, most clearly that leading to programmed cell death (apoptosis), leads to the generation of a complex time- and location-specific series of signaling molecules that regulate proliferation, migration, and differentiation of neural precursors, as well as the extension of their axons and dendrites to remote and appropriate locations. To what extent this process contributes to recovery from injury, to what extent it is capable of re-forming complex cytoarchitectonic arrangements (e.g., the six layers of the cerebral cortex), to what extent it can be manipulated to enhance recovery from injury or to mitigate degenerative disease, and to what extent neural precursor cells can be transplanted into specific regions of the brain to further aid recovery are all unknown and the subjects of intense research.

Neurohistology

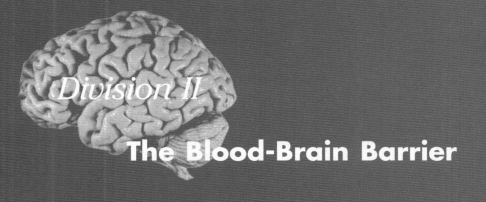

# Division II

# The Blood-Brain Barrier

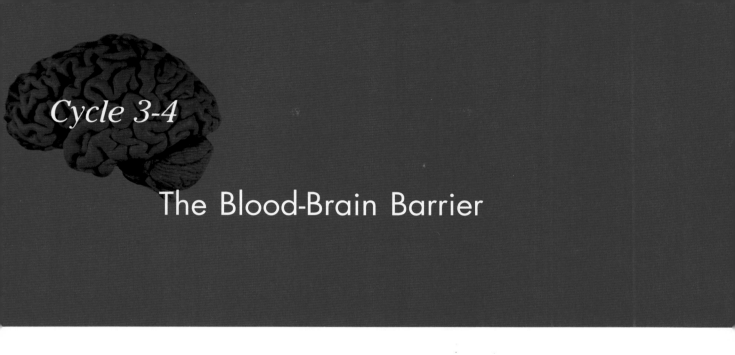

# Cycle 3-4

# The Blood-Brain Barrier

## Objectives

1. Be able to list the major components of the blood-brain barrier.

2. Be able to describe briefly the function of the blood-brain barrier and to provide experimental and clinical examples of blood-brain barrier effects.

3. Be able to list the "windows" in the blood-brain barrier.

4. Be able to describe briefly some clinical phenomena that reflect breakdown of the blood-brain barrier.

The blood-brain barrier (BBB) comprises three components characteristic of vasculature throughout the body: (1) a vascular basement membrane; (2) vascular endothelial cells; and (3) perivascular macrophages. It also exhibits three characteristics unique to the CNS: (1) tight junctions between vascular endothelial cells; (2) the coating of blood vessels and the pial surface of the brain by a syncytium of astrocytic foot processes; and (3) a complete absence of fluid-phase endocytosis and highly restricted receptor-mediated endocytosis (Fig. 3-16).

The BBB substantially isolates the CNS from the molecular and cellular constituents of the blood. Thus, as shown nearly a century ago by the German physiologist Paul Ehrlich, following the systemic injection of a vital dye such as Prussian blue, organs throughout the body are stained but not most of the CNS. Staining is observed in the choroid plexus and meninges, but there is no evidence of dye in the cerebrospinal fluid. However, if dye is injected directly into the CSF (intrathecal injection), the brain will be stained, indicating that the endothelial tight junctions and vascular basement membrane in the choroid plexus and meninges are responsible for excluding it. The relative isolation provided by the BBB is dramatically demonstrated by the normal composition of cerebrospinal fluid: a white blood cell count of ≤5/cu mm, no red blood cells, and a protein concentration of <45 mg/dL (compared with 6 to 8 g/dL in the blood).

There are four selective natural "windows" in the BBB:

1. Circumventricular organs (CVOs) (see Chapter 11) are regions of the brain characterized by particularly high vascularity and gaps between endothelial cells. This arrangement allows relatively free passage of large protein molecules into and out of these regions. The most important CVOs are in the general vicinity of the hypothalamus and pituitary gland. They permit the secretion of hypothalamic and pituitary hormones into the blood stream, and they allow exposure of hypothalamic and pituitary neurons to neuroendocrine proteins generated in response to the hypothalamic and pituitary signals.

2. There is a limited capacity for receptor-mediated endocytosis, for example, of insulin and leptin (a

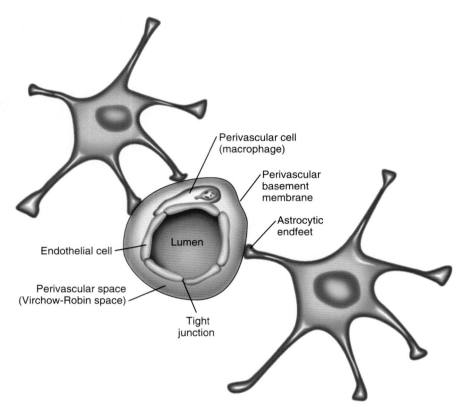

Perivascular cell
(macrophage)

Perivascular
basement
membrane

Astrocytic
endfeet

Endothelial cell

Lumen

Perivascular space
(Virchow-Robin space)

Tight
junction

**Figure 3-16** Structural components of the blood-brain barrier. The Virchow-Robin space is filled with cerebrospinal fluid.

hormone generated by adipocytes that is critical to regulation of body mass).

3. Lipid-soluble substances, such as corticosteroids, estrogen and testosterone, and certain drugs are capable of passing relatively freely into the CNS.

4. Active transport mechanisms exist for certain substances, most notably selected amino acids and glucose. The glucose transporter normally serves to maintain a cerebrospinal fluid glucose concentration that is about two thirds that of the blood glucose concentration.

The BBB can be broken down by infection as in viral, bacterial, or fungal invasion of the meninges (meningitis). The extent to which the breakdown contributes to the manifestations of these infections is unclear, but it is of some value in that it facilitates the passage of lipid-insoluble antibiotics into the CNS. Damage to the glucose transporter of the BBB by inflammation of the meninges or by infiltration of the meninges by cancer cells (meningeal carcinomatosis) often results in reduced cerebrospinal fluid glucose concentrations. The BBB is incomplete in many brain tumors (most notably there are gap junctions between the endothelial cells of the vasculature within these tumors). This fact is used to advantage in neuroimaging studies: iodine-containing compounds (in CT studies) and gadolinium (in MRI studies) pass across the faulty BBB in the tumors, causing them to have increased signal (appear white) on images. The same phenomenon occurs when the BBB is damaged, as in stroke. This feature will be apparent in many of the images reproduced in this text (see Figs. 2-23, 8-37).

# Cellular Organization of the Nervous System

Every region of the brain and spinal cord has its own distinctive cellular organization or cytoarchitecture. Although our understanding of the multicellular basis of neurologic function is limited, it is clear that these variations in cytoarchitecture are intimately related to the precise nature of the functions that neural structures and regions of the cerebral cortex perform. Our discussion will be limited to the most important structures.

# Brain (Cerebral Cortex, Hippocampus, and Cerebellum)

1. Be able to describe briefly the general cytoarchitectonic organization of the cerebral cortex and to indicate the particular roles of neurons in layers 3, 4, and 5.

2. Be able to distinguish between a projection neuron and an interneuron.

3. Be able to describe briefly the cytoarchitectonic structure of the hippocampus.

4. Be able to describe briefly the cytoarchitectonic structure of the cerebellum.

5. Be able to discuss how the hippocampus and cerebellum might fulfill their functions despite a far simpler structure than the cerebral cortex.

## CEREBRAL CORTEX

The cerebral cortex is uniformly composed of *six layers of neurons* (Figs. 3-17, 3-18, and 3-19). Variations in the thickness and cellular morphology of these layers provide the basis for the delineation of Brodmann's areas. Layers III and V, the outer and inner *pyramidal cell layers* (so-named because of the characteristic shape of the neurons in them), contain the majority of neurons that project long axons to other regions of the nervous system. The axons of *projection neurons* in layer III terminate on neurons in other regions of the

ipsilateral cerebral hemisphere. They also traverse the major commissures (mainly the corpus callosum and the anterior commissure) to terminate on neurons in the opposite hemisphere. The axons of projection neurons in layer V terminate on neurons in structures outside the cerebral cortex. These areas include subcortical cerebral structures, such as the basal ganglia and the thalamus, the brainstem, and the spinal cord.

The neurons of layer IV, the inner granular layer, comprise the major targets of afferent thalamocortical fibers. In regions of the brain, such as the calcarine cortex in the occipital lobes (subserving vision), the number of afferent fibers (from the lateral geniculate nuclei) is so large, and layer IV is so thick, that it is visible to the unaided eye. In other regions of the brain that are involved primarily in higher neural functions, such as the prefrontal cortex, there are far fewer afferent fibers, and layer IV is so thin that this cortex is sometimes referred to as "agranular."

The neurons in the cerebral cortex, as in many other portions of the nervous system, can be roughly grouped into two classes—projection neurons and *interneurons*. Projection neurons often have extensive dendritic arborizations that expose them to much of the information processing going on in their region of the brain, and they have the large cell bodies needed to support long axons. The pyramidal neurons of cortical layers III and V (Figs. 3-17, 3-18, 3-19) and the Purkinje cells of the cerebellar cortex (see later discussion) are exemplary. Interneurons, by contrast, typically have much smaller dendritic arborizations, a short axon that

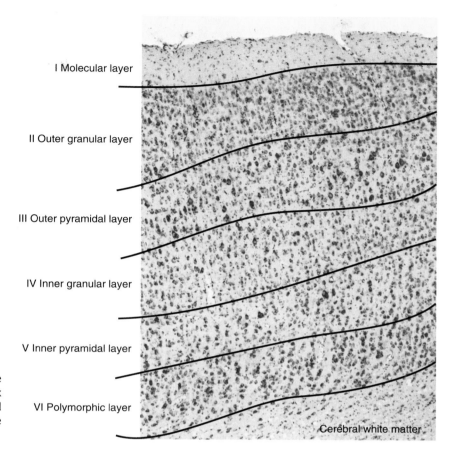

I Molecular layer

II Outer granular layer

III Outer pyramidal layer

IV Inner granular layer

V Inner pyramidal layer

VI Polymorphic layer

Cerebral white matter

**Figure 3-17** Micrograph of the cerebral cortex, demonstrating the six layers. The pial surface is at the top and the deep cerebral white matter is at the bottom. (Nissl, ×35)

projects locally, and a correspondingly small cell body. They go by a variety of names that reflect their particular cellular morphology. Projection neurons are involved in the local dynamics of neural information processing to varying degrees. In some cases, such as the caudate nucleus and putamen, the projection neurons, which make up 90 to 95 percent of the neurons in these structures, are also almost entirely responsible for information processing. Interneurons, however, are exclusively involved in local information processing. All layers of the cerebral cortex contain abundant glia and blood vessels.

## HIPPOCAMPUS

The cytoarchitecture of the hippocampus is demonstrated in Figures 3-20 and 3-21. This spectacular structure provides one of the best illustrations (together with the cerebellum) of the concept that cytoarchitecture

and function are intimately related. What is immediately apparent is that the structure of the hippocampus is vastly simpler than that of the cerebral cortex (though by no means simple in absolute terms!). This corresponds to the fact that the hippocampus, unlike the cerebral cortex, is involved in one single, unchanging function throughout the life span—encoding new memories of facts. The cells of the dentate, through their connections with overlying parahippocampal cortex, perform a single function: extracting nonoverlapping knowledge representations that represent the mathematical essence of very complex, detailed, and highly overlapping knowledge representations in the cerebral cortex. These mathematical distillations are then passed on to the pyramidal cells of the hippocampus proper. These pyramidal cells also have but a single function—to almost instantaneously form synapses (the process actually takes about 1 second) that will link (via a very long loop through the hippocampus) neurons in the cerebral cortex, thereby

Neurohistology

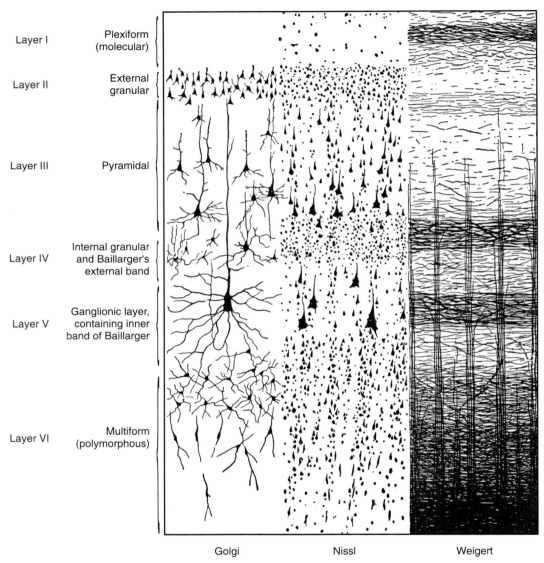

| Layer I | Plexiform (molecular) | | | |
| Layer II | External granular | | | |
| Layer III | Pyramidal | | | |
| Layer IV | Internal granular and Baillarger's external band | | | |
| Layer V | Ganglionic layer, containing inner band of Baillarger | | | |
| Layer VI | Multiform (polymorphous) | Golgi | Nissl | Weigert |

**Figure 3-18** Diagram of the cerebral cortex as revealed by various staining techniques: a Golgi silver stain, which demonstrates cell bodies, axons, and dendrites (*left*); a Nissl stain (e.g., cresyl violet), which primarily reveals cell bodies (*middle*); and a nerve fiber stain (*right*). As in Figure 3-17, the pial surface is at the top and the deep cerebral white matter is at the bottom. (After Brodmann.)

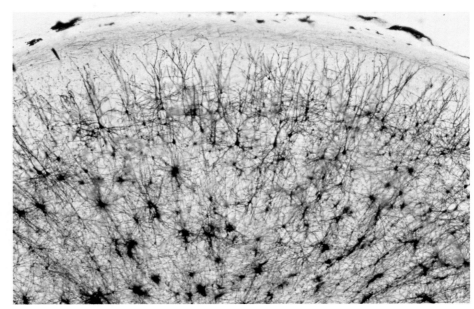

**Figure 3-19** Neurons and their processes in superficial layers of the cerebral cortex (Golgi stain). For poorly understood reasons, the silver impregnation methods of the Golgi stain label less than 1 percent of neurons. (×35)

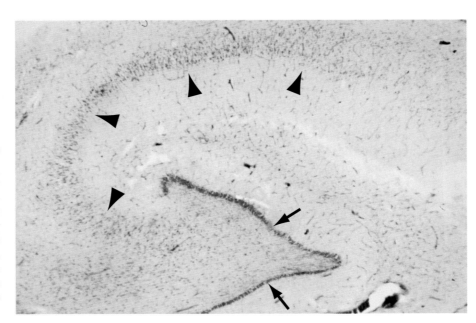

**Figure 3-20** A Nissl stain of the hippocampus, illustrating the relationship of the dentate gyrus (*arrows*) to the pyramidal neurons (*arrowheads*) of the hippocampus proper. The temporal horn of the lateral ventricle is immediately to the right, and the hippocampus is contiguous with cortex comprising the parahippocampal gyrus on the left. (×20)

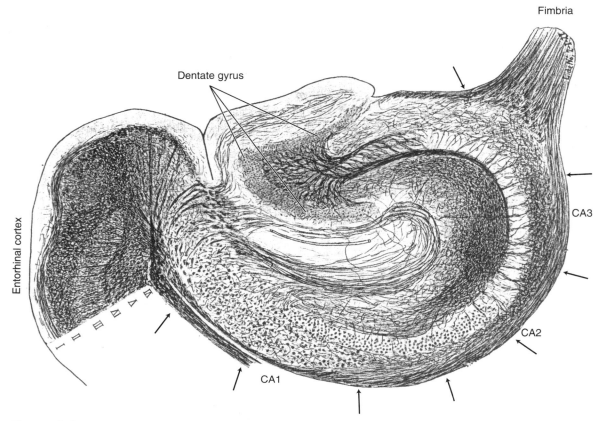

**Figure 3-21** Drawing from a silver stain of a horizontal section through the hippocampal formation of an adult mouse demonstrating the complex, but precisely organized neural fiber structure. Arrows delineate the actual hippocampus. The fimbria has a different spatial relationship to the hippocampus in the mouse. (Modified from Lorente de Nó R. Studies on the structure of the cerebral cortex. II. Continuation of the study of the ammonic system. J Psychol Neurol 46:113-177, 1934.)

establishing new fact knowledge. In the brain, the knowledge is in the connections. This single and unchanging function of the hippocampus can be contrasted with the function of the cerebral cortex, which differs from region to region, must constantly adapt to environmental circumstances, and changes throughout the life span—hence its far more complex structure. The consequences of loss of hippocampal function are illustrated in Case 3-4 (see page 147).

## CEREBELLUM

The cerebellar cortex consists of three layers: the granule cell layer, the Purkinje cell layer, and the molecular layer (Figs. 3-22, 3-23, 3-24). As with the hippocampus, its structure reflects its function. The function of the cerebellum is to define the space-time envelope of muscle contractions underlying

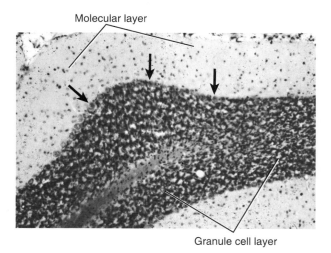

**Figure 3-22** Micrograph of the cerebellar cortex demonstrating the densely packed granule cells, Purkinje cells (*arrows*), and the much less cellular molecular layer. (Klüver-Barrera stain, ×45)

## Case 3-4

### Anterograde and Retrograde Amnesia due to Hippocampal Damage

*A 25-year-old man is found in bed, comatose, and brought to the emergency room. It is quickly determined that he has experienced carbon monoxide poisoning due to a poorly vented kerosene heater. He undergoes treatment with hyperbaric oxygen (breathing oxygen at an elevated pressure). He recovers consciousness, and ultimately regains most higher neural functions. However, he is permanently impaired in his ability to learn new facts and he has lost much of his memory of his personal life. He greets all his physicians as perfect strangers, even though he has seen them innumerable times. Automobiles manufactured over the last few years appear strange to him. He knows he is married, and he knows his wife's name, but he recalls nothing of the birth of his two children, and seems repeatedly surprised to learn that he even has children.*

**Comment:** *Carbon monoxide has a higher affinity for hemoglobin than does oxygen. Thus, with prolonged exposure to high concentrations (e.g., 1000 ppm), oxygen is displaced from a substantial portion of hemoglobin to the point that oxygen delivery to the CNS becomes inadequate to support cellular metabolism. The hippocampus is particularly susceptible to anoxic insults. The patient in this case has lost most of his hippocampal pyramidal neurons. Thus, he is severely impaired in his ability to acquire new pieces of information, and the connections representing his recall of many past facts, particularly autobiographic memories, have been destroyed.*

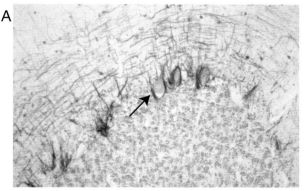

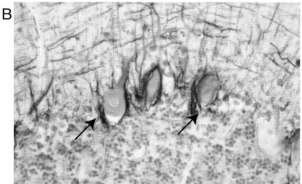

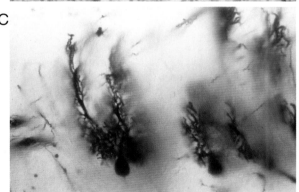

**Figure 3-23** The cerebellar cortex as seen with a neurofilament stain. In *A* and *B*, a few Purkinje cells are visible (*arrow*) extending their dendrites up into the molecular layer, where many parallel fibers arising from granule cells are evident. In *C*, the large, fanlike dendritic processes of Purkinje cells are better demonstrated. (*A, B,* Phosphorylated neurofilament, ×100 (*A*), ×200 (*B*); *C*, Golgi stain, ×180)

Neurohistology

movements involving multiple joints. The granule cell layer contains almost 50 billion neurons (half of all neurons in the CNS), which receive afferent projections from motor and premotor areas of the cerebral cortex and from the spinal cord. Each granule cell sends its axon up into the molecular layer, where the axon divides into two branches that run along the longitudinal axis of a cerebellar folium—the parallel fibers. The Purkinje cells are the projection neurons of the cerebellar cortex. Each Purkinje cell has an enormous fan-shaped dendritic arbor extending up into the molecular layer that is ideally designed and spatially oriented to make large numbers of synapses with the millions of parallel fibers traversing the molecular layer. The time it takes neural impulses to traverse the parallel fibers builds a temporal component into cerebellar processing. Thus, the cerebellar cortex incorporates a simple, two-cell, input-output arrangement that is structured to provide an ideal basis for learning to convert motor sequence input over space and time into output that is precisely tailored to the physical requirements of the situation. The consequences of loss of cerebellar function are illustrated in Case 3-5.

## Case 3-5

### Cerebellar Dysfunction due to Paraneoplastic Destruction of Cerebellar Purkinje Cells

*A 45-year-old woman develops a flulike illness. Over the next 3 weeks, as the acute symptoms subside, she notes an inability to control her arms. Her balance is so impaired that she cannot walk without a great deal of assistance from a family member. When asked to alternately touch her finger to her nose and then to the examiner's finger, she makes wild erratic swinging movements, and very nearly pokes herself in the eye. She totters dangerously when standing and will fall if not supported. She walks with her feet widely separated and more or less flings each leg forward, lurching from side to side, forward or backward.*

**Comment:** *This unfortunate patient has incurred severe loss of cerebellar Purkinje cells. This change has occurred because she has unsuspected ovarian carcinoma. A protein in the tumor cells shares an antigenic site (an epitope) with a Purkinje cell protein. As her body mounts an immunologic challenge to the cancer, Purkinje cells are killed as innocent bystanders.*

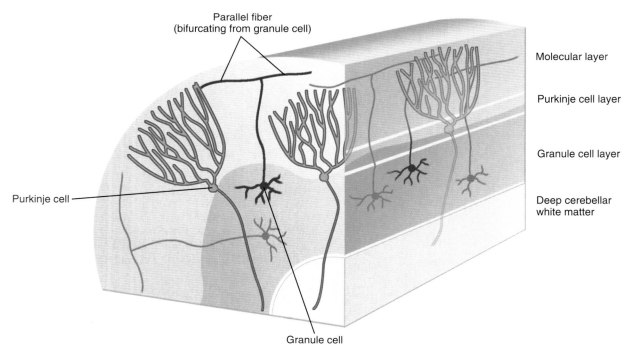

**Figure 3-24** Composite drawing of a folium of the cerebellar cortex illustrating the relationship of the granule cells, the parallel fibers, and the Purkinje cells.

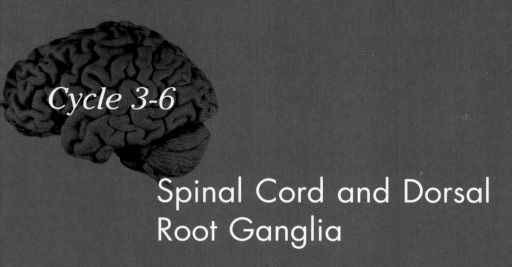

# Cycle 3-6

## Spinal Cord and Dorsal Root Ganglia

### Objective

Be able to describe briefly the cytoarchitectonic structure of the spinal cord and dorsal root ganglia.

Although cytoarchitectonic divisions have been delineated within the spinal cord (Rexed's lamina), this delineation is not nearly so obvious on microscopic examination as it is in the cerebral cortex. Rather, on a stained cross section of the spinal cord, the neurons appear to form a continuous sheet extending from the dorsal horns (site of sensory neurons), through the intermediate zone (the site of preganglionic autonomic neurons), through the ventral horn (site of motor neurons) (Figs. 3-25, 3-26). Neurons in the intermediate zone and the ventral horn at any given level in the spinal cord project via the respective ventral root to the spinal nerve at that level. Recall that clinicians commonly refer to spinal nerves as nerve roots and pathology of these nerves as radiculopathy. Spinal nerves emerge along the length of the spinal column from between each pair of vertebrae.

*Neurohistology*

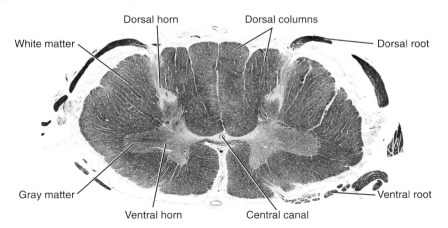

Dorsal horn    Dorsal columns

White matter    Dorsal root

Gray matter    Ventral root

Ventral horn    Central canal

**Figure 3-25** Cross-section of the spinal cord and dorsal and ventral roots.

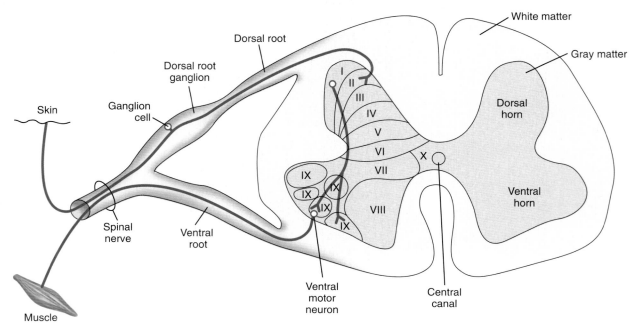

**Figure 3-26** Diagram of a spinal cord segment demonstrating the cytoarchitectonic lamination of the cord and the relationship of the dorsal and ventral roots and the dorsal root ganglia to the cord. At levels containing preganglionic autonomic neurons, lamina VI is vestigial and the intermediate zone consists of ventral portions of lamina V, the dorsal-most portions of lamina VII, and of lamina X.

The axons from intermediate zone cells terminate in autonomic ganglia. The axons from ventral horn cells terminate in muscles. Cells in the dorsal horn receive their input exclusively from cells in the dorsal root ganglion (Figs. 3-26, 3-27). The axons of *dorsal root ganglion* neurons bifurcate, one branch traveling distally via the dorsal root, spinal nerve, and peripheral nerve to terminate in a sensory receptor of some type, the other branch traveling proximally to either synapse on a neuron in the dorsal horn or to travel up the spinal cord to synapse on neurons in some more rostral structure. The dorsal root ganglion appears as an enlargement of the dorsal root. It is located near the intervertebral foramen where its spinal nerve will exit to the periphery (see Fig. 1-54); thus, the portion of the dorsal root between it and the spinal cord may be quite long in more caudal segments of the cord, where each cord level is quite rostral to its respective vertebral level (see Fig. 1-49).

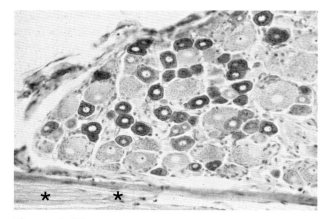

**Figure 3-27** Dorsal root ganglion and adjacent ventral root (*asterisks*). (GS-I B4 isolectin, ×70)

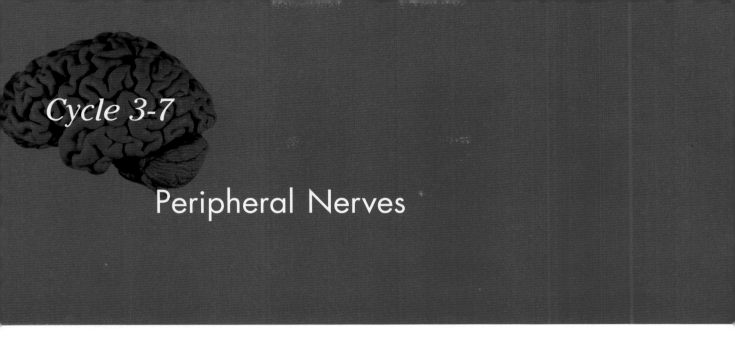
# Peripheral Nerves

**Objective**

Be able to describe briefly the structure of peripheral nerves.

Most peripheral nerves are mixed; that is, they contain both afferent and efferent fibers. These fibers lie in a matrix of connective tissue composed of fibroblasts and collagen known as the *endoneurium* (Fig. 3-28). Surrounding each bundle of nerve fibers and endoneurium is a connective tissue sheath known as *perineurium*. The entire bundle of perineurial sheaths and their contained nerve fibers and endoneurium is further enclosed, with adipocytes and blood vessels, in connective tissue sheath known as the *epineurium*. Peripheral nerves contain both myelinated and unmyelinated fibers (see Fig. 3-13).

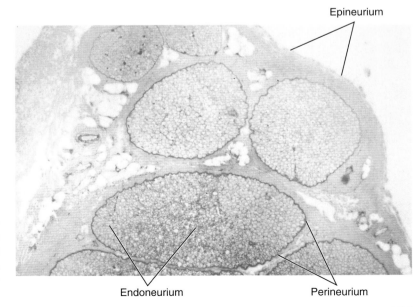

**Figure 3-28** Cross section of a peripheral nerve. Densely packed myelinated and unmyelinated axons lie within endoneurium, surrounded by perineurium. The entire bundle of nerve fascicles is surrounded by epineurium. (×24)

**Neurohistology**

151

Peripheral nerve fibers will readily regrow if they are cut. The epineurium forms a highly effective barrier that keeps growing nerve ends within the nerve and out of adjacent tissue. This phenomenon can be used to advantage in patients who experience accidental nerve injury, as Case 3-6 illustrates.

## Case 3-6

### Nerve Repair Following Injury

*A 23-year-old aspiring professional pianist and bassoonist notes the development of a small lump over her right shoulder. She consults a surgeon, who removes what turns out to be benign tissue. Unfortunately, he inadvertently severs her musculocutaneous nerve in the process, completely denervating her biceps and, it seems, ending her musical career. Four months later, she consults a neurosurgeon, who performs a second operation, trimming the two severed ends of the musculocutaneous nerve and carefully suturing the epineurium of the opposed ends together. Over the course of the following year, she recovers essentially normal function in her biceps and is able to resume her career.*

**Comment:** *This type of procedure can be performed on any peripheral nerve. The transected axons generate multiple sprouts or growth cones. These will be contained by the epineurium as they advance down the trajectory of the original nerve at a rate of 1 to 4mm per day. They are myelinated by Schwann cells along the way. Sensory axons that end up at neuromuscular junctions and motor axons that end up at sensory terminals form nonfunctional units or degenerate. Central nervous system plasticity enables sufficient central reorganization to correct for the completely novel somatotopic organization of the regenerated nerve.*

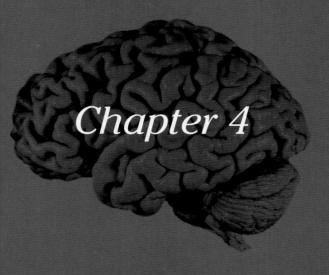

## Chapter 4

# CHEMICAL NEUROTRANSMISSION

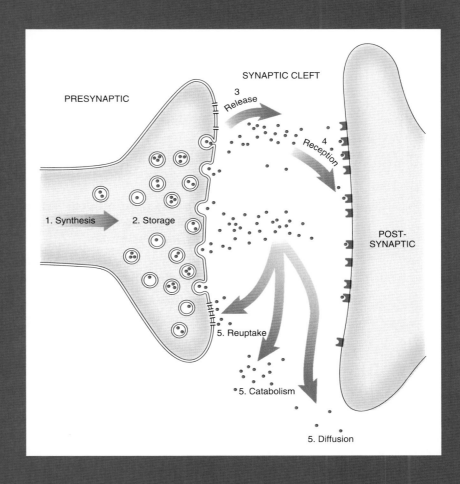

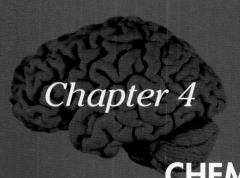

# Chapter 4

# CHEMICAL NEUROTRANSMISSION

# Introduction

The primary emphasis in this text is on the anatomy and function of major neural systems. However, to understand how these systems work and interact, it is necessary to understand how neurons communicate with each other. Neurons communicate primarily through the use of chemical neurotransmitters. In this chapter, we will review the neurotransmitters. In Chapter 5, Neurophysiology, we will review the mechanisms by which neurotransmitters exert their effects on neurons.

At some risk of oversimplification, neurotransmitters can be divided into three major groups: (1) those that mediate the communication of information between neurons (*neural signaling*), the most important being glutamate, gamma-aminobutyric acid (GABA), and glycine; (2) those that modulate (influence communication of information) by neurons within systems (*within-system modulators*), the most important being the neuropeptides, such as opioid peptides in the pain system; and (3) those that modulate the activity of large populations of target neurons that compose multiple systems (*trans-system modulators*), principally the biogenic amines dopamine, epinephrine (adrenaline), norepinephrine (noradrenaline), and serotonin (5-hydroxytryptamine, or 5-HT). For example, among the many functions of serotonin, most poorly defined, is modulation of the degree to which frontal lobe systems (which define goal-oriented behavior) are driven by the limbic system (which defines value and emotional feeling). Acetylcholine is distinctive in that it functions in information transfer at the neuromuscular junction, but it has a trans-system modulatory role in several cerebral systems (memory for skills, memory for facts, arousal, attention), and in the autonomic nervous system.

Just as neurotransmitters provide the means by which neurons interact, they also provide us with the primary means to manipulate the nervous system in disease states. The following examples will illustrate this point. The symptoms of Parkinson's disease are caused by a progressive deficiency of the trans-system modulatory neurotransmitter, dopamine, and can be effectively treated by providing patients with a drug that is converted to dopamine within the brain. Depression reflects dysfunction in parts of the brain that are supplied by the trans-system modulatory neurotransmitter serotonin and can be effectively treated with drugs that, in effect, increase brain serotonin. We have known since antiquity that morphine alleviates pain, but only relatively recently have we discovered that morphine acts on neural systems employing peptide neurotransmitters, the action of which is mimicked by morphine. We do not know of any disorder that involves a simple deficiency of a neurotransmitter, such as glutamate or GABA, that is involved in information transmission. However, there are circumstances such as seizures in which the delicate balance between neural excitation (mediated, for example, by glutamate) and inhibition (mediated by GABA) is tipped in the direction of excitation. We treat seizures using drugs that mitigate the effects of glutamate or potentiate the action of GABA.

Drugs used to manipulate neurotransmission are all developed to have fairly specific actions. However, they all have side effects, indicating that they act on more than one type of receptor or that a given neurotransmitter is employed by multiple neural systems subserving various functions. Furthermore, the response of individual patients to neurally active drugs, favorable or unfavorable, may vary substantially, depending on genetic differences in neurotransmitter receptors or in the distribution of receptor subtypes.

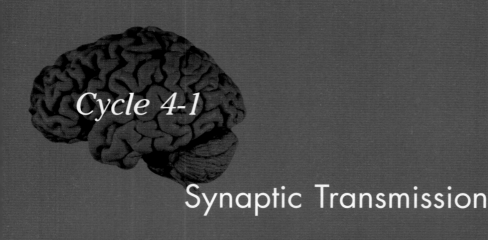

# Cycle 4-1

# Synaptic Transmission

## Objective

Be able to describe the five major steps in neurotransmitter processing.

The major steps in neurotransmitter processing are (1) synthesis, (2) storage, (3) release, (4) reception, and (5) inactivation (Fig. 4-1).

1. *Synthesis.* Neurotransmitters are synthesized within the brain from precursor substances. Enzymes involved in biogenic amine synthesis are concentrated within the axon terminal. Enzymes involved in neuropeptide synthesis are concentrated within rough endoplasmic reticulum in the cell body, and the neuropeptide must be transported down the axon to the axon terminal. Neurotransmitters such as glutamate, GABA, and glycine are by-products of intermediate metabolism.

2. *Storage.* Once neurotransmitters are synthesized, they are stored in 50- to 100-nm synaptic vesicles that are concentrated in the axon terminal, ready for release.

3. *Release.* The release process is triggered by an influx of calcium ions through *voltage-sensitive channels*, which are opened by membrane depolarization.[1] In response to the increase in intracellular calcium in the axon terminal, synaptic vesicles containing the neurotransmitter fuse with the plasma membrane, following which their contents are emptied into the synaptic cleft. Case 4-1 illustrates the consequences of loss of these channels.

4. *Reception.* The neurotransmitter passively diffuses across the synaptic cleft to the postsynaptic membrane where it binds to specific receptor proteins. A neurotransmitter or other compound that binds to a receptor is called a receptor *ligand*. What happens following receptor binding depends on the specific neurotransmitter and the specific receptor. The excitatory neurotransmitter glutamate illustrates the range of possibilities.

---

[1]Neurons normally have a resting membrane potential of approximately −70 mV. Any change in the transmembrane potential in the direction of greater positivity (e.g., to −50 mV) constitutes depolarization. Any change in the direction of greater negativity (e.g., to −80 mV) constitutes hyperpolarization. Restitution of a partially depolarized membrane to −70 mV constitutes repolarization. If a neuron is sufficiently depolarized, it will spontaneously undergo a series of ion channel events that leads to a transient reversal of membrane polarity, such that it actually becomes positive—something referred to as an action potential or neural firing. These phenomena will be discussed at greater length in the next chapter.

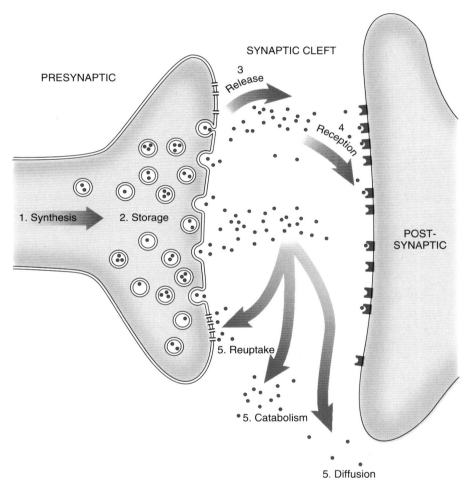

PRESYNAPTIC

SYNAPTIC CLEFT

3
Release

4
Reception

1. Synthesis

2. Storage

POST-
SYNAPTIC

5. Reuptake

5. Catabolism

5. Diffusion

**Figure 4-1** The major steps in neurotransmitter processing.

Chemical Neurotransmission

## Case 4-1

### Eaton-Lambert Syndrome

*A 60-year-old man with a history of many years of heavy smoking complains of several months of progressive generalized weakness, dry mouth, constipation, impotence, reduced sweating, and dizziness when he is standing or walking. On examination, he has relatively severe weakness primarily affecting the proximal muscles of his arms and legs as well as neck muscles, and he has orthostatic hypotension (blood pressure drops when he stands), indicating sympathetic autonomic dysfunction.*

*A nerve conduction study is carried out. A pair of stimulating electrodes is placed over a nerve and recording electrodes are placed over a muscle innervated by that nerve. With stimulation, the depolarization of the nerve normally results in depolarization of all the muscle fibers in the muscle, generating an electrical potential that can be measured. In this patient, this electrical potential is profoundly reduced (Fig. 4-2, top). However, after the patient vigorously contracts the muscle for 30 seconds and the nerve conduction study is repeated, a normal electrical potential is obtained (Fig. 4-2, bottom).*

*In the course of an extensive diagnostic evaluation, the patient is discovered to have a small cell carcinoma of the lung.*

**Comment:** *This patient has a rare disorder known as Eaton-Lambert syndrome. The small cell tumor of the lung derives from primitive neuroendocrine precursor*

*cells that express P/Q-type voltage-gated calcium channel proteins. These proteins engender an antibody response which then becomes directed at similar proteins in neural endings outside the central nervous system. Both acetylcholine-producing (cholinergic) neurons supplying the muscles of the body and the preganglionic cholinergic neurons projecting to the sympathetic and parasympathetic components of the autonomic nervous system are affected (hence the history of both weakness and a host of autonomic symptoms).*

*The nerve conduction results can be explained in the following way: In this patient, depolarization of a nerve ending leads to influx of a very small amount of calcium because most of the voltage-gated calcium channels have been destroyed. This leads to release of only a fraction of the normal amount of neurotransmitter. Only a few muscle fibers will be depolarized by this small amount to the point of firing. If the nerve is repeatedly stimulated very rapidly, enough calcium flows in (by small increments) sufficiently rapidly to outpace normal intracellular calcium uptake mechanisms, enabling release of a nearly normal quantity of neurotransmitter and depolarization of most, if not all, muscle fibers.*

*This patient's neurologic disorder may respond favorably, at least for a while, to treatment of the tumor. Unfortunately, this tumor is rarely cured and his prognosis is grave.*

---

Glutamate may bind to receptors on certain sodium channels (ionophores), inducing these channels to open for a period of time with resultant membrane depolarization. Channels such as these that are opened merely by binding of neurotransmitter to a receptor are called *ligand-gated ion channels*. The major glutamate ligand-gated ion channels are the AMPA[2] and kainate channels, named for the compounds that are the most specific ligands for these receptors (more specific than glutamate). Glutamate may bind to receptors on ligand-gated ion channels that also require partial

membrane depolarization to open (*voltage-sensitive ligand-gated ion channels*). The principal voltage-sensitive ligand-gated glutamate channel allows both sodium and calcium to enter the cell and is regulated by the *N*-methyl-D-aspartate, or NMDA receptor. Finally, glutamate may bind to *metabotropic* receptors which, following ligand binding, activate a G-protein, rather than opening up an ion channel. Activated G-proteins set in motion various intracellular events by activating such enzymes as phospholipase C or adenylate cyclase. Because ligand-gated channels are literally ion pores within barrel-shaped membrane protein complexes, they tend to operate very quickly. On

---

[2]α-Amino-3-hydroxy-5-methyl-4-isoxazide proprionic acid.

Response to a single supramaximal stimulus
before and after exercise

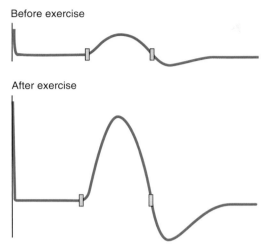

**Figure 4-2** Results of nerve conduction studies in Case 4-1.

the other hand, because activated G-protein-linked receptor proteins set in motion series of biochemical reactions, binding of neurotransmitter to these receptors tends to produce slower and longer lasting effects.

Each neurotransmitter has specific receptors, and as we have seen with glutamate, there may be more than one type of receptor for a given neuro-

transmitter. Some neurotransmitters, such as acetylcholine, have over 100 different types of receptors, and different receptor subtypes are distributed in different parts of the brain. A given neurotransmitter thus may have as many different functions as there are systems that utilize it and receptor subtypes within these systems that recognize it.

5. *Inactivation.* In order for a neuron to exert tight control over the amount of neurotransmitter at its synaptic clefts, that neurotransmitter must be rapidly inactivated. There are three ways by which this can be accomplished: (1) catabolism by an enzyme within the synaptic cleft (e.g., acetylcholine by acetylcholinesterase); (2) a mix of reuptake and catabolism, as with dopamine; and (3) a mix of diffusion out of the synaptic cleft and reuptake, as with glutamate.

## PRACTICE 4-1

**A.** Describe the five major steps in neurotransmitter processing.

**B.** Name two types of neurotransmitter receptors and describe how they work.  AMPA , NMDA.

**C.** What mechanisms are used to inactivate neurotransmitters?

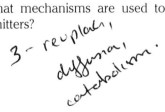

3 - reuptake, diffusion, catabolism.

# Division I

# Transmitters of Neural Signaling: Amino Acids

Glutamate, GABA, and glycine are the most widespread and important amino acid neurotransmitters and the only ones to be reviewed here. Others, including aspartate, proline, taurine, and β-alanine, play more limited roles in the central nervous system (CNS).

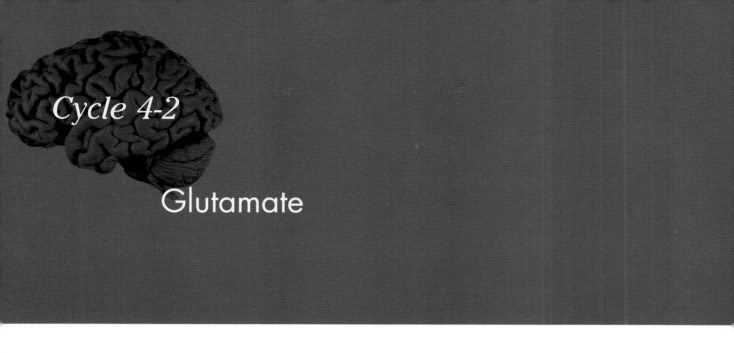

# Cycle 4-2

## Glutamate

### Objectives

1. Be able to describe the synthesis and catabolism of glutamate and the principal means by which its action is terminated.

2. Be able to define the major locations of glutamatergic neurons.

3. Be able to describe the two major neurotransmitter functions of glutamate and the receptors that subserve these functions.

4. Be able to describe the contributions of glutamate to the pathophysiology of seizures, migraine, and stroke.

Glutamate is the major excitatory neurotransmitter in the brain. It is synthesized from α-ketoglutarate, a component of the Krebs tricarboxylic acid cycle. It is normally catabolized by the reverse of the synthetic route but also may be decarboxylated to form GABA (Fig. 4-3). These enzyme systems are available in synaptic terminals. The action of glutamate is terminated by a specific carrier-mediated reuptake system as well as by simple diffusion.

## GLUTAMATE FUNCTION: NEURAL SIGNALING AND MODIFICATION OF NEURAL CONNECTIVITY

Glutamate is used by nearly all neurons in the cerebral cortex that send projections to other parts of the cortex (intra- and interhemispheric connections) and nearly all the cortical neurons sending projections to the brainstem (corticobulbar) and spinal cord (corticospinal). Glutamate actually fulfills two major functions: neural signaling and modification of neural connectivity (the basis for learning and memory).

Neural signaling is achieved principally through ligand-gated sodium channels. Glutamate released at synaptic endings binds to the receptors that gate these channels (most often AMPA and kainate receptors), opening the transmembrane protein channel or ionophore for a brief period of time and allowing sodium to enter and depolarize the postsynaptic membrane. If enough glutamate is released from enough axon terminals, depolarization will be sufficient to cause the postsynaptic neuron to fire and produce an action potential. The response of the postsynaptic neuron to presynaptic neuronal firing and glutamate release will depend on the number of glutamate-gated sodium channels on its membrane. If there is a

*161*

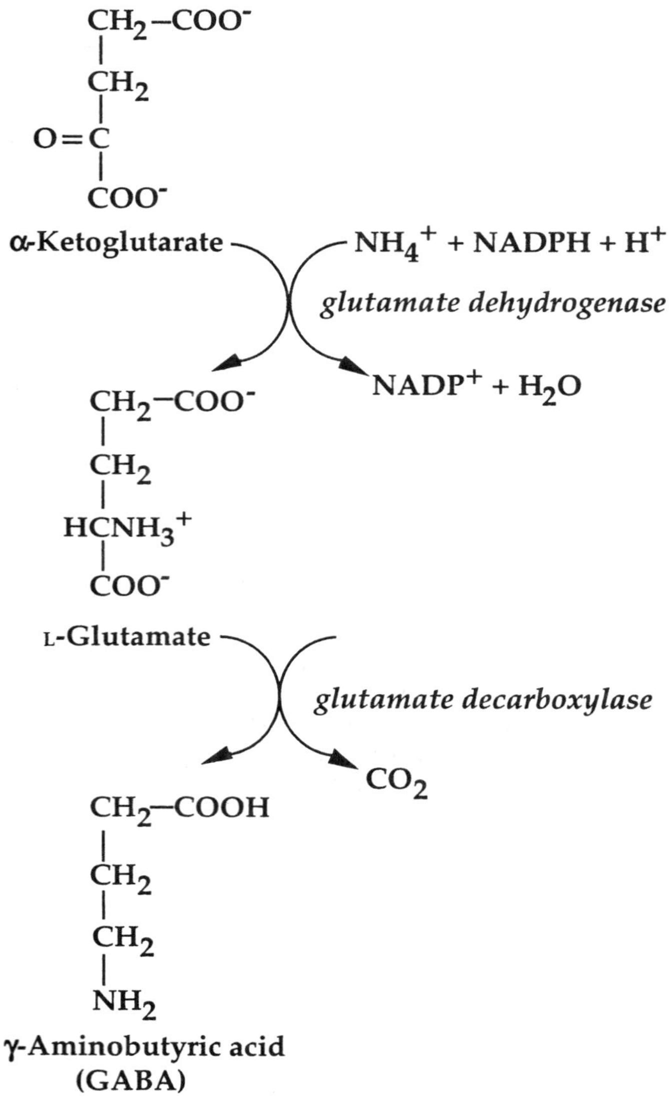

$$CH_2-COO^-$$
$$|$$
$$CH_2$$
$$|$$
$$O=C$$
$$|$$
$$COO^-$$

**α-Ketoglutarate** ⤵ $NH_4^+ + NADPH + H^+$

*glutamate dehydrogenase*

$NADP^+ + H_2O$

$$CH_2-COO^-$$
$$|$$
$$CH_2$$
$$|$$
$$HCNH_3^+$$
$$|$$
$$COO^-$$

**L-Glutamate** ⤵

*glutamate decarboxylase*

$CO_2$

$$CH_2-COOH$$
$$|$$
$$CH_2$$
$$|$$
$$CH_2$$
$$|$$
$$NH_2$$

**γ-Aminobutyric acid
(GABA)**

**Figure 4-3** The synthesis of glutamate and GABA.

sufficient number of receptors, the concurrent firing of presynaptic neurons will easily elicit an action potential in the postsynaptic neuron.

The number of postsynaptic receptors defines the strength of the neural connection. Connection strengths provide the major means by which the brain stores information, i.e., the basis for learning and memory. The modification of neural connectivity, that is, regulation of the number of receptors on the postsynaptic neural membrane, is a complex and poorly understood process. However, it is clear that voltage-sensitive ligand-gated ion channels possessing the NMDA type of glutamate receptor (which contain a sodium/calcium ionopore) play a major role in this process. Potent NMDA receptor blockers severely disrupt learning and memory.

## GLUTAMATE: CLINICAL IMPORTANCE

Although glutamate is a major work horse of normal CNS function, its clinical importance lies mainly in situations characterized by abnormal activity of glutamatergic neurons. For example, because glutamate is an excitatory neurotransmitter, excessively rapid and sustained firing of a relatively small group of glutamatergic neurons in one region of the brain may lead rapidly to successive excitation of ever larger numbers of glutamatergic neurons until major regions of the brain, or effectively the entire brain, is caught up in a paroxysmal discharge—a seizure. Case 4-2 exemplifies this situation.

### *Case 4-2*

#### Epilepsy

*A 23-year-old man begins experiencing spells during which he suddenly stops what he is doing, stares blankly, repeatedly smacks his lips, swallows, and picks absentmindedly at his shirt buttons. These spells last approximately a minute, following which he appears vaguely confused for another couple of minutes. He now experiences one of these spells almost daily. This morning he was in the midst of a typical spell when he suddenly uttered a cry, stiffened up in extreme extension, and seemed to stop breathing. Within 30 seconds he began violent, coarse, synchronous, rhythmic jerking movements, mainly involving his arms, and his breathing became labored and irregular. Bloody froth appeared in his mouth and he was incontinent of urine. After about 3 minutes he relaxed but remained somnolent and very confused. He went to sleep. An hour later he awoke and exhibited normal mental function but complained of feeling sore throughout his body. The magnetic resonance image (MRI) scan is normal except for a 3-mm diameter lesion of the anterior parahippocampal cortex on the right side. He is treated with phenytoin (Dilantin) and experiences no further convulsions but continues to have approximately one of his minor spells a week.*

**Comment:** *This patient is experiencing partial complex seizures ("partial" because they do not involve the entire brain, "complex" because they entail alteration of consciousness). The small lesion in the right parahippocampal cortex, a fundamentally benign*

*tangled mass of abnormal neuropil called a hamartoma, nevertheless predisposes to spontaneous depolarization of local functioning neurons (by complex and poorly understood mechanisms). Local excitatory neurons release glutamate, which in turn depolarizes other excitatory, glutamatergic neurons. If enough glutamatergic neurons in the vicinity of the hamartoma depolarize sufficiently synchronously, the wave of propagating excitation, mediated by glutamate release, will reach a "critical mass," which will overwhelm the countervailing influence of inhibitory interneurons. The paroxysmal discharge then spreads to involve large areas of the medial temporal region, first on the right, and ultimately bilaterally. Even when the epileptiform discharges finally subside, it takes some time for the neurons to reestablish normal ion gradients (intracellular-extracellular differences in ion concentrations), a time period during which they do not function normally. This entire sequence of paroxysmal spreading discharge and ultimate gradual recovery provides the basis for the complex partial seizures. Occasionally, the critical mass of the excitatory discharge is sufficiently great that it fails to be confined to the medial temporal regions, instead spreading to involve the entire brain. The result is a grand mal seizure.*

*The depolarization of neurons in this epileptic sequence is mediated by the action of glutamate on ligand-gated sodium channels (AMPA and kainate receptors) and sodium/calcium channels (NMDA*

**Chemical Neurotransmission**

## Case 4-2—cont'd

receptors). The actual firing of neurons is mediated primarily by a different group of sodium channels, which do not depend on a ligand and are opened only by membrane depolarization. The anticonvulsant phenytoin acts on these purely voltage-gated sodium channels. By prolonging the time that these channels are inactivated between openings, phenytoin reduces the probability that neurons will fire sufficiently rapidly

to propagate epileptiform discharges. These mechanisms will be discussed in greater detail in Chapter 5. We do not have drugs that control seizures by acting directly at the source of excitation—glutamate receptors. However, we do have drugs, such as phenobarbital and lorazepam, that control seizures by acting at GABA receptors to inhibit neuronal firing.

---

High concentrations of extracellular glutamate, whether due to prolonged seizures (Case 4-3) or stroke (Case 4-5), may have serious adverse effects on neurons.

## Case 4-3

### Prolonged Seizures and Excitotoxic Damage to Neurons

A 45-year-old man experiences a small intracerebral hemorrhage caused by a tiny vascular malformation of the brain, a cavernous angioma, located in the language cortex in the posterior portion of his left temporal lobe cortex. He acutely experiences some difficulty putting his thoughts into words (anomia) and reading (alexia). Ultimately he recovers without perceptible sequelae. One year later he suddenly develops severe impairment in language function. His anomia is so severe that he must struggle for minutes to express the simplest thought. Many of the words he does attempt come out as sequences of variously related speech sounds and syllables that together do not form acceptable English words (neologisms). For example: "Whenever I try to speat, steat. . . . I can't even wean the neppatl, the pepaple, the pep, the nessatl . . ." ("Whenever I try to speak . . . I can't even read the newspaper") (language disorders will be discussed more fully in Chapter 12). At first this language impairment fluctuates dramatically from minute to minute throughout the day. He consults a physician who performs an electroencephalogram (a recording of brain electrical activity), which demonstrates seizure activity involving the posterior left temporal cortex. The patient is treated with phenytoin. At first this seems to work, but soon the episodes resume. He is given progressively more phenytoin until he begins to show evidence of toxicity. A week later his

language impairment no longer fluctuates and remains severe.

**Comment:** Blood products in brain tissue commonly eventuate in epileptic foci. This process is thought to occur via iron-catalyzed chemical reactions that lead to the production of oxygen and hydroxyl free radicals, which are highly reactive species capable of damaging lipid membranes and other cellular constituents. In this case, the first evidence of seizure activity was in the form of repeated seizures occurring so quickly that there was not time for recovery between them. This condition is referred to as partial status epilepticus. In Case 4-2 we noted that glutamate released by repeatedly depolarizing neurons acts at both AMPA and kainate receptor-gated sodium channels and NMDA receptor-gated sodium/calcium channels. Action at the sodium channels is the primary drive to seizure propagation. However, the large amount of calcium that pours into cells through the NMDA receptor-gated channels may trigger a host of degradative intracellular enzymatic processes if it is not removed sufficiently quickly. Unfortunately, in this patient, the seizure discharges were so rapid and sustained that they exceeded the capacity of surrounding glia to take up extracellular glutamate and the capacity of neurons to reestablish normal intracellular calcium concentrations. Consequently, many of these neurons were irreversibly damaged and ultimately died, in a process known as apoptosis. This sequence of events is referred to as "excitotoxicity."

Glutamatergic neurotransmission is also a major contributor to the pathophysiology of several other common neurologic disorders, including migraine

headache and stroke, which are discussec 4-4 and 4-5.

## Case 4-4

### Migraine

In the early 1940s, a famous Harvard experimental psychologist, Karl Lashley, published a paper describing his own migraine headaches. These headaches were heralded, as in many migraineurs, by a visual "aura" characterized by a pulsing figure in the center of his vision that slowly expanded from pinpoint size until it encompassed the entirety of a visual field (Fig. 4-4). Lashley reasoned correctly that this reflected something happening in his visual cortex. Because he knew the dimensions of the calcarine cortex, by plotting the diameter of the jiggling figure over time, he was able to compute the rate of progression of this process along the calcarine fissure. He estimated 3 mm/minute.

Two years later, a Brazilian neurophysiologist, Leao, then also working at Harvard, reported an annoying but interesting phenomenon he had encountered in his experimental work with animals. Sometimes the application of small amounts of certain ionic solutions to the cortex of cats elicited a sudden temporary but profound depression of cortical neuronal activity that slowly expanded across the cortex like a ripple caused by a stone thrown into a pond. The rate of expansion was 3 mm/minute. This phenomenon has since been known as "spreading depression of Leao." Leao actually speculated that it might be the mechanism underlying migrainous aura. The ion channel processes underlying spreading depression of Leao are not yet well understood.

In the early 1970s, investigators in Scandinavia perfected a means to measure cerebral blood flow by injecting radioactive xenon into a carotid artery and measuring the ultimate distribution of radioactivity over

the hemisphere, using a large number of scintillation counters mounted in a helmet placed over the head. Because cerebral blood flow is determined by synaptic activity, this promised to be a means for defining the particular regions of the brain engaged by specific tasks. Hundreds of laboratories are now involved in this type of research. These Scandinavian investigators quickly discovered that inserting a needle into a carotid artery of a migraineur was a very effective way of precipitating a migraine. They found that the aura phase of migraine began with a profound reduction of cerebral blood flow in the occipital regions of the brain that slowly expanded anteriorly until it encompassed the entire hemisphere. The rate of forward expansion was 3 mm/minute.

**Comment:** It is now generally accepted that migrainous aura is caused by spreading depression of Leao. Further research has shown that the transient profound depression of neural activity is caused by massive glutamate release that depolarizes cortical neurons and temporarily renders them incapable of repolarizing sufficiently to resume firing. Furthermore, when spreading depression is induced in animals, it triggers activity in the spinal nucleus of cranial nerve V, strongly suggesting that these animals are experiencing headache. The spinal nucleus of cranial nerve V contains neurons subserving pain and temperature sensation for the face and much of the meninges (pia, arachnoid, and dura). The mechanism by which this occurs is not known.

Chemical Neurotransmission

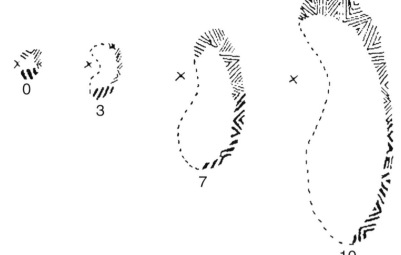

**Figure 4-4** The development of Karl Lashley's migrainous visual aura over time. The more or less elliptical shaded patterns are Lashley's sketches of what he actually saw over time (in minutes, as indicated below the patterns). The x's mark the point at which he was fixating his vision. (From Lashley KS. Patterns of cerebral integration indicated by the scotomas of migraine. Arch Neurol Psychiatry 46:331-339, 1941.)

## Case 4-5

### Stroke

A 75-year-old man with an abnormal heart rhythm (atrial fibrillation), which predisposes to the formation of blood clot in the heart, experiences a stroke when a fragment of clot from the heart lodges in the proximal portion of his left middle cerebral artery. He immediately loses his ability to talk (aphasia) and experiences paralysis of his right arm and leg. He undergoes positron emission tomography (PET) to map his cerebral blood flow. Blood flow throughout the right hemisphere is 55 mL/100 g/minute (normal). A small portion of the cortex of the left hemisphere has blood flow that is less than 10 mL/100 g/minute—too low to support even basic neuronal metabolic activity. This region of the brain promptly undergoes irreversible damage. In a much larger region of the brain with blood flow between 10 and 18 mL/100 g/minute, irreversible change occurs more gradually, over minutes to hours.

**Comment:** Animal studies have shown that, during a stroke, repeated waves of spreading depression of

Leao travel across the region of moderately reduced blood flow. The massive glutamate release associated with these waves opens up glutamate-gated sodium and calcium channels. Unfortunately, unlike in the migraineur with spreading depression of Leao, these neurons do not have enough glucose and oxygen (because of lack of blood flow) to run their sodium-potassium pumps and reestablish normal ion gradients. These osmotically active cations bring water with them, causing the neurons to swell and even lyse. Large concentrations of intracellular calcium activate a host of degradative enzyme systems and the neurons die. Intensive research is under way to find drugs capable of either blocking glutamate release or glutamate receptors in an effort to mitigate the damage caused by stroke-induced spreading depression of Leao in humans. When injected in experimental animals at the time of stroke induction, such drugs have been shown to reduce stroke size by as much as 50 percent.

# PRACTICE 4-2

**A.** From what is glutamate primarily synthesized? How is it catabolized? Is the termination of its action mainly dependent on catabolism? Why or why not?

**B.** Why is the action of glutamate on ligand-gated channels quicker and briefer than its action on metabotropic receptors?

**C.** Locate the major glutamatergic systems in the cerebrum.

**D.** What are the two major functions subserved by glutamate? What receptor types support these functions?

**E.** Describe the principles of action of phenytoin on glutamate-gated ion channels.

**F.** An NMDA-glutamate receptor blocker would provide an ideal way to minimize brain damage caused by stroke. Explain both why this is the case and why such a drug could not be given chronically to patients at high risk for experiencing stroke.

**G.** Until recently, grand mal status epilepticus was often treated in substantial part simply by paralyzing the patient with a neuromuscular blocker. In the absence of the violent jerking, the patient could be maintained easily on a respirator (achieving good systemic oxygenation) and provided appropriate nursing care. Explain why this is not good care. What should be the first priority in treating grand mal status epilepticus? What about partial status epilepticus? Why?

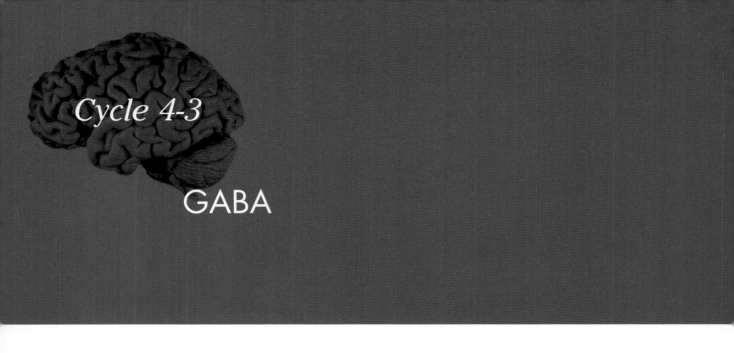

# Cycle 4-3

# GABA

### Objectives

1. Be able to describe the synthesis and catabolism of GABA and the principal means by which its action is terminated.

2. Be able to describe the major function of GABA and how it is mediated by the various GABA receptors.

3. Be able to indicate where GABAergic neurons are primarily located.

4. Be able to describe why GABA-mimetic drugs are effective anticonvulsants.

5. Be able to describe the basis for the alcohol withdrawal syndrome and the rationale for use of GABA-mimetic drugs in treating it.

GABA is the principal neurotransmitter of interneurons throughout the brain. It is also the neurotransmitter of the predominant neurons in the striatum and globus pallidus and the Purkinje cells of the cerebellum. It is the major inhibitory neurotransmitter. It is synthesized from glutamate via the enzyme glutamic acid decarboxylase (GAD) (Fig. 4-3). It is catabolized by GABA-transaminase to yield glutamate and succinate semialdehyde, which is then converted to succinate, a component of the Krebs tricarboxylic acid cycle. These enzyme systems are available in synaptic terminals. The action of GABA is terminated by a specific carrier-mediated presynaptic reuptake system as well as by simple diffusion.

The function of GABA is to mediate neural signaling. GABA acts at $GABA_A$ and $GABA_C$ receptors to potentiate chloride conductance and at $GABA_B$ receptors to potentiate potassium conductance.[3] Both these actions hyperpolarize the postsynaptic neuron and thus reduce its ability to fire an action potential—the neurophysiologic basis of inhibition. In the normal brain, glutamate and GABA neurons provide the major substrate for information processing. GABA is clinically important chiefly in pathologic states characterized by the development of a significant generalized imbalance between excitatory and inhibitory influences in the brain, that is, between glutamate- and GABA-mediated neuronal signaling. GABA-mimetic drugs are also used to induce sleep and to treat anxiety; the precise mechanisms underlying these effects are uncertain. Case 4-6 illustrates the use of a GABA-mimetic drug, lorazepam, to address a generalized imbalance between excitatory and inhibitory processes in the brain.

---

[3]Conductance is a measure of the ease with which an ion is able to pass through channels in the neural membrane. It will be discussed in greater detail in Chapter 5.

## Case 4-6

### Alcohol Withdrawal

*A 35-year-old chronic alcoholic, after consuming up to 2 quarts of vodka a day for several weeks, runs out of money and presents to the emergency room in acute alcohol withdrawal. He is extremely agitated, trembling violently, and an hour after arriving at the emergency room, experiences the first of several grand mal seizures. He is given a loading dose of phenytoin, which controls his seizures, and then is administered lorazepam, as much as 10mg every 4 hours (a high dose), to control his agitation and tremulousness.*

**Comment:** *Alcohol has complex effects on the nervous system, many of which we are only beginning to understand. One effect appears to be to augment GABA-mediated inhibition. This chronic potentiation of GABAergic neurotransmission leads to downregulation of GABA receptors. Thus, when an alcoholic suddenly stops drinking, a deficiency in GABA-mediated inhibition rapidly develops, leading to seizures and such behavioral manifestations as agitation and tremulousness. Lorazepam, a benzodiazepine, potentiates the action of GABA at $GABA_A$ receptors, increasing the frequency of chloride channel opening, and in this way, alleviates the symptoms of alcohol withdrawal. The control of seizures requires, in addition, the moderation of glutamatergic effects on sodium channels by drugs such as phenytoin.*

## PRACTICE 4-3

**A.** From what is GABA primarily synthesized? How is it catabolized? How is its action terminated?

**B.** Where are GABAergic neurons primarily located?

**C.** What is the major neurotransmitter function of GABA and how is it mediated by GABA receptors?

**D.** Why are GABA-mimetic drugs effective anticonvulsants?

**E.** Why are GABA-mimetic drugs useful in the treatment of alcohol withdrawal syndrome?

**F.** Refer to Cases 4-2 and 4-3. In light of what you have learned in this cycle, can you suggest any other ways of treating these patients?

Chemical Neurotransmission

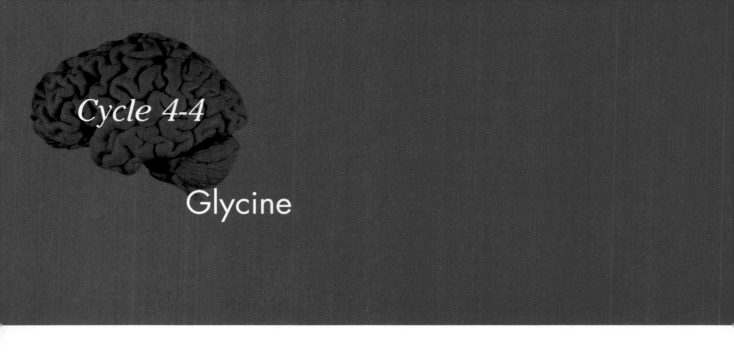

# Glycine

## Objectives

1. Know the predominant location of glycinergic neurons and be able to describe their major function.
2. Be able to describe the consequences of interference with glycinergic neural transmission, as in tetanus and strychnine poisoning.

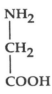

$$
\begin{array}{c}
NH_2 \\
| \\
CH_2 \\
| \\
COOH
\end{array}
$$

**Glycine**

**Figure 4-5** Glycine.

Glycine (Fig. 4-5) is the second most widespread inhibitory neurotransmitter in the CNS. Glycine is present in the diet but can also be synthesized from serine. Like GABA, it is primarily a neurotransmitter of interneurons, and it acts by opening chloride channels. Glycinergic neurons are present throughout the brain, but are particularly prevalent in the brainstem and spinal cord. Like other neurotransmitters involved in neuronal signaling, glycine normally functions in CNS information processing. Clinical disorders involving glycine arise only when a toxin inhibits release of glycine from synaptic endings (e.g., tetanus—Case 4-7) or blocks glycine receptors (e.g., strychnine) and fundamentally shifts the excitatory-inhibitory balance among large populations of neurons.

## Case 4-7

**Tetanus**

*A 60-year-old man living in a cabin in the Ocala National Forest cuts his foot. Self-reliant as always, he tends to it himself. A week later he presents to an emergency room. The wound is obviously infected. He complains of stiffness and soreness in his neck, tightness in his jaw, difficulty swallowing, and pain between his shoulder blades. He opens his jaw only with great difficulty and his face is fixed in a tight, tortured smile (risus sardonicus). His limbs are very stiff. His abdomen has boardlike rigidity. When a nurse drops an instrument tray, his arms and legs stiffen in extreme extension, his back arches, and his*

*Continued*

## Case 4-7—cont'd

*neck hyperextends (opisthotonus). He cries out in pain. He sweats profusely.*

**Comment:** *This patient's cut is infected with Clostridium tetani. The bacterium produces a toxin that ultimately may cause widespread neuronal injury and death throughout the CNS. However, at lower concentrations, it inhibits the release of glycine and GABA. This results in marked increases in muscle tone due to uninhibited firing of motor neurons. Bulbar muscles (muscles innervated by cranial nerves) tend to be most affected, hence the risus sardonicus and the term "lockjaw," but with severe intoxication, muscles throughout the body are affected. Minor stimuli, such as noises or touching the patient, tend to precipitate generalized muscle spasms. The intense muscle contractions increase body temperature, leading to compensatory sweating. CNS disinhibition may be so extreme as to precipitate epileptic seizures. Treatment consists of placing the patient in a quiet room, free from as many sources of stimulation as possible, cleaning the wound, giving antibiotics, administering tetanus immune globulin, which eliminates the tetanus toxin by forming antigen-antibody complexes, and administering a benzodiazepine such as lorazepam, which potentiates the action of GABA at its receptors.*

## PRACTICE 4-4

**A.** Where are glycinergic neurons predominantly located?

**B.** What is the major function of glycinergic neurons?

**C.** Describe the consequences of interference with glycinergic neurotransmission.

Chemical Neurotransmission

# Division II

## Within-System Neural Modulators

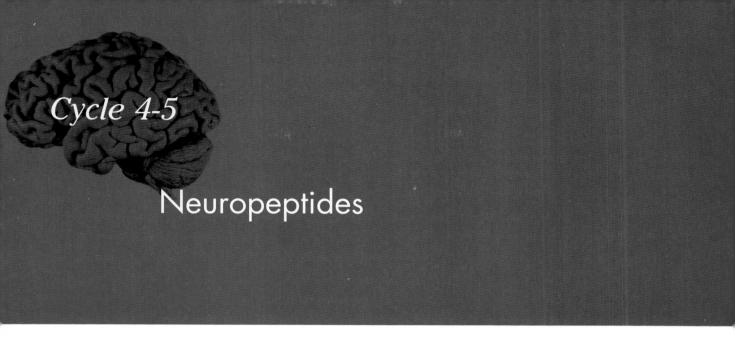

## Cycle 4-5

# Neuropeptides

### Objectives

1. Be able to describe how and where peptide neurotransmitters are synthesized, transported, and degraded.
2. Be able to describe what is meant by receptor downregulation and give a clinical example.
3. Be able to describe what is meant by ligand non-specificity and give a clinical example.

In general, neurotransmitters involved in within-system neural modulation act only to modify the actions of transmitters involved in neural signaling, and they exert this modulatory effect within single neural systems. The most important class of within-system modulatory neurotransmitters is the neuropeptides.

There are a host of peptide neurotransmitters. One large group is implicated in hypothalamic function (angiotensin, corticotropin releasing hormone [CRH], luteinizing hormone releasing hormone [LHRH], oxytocin, vasopressin [antidiuretic hormone, or ADH], thyrotropin releasing hormone [TRH], growth hormone releasing hormone [GHRH], and neuropeptide Y [NP-Y]). Another group is involved in central pain systems (β-endorphin, enkephalins). Other peptide neurotransmitters, such as somatostatin and NP-Y, are widely distributed throughout the cerebral cortex, where they modulate neuronal intercommunication involved in information processing in higher neural functions. Some neuropeptides are identical to hormones found in the gut (e.g., cholecystokinin and vasoactive intestinal polypeptide [VIP]). Peptide neurotransmitters may constitute the exclusive neurotransmitter released by a neuron or they may be co-released with another neurotransmitter (e.g., somatostatin and GABA, substance P and serotonin).

The neuropeptides are produced by proteolytic cleavage of large precursor proteins. These proteins are synthesized by rough endoplasmic reticulum in the neuron cell body and then transported to presynaptic terminals. Following their release, neuropeptides are degraded by extracellular proteases.

The actions of these neurotransmitters are as various as the systems that utilize them. We will consider only endorphins and enkephalins, which are among the major neurotransmitters employed by pain systems.

## ENDORPHINS (ENDOGENOUS OPIOIDS)

Discounting alcohol consumption, the use of opium for analgesia probably constituted the first manipulation of a neurotransmitter system for therapeutic purposes. However, only quite recently was it discovered that opiate derivatives such as morphine, which are not peptides, act at the target sites of two classes of endogenous peptide neurotransmitters, the endorphins and the enkephalins. Although these neurotransmitters are utilized at many loci in the CNS and peripheral nervous system (PNS), only their role in pain systems is understood in any detail. Central pain systems will be discussed in detail in the chapter on somesthesis. Here we consider only two aspects of endorphins and enkephalins: *receptor regulation effects* (tolerance and dependence), and *ligand nonspecificity*.

By *receptor regulation effects*, we mean the impact of tonic levels of endorphins, enkephalins, and their functional analogs, such as morphine, on receptor density at postsynaptic sites. As we noted in Case 4-6, chronic intensive stimulation of neurotransmitter receptors may induce a reduction in the density of receptors, something often referred to as downregulation. Downregulation reduces the sensitivity of target neurons to the neurotransmitter and it sets the stage for inadequate stimulation of target neuronal populations if there is a sudden reduction in the neurotransmitter or a functional analog, as exemplified in Case 4-8.

## Case 4-8

### Opioid Tolerance and Dependence

*A 35-year-old man is involved in a serious automobile accident in which he shatters several lumbar vertebrae. He undergoes surgical stabilization and escapes significant neurologic injury. However, he is left with severe, chronic low back pain. His pain is initially controlled on a regimen of oxycontin (a slow release form of a potent opioid analgesic, oxycodone), 40 mg every 8 hours. However, within a month, his pain again starts to become unbearable. Without consulting his physician, he gradually increases the dose, ultimately to 80 mg every 6 hours, always just barely keeping the pain under control. Unfortunately, because he is using far more medication than planned, he runs out before his next clinic visit. He comes to the emergency room in severe pain. He has been unable to sleep for 24 hours and complains of hot and cold flashes, nausea, abdominal pain, cramps, and diarrhea. He is agitated, extremely restless, obviously in pain, sweats profusely, constantly yawns, and has a runny nose and watery eyes. He is mildly febrile and has a heart rate of 120 bpm and a respiratory rate of 32.*

**Comment:** *This patient developed opiate tolerance as constant high levels of a drug, oxycodone (which emulates the action of endorphins and enkephalins) led to downregulation of opioid receptors, reducing the impact of the current dose of medication and requiring constant increases in dosage to achieve the same analgesic effect. When he ran out of medication, the action of endogenous opioid neuropeptide systems on the reduced number of receptors was insufficient, leading to a withdrawal syndrome and a marked increase in pain. This withdrawal syndrome, indicating opioid dependence, ended days later as the number of*

*receptors normalized, at which point pain levels returned to baseline.*

*Although the mechanisms of tolerance and dependence described here seem relatively straightforward, actual human behavior is considerably more complicated. Not every patient who is placed on around-the-clock opioid analgesics develops tolerance and dependence. Patients with pain due to cancer are least likely to develop tolerance and dependence. The reason for this is unknown.*

*Drug dependence may be driven both by desire to avoid suffering due to withdrawal symptoms precipitated by functional neurotransmitter deficiency, as described here, and desire for the pleasure derived from drug ingestion. The sense of both suffering and pleasure is defined by the limbic system, which provides the basis for the subjective value we attach to all experiences and perceptions (see Chapter 12). In the case of opioids, the aversiveness of withdrawal symptoms appears to depend substantially on neural systems involving the periaqueductal gray, an endorphinergic center in the midbrain with extensive limbic connections. On the other hand, the pleasure of opioid use appears to be critically dependent on opiate receptors on dopaminergic cells in the ventral tegmental area of the midbrain, which project both to the limbic system and to the nucleus accumbens, a structure lying immediately below the head of the caudate nucleus that is heavily interconnected with the limbic system.*

*Neural systems incorporating the nucleus accumbens are also strongly implicated in addictive behavior involving sympathomimetic substances such as amphetamine and cocaine. Addictive behavior is associated with drug craving so intense that humans*

## Case 4-8—cont'd

(and animals) will go to almost any lengths, forgo almost any other behavior (sex, eating, sleep), suffer almost any loss (employment, family, financial well-being), or incur great risk (serious physical illness,

death, apprehension for illegal activity) to get it. The absence of reward is apparently more important than the threat of withdrawal in driving addictive behavior.

By *ligand nonspecificity*, we refer to the fact that opioid drugs (the ligands) bind to endorphin and enkephalin receptors throughout the nervous system, only some of which are implicated in analgesic mechanisms. These nonspecific effects account for "side effects" of the medication, such as constipation, nausea, itching, slurring of speech, imbalance, incoordination, drowsiness, confusion, and with very high doses, respiratory depression. Many of these unwanted effects are related to specific receptor subtypes, raising the possibility of developing drugs with greater affinity for receptors in systems responsible for analgesia and little affinity for receptors in systems responsible for these side effects, as well as such phenomena as tolerance, dependence, and addictive behavior. Butorphanol (Stadol) is a β-endorphin antagonist/ kappa-enkephalin agonist that was developed with the aim of providing analgesia without the "high" thought to contribute to addiction. It is commonly used in the treatment of migraine. Unfortunately, butorphanol has proved sufficiently prone to abuse that the Food and Drug Administration recently made it a controlled substance. Thus, we have not yet had a major clinical success in selectively targeting opioid receptor subtypes. One consequence of ligand nonspecificity is illustrated in Case 4-9.

## Case 4-9

### Opiate Overdose
A 25-year-old heroin addict unwittingly purchases an unusually pure form of heroin, injects himself, and collapses. A friend finds him shortly thereafter, barely

## Case 4-9—cont'd

breathing. He is left at a local emergency room where medical personnel immediately recognize the situation and give him a dose of naloxone (Narcan), a nonspecific opiate receptor antagonist. The patient almost immediately begins breathing normally and shortly thereafter, begins to exhibit signs of severe opiate withdrawal.

**Comment:** Naloxone is a valuable drug in treating opiate overdose, whether self-administered or iatrogenic (resulting from medical treatment). However, its unfortunate lack of specificity is amply revealed in this case, in which respiratory depression cannot be reversed without precipitating the multisystem opioid dysfunction that generates withdrawal symptoms.

## PRACTICE 4-5

**A.** How and where are peptide neurotransmitters synthesized, transported, and degraded?

**B.** What is receptor downregulation? Give a clinical example of its ramifications.

**C.** What is meant by ligand nonspecificity? Give a clinical example.

Chemical Neurotransmission

# Division III

# Trans-System Neural Modulators: The Biogenic Amines: Catecholamines and Indoleamines

In general, trans-system modulators, like within-system neuromodulators, act only to modify the actions of transmitters involved in neural signaling. However, unlike within-system modulators, they appear to regulate the balance of actions *between* systems.

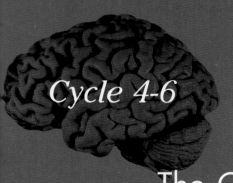

## *Cycle 4-6*

# The Catecholamines: Dopamine, Norepinephrine, Epinephrine

Without reproducing detailed chemical structures, be able to describe the synthesis and degradation of catecholamines and the way in which their action in the synaptic cleft is terminated.

The synthetic pathway of the catecholamines is depicted in Figure 4-6. The rate-limiting step is defined by tyrosine hydroxylase. Whether a particular neuron is dopaminergic, noradrenergic, or adrenergic depends on whether it contains the critical enzymes needed to produce these end products (e.g., dopamine-β-hydroxylase, phenylethanolamine-N-methyltransferase). All catecholamines are initially degraded by the same two intracellular enzymes, monoamine oxidase (MAO) and catechol-O-methyltransferase (COMT). MAO is found in both neurons and glia. COMT is found in glia and in plasma. Figure 4-7 illustrates the effect of these enzymes on dopamine. Because in the CNS these enzymes are intracellular, they perform but a minor role in terminating the actions of catecholamines, which is achieved primarily through neurotransmitter reuptake by specific transporter systems. A cascade of further enzymes ultimately degrades the products of MAO and COMT to simple aromatic acid and alcohol catecholamine derivatives, much of which are eliminated in the urine.

## PRACTICE 4-6

**A.** What feature distinguishes noradrenergic from dopaminergic neurons?

**B.** Which would have a greater impact on catecholamine neurotransmission, a drug that inhibited reuptake or a drug that blocked MAO and COMT? Why?

Chemical Neurotransmission

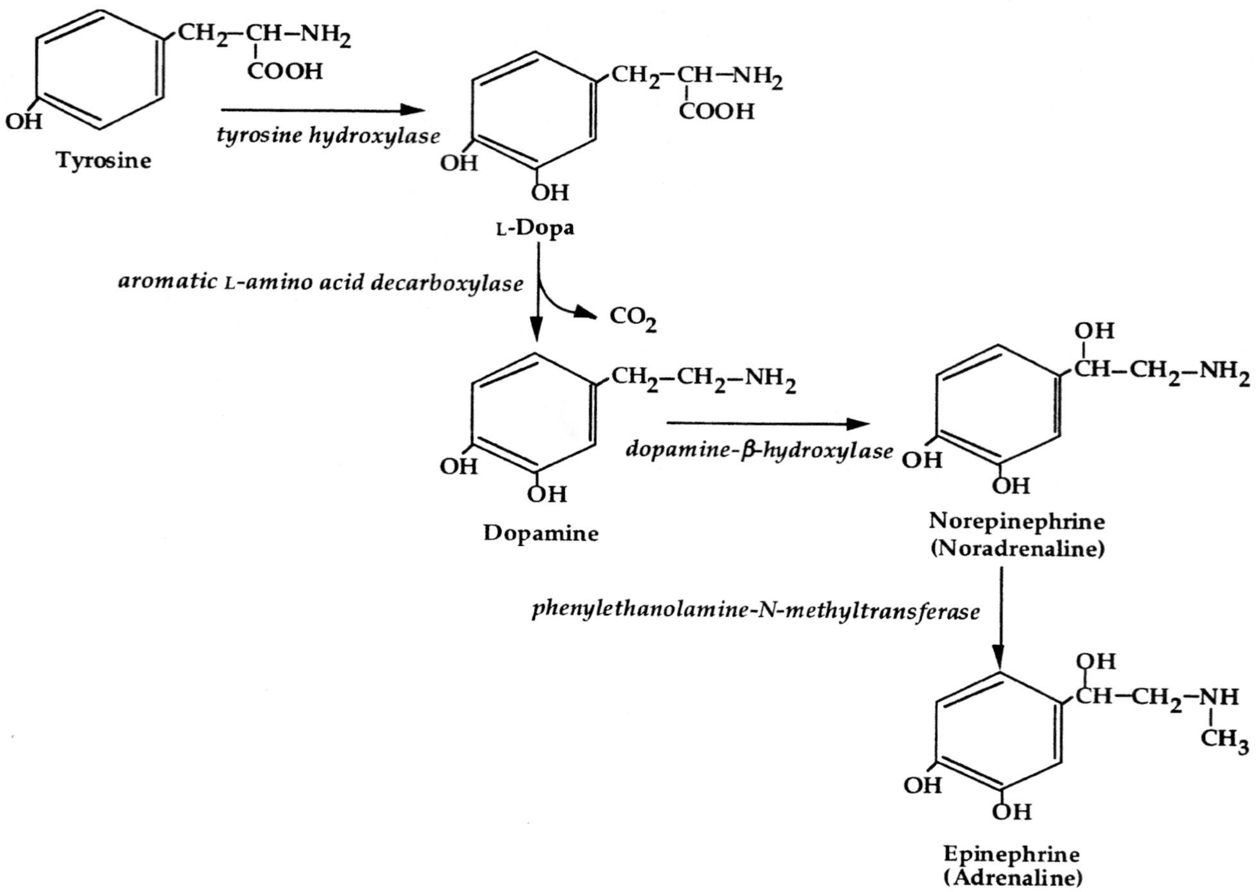

**Figure 4-6** Catecholamine synthesis.

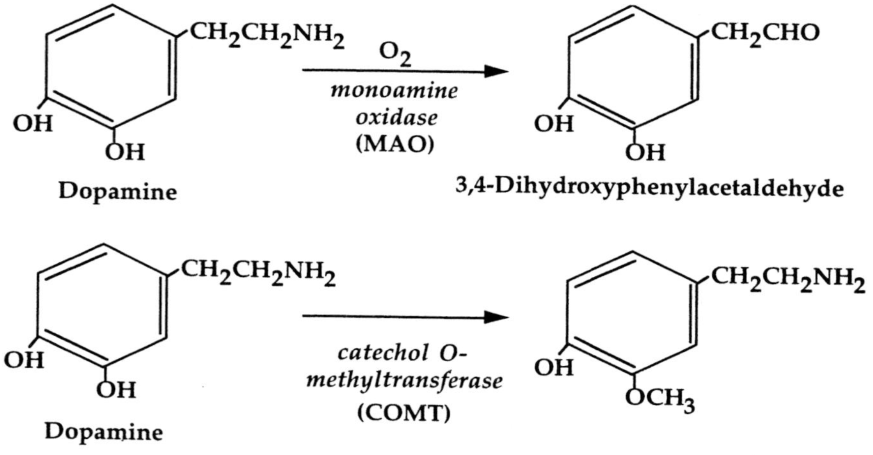

**Figure 4-7** Catecholamine degradation.

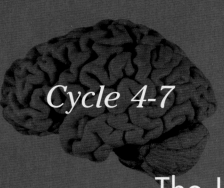

# Cycle 4-7

# The Indoleamine Serotonin (5-Hydroxytryptamine)

## Objective

Without reproducing detailed chemical structures, be able to describe the synthesis and degradation of serotonin and the way in which its action in the synaptic cleft is terminated.

The synthetic pathway of 5-hydroxytryptamine (5-HT) is depicted in Figure 4-8. Comparison of Figure 4-8 with Figure 4-6 will show that the synthesis of 5-HT precisely parallels that of the catecholamines. The rate-limiting step is defined by tryptophan hydroxylase. Serotonin is initially degraded by MAO only. A cascade of further enzymes ultimately degrades the products of MAO to simple aromatic acid and alcohol indoleamine derivatives, most of which are eliminated in the urine.

**Figure 4-8** Synthesis of serotonin.

179

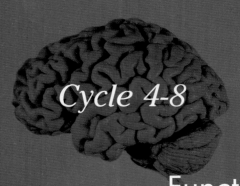

# Cycle 4-8

# Functions of the Biogenic Amines

## Objectives

1. Be able to describe the two major dopamine systems in the brain and the subdivisions of the system originating in the midbrain.

2. Be able to describe how a very specific dopamine receptor blocker (as opposed to a nonspecific blocker) could improve the balance of beneficial and adverse effects of receptor blockade.

3. Be able to describe the major properties of biogenic amine neurotransmitters that define them as modulatory rather than signaling systems.

4. Be able to describe the ways in which dopamine systems can be manipulated to treat Parkinson's disease, dyskinesias, and psychosis.

5. Be able to describe the ways in which noradrenergic and serotonergic systems can be manipulated to treat depression.

6. Be able to describe why a serotonin receptor blocker is effective in the treatment of migraine.

## DOPAMINERGIC, NORADRENERGIC, AND SEROTONERGIC FUNCTIONS: AN OVERVIEW

The biogenic amines function as neurotransmitters in a multitude of systems in the CNS and PNS and 5-HT functions in a number of CNS systems. To a degree, the various catecholamine and 5-HT systems are anatomically distinct. However, the impact of these neuro-transmitter systems on their target structures is further differentiated by the distributions of a large number of different receptor types. These attributes of biogenic amine systems are illustrated in the following sections.

### Dopamine Systems

There are two major dopamine systems in the brain. One, the tuberoinfundibular system, originates in the hypothalamus and inhibits the pituitary secretion of prolactin, which promotes lactation. The second originates in a W-shaped wedge of cells extending across the entire ventral midbrain immediately adjacent to the cerebral peduncles (Fig. 4-9). The cells making up the lateral portions of the W, directly above the cerebral peduncles (called the substantia nigra because of its dark color), project to the caudate nucleus (mainly interconnected with prefrontal cortex) and the putamen (mainly connected to motor and premotor cortices), referred to collectively as the dorsal striatum. The cells making up the middle portion of the W, directly above the interpeduncular fossa (the ventral tegmental area), project to the nucleus accumbens (the ventral striatum), to a number of structures in the limbic system connected to nucleus accumbens (the mesolimbic system), and to much of the cerebral cortex (the mesocortical system). Case 4-10 illustrates the clinical value of stimulating the tuberoinfundibular system, and Case 4-11 illustrates the value of selectively blocking certain dopamine receptors in the nigrostriatal/mesolimbic systems.

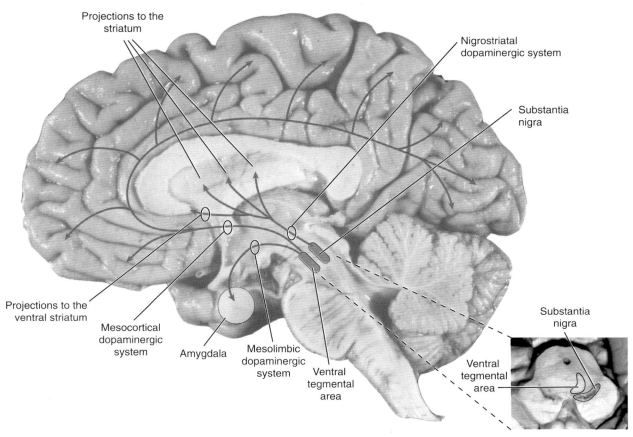

**Figure 4-9** The dopaminergic systems. Midline sagittal section demonstrating the projections. *Inset:* Axial section of the midbrain demonstrating the location of the dopaminergic neurons.

## Case 4-10

### Prolactinoma

*A 35-year-old woman consults her gynecologist because she has not had a menstrual period for 4 months (amenorrhea) and for the last 2 months she has experienced watery secretion from her breasts (galactorrhea). A pregnancy test is negative. Diagnostic evaluation reveals a 1-cm pituitary tumor. Serum prolactin levels are markedly elevated. She is treated with a dopamine receptor agonist, bromocriptine. Her galactorrhea rapidly subsides, she eventually resumes her menstrual periods, and a follow-up MRI scan of the brain reveals that the tumor has markedly diminished in size.*

**Comment:** *This patient has a prolactinoma, a tumor composed of a clonal expansion of prolactin-secreting cells in the pituitary. It is producing excessive quantities*

*of prolactin, hence the galactorrhea, and it is interfering with the normal hypothalamic-driven pituitary secretion of luteinizing hormone (LH) and follicle-stimulating hormone (FSH), hence the amenorrhea. Although the growth of these cells and their production of prolactin can no longer be inhibited by the relatively small amounts of dopamine that can be produced by the hypothalamus, they can fortunately be inhibited by the provision of a larger, exogenous source of dopaminergic stimulation, such as bromocriptine. This drug can be administered indefinitely, shrink the tumor by inhibiting prolactin-secreting cells, and thus obviate the need for neurosurgical excision. The effects of small amounts of bromocriptine on the other major dopamine system in the brain are imperceptible.*

**Chemical Neurotransmission**

## Case 4-11

### Schizophrenia

*A 21-year-college senior rapidly becomes withdrawn and paranoid and develops delusions that her mind is being controlled by extraterrestrial beings. More and more she hears voices that seem to be telling her to do something. Eventually she is brought to the emergency room by her parents. She is extremely agitated, incoherent, and combative. A diagnosis of acute paranoid schizophrenia is made and she is placed on haloperidol, a dopamine receptor antagonist. Her agitation, hallucinations, and delusions very quickly dissipate but she develops muscular rigidity, becomes quite akinetic (exhibits little or no spontaneous behavior and minimal responses to stimulation), and from time to time exhibits dystonic postures such as extreme protrusion of the tongue or bending uncontrollably at the waist. She is switched to olanzepine. On this drug, her hallucinations, delusions, and agitation remain under control but her motor symptoms subside.*

**Comment:** *Until recently, it appeared that all drugs that control psychosis (neuroleptics) blocked $D_2$ dopamine receptors (the role of $D_1$ receptors is complex and remains unclear). Haloperidol is a nonspecific $D_2$ blocker. Thus, it blocks $D_2$ receptors in the mesolimbic system, effectively ameliorating psychosis, but it also blocks $D_2$ receptors in the dorsal striatum, producing prominent and often very debilitating motor side effects, as seen in this patient. Newer neuroleptics have been developed (e.g., olanzepine, risperidone) that effectively control psychosis without causing debilitating motor side effects. The mechanism of their action is not yet clear. They may bind selectively to mesolimbic $D_2$ receptors without affecting striatal $D_2$ receptors, or they may bind to other dopamine receptors ($D_3$, $D_4$, or $D_5$) that may be important in modulating the activity of the mesolimbic system.*

There are even dopamine receptors outside the CNS. Although dopamine is produced in small quantities by the adrenal medulla, its role in normal physiology outside the CNS is unclear. However, peripheral dopamine receptors are engaged to good advantage by intensive care physicians seeking to increase blood pressure in a way that produces vasoconstriction in organ systems, such as muscle, that are relatively tolerant of low blood flow, but minimally affects blood flow to such vital organs as the heart, kidneys, and brain, at least at low to moderate doses.

### Noradrenergic Systems

Most of the noradrenergic projections to the cerebrum originate in a compact, darkly colored nucleus in the lateral pontine tegmentum, the locus ceruleus (Fig. 4-10). This nucleus projects diffusely to essentially every part of the cerebrum with the exception of the dorsal striatum. It is therefore even more difficult to delineate subsystems within this system than in the dopaminergic system. There is a small ventral noradrenergic system that originates in neurons in the lateral pontomesencephalic tegmentum and projects to the hypothalamus as well as to the brainstem and

spinal cord. Norepinephrine is also the neurotransmitter of the sympathetic autonomic nervous system, which will be reviewed in Chapter 11. There are two major families of noradrenergic receptors, $\alpha$ and $\beta$, each of which has a number of subtypes: $\alpha_1$ and $\alpha_2$, and $\beta_1$, $\beta_2$, and $\beta_3$.

### Serotonergic Systems

Serotonergic projections originate in a series of compact nuclei, known as the raphe nuclei, that lie in the midline of the brainstem tegmentum (Fig. 4-11). The most rostral of these, the dorsal raphe nucleus, projects to all structures in the cerebrum as well as to the cerebellum. More caudal raphe nuclei project to the spinal cord. At latest count, there are a total of seven families of 5-HT receptors, including 14 separate types.

## PRINCIPLES OF FUNCTION

Although the exact function of biogenic amine systems still remains uncertain, they exhibit several peculiar properties that provide important clues. First, we have already noted that they project widely to a host of func-

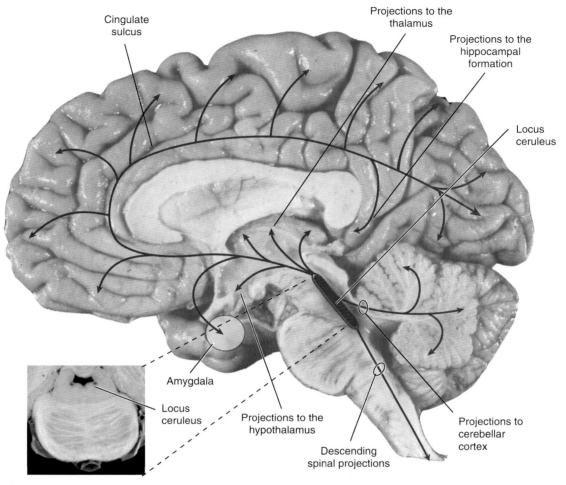

Cingulate
sulcus

Projections to the
thalamus

Projections to the
hippocampal
formation

Locus
ceruleus

Amygdala

Locus
ceruleus

Projections to the
hypothalamus

Descending
spinal projections

Projections to
cerebellar
cortex

**Figure 4-10** The central noradrenergic systems. Midline sagittal section demonstrating the projections. *Inset:* Axial section of the pons demonstrating the location of the noradrenergic neurons.

tionally disparate targets, a dramatic contrast to the neurotransmitter systems involved in neural signaling (e.g., glutamate), which are characterized by sharply focused projections. Second, each biogenic amine neuron may have over a million synaptic contacts, which is over one order of magnitude greater than for neurons in any signaling system. Finally, there is substantially less variability in the firing rates of biogenic amine neurons, suggesting that they tend to exert tonic influences rather than mediate information exchange. All these observations suggest that biogenic amine systems function as modulators of their target systems, perhaps serving to regulate the balance of functions between these systems.

Quite consistent with this concept, neurophysio-

logic studies have shown that biogenic amine systems act to regulate signal-to-noise ratio. This means that they increase or decrease the rate at which a neuron fires in response to an input, compared to the rate at which that neuron fires in response to background noise. Thus, biogenic amine systems might be viewed as serving to optimize the function of target systems. However, we are beginning to see that this is a simplistic view. You probably already have the sense that there are almost innumerable neural systems in the brain and perhaps you have wondered what maintains order in this "organ of Babel." Some evidence suggests that biogenic amine systems are among a number of systems that serve to maintain order, shifting the relative efficiency of different, potentially competing neural

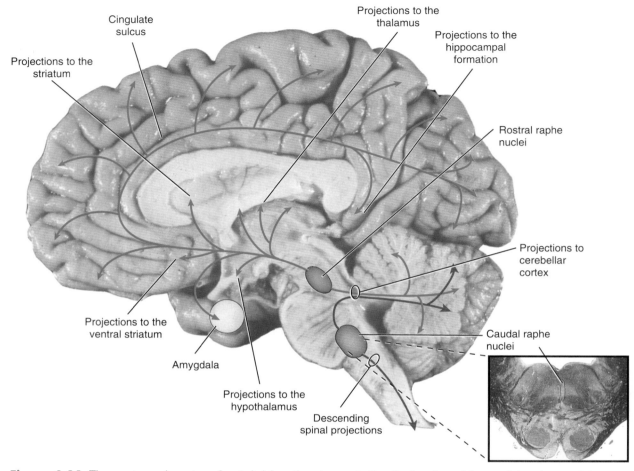

**Figure 4-11** The serotonergic system. *Inset:* Axial section demonstrating the location of the caudal raphae nuclei.

systems as the situation demands (see Chapter 12). The precise role of the host of different biogenic amine receptors remains very unclear, but these different receptor subtypes provide us enormous opportunity to manipulate the balance between competing cerebral systems from without through various drugs.

## PHARMACOLOGIC MANIPULATION

We conclude this section with some specific examples of pharmacologic manipulation of biogenic amine systems to treat certain disorders that illustrate the behavioral impact of these systems.

### *Case 4-12*

#### Parkinson's Disease
*A 60-year-old man develops a rotatory (pill rolling) tremor of his right arm, progressive stiffness of the arm (dystonia), and difficulty arising from a seated position. His writing has become very small (micrographia). He speaks much more softly (hypophonia). His physiognomy has become much less expressive (hypomimia or "masking of facies"). His stride has diminished (petit pas), and it takes him several steps to*

*make a turn while walking. He feels that his legs are stiff and weak. He tends to fall backward. A neurologist makes a diagnosis of Parkinson's disease and begins the patient on L-dopa. Within days, nearly all the patient's symptoms have resolved.*

**Comment:** *The cardinal manifestations of Parkinson's disease are caused by progressive loss of dopaminergic neurons in the substantia nigra. The*

## Case 4-12—cont'd

resulting reduction in dopamine levels in the putamen causes neurons in this structure to function in suboptimal fashion. As the putamen projects via a multisynaptic route to the supplementary motor area, premotor and motor cortex, the result is the motor dysfunction described (see Chapter 6). Dopamine administered systemically will not cross the blood-brain barrier. However, L-dopa readily crosses the blood-

brain barrier and, within the CNS, it is converted by aromatic L-amino acid decarboxylase to dopamine. Because dopamine has a more or less tonic influence on the putamen, the lost function of the endogenous source of dopamine in the substantia nigra can fairly readily be emulated through the exogenous supply of a dopamine precursor through pills.

## Case 4-13

### Depression

In the course of an annual physical, an internist notes that a 65-year-old woman appears depressed. She admits to persistent feelings of hopelessness. She feels she is nothing but a burden to her husband. She doesn't seem to enjoy anything anymore and finds that she is not looking forward to Christmas, even though she will be seeing her grandchildren then. She sleeps poorly, tending to wake up at 3 or 4 AM. Her appetite is diminished and she has lost 10 lb over the past 2 months. She has frequent crying spells. She denies suicidal ideation but wishes she could just quietly die. Her physician provides her a prescription for fluoxetine (Prozac), a drug that inhibits the reuptake of serotonin, thus increasing the concentration of this neurotransmitter

within the synaptic cleft and prolonging its action on postsynaptic neurons. When he sees her a month later, she is dramatically improved. She chats excitedly about travel plans she and her husband are making.

**Comment:** The precise mechanisms underlying depression continue to elude us (see Chapter 12). However, depression clearly implicates the limbic system, which receives heavy serotonergic and noradrenergic projections. Drugs that act to increase the synaptic concentrations of these neurotransmitters apparently ameliorate depression by altering the pathologic function of this system. These drugs include the tricyclic antidepressants and the newer serotonin-selective-reuptake inhibitors (SSRIs), such as fluoxetine.

## Case 4-14

### Migraine

A 23-year-old graduate student is seen in a neurology clinic for further evaluation of headaches. Headaches typically begin with the appearance of jagged yellow and black lines in her right visual field. Within 20 minutes, this visual aura gives way to a severe, pounding left hemicranial headache associated with nausea, vomiting, photophobia (aversion to light), and phonophobia (aversion to noise). She is unable to function in this state and seeks relief by lying down in the quiet and dark of her bedroom. Her physician provides her with a prescription for sumatriptan (Imitrex) and advises her to take two tablets as soon as the visual symptoms develop. She finds that she is able to prevent 90 percent of her headaches using this medication.

**Comment:** It has been shown in animal studies that spreading depression of Leao (see again Case 4-4), thought to be responsible for migrainous aura, is associated (by unknown mechanisms) with activation of the spinal nucleus of cranial nerve V, which subserves pain and temperature sensation to the face and most of the cranial cavity. This activation is linked to increased activity of trigeminal sensory neurons in the gasserian ganglion within the cavernous sinus and is associated with headache pain. As these neurons fire, they release a variety of vasoactive substances from their endings, which produce vasodilatation and increase the permeability of local microvasculature. The subsequent leakage of plasma constituents into the interstitial space stimulates further trigeminal neural firing, setting in motion a vicious circle. Remarkably,

*Continued*

Chemical Neurotransmission

## Case 4-14—cont'd

there are 5-HT$_{1D}$ receptors on these neural afferent terminals. Sumatriptan binds selectively to these terminals and inhibits release of the vasoactive proteins, thus preventing the vicious cycle from developing. The natural ligand for these receptors is not known and may not even exist. There may be hundreds or thousands of such "ligandless" receptor systems throughout the brain that have been left as the brain evolved new solutions to environmental demands. The migraine phenomenon illustrates, however, that they can be engaged to good advantage in the treatment of human disease.

## PRACTICE 4-8

**A.** Reserpine is a drug used to treat high blood pressure (hypertension) that is distinctive for its effectiveness and low cost ($0.01 per day). It can also be given as a single daily dose, which improves patient compliance. Reserpine acts by interfering with the storage of neurotransmitter within the synaptic vesicles of neurons employing biogenic amines. What major side effect might you expect with this drug? What effect would it have on patients with Parkinson's disease?

**B.** Review the synthesis and metabolism of dopamine. Suggest an alternative to the use of L-dopa or dopaminergic drugs in the treatment of Parkinson's disease. Could the same mechanism be employed to therapeutic advantage in depression? Blockade of neurotransmitter reuptake constitutes the primary current means for treating depression. Could an analogous approach be used to treat Parkinson's disease?

**C.** Aromatic L-amino acid decarboxylase, which among other things converts L-dopa to dopamine, is widely distributed in the body as well as in the catecholaminergic neurons of the CNS. Thus, when L-dopa is administered as pills, dopamine levels rise in the peripheral blood. Although systemic dopamine generally is not able to cross the blood-brain barrier, it does cross in a region of unusual permeability in the area postrema of the medulla, where it has the unfortunate effect of producing loss of appetite and nausea. In many patients with Parkinson's disease, this severely limits the amount of L-dopa that can be administered. Can you come up with a solution to this problem?

**D.** Tourette's syndrome is a disorder that typically first presents in childhood and is characterized by a propensity for making involuntary jerking movements of the extremities, facial grimaces, grunts (dyskinesias), and in a minority, coprolalia (involuntary expletives). Think carefully about the major features of Parkinson's disease and their response to dopaminergic agonists and the side effects of drugs used to treat schizophrenia, and suggest some potential treatments for Tourette's syndrome. What effect would L-dopa have on this disorder?

**E.** A 65-year-old man is found to have a large nonprolactin secreting pituitary tumor. Nevertheless, his serum prolactin levels are somewhat elevated. Explain why. (Hint: What effect did the tumor in Case 4-10 have on LH and FSH production?)

**F.** What are the major properties of biogenic amine systems that define them as modulatory rather than signaling systems?

**G.** List the ways in which dopaminergic systems could be manipulated to treat Parkinson's disease, dyskinesias, and psychosis.

**H.** Describe other ways in which noradrenergic and serotonergic systems could be manipulated to treat depression.

# Division IV

# A Transmitter Subserving Both Trans-System Modulatory and Neural Signaling Functions

# Cycle 4-9

# Acetylcholine

## Objectives

1. Be able to describe the synthesis and catabolism of acetylcholine.

2. Be able to locate the major concentrations of cholinergic neurons within the CNS.

3. Be able to describe the major disorders of the neuromuscular junction: myasthenia gravis, Eaton-Lambert syndrome, and botulism.

4. Be able to explain why anticholinergic drugs interfere with memory formation and why cholinomimetic drugs might alleviate symptoms of Alzheimer's disease.

Most choline comes from the hydrolysis of phosphatidylcholine (lecithin), a common lipid in cell membranes. Phosphatidylcholine can be synthesized in the brain but much of it is taken up by the brain from the plasma. Choline in the brain is acetylated by the enzyme choline-O-acetyltransferase (CAT), in conjunction with acetyl coenzyme A, to produce acetylcholine (Fig. 4-12). Acetylcholine is degraded within the synaptic cleft by acetylcholinesterase (AChE), regenerating choline, which is then taken up by the nerve endings by a specific, high-affinity system that serves as the rate-limiting step in acetylcholine synthesis.

Acetylcholine is employed primarily as a trans-system modulatory neurotransmitter within the CNS and as both a signaling and a trans-system modulatory neurotransmitter outside the CNS.

## CENTRAL NERVOUS SYSTEM FUNCTION

Within the CNS, there are high concentrations of cholinergic neurons within (1) the midbrain reticular formation (responsible for our level of wakefulness); (2) the basal ganglia (where their function is unclear); and (3) the basal forebrain (an area at the base of the frontal lobes just anterior to the hypothalamus, including the medial septal nuclei and the nucleus basalis of Meynert). The medial septal nuclei supply acetylcholine to the hippocampus, and the nucleus basalis supplies acetylcholine to the entire cerebral cortex. Through these projections, acetylcholine appears to play a crucial role in the alteration of neural connectivity in the cerebral cortex to form new memories. These memories include both facts (in which the hippocampus is critically involved) and motor skills. These aspects of cholinergic function will be discussed at greater length in Chapter 12. The effects of blocking CNS acetylcholine receptors are illustrated in Case 4-15.

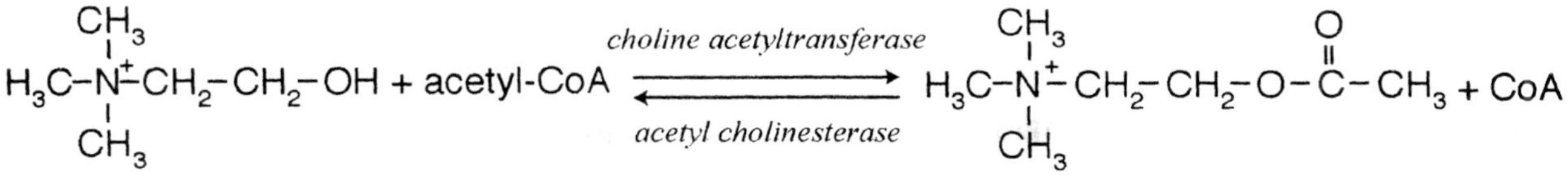

$$H_3C-\overset{CH_3}{\underset{CH_3}{N^+}}-CH_2-CH_2-OH + acetyl\text{-}CoA \underset{acetyl\ cholinesterase}{\overset{choline\ acetyltransferase}{\rightleftharpoons}} H_3C-\overset{CH_3}{\underset{CH_3}{N^+}}-CH_2-CH_2-O-\overset{O}{\overset{\|}{C}}-CH_3 + CoA$$

Choline                                   Acetylcholine

**Figure 4-12** Synthesis of acetylcholine.

## Case 4-15

### Memory Impairment due to Anticholinergic Drugs

*A 59-year-old man was found one evening in a 7–11 store, disoriented and apparently hallucinating, unable to say what he was doing there. He was brought to the emergency room. A drug patch was noted behind his right ear. On neurologic examination, he was somewhat inattentive and slightly drowsy, but he was cooperative and followed most commands. He did not know the date or where he was. He could repeat three words but recalled none of them after several minutes of distraction (indicating severely impaired memory acquisition). The remainder of the neurologic examination was normal. The drug patch was removed and he was admitted for observation.*

*The next morning he appeared better. He said he had flown to Gainesville from Buffalo, New York, the previous morning, to look for a place to live. He could recall little about the remainder of that day, but his recall was now three of three words. His son was*

*contacted in Buffalo and confirmed the patient's story. He reported that his father was a reformed alcoholic but had no other medical problems. On further questioning, the patient denied recent alcohol use. He did mention that he had severe motion sickness and had applied a scopolamine patch before he boarded the airplane the previous day.*

**Comment:** *Scopolamine is a potent anticholinergic drug both in the CNS and peripherally. In this patient, it affected receptors in the midbrain reticular formation, causing drowsiness and inattention, and in the hippocampus, causing impairment in recent memory and disorientation. This patient's history of alcohol abuse, which is commonly associated with damage to hippocampal memory systems (because of thiamine deficiency), may have made him particularly susceptible to these CNS effects of scopolamine (see Chapter 12). The elderly are also very susceptible, for poorly understood reasons.*

In patients with Alzheimer's disease, there is usually severe loss of acetylcholinergic neurons in the medial septal nuclei and in the nucleus basalis of Meynert. The resultant reduction in acetylcholine concentrations in the hippocampus and the cerebral cortex impairs the ability of these patients to learn. Increasing acetylcholine in these target structures, for example, by giving them an acetylcholinesterase inhibitor such as donepezil (Aricept) that penetrates the CNS, slows the decline in function in these patients, presumably by facilitating learning even as they lose knowledge in the course of the neurodegenerative process.

## PERIPHERAL FUNCTION

Outside the CNS, acetylcholine is a key neurotransmitter in the autonomic nervous system (discussed in Chapter 11), where its role might reasonably be viewed as modulatory. It is also the neurotransmitter at the neuromuscular junction, the point of synapse of motor neurons on muscle fibers, where its role is clearly one of neural signaling.

The two major classes of acetylcholine receptors are muscarinic and nicotinic (scopolamine is a muscarinic receptor blocker). Both are present in the CNS.

Chemical Neurotransmission

Acetylcholine receptors at the postsynaptic terminals of the parasympathetic autonomic nervous system are muscarinic and those at the postsynaptic terminals of the neuromuscular junctions and autonomic ganglia are nicotinic. There are five subtypes of muscarinic receptor and over 100 types of nicotinic receptor.

The neuromuscular junction is affected in a variety of disorders, as illustrated in Cases 4-16 and 4-17.

The history of medicine is replete with examples of toxins produced by various organisms, most notably bacteria and fungi, that are used to therapeutic advantage. The best examples are antibiotics and the potent immunosuppressive drug, cyclosporin, used to facilitate survival of organ transplants. Botulinum toxin is no exception, as Case 4-18 illustrates.

## Case 4-16

### Myasthenia Gravis

*In the early 1930s, Dr. Mary Walker, a Registrar (resident) at a hospital in London, admitted a patient with ptosis (drooping of the eyelids), diplopia (double vision), dysarthria (slurred speech), and weakness of proximal limb muscles. On the basis of the clinical findings, she suspected that the patient had myasthenia gravis. In reading about myasthenia, she found that the symptoms resembled those that had been reported in curare poisoning. She looked up the treatment of curare poisoning and found that physostigmine, an acetylcholinesterase inhibitor, was recommended. Her mentor, Derek Denny-Brown, strongly discouraged her from this line of thinking, insisting that the resemblance was only superficial. Nevertheless, she persevered and treated her patient with physostigmine. His strength improved dramatically. This attempt was the first successful treatment of a patient with myasthenia gravis.*

**Comment:** *Curare irreversibly blocks nicotinic acetylcholine receptors at the neuromuscular junction. In myasthenia gravis, these receptors are destroyed by an autoimmune mechanism. In either circumstance, the amount of acetylcholine normally released by the neuron at neuromuscular junctions is no longer sufficient to absolutely assure that sufficient membrane depolarization will occur in the muscle cell to precipitate an action potential and muscle contraction. Physostigmine is a reversible acetylcholinesterase inhibitor. By blocking acetylcholinesterase, it prolongs the duration of high concentrations of acetylcholine in the neuromuscular junction, increasing the probability that sufficient depolarization will occur in the muscle cell to assure an action potential. A congener of physostigmine, pyridostigmine is a mainstay in the treatment of patients with myasthenia gravis to this day.*

## Case 4-17

### Botulism

*A 42-year-old woman complains of several days of constipation, difficulty urinating, blurred vision, and double vision. She was previously in good health, independent, living alone on a small farm. Examination reveals decreased bowel sounds, mild abdominal distention, a normal mental status, and dilated pupils that react poorly to light or accommodation (as we look at something very close, our eyes become slightly crossed and our pupils constrict, i.e., we accommodate). Her visual acuity is normal, but extraocular movements are limited. There is bilateral*

*facial weakness and mild weakness of proximal extremity muscles. She is diagnosed with possible Guillain-Barré polyradiculoneuropathy (a disorder in which the myelin enveloping peripheral nerves and nerve roots is damaged via immune-mediated mechanisms), and is treated with plasmapheresis (a procedure by which immunoglobulins can be somewhat selectively removed from the blood). Over the first few days she gets weaker, but then she gradually recovers. After discharge, she expresses her gratitude by sending you a can of her home-grown string beans.*

## Case 4-17—cont'd

**Comment:** *Do not eat those beans! They are contaminated with Clostridium botulinum, an anaerobic bacterium that thrives in the low oxygen environment of canned food. It produces a potent toxin that disrupts the apparatus that captures acetylcholine vesicles in the cholinergic neuron terminal and fuses them to the membrane, leading to release of their contents into the synaptic space. Synapses with both nicotinic and muscarinic postsynaptic receptors are affected. Thus, patients experience weakness of ocular and systemic*

*muscles and a variety of autonomic effects (loss of pupillary reactivity and bowel motility, urinary retention). The disease may be fatal if not treated promptly with antibodies to the toxin. Quite remarkably, infants given "natural" or "raw" (unpasteurized) honey, which sometimes is contaminated with Clostridium botulinum, may colonize their bowels with the bacterium. By producing small amounts of toxin over weeks and months, it produces chronic weakness.*

## Case 4-18

### Spasmodic Dysphonia

*Over several years, a 38-year-old minister has experienced progressive difficulty with his voice, which sounds strained and high pitched, without resonance or volume. His general physical and neurologic examinations and all laboratory tests have been normal, and he has not benefited from prolonged psychotherapy. He feels that his career is in jeopardy and is extremely discouraged. An ear, nose, and throat physician finds normal-appearing vocal cords at rest. She diagnoses spasmodic dysphonia and injects a minuscule amount of botulinum toxin into each thyroarytenoid muscle. Two days later, the minister's voice is normal.*

**Comment:** *This patient has one of a large variety of focal dystonias, disorders characterized by excessive activity in certain muscle groups and cocontraction of agonists and antagonists. In this case, however, the excessive tone is predominantly in the cricoarytenoid*

*muscles, which tend to maintain the vocal cords in excessive adduction, narrowing the space through which air passes and causing the voice to be high pitched and "tight" sounding. Weakening these muscles with botulinum toxin injections helps to restore the normal balance between vocal cord abductors and adductors, with corresponding normalization of the voice. Focal dystonias were until quite recently almost uniformly ascribed to psychiatric disease. We now know they are neurologic disorders. They most often develop with extremely sustained repetitive use of a muscle, as is often seen with professional pianists and violinists (finger flexors and intrinsic hand muscles), but may be seen in public speakers and even in association with extensive handwriting (writer's cramp). Their neurologic basis is poorly understood but will be discussed in Chapter 6. The reason for the persistence of the therapeutic effects of botulinum toxin injection are also poorly understood.*

**Chemical Neurotransmission**

## PRACTICE 4-9

**A.** Acetylcholine is unique among the nonpeptide neurotransmitters in the way that its action is terminated. Why?

**B.** Where are the major concentrations of acetylcholine in the nervous system?

**C.** Describe the major disorders of the neuromuscular junction.

**D.** Over-the-counter remedies for symptoms of the common cold contain antihistamines, which have prominent anticholinergic effects. Explain why you should simply endure your cold symptoms when studying for a test.

**E.** Would you predict that patients with myasthenia gravis, Eaton-Lambert syndrome, and botulism would have memory and cognitive impairment? Why?

**F.** Edrophonium (Tensilon) is an acetylcholinesterase inhibitor that has an approximately 2-minute duration of action. Can you think of a use for this drug in myasthenia gravis?

**G.** Myasthenia gravis is caused by the genesis of circulating antibodies to nicotinic acetylcholine receptors at the neuromuscular junction. There are also nicotinic acetylcholine receptors at the autonomic ganglia.

Predict the results of an autoimmune disease characterized by the genesis of antibodies to these receptors. How would you treat this disease?

**H.** Now that you have had a chance to gain an overview of chemical neurotransmission, describe the differences between neural signaling, within-system neural modulation, and trans-system neural modulation, and give examples of each.

## CYCLE 4-1

**A.** Synthesis, storage, release, reception, inactivation.

**B.** Ligand-gated ionophores, ligand-gated voltage-dependent ionophores, voltage-dependent ionophores, metabotropic (G-protein-linked) receptors.

**C.** Reuptake, catabolism, diffusion.

## CYCLE 4-2

**A.** Synthesis: a-ketoglutarate. Catabolism: reverse of synthesis; decarboxylation to GABA. Termination by reuptake, diffusion. Catabolic enzymes are intracellular.

**B.** Ligand-gated channels are ionophores that are opened by the ligand and then automatically close a short time later. Metabotropic receptors activate G-proteins, which set in motion sequences of biochemical reactions.

**C.** Cerebral neurons providing corticocortical, corticobulbar, and corticospinal projections.

**D.** Neural signaling and altering the strength of neural connections in the signaling systems, the basis for learning and memory. Signaling is achieved primarily through ligand-gated sodium channels (AMPA and kainate). Learning is accomplished primarily through NMDA receptor-gated sodium/calcium channels.

**E.** Phenytoin, carbamazepine, and lamotrigine block voltage-gated sodium channels that are not dependent on ligand binding in a rate-dependent way. This inhibits high frequency discharges contributing to seizures, but permits the lower frequency discharges of normal neuronal function.

**F.** It would block the uncontrolled calcium influx that ultimately activates degradative intracellular enzyme systems. Chronic administration would seriously disrupt learning and memory formation.

**G.** Even in the presence of normal oxygenation, the excitotoxic effects of sustained epileptiform discharges rapidly eventuate in brain damage. It is generally thought that this begins to occur with 30 to 40 minutes of continuous seizures. Therefore, both generalized and partial status epilepticus are treated as medical emergencies. GABA agonists, such as lorazepam, which very rapidly achieve therapeutic concentrations in the CNS and inhibit neural firing, are given acutely. Unfortunately, seizures will rapidly recur unless longer-acting anticonvulsants, such as phenytoin, are also administered. Phenytoin effectively reduces the rate of neuronal discharge associated with massive glutamate release and thus inhibits the spread of seizure discharges.

## CYCLE 4-3

**A.** Synthesis from glutamate via glutamic acid decarboxylase. Catabolism via GABA-transaminase. Termination of action through reuptake via a specific carrier-mediated transport mechanism.

**B.** Interneurons throughout the brain. The basal ganglia (the majority of neurons) and the cerebellum (Purkinje cells).

**C.** Inhibitory neural signaling. Mediated via potentiation of chloride channel conductance or potassium channel conductance, both of which hyperpolarize the postsynaptic neurons and inhibit the generation of an action potential.

**D.** By hyperpolarizing neurons, they inhibit the rapid neuronal discharges underlying seizure activity.

**E.** Because alcohol is GABA-mimetic, chronic use leads to downregulation of GABA receptors. Cessation of alcohol consumption then leads to a generalized state of insufficient inhibition within the CNS that can be corrected in part by potentiating GABA effects at remaining GABA receptors.

**F.** Potentiate inhibitory GABAergic neurotransmission. Acutely this can be done with agents like lorazepam. Lorazepam is in fact the first line of treatment in status epilepticus, rapidly bringing seizures under control so that the patient can be intubated, blood drawn for further studies, and intravenous lines placed. Unfortunately, lorazepam has a very short duration of action, probably because it is rapidly redistributed such that effective concentrations are no longer maintained in the vicinity of neurons caught up in the epileptic process. Thus, for long-term management, drugs such as phenobarbital that provide more sustained potentiation of GABA actions may be used.

## CYCLE 4-4

**A.** Interneurons in the brainstem and spinal cord.

**B.** Inhibitory neural signaling.

**C.** Marked generalized increase in muscle tone, further potentiated by any stimulus.

## CYCLE 4-5

**A.** Peptide neurotransmitters are formed through proteolytic cleavage of precursor proteins synthesized by rough endoplasmic reticulum in the cell body, transported down the axon to synaptic endings, released in the course of synaptic transmission, and degraded by extracellular proteases.

**B.** Chronic high-intensity stimulation of neurotransmitter receptors leads to a reduction in the number of receptors. When that high level stimulation ceases, an acute state of understimulation occurs. When inhibitory receptors are downregulated, a withdrawal syndrome characterized by excessive excitation occurs: severe anxiety, tremulousness, and seizures in the case of GABA receptors (following alcohol or barbiturate withdrawal); agitation and severe autonomic hyperactivity in the case of opioid receptors.

**C.** A ligand is said to be nonspecific when it binds to a given type of receptor within multiple different systems. Thus, naloxone administered to alleviate respiratory depression in opiate overdose also blocks opiate receptors throughout the nervous system, precipitating severe symptoms of opiate withdrawal in the drug-dependent patient. Much neuropharmacologic research involves efforts to develop ligands of greater specificity, hence a narrow range of actions.

## CYCLE 4-6

**A.** The presence of dopamine-β-hydroxylase.

**B.** A reuptake inhibitor, because reuptake is the primary means by which catecholamine activity at

receptors is terminated. Contrast, for example, the dramatic effects of cocaine, a drug that blocks the dopamine reuptake transporter, with the rather subtle effects of MAO and COMT inhibitors that are used in the treatment of Parkinson's disease.

## CYCLE 4-8

**A.** Approximately 20 percent of patients given reserpine develop depression, at least partially as a result of depletion of serotonin. Because reserpine also depletes dopamine, it aggravates symptoms of Parkinson's disease.

**B.** Dopamine is metabolized by MAO and COMT. Therefore, drugs that inhibit these enzymes should, at least theoretically, increase the amount of available dopamine in the synaptic cleft. The drug selegiline (also known as deprenyl or Eldepryl) selectively inhibits the subtype of MAO found at dopaminergic synapses, MAO-B, and improves symptoms of Parkinson's disease. The COMT inhibitor entacapone (Comtan) also appears to be clinically beneficial. MAO also metabolizes serotonin and MAO inhibitors have been used for many years as effective antidepressants. Unfortunately, MAO metabolizes a large number of different biogenic amines and when it is inhibited, these amines may build up to toxic concentrations, causing potentially serious side effects such as hypertensive crises. Patients taking MAO inhibitors must avoid consuming such things as alcoholic beverages, cheese, yogurt, and preserved meats such as delicatessen meat (presumably because they contain tyramine, which is thought to mediate these toxic effects), and they must limit chocolate and caffeine intake.

Blockade of neurotransmitter reuptake theoretically would be a very effective way of treating Parkinson's disease. Unfortunately, the only drug available that blocks the dopamine reuptake transporter is cocaine, clearly not a viable therapeutic agent.

**C.** The solution is to combine L-dopa with an inhibitor of aromatic L-amino acid decarboxylase that does not cross the blood-brain barrier. In this way, L-dopa is not converted to dopamine until it gets into the brain. L-Dopa is now universally administered in combination with just such an inhibitor, carbidopa (which cannot cross the blood-brain barrier). This reduces the total amount of L-dopa that must be given, as most of the administered dose is sequestered in the brain as dopamine, and it increases the amount of dopamine that can be tolerated before nausea and anorexia develop.

**D.** Akinesia in Parkinson's disease is caused by dopamine deficiency in the putamen. The treatment of schizophrenia with dopamine receptor blockers such as haloperidol produces akinesia as a side effect. Thus, a good guess would be that drugs that interfere with dopaminergic transmission might be of benefit in patients with dyskinesia. In fact, both pimozide, a dopaminergic receptor blocker, and reserpine, which depletes dopamine from neural endings, have been used to good effect in the treatment of Tourette's syndrome. L-Dopa would worsen the symptoms of Tourette's syndrome.

**E.** The tumor has damaged the dopaminergic projections from the hypothalamus that normally inhibit prolactin secretion by the pituitary just as the tumor in Case 4-10 interfered with hypothalamic stimulation of pituitary LH and FSH production.

**F.** (1) Wide projection to functionally disparate targets; (2) very large number of synaptic contacts per neuron; (3) less variability in firing rates than signaling neurons.

**G.** Parkinson's disease: give L-dopa to directly increase dopamine; use a dopamine receptor agonist, such as bromocriptine; inhibit dopamine catabolism using MAO or COMT inhibitors; block dopamine reuptake with cocaine.

Dyskinesias, psychosis: block dopamine receptors with neuroleptics such as haloperidol or olanzepine, deplete synaptic vesicles of dopamine with reserpine or inhibit release of dopamine (not possible at this time).

**H.** Inhibit norepinephrine and serotonin reuptake using tricyclic antidepressants or SSRIs, inhibit MAO, directly stimulate appropriate norepinephrine and serotonin receptors (not possible at this time), potentiate release of norepinephrine with amphetamine (usually undesirable because of side effects).

## CYCLE 4-9

**A.** The action of all the other major nonpeptide neurotransmitters is terminated primarily by reuptake and to some extent by diffusion. The action of acetylcholine is terminated by catabolism by an extracellular, intrasynaptic enzyme, acetylcholinesterase.

**B.** Midbrain reticular formation, basal ganglia, medial septal nuclei, nucleus basalis, anterior horn cells of spinal cord (which innervate muscles), first-order neurons in the autonomic nervous system, which project from the CNS to the autonomic ganglia, and second-order neurons of the parasympathetic nervous system.

**C.** Blockade of acetylcholine release through binding to the synaptic vesicle mobilization mechanism (botulinum toxin) or immunologic destruction of voltage-sensitive calcium channels on nerve endings (Eaton-Lambert syndrome—review Case 4-1).

Blockade of nicotinic neuromuscular acetylcholine receptors (curare poisoning, muscle relaxation during general anesthesia with succinyl choline), or immunologic destruction of these receptors (myasthenia gravis).

Inactivation of acetylcholinesterase (organophosphate poisoning).

**D.** These drugs penetrate the CNS and block acetylcholine receptors in the hippocampus, thus interfering with recent memory formation. Scopolamine is often given to women during labor and delivery for sedative effect and to prevent them from later recalling the suffering associated with childbirth.

**E.** In principle, these disorders could be associated with cognitive and memory impairment. However, fortunately, neither botulinum toxin nor the antibodies that cause myasthenia gravis and Eaton-Lambert syndrome are capable of crossing the blood-brain barrier.

**F.** The duration of action of edrophonium is far too short for it to have value in the treatment of myasthenia. However, it provides a very handy diagnostic tool. A number of disorders can mimic myasthenia gravis. A dramatic response to edrophonium injection can be very helpful in distinguishing myasthenia from these other disorders.

**G.** Patients with this disorder have symptoms of generalized autonomic dysfunction—orthostatic hypotension, severe constipation, dry mouth, impotence, and reduced sweating (as in Case 4-1). They can be treated in precisely the same manner as patients with myasthenia gravis—with acetylcholinesterase inhibitors.

The existence of these two distinct diseases is explained by the fact that nicotinic receptors are composed of multiple subunits (2 $\alpha$, a $\beta$, a $\delta$, and a $\gamma$). The nicotinic receptors at the neuromuscular junction have $\alpha_1$ subunits whereas those at the autonomic ganglia

*Chemical Neurotransmission*

have $\alpha_3$ subunits. The antibodies generated in these two diseases are specific to one type of $\alpha$ subunit. Many patients with autoimmune ganglionopathy have an occult (inapparent) underlying cancer. Evidently, the cancer cells express an epitope quite similar to a site on the $\alpha_3$ subunit. Remarkably, just as there were tribes of South American Indians (originally discovered by Sir Walter Raleigh) that coated their arrow tips with curare (an alkaloid derived from plants of the genus Strychnos that binds irreversibly to neuromuscular acetylcholine receptors), there was also a tribe that used epibatidine, a toxin derived from a frog (the "poison arrow" frog) that irreversibly binds to autonomic acetylcholine receptors.

**H.** See Introduction to this chapter. Neural signaling underlies the communication of information from one set of neurons to another. Transmitters involved in neural signaling are uniformly capable of eliciting (e.g., glutamate) or suppressing (e.g., GABA, glycine) action potentials in postsynaptic neurons (depending on the part of those neurons contacted by the synapse—to be discussed in the next chapter). In some neural systems (e.g., the thalamus) the transmission of information may be so complete that under certain circumstances, there is nearly a one-to-one relationship between input and output neural discharges. Neurotransmitters involved in within-system neural modulation (e.g., neuropeptides) tend to have less specific effects (they have longer half-lives and tend to diffuse further), and they are generally not capable of eliciting action potentials in postsynaptic neurons, only of modulating the effects of neural signaling transmitters. Neurotransmitters involved in trans-system neural modulation (e.g., dopamine, norepinephrine, serotonin) share properties with those involved in within-system neural modulation. However, they are produced by tiny concentrations of cells located mainly in the brainstem (dopamine: substantia nigra/ventral tegmental area and hypothalamus; norepinephrine: locus ceruleus; serotonin: raphe nuclei), each of which projects to extensive regions within the cerebrum, if not to the entire cerebrum. They apparently serve to regulate the balance of functions between these systems.

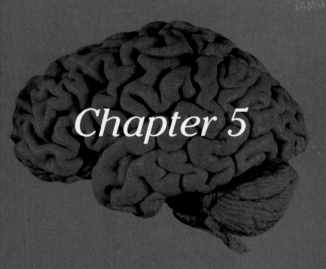

# Chapter 5

# NEUROPHYSIOLOGY

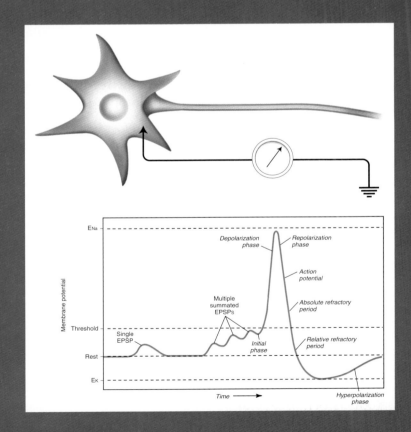

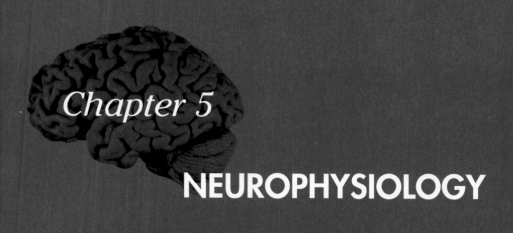

# *Chapter 5*

# NEUROPHYSIOLOGY

# Introduction

In Chapter 4 we introduced concepts such as excitation, inhibition, neural depolarization, and action potentials. We discussed in general terms how neurons intercommunicate through the release of neurotransmitters, which interact with receptors linked either to ion channels or to enzyme-linked secondary messenger systems (e.g., cyclic AMP). In this chapter we will describe the principles underlying the electrical events set in motion by chemical neurotransmission.

Table 5-1 provides a list of definitions that may be useful to you as you read this chapter. In Cycle 5-1, a number of equations are introduced as an aid to understanding, and as a demonstration that neural membrane events are sufficiently well understood to be definable in precise, mathematical terms. However, you will be expected to understand the material in this chapter only at the conceptual level.

## TABLE 5-1 Definitions

*Membrane potential:* An electrical potential across the cell membrane. All live cells possess a membrane potential.

*Excitable cell:* A cell that, in vivo, can use rapid changes in the membrane potential as a means for signaling or work, e.g., neurons, muscle cells.

*Potential:* When applied to electrical systems, refers to a difference in charge between two points in a circuit, usually across a resistor. This difference creates a "potential" for movement of the charge (current), which is also a "potential" for work.

*Current:* The movement of electrical charges (see also ions).

*Resistor:* A material that offers resistance to the movement of charge. This term is usually applied to a part of a circuit that is designed to use the potential across it, and the current that moves through it as a result of the potential, to do work. A material with infinite resistance is an insulator or dielectric.

*Capacitor:* A material that can store charge. It usually has two very closely apposed parts of the same circuit separated by a dielectric (insulator).

*Ions:* Charged atoms. Ions are biologic charge carriers. Electrons are charge carriers in electrical systems. Movement of charges (current) in biologic systems is movement of ions.

*Hyperpolarization/depolarization:* The change in membrane potential of a neuron is labeled in reference to the resting membrane potential, not in reference to electrical neutrality or zero volts.
   Hyperpolarization: To be made more negative than the resting potential.
   Depolarization: To be made more positive than the resting potential.

*Concentration gradient:* A difference in concentration of a substance across a space. The laws of diffusion state that the material will move to become equally distributed in the whole of the space.

*Electrical potential:* A capacity for work produced by the drive of charges in an electrical gradient to move down the gradient until they are equally distributed and the gradient disappears.

*Permeability:* The readiness with which a membrane allows the movement of atoms or molecules, charged or uncharged, through it.

*Conductance:* The readiness with which an ion is able to pass through a membrane. The inverse of resistance.

*Action potential:* The rapid reversal of the membrane potential in an area of a cell or axon caused by change in the permeability of the membrane to sodium and potassium ions over a short period of time.

*Threshold:* The membrane potential at which voltage-gated sodium channels undergo the conformation shift that markedly enhances the permeability of the membrane to sodium ions and thereby initiates the cascade of events underlying the action potential.

*Equilibrium potential:* The potential at which the electrical force produced by charge separation across a membrane exactly counterbalances the chemical diffusion force exerted on a specific ion due to the concentration gradient of that ion across the membrane. At the equilibrium potential, there is no net flux of the ion across the membrane.

*Driving force:* The cumulative force exerted on an ion by both diffusion and electrical forces. The driving force varies as the membrane potential changes, and it is zero at the equilibrium potential of an ion.

# The Neural Membrane Potential

### Objective

Be able to understand and explain the mechanisms underlying the neural membrane potential.

Let us begin with the simplest possible conceptualization of a neuron: a balloon full of a dilute ionic solution that is immersed within a somewhat different ionic solution. The walls of the balloon consist of a membrane composed of a bilayer of phospholipid molecules. In the most thermodynamically stable configuration, the phospholipid molecules are aligned with their hydrophobic lipid components in the center of the membrane and their hydrophilic phosphate groups facing outward to contact the ionic solutions inside and outside the cell (Fig. 5-1).

Let us also assume that the ionic solution within the neuron has a potassium concentration [K⁺] of 155 millimolar (mM) and a [Cl⁻] of 4 mM. The ionic solution outside the neural balloon has a [K⁺] of 4 mM and a [Cl⁻] of 120 mM. We will assume the additional presence of sufficient appropriately charged particles other than K⁺ and Cl⁻ inside the cell (151 mM net concentration of negative charges) and outside the cell (116 mM net concentration of positive charges) that there is no net charge either inside or out.

Because a phospholipid bilayer is impermeable to all ions, the primitive neuron we have constructed will have no transmembrane potential, that is, there will be no voltage difference between the inside and the outside of the neural membrane. Using Ohm's law,

$$V = IR$$

where $V$ = voltage, $I$ = current, and $R$ = resistance, we see that with $I = 0$, $V$ will be 0.

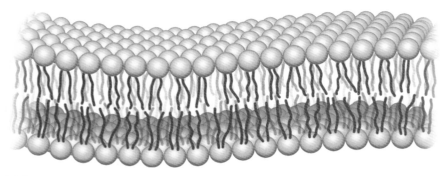

**Figure 5-1** A phospholipid bilayer membrane.

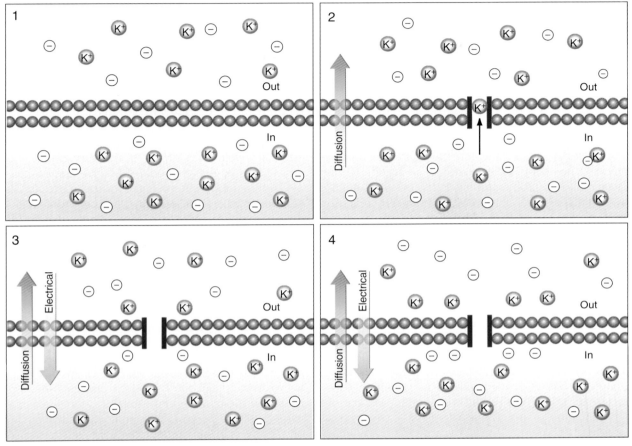

**Figure 5-2** Ionic environment in the immediate vicinity of the neural membrane following the insertion of channels permeable to potassium. In panel 1, the membrane is impermeable to potassium, with more potassium ions located inside the cell. Following the insertion of a potassium-permeable channel (2), the diffusion force moves the potassium out of the cell, creating an electrical force (3) directed toward the inside of the cell. Equilibrium is reached (4) when the force created by diffusion equals the electrical force.

Suppose, however, that we insert in the bilayer some barrel-shaped multiunit protein complexes that form channels through the membrane that allow the passage of potassium ions with relatively low resistance (high conductance). These ions will then begin to flow down their concentration gradient from inside the cell to outside the cell. However, very soon after this flow begins, it will be halted because the movement of positively charged ions from inside to outside begins to generate a net negative charge within the cell. At this point, the force generated by the concentration gradient (pushing K$^+$ ions out) is exactly balanced by the electrical gradient (pulling K$^+$ ions in). Look at what has happened to the ionic environment in the immediate vicinity of the neural membrane as these events take place (Fig. 5-2).

The incipient flow of potassium ions down their concentration gradient has generated a charge separation at the membrane. This occurs only at the membrane—the electrical gradient that is immediately generated by this ion movement prevents the flow of sufficient ions to cause an imbalance in charge between the inside and the outside of the cell. Because the number of ions that moves is very small and because the movement is restricted to the immediate vicinity of the membrane, there is no measurable change in ion concentrations within either the intracellular or the extracellular fluid. The charge separation present at the membrane generates the *equilibrium potential*. The size of the equilibrium potential can be calculated using an equation derived by Nernst, a German electrochemist:

$$E_K = \left(2.306 \frac{RT}{zF}\right)\log_{10}\left(\frac{[K^+]_o}{[K^+]_i}\right)$$

where $R$ is the ideal gas constant, $T$ is the temperature in degrees Kelvin, $F$ is the Faraday constant, $z$ is the ionic valence (=1 for potassium), $[K^+]_o$ is the concentration of potassium outside the cell, and $[K^+]_i$ is the concentration of potassium inside the cell. The quantity $2.306RT/zF$ is equal to $61\,mV$ at body temperature. Given $[K^+]_o = 4$ and $[K^+]_i = 155$, $E_K = -97\,mV$. That is, the potential inside the cell produced by the potassium concentration gradient is negative relative to outside the cell. The Nernst equation defines in mathematical terms the point at which electrical forces across the membrane, generated by charge separation, are exactly balanced by chemical forces, generated by the difference in ion concentration between the inside and the outside of the cell.

This highly simplified "neuron" actually more closely resembles a glial cell because in glia, the membrane potential is defined mainly by potassium conductance. Glia have a resting membrane potential of approximately $-90\,mV$. The situation in a real neuron is somewhat more complicated because there are three major ions—potassium, sodium, and chloride—and the membrane is more or less permeable to all three of these ions at any given time. Consequently, the actual membrane potential of a real neuron is never able to actually reach the equilibrium potential of any one ion. Rather, a steady-state *resting membrane potential* is produced that is jointly defined by all three ions. The degree to which a particular ion contributes to the

membrane potential depends on how permeable the membrane is to that ion, that is, how many ionophores specific to that ion are open. In neurons in their resting state, the membrane is most permeable to potassium, far less so to sodium. Thus, the resting membrane potential is far closer to the equilibrium potential of potassium than that of sodium. The neural membrane is also permeable to chloride. However, if we used the Nernst equation to calculate the equilibrium potential generated by chloride ions (see Table 5-2), we would arrive at a value of $-90\,mV$, that is, very close to the equilibrium potential of potassium. We can calculate the resting membrane potential for this more realistic neuron in which the resting membrane potential is defined jointly by three ions, each with its own permeability, using the Goldman-Hodgkin-Katz equation:

$$E_M = \left(2.306 \frac{RT}{zF}\right)\log_{10}\left(\frac{P_K[K^+]_o + P_{Na}[Na^+]_o + P_{Cl}[Cl^-]_i}{P_K[K^+]_i + P_{Na}[Na^+]_i + P_{Cl}[Cl^-]_o}\right)$$

This equation says that the resting membrane potential is, in effect, the permeability-weighted average of the equilibrium potentials for the three ions. Using the values in Table 5-2 and filling in the relative permeabilities of the three ions, $E_M$ can be calculated to be approximately $-70\,mV$. Potassium and chloride, with their high membrane permeabilities, strongly push $E_M$ toward $-90\,mV$. Sodium, with an equilibrium potential of $+66\,mV$ but low membrane permeability, weakly pushes $E_M$ in the opposite direction, leaving us with a net $E_M$ of $-70\,mV$.

## PRACTICE 5-1

**A.** Assume that the very simple neuron we introduced at the beginning of this cycle is highly permeable to

---

**TABLE 5-2 Concentration and Equilibrium Potentials of Three Major Ions***

| Ion | Extracellular Concentration (mM) | Intracellular Concentration (mM) | Equilibrium Potential (mV) |
|---|---|---|---|
| Na$^+$ | 145 | 12 | +66 |
| K$^+$ | 4 | 155 | −97 |
| Cl$^-$ | 120 | 4 | −90 |

*These concentrations and equilibrium potentials were calculated using the Nernst equation and are for major ions involved in neuronal electrochemical activity. Both inside and outside the cell, there are anions (negatively charged ions) such as amino acids, inorganic phosphate, and proteins, that cannot pass through the membrane and serve to exactly balance the apparent excess of positive charges supplied by sodium and potassium ions. Thus, *there is no net charge either inside or outside the cell.*

chloride, but not to potassium. Also assume the ion concentrations listed in Table 5-2. Draw the neural membrane, indicate the direction of the ion gradient, and illustrate the transmembrane charge separation induced by the force of the chloride concentration gradient. Use the Nernst equation to confirm that the equilibrium potential for this neuron is indeed approximately −90 mV, as noted earlier in this cycle. Is the potential inside the membrane positive or negative relative to the outside? Why?

**B.** In the last paragraph of Cycle 5-1, we said that for a neuronal membrane permeable to multiple ions, the resting membrane potential will be closest to the equilibrium potentials of the ions with the greatest conductance. This intuitively makes sense, but in this problem you are going to demonstrate this mathematically. Let us assume that the neural membrane is permeable only to sodium and potassium. Start with Ohm's law:

$$V = IR$$

It turns out to be easier to conceptualize the problem if we think in terms of conductance $(g)$, which is the inverse of resistance $(R)$. Thus:

$$V_{Na^+} = I_{Na^+}\left(\frac{1}{g_{Na^+}}\right) = \frac{I_{Na^+}}{g_{Na^+}}$$

$$V_{K^+} = I_{K^+}\left(\frac{1}{g_{K^+}}\right) = \frac{I_{K^+}}{g_{K^+}}$$

What is the voltage (or force) driving Na⁺ ions or K⁺ ions? At the Na⁺ equilibrium potential (+66 mV), there is zero net force on Na⁺ ions because the force derived from the concentration gradient is exactly counterbal-

anced by the force derived from the electrical gradient. However, at the resting membrane potential of −70 mV, Na⁺ ions are driven inward, both by the force derived from their concentration gradient and the force derived from the strong electrical gradient, as Na⁺ ions are attracted to the negative charge on the inside of the membrane. The strength of this combined force will be equal to the difference between the resting membrane potential and the Na⁺ equilibrium potential. Thus,

$$V_{Na^+} = E_M - E_{Na^+}$$

And therefore:

$$E_M - E_{Na^+} = \frac{I_{Na^+}}{g_{Na^+}}$$

And by the same token:

$$E_M - E_{K^+} = \frac{I_{K^+}}{g_{K^+}}$$

At the resting membrane potential $(E_M)$, will there be a net flow of charge across the membrane? Remember, at the resting membrane potential, the cell is in a steady state. What does this tell you about the sum of the inward and outward currents, $I_{Na^+} + I_{K^+}$ at $E_M$? State your answer to this question as an equation involving $I_{Na^+}$ and $I_{K^+}$. Now solve the two equations immediately above for $I_{Na^+}$ and $I_{K^+}$, respectively, and plug the results into your equation involving $I_{Na^+}$ and $I_{K^+}$. Solve this equation for $E_M$. What does this equation tell you about which ion will be the chief determinant of $E_M$? If $g_{K^+} = 20g_{Na^+}$ (the normal situation in a neural membrane at rest), will $E_M$ be closer to $E_{K^+}$ or to $E_{Na^+}$?

# Cycle 5-2

## Neural Transmission and the Action Potential

### Objectives

1. Describe the sequence of molecular and ionic events underlying the action potential.
2. Be able to explain why action potentials are necessary for neural transmission.

The neuron we have envisaged so far provides a reasonable accounting for the resting membrane potential. However, it does not provide any obvious mechanisms by which neurons might communicate with each other. The problem lies in our assumptions about the protein structures, ionophores, that provide the basis for ion conductance. We have so far viewed them simply as holes in the membrane that allow the selective passage of certain ions. In fact, ionophores are extraordinarily complex structures. The detailed understanding that we now have of some of them represents one of the major triumphs of molecular biology.

In Chapter 4, Chemical Neurotransmission, we introduced the concept that the permeability of ion channels is variable and can be regulated. For example, certain sodium channels are "opened"—they undergo a change in conformation that markedly increases sodium conductance—when glutamate binds to its receptors on these channels. These are called *ligand-gated channels*. Other channels are opened solely by a critical change in the membrane voltage. A good

example of a *voltage-gated channel* is the N-type calcium ionophore on axonal endings that, in response to membrane depolarization, allows the influx of calcium needed to mediate the release of neurotransmitter (see Case 4-1 for an example of a disease, Eaton-Lambert syndrome, in which such channels are destroyed by the immune system). Still other channels require both the presence of a neurotransmitter and a critical change in membrane voltage—*voltage-sensitive ligand-gated channels*. A good example is the glutamate-gated NMDA sodium-calcium channel (discussed in Chemical Neurotransmission as critical both to neural transmission and to the alteration of neuronal connection strengths underlying learning).

## NEUROPHYSIOLOGY OF THE ACTION POTENTIAL

We are now prepared to consider the sequence of chemical and electrical events underlying neural transmission. The sequence begins with the release of an excitatory neurotransmitter (e.g., glutamate) by presynaptic neurons. Each vesicle of released neurotransmitter delivers a quantity of neurotransmitter to the postsynaptic membrane that binds to ligand-gated sodium channel receptors. The conductance of these channels is transiently increased, allowing Na$^+$ to flow into the cell, down its electrical and concentration gradients. This flow slightly drives the membrane potential toward the sodium equilibrium potential (+66 mV) (see

**TABLE 5-3** Summary of Postsynaptic Potentials

| Feature | Excitatory Postsynaptic Potentials | Inhibitory Postsynaptic Potentials |
|---|---|---|
| Action on membrane | Depolarization | Hyperpolarization |
| Current flow | Inward flow of cations | Outward flow of cations or inward flow of anions |
| Ions commonly involved | $Na^+$, $Ca^{2+}$ | $K^+$, $Cl^-$ |
| Major neurotransmitters mediating effect | Glutamate | GABA, glycine |

Table 5-1) and partially depolarizes the membrane by making it more positive. The degree of depolarization elicited by the binding of the contents of all the vesicles released by a presynaptic terminal is called an *excitatory postsynaptic potential (EPSP)*. An inhibitory neurotransmitter, such as GABA, would hyperpolarize the membrane by eliciting an *inhibitory postsynaptic potential or IPSP* (Table 5-3). Note: A neurotransmitter is not intrinsically excitatory or inhibitory. Rather, it is the effect that a neurotransmitter has on postsynaptic membrane receptors that defines it as excitatory or inhibitory. Thus, glutamate is excitatory because it happens to bind to channels ($Na^+$ or $Ca^{2+}$) that, when opened, will depolarize the membrane.

Figure 5-3 illustrates a single EPSP, which depolarizes the membrane by approximately 10 mV (actual EPSPs are much smaller). Notice that the EPSP is transient because the sodium channels only open briefly (i.e., change their conformation only briefly). If a sufficient number of EPSPs occurs sufficiently synchronously, the individual depolarizations will summate, producing a much larger depolarization (Fig. 5-3, multiple summated EPSPs). If this larger depolarization exceeds the critical *threshold* necessary to change the conformation of *voltage-sensitive sodium channels* (about −55 mV or 15 mV above the resting membrane potential), they will open as a group for about 0.5 ms. This period is the *initiation phase* of the action potential. The tremendous increase in sodium conductance associated with these events will allow sodium ions to flow down both their chemical concentration and electrical gradients and strongly drive the membrane potential toward the sodium equilibrium potential of +66 mV (see Fig. 5-3). This is the *depolarization phase* of the action potential. The action potential is transient for two reasons: (1) the rapid accumulation of positive charge inside the membrane induces a change in the sodium channel protein that inactivates it and prevents further

sodium ion flow; and (2) the large membrane depolarization, after a slight delay, also opens up voltage-sensitive potassium channels. These channels are sensitive to depolarization, like voltage-sensitive sodium channels, but as a group they have slower kinetics. The decrease in sodium conductance, due to sodium channel inactivation, coupled with the increase in potassium conductance, then strongly drives the membrane potential toward the potassium equilibrium potential of −97 mV (the *repolarization phase* of the action potential). The inactivation of sodium channels generates an *absolute refractory period* (corresponding to a transmembrane potential between 0 and −55 mV) during which no quantity of EPSPs will elicit another action potential. As the transmembrane potential becomes more negative than −55 mV (as a result of $K^+$ channels opening and driving the $E_M$ toward the $K^+$ equilibrium potential), the membrane enters a relative refractory period. This period continues through a period of after-hyperpolarization (Fig. 5-3) caused by transient excessive $K^+$ channel permeability. Eventually $K^+$ channel permeability returns to baseline, ending the after-hyperpolarization and the relative refractory period. During the relative refractory period, an action potential can be elicited, but only by a large stimulus. These events are summarized in Figure 5-4.

In the still simplistic neuron we have so far developed, we have incorporated membrane ion channels with variable permeability that enable us to explain how the release of neurotransmitter by presynaptic neurons is able to elicit a dramatic electrical event, the action potential. One might well ask at this point, why are action potentials necessary? The essential explanation is this: In order to communicate with one another, neurons must relay electrical impulses from one part, such as a dendrite, to an axonal ending that may be as much as a meter away in a human (10 m in a whale!). The small inward sodium current generated by an EPSP

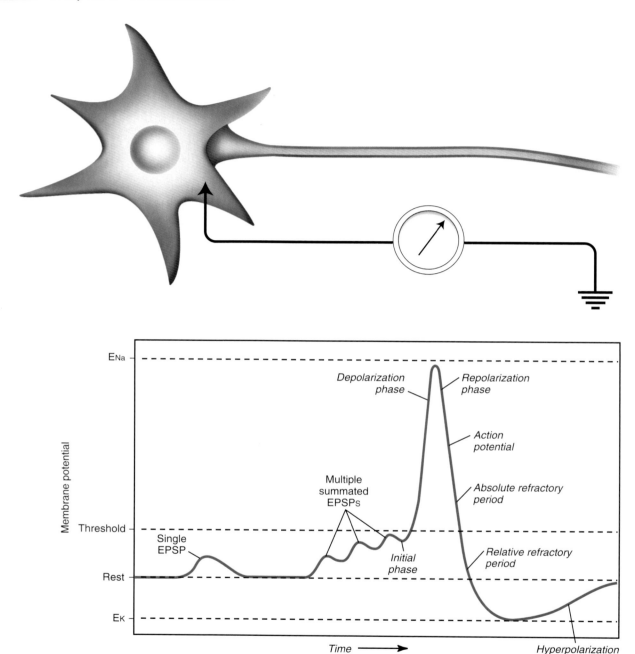

**Figure 5-3** Response of the neuron to the release of excitatory neurotransmitter by presynaptic neurons. The membrane potential (ordinate) transiently becomes more positive as the binding of neurotransmitter released by firing of the presynaptic neuron increases sodium permeability through ligand-gated sodium channels, producing an excitatory postsynaptic potential (EPSP). One EPSP of exaggerated amplitude is shown, following which sufficient EPSPs occur in quick succession to summate and elicit enough membrane depolarization to open up voltage-sensitive sodium channels. This strongly drives the membrane toward the sodium equilibrium potential of +66 mV, producing an action potential. The action potential is terminated as the various sodium channels are inactivated and voltage-sensitive potassium channels open and not only repolarize the membrane but actually transiently hyperpolarize it as they briefly drive the membrane potential toward the potassium equilibrium potential of −97 mV.

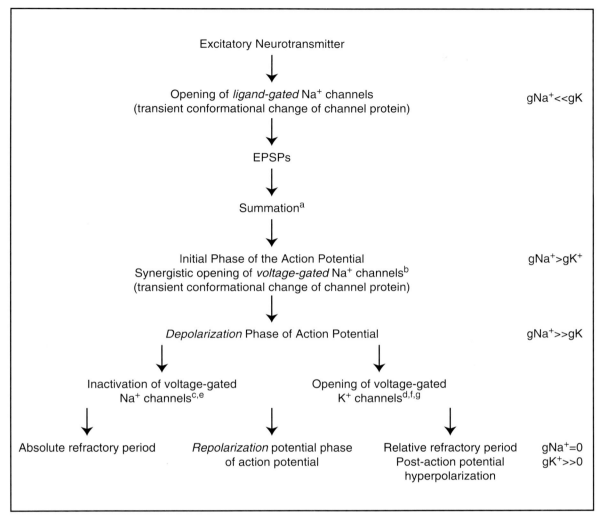

**Figure 5-4** Sequence of events underlying the action potential. Sites of dysfunction in human disease: myasthenia gravis (Case 5-1)[a]; hypo- and hypercalcemia (Practice 5-2D)[b]; hyperkalemic periodic paralysis (Case 5-2)[c]; benign familial neonatal convulsions (Case 5-3).[d] Sites of action of phenytoin, carbamazepine, and local anesthetics (Cases 5-4, 5-5),[e] baclofen (Practice 5-2E),[f] and 4-aminopyridine (Practice 5-4D).[g]

or even hundreds of EPSPs will not be transmitted these long distances because of resistance to current flow inside neural processes (which do not conduct nearly so readily as a copper wire), the tendency for current to leak through the neural membrane, and the tendency of current to be stored along neural membranes (i.e., capacitance). In fact, any ion flows elicited by a change in membrane voltage will be attenuated by a factor of 2.7 for every 0.2 mm distance along a 1-mm diameter nerve fiber. This means that only 1 mm along such a nerve fiber, the voltage change will only be 0.7 percent the size of the original voltage change. The

degree of attenuation is inversely proportional to fiber diameter. This problem can be circumvented by employing a mechanism through which the membrane depolarization becomes self-propagating as the action potential. Once generated, the large depolarization corresponding to the action potential opens up voltage-gated sodium channels in the immediately adjacent membrane, leading that membrane to generate an action potential in turn. Thus, through the generation of a nearly infinite succession of action potentials, the original action potential effectively travels down the neural membrane without any loss of amplitude. When it reaches the axon terminal, the large membrane depolarization opens N-type voltage-sensitive calcium channels and the influx of calcium triggers release of neurotransmitter, enabling the neuron to communicate across its synapses with other neurons.

## Case 5-1

### Myasthenia Gravis

*Myasthenia gravis provides us with a particularly clear view of the events underlying action potential generation through neurotransmitter reception. As we have noted (see Case 4-16), myasthenia gravis is caused by immune-mediated destruction of acetylcholine receptors on the muscle side of the neuromuscular junction. Because a muscle fiber has no axons or dendrites, it rather resembles the very simple saccular neuron we have developed thus far in this chapter. It is innervated by a single axon terminal which, when it depolarizes, releases many vesicles of acetylcholine. When the contents of each vesicle bind, they elicit a miniature end plate potential (MEPP). At a normal neuromuscular junction, so much acetylcholine is released and binds to postsynaptic receptors that the large number of MEPPs generated immediately summates to produce an end plate potential that exceeds threshold and triggers a muscle action potential every time the nerve fires (in much the same way that a large number of EPSPs generated by the multiple excitatory afferent terminals on a CNS neuron is able to elicit an action potential) (Fig. 5-5, top). That is, there is a large safety factor in normal neuromuscular transmission. However, at the myasthenic neuromuscular junction, so many receptors have been destroyed that sometimes the MEPPs do not summate to produce an end plate potential that will exceed threshold and trigger a muscle action potential (Fig. 5-5, bottom, trace 4). Moreover, rather than almost instantly summating to threshold, as in a normal junction, the time over which the MEPPs eventually add up to threshold becomes quite variable (Fig. 5-5, bottom, traces 1-3). This irregularity in timing is reflected in a phenomenon called jitter.*

The electromyographic assessment of jitter provides an exceptionally sensitive test for myasthenia gravis. However, imagine the consequences when thousands or millions of muscle fibers fail to reach threshold for firing when the axons supplying them fire. Now you understand quite precisely the basis for weakness in the myasthenic patient.

## CONSEQUENCES OF ION CHANNEL DYSFUNCTION

The ability of a muscle or nerve membrane to generate action potentials is clearly dependent on normally functioning sodium and potassium channels. There are a number of disorders caused by mutations in these channels, as illustrated in Cases 5-2 and 5-3.

## Case 5-2

### Familial Hyperkalemic Periodic Paralysis

*A 12-year-old boy is brought in by his parents because of recurrent episodes of weakness. These periods have been occurring during much of his life and always seem to appear when he relaxes after brisk exercise. However, they were relatively mild until he recently began training for football. After practice, he may be unable to walk or lift his arms for as long as 2 hours and occasionally his speech is slurred. His mother thinks they might be "hypoglycemic attacks" and for years has treated them by giving her son something sweet to eat or drink. This approach has usually worked, but the severity of the recent attacks has his parents worried.*

**Comment:** *In this disease, a single point polymorphism in a muscle voltage-sensitive sodium channel gene leads to a dysfunctional amino acid substitution at a critical locus in the channel protein. In the presence of high extracellular potassium concentrations, sodium channels fail to close entirely or they open for far too long, thereby causing persistent muscle membrane depolarization. As long as the muscle membrane remains depolarized, it is inexcitable (the absolute refractory period is extremely prolonged). Because the calcium release (achieved via transient channel openings) that is necessary to trigger muscle contraction depends on repeated muscle firing (because normal voltage-sensitive calcium channels open only transiently), this sustained muscle membrane depolarization produces paralysis. The spells of weakness tend to occur after exercise because exercise induces release of potassium from muscle and an increase in serum potassium concentration. The boy's mother has employed a scientifically valid approach to treating the spells: glucose ingestion triggers insulin release, and the two in combination induce cells to take up potassium, thus lowering the serum potassium. This method is also a standard treatment for patients who have life-threatening hyperkalemia.*

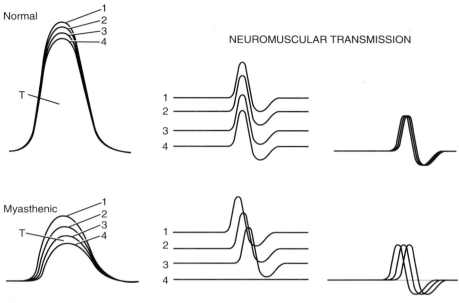

**Figure 5-5** *Top,* Neuromuscular transmission in normal muscle. *Bottom,* Jitter and occasional complete failure of neuromuscular transmission in a myasthenic patient. *Left column,* Four superimposed end plate potentials. Note in myasthenia their amplitude is diminished and more variable because many muscle ACh receptors are blocked or destroyed by antibodies. It also takes longer for potential 3 to reach the threshold (*T*) for activating a muscle fiber action potential than potential 1 or 2, and this difference is much greater in myasthenic patients than in normal subjects. In the myasthenic end plate potential, 4 never reaches threshold. *Middle and right columns,* Muscle fiber action potentials corresponding to the end plate potentials shown to the left. These are shown sequentially in the middle column and superimposed on the right. Notice the variability in timing of the muscle action potentials, called "jitter," is increased in myasthenia due to the variability in time of the end plate potential to reach threshold (*left column*). End plate potential 4 does not reach threshold, hence there is a "blocking" of the muscle action potential.

## Case 5-3

### Benign Familial Neonatal Convulsions

*Thirty-six hours after being born, a baby has his first seizure. The seizure begins with a shrill cry, stiffening of his arms and legs, and shallow breathing. He then lies quietly, staring, unresponsive to gentle stimulation. Following this, eye blinking and jerking of the limbs are observed, culminating in another period of stiffening and staring that appears to end the seizure. He initially experiences three to six seizures a day. However, within a few weeks seizure activity declines and ultimately stops. Both the child's parents are from Newfoundland. His father reports that he and other members of his family had similar seizures when they were young and some experience seizures as adults.*

**Comment:** *This infant has an epileptic syndrome known as benign familial neonatal convulsions. It is inherited in autosomal dominant fashion and is prevalent only in Newfoundland. Affected patients are otherwise normal. However, there is a 16 percent chance they will develop epilepsy as adults. This disorder has been linked to a variety of abnormalities affecting two genes, one on chromosome 8 and one on chromosome 20, which code for the two components of a heteromeric voltage-gated potassium channel. The precise mechanisms underlying the seizures have not been defined and it is not understood why the seizure disorder so rapidly resolves in most cases. However, if you refer to Figure 5-3, you can appreciate the potential impact of a defect in voltage-sensitive potassium channels. If these channels are partially defective, and the permeability of the neural membrane to potassium is reduced, the*

*Continued*

Neurophysiology

## Case 5-3—cont'd

*membrane will not hyperpolarize after the action potential. Thus, it will be more easily depolarized to firing threshold by new EPSPs. This, in turn, leads to more rapid firing, the basic event underlying seizures.*

## MANIPULATING ION CHANNELS FOR THERAPEUTIC PURPOSES

The two preceding cases illustrate the consequences of inborn defects in sodium and potassium channels. There are occasions, on the other hand, when it is useful to induce an abnormality in the function of these channels, as in the treatment of epilepsy (Case 5-4) and the induction of local anesthesia (Case 5-5).

## Case 5-4

### Epilepsy

*Within the central nervous system, sodium channel conductivity and potassium channel conductivity define a crude balance: sodium channel conductivity favoring neuronal depolarization and the generation of action potentials, potassium channel conductivity favoring membrane hyperpolarization and neuronal silence. In Case 5-3 we saw how a defect in potassium channels might tip this balance toward unwanted action potentials, hence seizures. In the far more common forms of epilepsy that affect approximately 2 percent of the population, sodium and potassium channels are normal but an area of damage in the cerebral cortex leads to the spontaneous generation of rapidly repeated neuronal depolarizations. When these generate widespread depolarizations throughout the brain, seizures result (see Cases 4-2 and 4-3). In such patients, it is useful to tip the balance between sodium and potassium conductance in favor of potassium by inducing a defect in sodium channels. This can be done by administering the drug phenytoin (Dilantin), which prolongs the time during which voltage-gated sodium channels are inactivated between openings by preferentially binding to the inactivated conformation of the sodium channel membrane complex. Carbamazepine (Tegretol), another commonly used anticonvulsant, works via a similar mechanism. This slows the rapid discharges, providing inhibitory neurons a greater opportunity to inhibit the spread of these discharges.*

## Case 5-5

### Local Anesthesia

*A great variety of surgical procedures, ranging from dental care to such major operations as repair of shoulder rotator cuff tears, carotid endarterectomy, and many neurosurgical procedures, are done substantially or exclusively with local anesthesia. Local anesthetics such as lidocaine (Xylocaine) and bupivicaine (Marcaine) act by substantially the same mechanism as phenytoin, that is, by binding preferentially to the inactivated conformation of voltage-sensitive sodium channels. However, when applied in high concentrations, these agents do not simply prevent pathologically rapid discharges—they prevent the generation of all action potentials. They actually bind to a site inside the neural membrane. They act preferentially on the small sensory fibers that transmit pain because these fibers tend to have long duration action potentials that provide maximal opportunity for these anesthetic molecules to pass through open sodium channels into the cell.*

## PRACTICE 5-2

**A.** Describe the sequence of events underlying the action potential.

**B.** Why is an action potential necessary?

**C.** The effect of local anesthetics (Case 5-5) derives from their preferential binding to the inactive conformation of the voltage-gated sodium ionophore. Predict what would happen within the CNS if these drugs acted in a similar way but had some selectivity in their action for GABAergic neural processes.

**D.** A 60-year-old woman undergoes surgical removal of the thyroid gland for treatment of hyperthyroidism associated with Graves' disease. Although the surgeon strives to preserve adequate parathyroid tissue, the parathyroid glands undergo infarction and fibrosis in the perioperative period. Parathyroid hormone is critical to the absorption of calcium from the gut and to mobilizing sufficient calcium from bone to maintain normal serum calcium levels. Extracellular calcium concentrations influence the threshold at which voltage-gated sodium channels are opened. High concentrations increase the threshold, making it harder to generate an action potential, whereas low concentrations reduce the threshold, making it easier to generate an action potential, both within and outside the CNS. Predict the clinical consequences of the hypocalcemia in this case.

**E.** Explain what value drugs that potentiate the opening of chloride channels or of voltage-gated potassium channels might have in medicine and why.

**F.** Refer back to Figure 5-4. Predict the manifestations of diseases characterized by accelerated inactivation of voltage-gated sodium channels or prolonged opening of voltage-gated potassium channels.

**G.** Each time an action potential traverses a synaptic ending (bouton), N-type calcium channels open,

enabling the release of synaptic vesicles. There are a variety of calcium reuptake mechanisms. However, if action potentials occur sufficiently rapidly, calcium may be allowed to enter at a rate that exceeds the capacity of these reuptake mechanisms. The extraordinarily large amounts of calcium that accumulate within the synaptic endings under these circumstances then lead to the release of greater than normal amounts of neurotransmitter. This in turn increases the size of the EPSP evoked in the postsynaptic neuron. This process is called *post-tetanic potentiation*. Predict the consequences of post-tetanic potentiation in the CNS. How would you stop it?

# Cycle 5-3

## The Neuron as an Integrative Structure

### Objective

Be able to explain the principal factors underlying spatiotemporal summation by neurons.

The neural model we have developed so far might look like a long slender tube formed by a phospholipid bilayer, perforated by some complex proteins forming ionophores for a number of different ions. The permeability of the membrane due to the different ionophores is such that it leads to the formation of a resting membrane potential. The permeability can be transiently altered by the chemical and electrical events precipitated by the release of excitatory neurotransmitter by a presynaptic neuron, leading to the generation of action potentials. In this model, action potentials can be generated anywhere and their self-generative property leads them to travel down the neuron to one end, where the opening of N-type voltage-sensitive calcium channels leads to neurotransmitter release.

In this section, we will sketch the possibilities that emerge when we go from this still simplistic model to a more realistic model approaching the complexity of the neuron pictured in Figure 5-6, replete with an enormous and complex dendritic tree and a nonuniform distribution of ion channels. The responses of a neuron like this reflect the principles of *spatiotemporal summation*. Such a neuron receives thousands or tens of

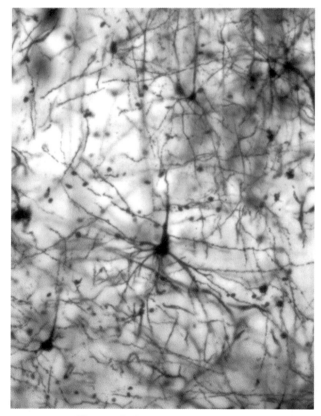

**Figure 5-6** A pyramidal neuron.

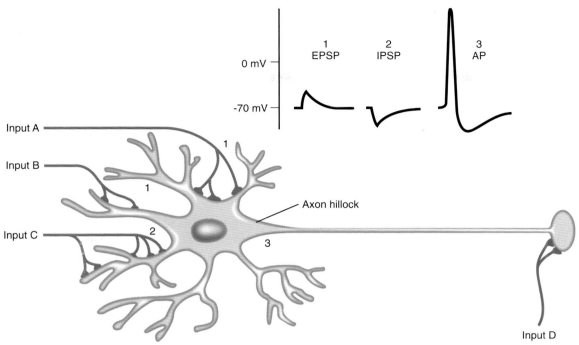

**Figure 5-7** The anatomic and physiologic basis for the variable effects of synaptic inputs to a neuron and the phenomenon of spatiotemporal summation. See text for details. AP = action potential, EPSP = excitatory postsynaptic potential, IPSP = inhibitory postsynaptic potential.

thousands of synaptic contacts distributed over its entire dendritic tree, the cell body, and on the axon near terminal boutons (Fig. 5-7). The voltage-sensitive sodium channels critical to the initiation of an action potential are preferentially distributed in a region at the base of the axon known as the *initial segment*, which is immediately adjacent to the axon hillock. The transmission of electrical impulses along the axon (and in some neurons, the stems of large dendrites), is "all or none" because it takes advantage of the self-perpetuating dynamics of the action potential: once an action potential is generated at the axon hillock, it regenerates itself all the way down the axon (3 in Fig. 5-7). However, transmission of impulses along dendritic branches is passive and therefore subject to the attenuating effects of fiber resistance and capacitance that we discussed earlier. Therefore, synaptic contacts that are on large dendritic branches (low resistance) are going to have more influence on the neuron than synaptic contacts on small branches (high resistance), and synaptic contacts near the cell body (or even better, the initial segment near the axon hillock) (input A, Fig. 5-7) are going to have more influence than synaptic contacts distant in the dendritic tree (input B, Fig. 5-7).

To complicate matters further, synaptic contacts may be excitatory (e.g., glutamate, generating EPSPs) or inhibitory (e.g., GABA, generating IPSPs) (as in input C, Fig. 5-7). Synaptic contacts on the axon terminal are capable of modifying the amount of neurotransmitter emitted by an action potential, something referred to as presynaptic excitation or inhibition (input D, Fig. 5-7).

It also takes time for membrane depolarizations distal in the dendritic tree to be transmitted to the cell body. We see this manifested in the electroencephalogram (EEG), in which the voltage fluctuations we measure via scalp electrodes actually reflect the voltage differences that develop between the dendritic trees and the cell bodies of cortical pyramidal cells as afferent input (e.g., from the thalamus) depolarizes the dendritic tree of large numbers of these neurons. Membrane depolarizations initiated at various points in the dendritic tree are going to contribute to action potential generation at the axon hillock only to the extent that the currents generated by them arrive at the axon hillock simultaneously.

Any given neuron produces action potentials at a rate that reflects a spatially weighted integral of all its inputs over time—that is, *spatiotemporal summation*.

Neurophysiology

Although this arrangement seems to provide neurons with the potential for enormous information processing sophistication, the details of this capability and the extent to which it is utilized by different types of neurons are largely unknown.

## PRACTICE 5-3

Explain the principal factors underlying spatiotemporal summation.

# Cycle 5-4

## Axonal Conduction and the Role of Myelin

### Objectives

1. Be able to explain why the slow propagation of an action potential along an unmyelinated axon would present a serious problem in animals such as vertebrates for which the capability for rapid movement is often critical to survival.

2. Be able to explain the mechanism by which myelin accelerates the propagation of action potentials down an axon.

3. Be able to explain why myelin destruction may produce conduction block.

Although the capability for generating action potentials provides a neuron with great reliability in electrical transmission down the axon, leading ultimately to the release of neurotransmitter, the process suffers from being slow: action potentials are propagated at approximately 1 m/sec. At this rate, it would take over 2 seconds for you to remove your hand from contact with a hot stove! In the evolution of the vertebrate nervous system, this problem has been solved through myelination. Axons are wrapped in multiple concentric layers of myelin incorporated in the cell membrane of myelin-producing cells—*oligodendrocytes* in the CNS, *Schwann cells* in the peripheral nervous system. This continuous investment of axons by myelin is interrupted at highly regular intervals known as *nodes of*

*Ranvier*. Portions of the axon that are wrapped in myelin are highly resistant to the transmembrane flow of ions. Nodes of Ranvier are equipped with voltage-sensitive ion channels that make them fully capable of generating an action potential, much like the axon hillock (Fig. 5-8) .

We will now consider how action potentials are transmitted in a myelinated axon. An action potential generated in the axon hillock cannot be propagated in the normal fashion down the axon because it immediately runs into myelinated portions of the axon that will not permit any ion flow across the membrane. However, the current generated by the action potential is passively conducted via the dilute electrolyte solution within the axon. Ions are shunted through the myelin-encased segments (rather than passively diffusing), in the same way that electrons are shunted down a wire conducting electricity, enabling extremely fast conduction. This current will be attenuated by resistance and capacitance, as we discussed earlier (but not by trans-membrane leakage as in the unmyelinated axon). However, because the action potential generated a very large voltage change to begin with, and because the capacitance of a myelinated axon is substantially less than that of an unmyelinated one, a depolarization is generated at the first node of Ranvier that is sufficiently large to open voltage-sensitive sodium channels and trigger another action potential (i.e., it is supra-threshold). This same process is repeated from one node of Ranvier to the next. Thus, the action potential "jumps" from one node of Ranvier to the next, a

Neurophysiology

*215*

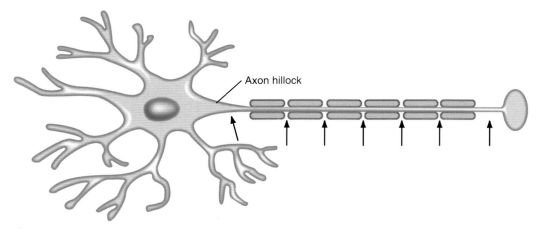

**Figure 5-8** A neuron with myelin sheathing of its axon. The interruptions in the myelin sheath are the nodes of Ranvier. The arrows indicate regions of high-density, voltage-sensitive sodium channels, current flow, and action potential generation.

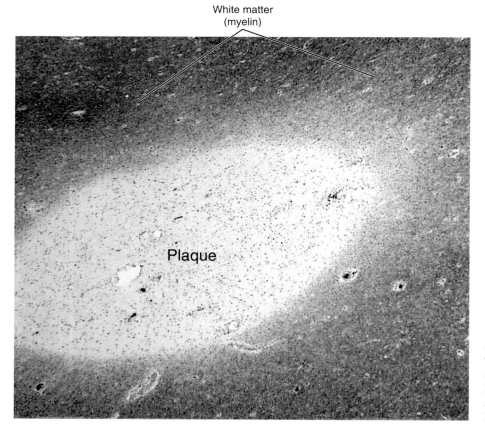

**Figure 5-9** A myelin-stained section of brain from a patient with multiple sclerosis demonstrating the nearly complete loss of myelin in a "plaque"—a site of old inflammation, now healed.

process known as *saltatory conduction*. Saltatory conduction enables conduction velocities of up to 150 m/sec, velocities that are crucial to satisfying the neuronal processing requirements of large, complex organisms.

Unfortunately, the enormous value of myelin in enabling saltatory conduction brings with it a serious liability in situations in which disease processes damage the myelin. The lesions produced by these diseases may markedly increase the amount of current stored as capacitance charge, leading to loss of sufficient current to trigger an action potential at the next node of Ranvier, hence failure of the impulse to be propagated all the way to the axonal endings. Case 5-6 (multiple sclerosis) and Case 5-7 (Guillain-Barré syndrome) illustrate the effects of this breakdown, known as conduction block.

## Case 5-6

### Multiple Sclerosis

*A 19-year-old college student experiences progressive painless loss of vision in her right eye over the course of a couple of days. She is able to detect light but not much else for about a week, following which her vision starts to recover. Eventually she achieves vision with 20/40 acuity. Eight months later she develops rapidly progressive generalized weakness. Again, she experiences dramatic recovery to the point that she is left with only subtle abnormalities of gait and some urinary urgency. One evening, a month later, after an exhausting day, she luxuriates in a hot bath. However, to her horror, she becomes too weak to climb out of the tub. Fortunately, her roommate returns and rescues her.*

**Comment:** *This history is fairly typical of multiple sclerosis—first a bout of optic neuritis, then a transient quadriparesis produced by a lesion high in the cervical spinal cord. These lesions are caused by a recurrent autoimmune inflammatory attack directed at myelin (Figs. 5-9, 5-10). As the lesions heal, oligodendrocytes partially repair the myelin. This remyelination reduces the capacitance and the leakiness of the bare axonal membrane passing through the area of the lesion, thus reducing the fraction of the axonal current generated by action potentials that is lost. Furthermore, the axon increases the number of voltage-sensitive sodium channels, increasing the probability that even a reduced axonal current will succeed in generating sufficient depolarization to trigger action potentials at nodes of Ranvier. Unfortunately, neither of these compensatory responses may be adequate. Conduction through the axon then becomes quite tenuous and exquisitely sensitive to a number of factors, body temperature among them. A small rise in body temperature may significantly reduce the probability that the neural membrane within the lesion will be depolarized to threshold, leading to conduction block. This phenomenon provided the basis for the hot bath test, once used mainly in Great Britain as an aid to the diagnosis of multiple sclerosis. You can appreciate the serious consequences it might have for a patient such as the one described here, in which it reinstated the quadriparesis. Patients with multiple sclerosis routinely do worse in summer months and are intolerant of brisk exercise, which raises body temperature. Fortunately, we now have some effective treatments, such as β-interferon, that help to prevent the development of new lesions in these patients by suppressing the immune processes that cause them.*

Conduction block can be demonstrated electrophysiologically in both the CNS and the peripheral nervous system (PNS), but its electrophysiologic effects are most clear-cut in patients with disorders affecting peripheral nerve myelin, such as Guillain-Barré syndrome.

Neurophysiology

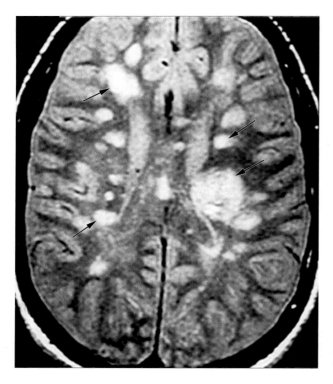

**Figure 5-10** Magnetic resonance image (MRI) of the brain of a patient with multiple sclerosis, demonstrating multiple demyelinated plaques (*arrows*).

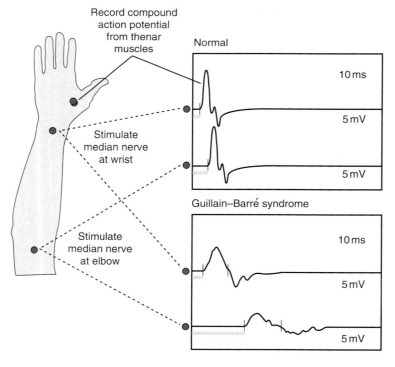

**Figure 5-11** Results of nerve conduction studies in a normal subject (*above*) and in a patient with Guillain-Barré syndrome (*below*). See text for more details.

## Case 5-7

### Guillain-Barré Syndrome

*A 19-year-old college student acutely develops nausea, some vomiting, diarrhea, and a great deal of malaise. He recovers in 3 days. However, 10 days later, during a routine workout at his physical fitness center, he discovers that he is unable to lift even 50 percent of his customary weights. He reports to the Infirmary in a panic. The physician there sets up a Neurology Clinic appointment in 2 weeks. The next day the student finds himself barely able to walk to class and presents to the Emergency Room. There he exhibits some weakness of facial muscles (air leaks from his mouth as he attempts to inflate his cheeks). He has weakness involving muscles throughout his body, particularly those of his proximal lower extremities. A diagnosis of Guillain-Barré syndrome is suspected. Nerve conduction studies are carried out to confirm the diagnosis and thereby rule out alternatives.*

*A right median motor nerve conduction study is carried out by stimulating the median nerve first at the wrist and then at the cubital fossa and measuring the electrical potential elicited in median innervated muscles in the thenar eminence (the compound muscle action potential, or CMAP) (Fig. 5-11). Two things are noteworthy. First, the time from stimulation in the anticubital fossa to the appearance of the CMAP is prolonged—that is, the conduction velocity is reduced. Second, the amplitude of the CMAP elicited from the anticubital fossa is less than that elicited from behind the wrist.*

**Comment:** *This patient does indeed have Guillain-Barré syndrome (GBS)—also called acute inflammatory demyelinating polyradiculoneuropathy. GBS classically occurs after a minor infectious illness. It appears that*

*an immune response develops to a specific antigenic site (an epitope) on myelin that resembles an epitope on one of the proteins of the infectious organism. The result is inflammatory damage to myelin throughout the PNS, involving both nerves and nerve roots ("radicals"). This destruction undermines the role of myelin in enabling saltatory conduction, thereby reducing nerve conduction velocities. It may be sufficiently severe to produce conduction block, as seen with multiple sclerosis in the CNS. The nerve conduction studies depicted in the lower box in Figure 5-11 illustrate conduction block. Supramaximal electrical stimulation within the anticubital fossa depolarizes all axons within the median nerve. The induced action potentials travel down the nerve. However, at one or more points in the forearm, conduction is blocked in some axons as a result of demyelination. Beyond these points, action potentials continue to travel down only a fraction of the axons in the nerve, those unaffected by demyelination, hence the small CMAP elicited from the anticubital fossa. Stimulation at the wrist excites nerve that is nearly normal (albeit partially demyelinated more proximally)—hence, a nearly normal CMAP. Conduction block causes weakness by reducing the ability of neural firing to elicit muscle contraction.*

*Guillain-Barré syndrome may be sufficiently severe to cause quadriparesis and respiratory arrest (from involvement of the phrenic nerves). The course of the disease can now be substantially attenuated using therapies, such as the administration of high-dose immunoglobulins (IV Ig) or the removal of substantial amounts of the patient's own immunoglobulins (plasmapheresis). Rarely do patients die and nearly all eventually recover nearly normal neurologic function.*

Neurophysiology

## PRACTICE 5-4

**A.** Explain the need of vertebrates for rapid axonal conduction.

**B.** Explain the mechanism by which myelin accelerates the propagation of action potentials.

**C.** Why does myelin destruction sometimes produce conduction block?

**D.** 4-Aminopyridine blocks voltage-sensitive potassium channels. Explain why this drug might be useful in the treatment of manifestations of multiple sclerosis. Would you expect any adverse effects?

# Maintenance of Ion Gradients: Neuronal Housekeeping

## Objective

Be able to explain why the sodium-potassium pump is so important to neurons.

In the first cycle of this chapter, we developed a primitive model of a neuron as a phospholipid bilayer membranous sack of dilute ionic solution immersed in another dilute ionic solution of somewhat different composition. Since then, we have discussed at some length the perforation of the lipid membrane by numerous ion-conducting channels. These channels make the membrane leaky. The resting membrane potential and the various changes it undergoes in the course of chemical neurotransmission, action potential generation, and propagation, and the release of neurotransmitter by the postsynaptic neuron, are all based upon changes in membrane permeability, not redistribution of ions. Nevertheless, with each of the millions of EPSPs that may occur in any given neuron in a second and the up to 1000 action potentials a neuron might produce in

a second, a small amount of ion redistribution does take place. Furthermore, unlike the neuron of Cycle 5-1, in which the membrane was permeable only to potassium, the multi-ion permeability of real neurons means that outflow of potassium can be electrically balanced by inflow of sodium or outflow of chloride ions. Thus, electrical gradients are not quite as constraining in real neurons. As a result, within the cell, the concentrations of sodium and chloride rise and the concentration of potassium falls. To maintain the ion gradients necessary for normal function, neurons are equipped with a number of ion exchange pumps, the most important being the sodium-potassium pump. These pumps all require energy to operate because they are pumping ions against their concentration gradients. This energy is derived from hydrolysis of adenosine triphosphate (ATP) to adenosine diphosphate (ADP). Even though the ion exchange occurring in the course of neural transmission is minute, neurons are so electrically active that they ultimately require the expenditure of enormous energy to run the ion exchange pumps—more than 50 percent of all energy produced by intermediate metabolism. Case 5-8 illustrates the difference that functioning sodium-potassium pumps can make in certain pathological situations.

## Case 5-8

### Migraine and Stroke

*Review Cases 4-4 and 4-5. Spreading depression of Leao appears to occur in both migraine, in which it accounts for the aura, and in stroke, in which it is not clinically evident in most cases, for poorly understood reasons. Spreading depression of Leao is primarily driven by depolarization of excitatory, glutamatergic neurons. The resultant high extracellular concentrations of glutamate open glutamatergic ligand-gated sodium channels (AMPA and kainate) and glutamatergic voltage-sensitive ligand-gated sodium/calcium channels (NMDA). Consequently, sodium and calcium pour into cells throughout the cortex.*

*Migraine is a fundamentally benign condition. Stroke corresponds to permanent damage to the brain.*

*The difference in the outcome of these two disorders appears, in good part, to be attributable to the fact that in migraine, cells have the glucose and oxygen supply necessary to run their ion exchange pumps and maintain normal ion gradients, whereas in stroke, glucose and oxygen supply are interrupted by vascular occlusion. Sodium and chloride ions enter cells in stroke, bringing with them osmotically obligated water, and the cells swell, producing "cytotoxic" edema (visible on CT scans and MRIs). Calcium entering cells activates a number of degradative enzyme systems, leading to cell death.*

## PRACTICE 5-5

Explain the need for the sodium-potassium pump. Why does it consume energy?

### CYCLE 5-1

**A.** See Figure 5-12.

$$E_{Cl^-} = (61)\log\frac{[Cl^-]_{In}}{[Cl^-]_{Out}}$$

$$= -90\,mV$$

The potential inside the cell is negative because there is an excess of negative charges on the inner surface of the membrane produced by the flow of chloride ions down their chemical gradient.

**B.** At $E_M$, there will be no net flow of charge across the cell membrane. Therefore, the sum of the inward current $(I_{Na^+})$ and the outward current $(I_{K^+})$ must be 0:

$$I_{Na^+} + I_{K^+} = 0$$

Substituting for these currents using the two equations provided, we have:

$$g_{Na^+}(E_M - E_{Na^+}) + g_{K^+}(E_M - E_{K^+}) = 0$$

$$E_M = \frac{g_{Na^+}E_{Na^+} + g_{K^+}E_{K^+}}{g_{Na^+} + g_{K^+}}$$

From this equation, it is clear that $E_M$ reflects the combined influence of all the ions to which the membrane is permeable, the permeability of the membrane to

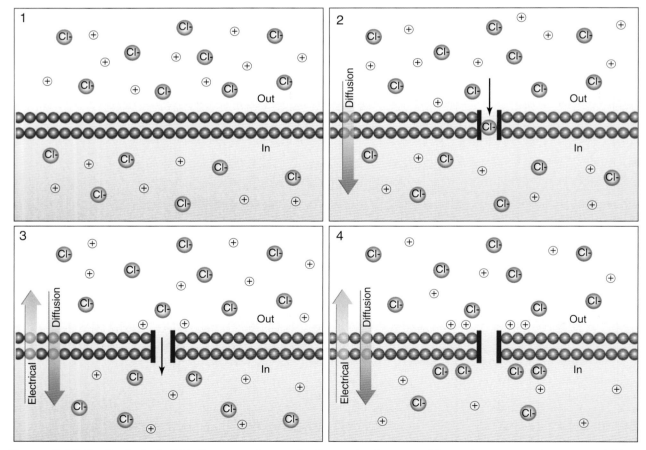

**Figure 5-12** Feedback: Cycle 5-1A. Sequence of events leading to development of the resting transmembrane potential in a highly simplified neuron with a membrane permeable only to chloride ions.

these various ions (i.e., their conductances), and the equilibrium potentials of these ions. It is a steady-state potential because it is the potential at which inward current exactly equals outward current. The equation tells you that an increase in sodium conductance will shift $E_M$ in the positive direction; this corresponds to the fact that increased inward flow of positively charged sodium ions will decrease the net amount of negative charge on the inside of the membrane. The equation tells you that an increase in potassium conductance will shift $E_M$ in a negative direction (because outward current is negative); this corresponds to the fact that increased outward flow of positively charged potassium ions will increase the net amount of negative charge on the inside of the membrane. $E_M$ will be pulled toward the equilibrium potential of the ion for which the membrane is most permeable, that is, for which $g$ is the highest. If $g_{Na^+}$ were zero, $E_M$ would become simply the equilibrium potential for potassium. If $g_{K^+} >> g_{Na^+}$, the resting membrane potential will be close to the equilibrium potential for potassium.

# CYCLE 5-2

**A.** See Figures 5-3 and 5-4. If there is any element of these figures that you do not understand, you should seek help.

**B.** The action potential is necessary because, regardless of the number of EPSPs produced on the neural membrane, the inward flow of current through the membrane and then down a neural process is rapidly dissipated because of the resistance to the flow of current through the dilute intracellular electrolyte solution, and by the deposition of charges along the neural membrane (capacitance). The action potential circumvents this dissipation because it is self-regenerating.

**C.** The suppression of action potentials in inhibitory neurons would lead to seizures. In fact, high serum levels of lidocaine do cause seizures, presumably by this mechanism.

**D.** Generalized seizures due to CNS effects. Peripheral and perioral paresthesias, carpal and pedal spasm, Chvostek's and Trousseau's signs, and other evidence of an increased tendency to muscle spasms due to increased excitability (lower threshold for action potential generation) in the PNS. In carpal spasm, the wrists are strongly flexed, the thumb is strongly adducted, and the fingers are stiff, slightly flexed at the metacar-

pophalangeal joints, and gathered about the thumb. This posture reflects the result of extreme contraction of all the muscles of the forearm and hand and the dominant force of flexor muscles. In pedal spasm, there is extreme extension at the ankles and flexion of the feet. Chvostek's sign consists of unilateral spasm of facial musculature elicited by a tap of the facial nerve at the point where it emerges from the parotid gland. Trousseau's sign consists of the elicitation of carpal spasm by the sustained inflation of a blood pressure cuff on the upper arm.

**E.** Drugs such as barbiturates and benzodiazepines act at GABA$_A$ receptors to potentiate chloride conductance. This change tends to drive the neural transmembrane potential to the chloride equilibrium potential of $-90\,\text{mV}$, hyperpolarizing the cell membrane. This reduces the likelihood of membrane depolarization reaching the threshold for action potential generation. Both classes of drugs are thus useful in the treatment of seizures, and benzodiazepines are effective in reducing the excessive activity in central motor systems associated with spasticity (marked muscle stiffness) after stroke and spinal cord injury. Baclofen acts on GABA$_B$ receptors to potentiate potassium conductance. This also tends to hyperpolarize the neural membrane and reduce the probability of action potential generation. Baclofen is not a useful anticonvulsant but it is effective in treating spasticity and in attenuating the rapid neuronal discharges that produce excruciating pain in such disorders as trigeminal neuralgia.

**F.** Neither of these disorders has been described. Accelerated inactivation of voltage-sensitive sodium channels would lead to excessively brief action potentials, reduction in the amount of calcium taken up by neural endings during depolarization, and hence reduction in the amount of neurotransmitter released, centrally and peripherally. Prolonged activation of voltage-sensitive potassium channels would reduce the probability of generating action potentials—hence reduced neurotransmitter release as well. Centrally, we might expect lethargy, stupor, or coma and paralysis as neuronal intercommunication declines. This is in fact what we do see with severe hypercalcemia, which increases the threshold for opening of voltage-gated sodium channels (see preceding problem) or very toxic levels of phenytoin or carbamazepine, which, by binding selectively to the inactivated state of voltage-gated sodium channels, ultimately prevent them from opening at all. Prolongation of the opening of potassium channels by drugs such as baclofen, as we have already noted, may be very effective in reducing spasticity, but sometimes at the cost of inducing weakness.

Peripherally, one might expect weakness and sensory loss with these theoretical disorders, due to loss of peripheral sensory and motor transmission. Such effects are induced by drugs like local anesthetics that selectively bind to the inactivated state of voltage-gated sodium channels. Interestingly, although phenytoin and carbamazepine do not induce numbness, they may be effective in reducing the high frequency discharge of sensory neurons associated with excruciating pain following nerve injury or in trigeminal neuralgia.

**G.** Because post-tetanic potentiation increases the amplitude of EPSPs, it increases the likelihood that action potentials in afferent neurons will elicit action potentials in postsynaptic neurons, that is, it increases the likelihood of spread of discharges. This mechanism is thought to be important in the spread of seizure discharges. Anticonvulsants like phenytoin and carbamazepine that act to reduce the maximum rate of action potential generation are effective in preventing post-tetanic potentiation.

## CYCLE 5-3

At least four factors can be cited:

1. EPSPs on distal portions of the dendritic arborization have the least impact on action potential generation because the intracellular currents generated are most likely to be completely attenuated over the long distance to the axon hillock.

2. Intracellular currents generated by EPSPs in small dendritic fibers are more likely to be completely attenuated before they get to the axon hillock because the degree of attenuation of these currents is inversely proportional to fiber diameter.

3. Ion currents generated by EPSPs must reach the axon hillock in sufficient temporal contiguity to summate to the point that the threshold for action potential generation is reached. Thus, a neuron is a very effective noise filter, making no response to random, nonsynchronous EPSPs.

4. EPSPs and IPSPs will tend to cancel each other's effects on transmembrane and intraneuronal ion currents.

## CYCLE 5-4

**A.** Even so simple a task as standing requires postural reflexes that depend on conduction of impulses from the vestibular system in the brainstem down the spinal cord and then, after synapse, to appropriate muscles—a total distance of up to 1 m. Given maximum nerve conduction velocities of 1 m/sec in unmyelinated neurons, it would take a full second for a human to begin to produce the muscle contractions needed to prevent a fall—obviously far too slow a response. Timely withdrawal from noxious stimuli, response to threat, and the performance of rapid complex movements, not to mention the complex cerebral processes that underlie cognitive activity, all require fast neural conduction—a requirement met by myelinated nerves, which are able to conduct at up to 150 m/sec.

**B.** Myelin is able to accelerate conduction because it enables action potentials to "jump" almost instantaneously from node of Ranvier to node of Ranvier, as ions are shunted down myelinated axon segments like electrons in a wire.

**C.** Myelin destruction may produce conduction block because of the associated increase in axonal membrane capacitance—the storage of charge along the membrane. An action potential produces a sudden transient influx of positive charges that passively flow through the axon. Normally, this should generate sufficient depolarization to trigger an action potential at the next node of Ranvier. However, if much of this positive current is dissipated through deposition along substantially demyelinated membrane, there may not be enough left to generate the threshold voltage change needed to elicit an action potential.

**D.** By blocking voltage-sensitive potassium channels, 4-aminopyridine prevents hyperpolarization of the neural and axonal membranes. This means that a much smaller current is necessary to depolarize the membrane sufficiently to elicit an action potential. In axons in which ion currents are partially dissipated by the increased capacitance along demyelinated membrane, the presence of 4-aminopyridine may thus preserve the ability to generate an action potential at the demyelinated segment or at the next node of Ranvier. Unfortunately, blocking potassium current-induced hyperpolarization may increase the likelihood of neural discharges and hence, the likelihood of seizures. This is in fact the major side effect of 4-aminopyridine, one so serious that, until recently, it prevented the approval of this drug by the Food and Drug Administration. You might also recall that earlier we spoke of the use of baclofen to potentiate potassium conductance in order to reduce the excessive neural activity in motor systems of patients with CNS injury associated with spasticity. Thus, 4-aminopyridine might improve strength and reduce sensory symptoms caused by conduction block, but it might also increase spasticity.

## CYCLE 5-5

There is a constant leak of ions down their concentration gradients, episodically increased during action potentials. In order for a neuron to maintain its ability to respond to input EPSPs and generate action potentials, it must be able to maintain normal ionic gradients. The Na-K pump that does this is energy-consuming because it is pumping ions against their concentration gradients. In a very active neuron, a great deal of energy is consumed in this process.

Neurophysiology

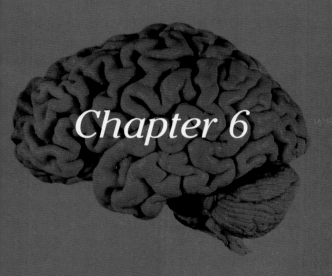

# Chapter 6

# THE MOTOR SYSTEM

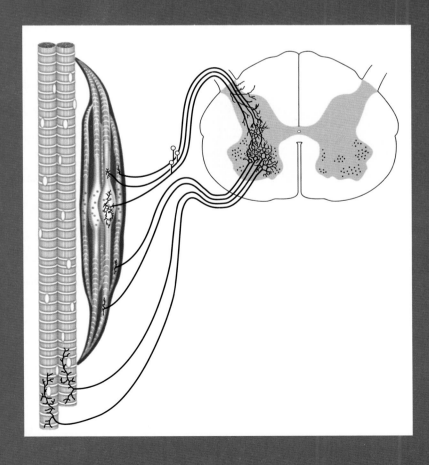

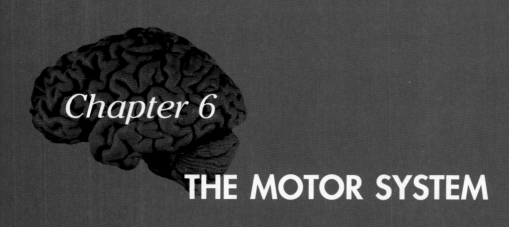

# *Chapter 6*

# THE MOTOR SYSTEM

# Introduction

The central nervous system (CNS) has two major output systems: the motor system and the efferent component of the autonomic nervous system. Only the function of the motor system is openly revealed to us as behavior. The motor system has a hierarchical structure, the major components of which are located at either end of the neuraxis (cerebral cortex and muscle), as well as at multiple loci in between, in the deep gray matter of the cerebrum, the brainstem, and the spinal cord. Because of the visibility of the motor system in health and disease, and because it spans the neuraxis in its hierarchical organization, the motor examination is the single most important component of the neurologic examination. In this chapter we will enable you to understand the scientific principles that make it possible to have a dialogue with this system through the neurologic examination. The autonomic nervous system will be considered in Chapter 11.

We will approach the motor system from the bottom up, beginning with the motor unit, composed of an α-motoneuron and the muscle fibers it innervates, and ascending the CNS by stages, building the hierarchy of motor control systems until we end up at the cerebral cortex. Near the end of the chapter, we will review two consultant systems to cerebral motor cortices, the basal ganglia and the cerebellum.

# The Motor Unit—Anatomy

## Objectives

1. Be able to define a motor unit.
2. Be able to describe the location and distribution (somatotopic organization) of α-motoneurons supplying a muscle.
3. Be able to describe what is meant by the trophic influence of an α-motoneuron on its respective muscle and the consequences of α-motoneuron death or axonal injury for the muscle.

*Alpha-motoneurons* are located in the ventral horn of the spinal cord. Their dendritic trees spread through parts of the ventral horn and the junctional zone between the ventral and dorsal horns. Their axons pass out through the ventral roots and successively pass through the spinal nerves[1] and the peripheral nerves until they exit to form multiple axon branches, which innervate multiple muscle fibers (Fig. 6-1). A single α-motoneuron may innervate as few as 35 muscle fibers (e.g., in one of the extraocular muscles) or as many as 2000 muscle fibers (e.g., in the quadriceps femoris muscle of the thigh). Generally, the finer the level of control required of a muscle, the lower the ratio of muscle fibers to α-motoneurons. Each muscle fiber is innervated by only one α-motoneuron. The combination of an α-motoneuron and the muscle fiber it supplies is referred to as a *motor unit*.

The several hundred α-motoneurons that innervate one muscle form a cigar-shaped column of cells within the ventral horn that may span several spinal cord segments. For example, the α-motoneurons innervating the quadriceps femoris span the spinal cord between the L2 and L4 levels, and their axons exit through the L2, L3, and L4 nerve roots. The α-motoneurons supplying axial and limb girdle muscles tend to be located in the medial portion of the ventral horn at any given spinal level, whereas those innervating peripheral limb muscles tend to be located in the lateral region. The α-motoneurons supplying flexor muscles tend to be located in the portion of the ventral horn nearest the center of the cord, while those innervating extensor muscles tend to be located in the more peripheral portions of the ventral horn (Fig. 6-2).

Alpha-motoneurons exert a trophic influence on the muscle fibers they innervate. When an α-motoneuron dies or when its axon is destroyed by injury or disease (e.g., damage to nerve roots—radiculopathy, or damage to nerves—neuropathy), the

---

[1]Clinicians somewhat misleadingly use the shorthand "nerve root" to refer to spinal nerves. For example, the C5 nerve root corresponds to the spinal nerve comprising both dorsal and ventral roots. The term "radicular" is also used to refer to nerve roots (in the clinical sense). Thus, someone with excruciating pain radiating down the back of one leg due to a herniated L5-S1 disk with compression of the S1 nerve root is said to have an S1 radiculopathy.

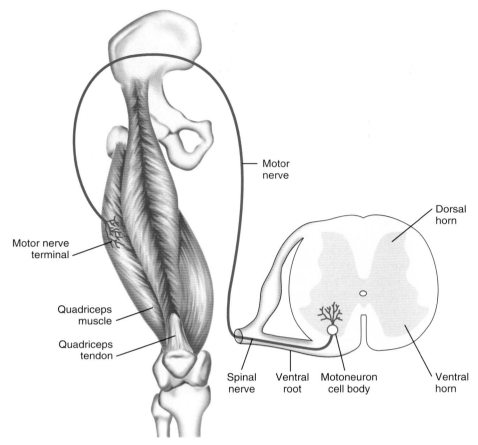

**Figure 6-1** The location of an α-motoneuron and the pathway of its axon.

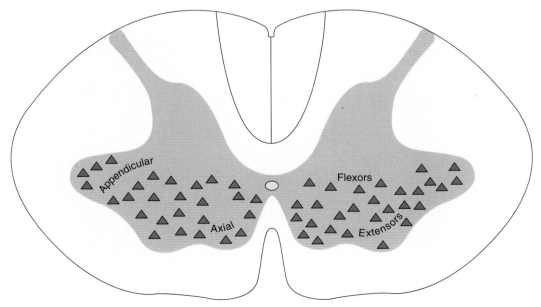

**Figure 6-2** Cross section of the spinal cord at the C7 level, showing the somatotopic organization of α-motoneurons.

axons of neighboring α-motoneurons may generate growing branches (sprouts) to innervate the muscle fibers it once supplied. However, if this does not occur, the muscle fibers will atrophy and eventually disappear because of loss of trophic support. If a sufficient number of α-motoneurons or axons is lost, the result is muscle wasting, as illustrated in Case 6-1.

## Case 6-1

### Ulnar Neuropathy

*A 55-year-old man consults a physician for the first time in years for a "routine checkup." On examination, the physician notices that in the man's left hand, there is wasting of the first dorsal interosseus muscle (abducts the index finger), the abductor digiti quinti (abducts the little finger), and less conspicuously, other interosseus muscles (spread the fingers) of the left hand. There is modest weakness of these muscles as well. Strength and bulk in the abductor pollicis brevis (pulls the adducted thumb away from the palm) and the opponens pollicis (pulls the thumb toward the little finger) are completely normal.*

**Comment:** *This patient has an ulnar neuropathy. The ulnar nerve innervates the interossei and the abductor digiti quinti. The most common cause is the cubital tunnel syndrome, in which the nerve is compressed in a musculotendinous groove just after it passes through the ulnar groove at the elbow. All the muscles mentioned are innervated by the C8 and T1 nerve roots. However, the abductor pollicis brevis and opponens pollicis are innervated by fibers from the C8 and T1 roots supplying the median nerve. The fact that muscles innervated by the median nerve are normal provides evidence that this patient has an ulnar neuropathy and not a C8 or T1 radiculopathy. The cause of the cubital tunnel syndrome is unknown. Most of us can function remarkably well with very weak ulnar-innervated hand muscles, but if a cubital tunnel syndrome threatens disability, as it might in a musician, the nerve can be surgically decompressed.*

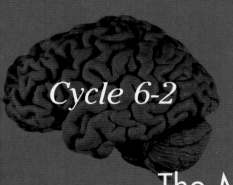

# Cycle 6-2

## The Motor Unit—Function

### Objectives

1. Be able to describe the process of recruitment.
2. Be able to describe and explain the electro-myographic findings associated with chronic denervation, including increased motor unit potential, amplitude, and duration, and decreased recruitment.

Figure 6-3 summarizes the sequence of events that occur as an $\alpha$-motoneuron induces muscle contraction.

When we voluntarily contract a muscle, steadily producing greater and greater force, we progressively engage the entire cigar-shaped spinal $\alpha$-motoneuron pool for that muscle. This innervation occurs in an orderly fashion: small $\alpha$-motoneurons fire before large $\alpha$-motoneurons. In small $\alpha$-motoneurons, because there is less total membrane, a relatively smaller proportion of the current generated by an excitatory post-synaptic potential (EPSP) is stored along the membrane (i.e., dissipated as capacitance current). Therefore, a given EPSP achieves a relatively greater depolarization at the initial segment (axon hillock). For this reason, the smallest $\alpha$-motoneurons are the first to fire, all other things being equal, and at any given force level, the smallest neurons will fire at a higher rate than large motoneurons. When the muscle is contracted with minimal force, only small $\alpha$-motoneurons will fire and they fire slowly (e.g., at 10 to 20 Hz). As increasing force is generated, the firing rate of these same neurons increases to 30 to 40 Hz at the same time that increasing numbers of larger $\alpha$-motoneurons begin to fire (they are *recruited*), first at slow rates, ultimately at high rates (e.g., 60 to 70 Hz) when maximal force is generated.

The amplitude and duration of motor unit potentials and the recruitment pattern can be assessed using the technique of *electromyography*. Electromyography allows the neurologist to achieve an intimate view of the state of the motor units in various muscles, as illustrated in Case 6-2.

The Motor System

233

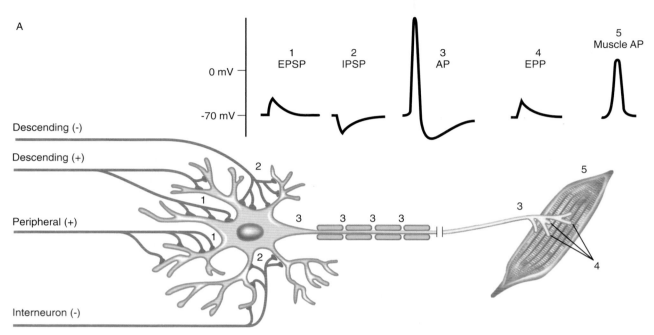

**Figure 6-3** Physiology of the motor unit. *A,* The sequence of events during contraction.

• Descending input from the cerebral cortex, brainstem, and spinal cord, together with sensory afferents from the periphery, synapse on the dendrites and cell body of the α-motoneuron (1, 2). These induce excitatory and inhibitory postsynaptic potentials (EPSPs and IPSPs) in the α-motoneuron cell membrane (see Chapter 5).

• When the algebraic sum of EPSPs and IPSPs at the initial segment of the axon of the α-motoneuron (the axon hillock) exceeds threshold, voltage-sensitive sodium channels open in synergistic fashion, rapidly driving the transmembrane potential to the sodium equilibrium potential (+66 mV), thus generating an action potential, or AP (3).

• The action potential is conducted down the axon to its terminal fibers (3). The axons of α-motoneurons are myelinated, so the action potential is conducted very rapidly, in saltatory fashion, as it "jumps" from one node of Ranvier to another, achieving conduction velocities of up to 120 m/sec.

• As the action potential invades each axon terminal, the membrane depolarization opens voltage-gated calcium channels. The influx of calcium induces the release of neurotransmitter, acetylcholine, into the synaptic cleft at the *neuromuscular junction* (4).

• The neurotransmitter traverses the synaptic cleft. Each packet of acetylcholine released into the cleft elicits a small depolarization of the muscle membrane (a miniature end plate potential) as neurotransmitter molecules bind to receptors (4). At the same time, acetylcholine is rapidly metabolized within the synaptic cleft by choline acetyltransferase. This assures that the chemical signal is tightly linked temporally to the neural signal.

• Miniature end plate potentials (EPP) summate to generate an action potential in the muscle cell membrane (5). The action potential "penetrates" each muscle fiber via the T-tubule system, arrays of channels perpendicular to the long axis of the muscle that penetrate the muscle at regular intervals along this axis. The T-tubule system is open to the extracellular space but also intimately linked to the intracellular sarcoplasmic reticulum, which is specially adapted for the storage and release of calcium.

• As the action potential invades the T-tubule system, large quantities of calcium are released from the sarcoplasmic reticulum. The large quantity of cytosolic calcium then leads to the successive formation and breakage of cross-bridges between actin and myosin, leading to muscle shortening.

• The spatially integrated sum of all the muscle fiber action potentials generated by the firing of a single α-motoneuron is referred to as a *motor unit potential (MUP).*

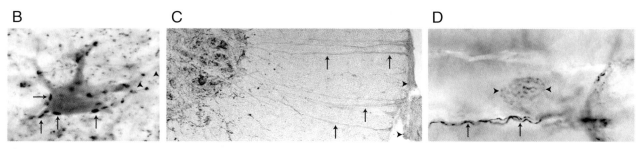

**Figure 6-3**, cont'd. Physiology of the motor unit. *B,* Photomicrograph of a ventral horn motoneuron. Synaptic densities are indicated by the arrows and the axon is indicated by the arrowheads. *C,* Low-power photomicrograph of a spinal ventral quadrant labeled to show motor axons coalescing (*arrows*) to form a ventral root (*arrowheads*). *D,* Photomicrograph of muscle with motor axon (*arrows*) and a neuromuscular junction (between *arrowheads*).

## *Case 6-2*

### Amyotrophic Lateral Sclerosis (Lou Gehrig's Disease)

*A 60-year-old man complains of a 6-month history of progressive weakness. He first noticed weakness in his right leg. He tripped repeatedly and found he had trouble dorsiflexing his right ankle. Subsequently the weakness of the right leg became more pervasive and about 2 months ago he noted weakness in the left leg. He now has to push with his arms to get out of chairs. He has noted some twitching of muscles in his legs and his hands. He frequently experiences cramps in his calves. On neurologic examination, there is wasting of the intrinsic hand muscles bilaterally, with mild associated weakness. In the lower extremities, there is mild weakness of the hip flexors and quadriceps femoris bilaterally, more so on the right, and there is more marked weakness of the right tibialis anterior. Fasciculations (muscle twitches) are visible or palpable in the right tibialis anterior and in the gastrocnemius muscles bilaterally.*

*An electromyographic (EMG) examination is performed on multiple proximal and distal muscles in the right arm and leg. In each muscle, a very fine, Teflon-coated needle is inserted into the muscle belly and the firing of muscle fibers is electronically recorded. In nearly every muscle examined, while the muscle is at rest, there are fasciculation potentials (irregular, broad, high amplitude, multiphasic potentials). When the patient is asked to contract the muscle, the amplitude and duration of the motor unit potentials (MUPs) are increased (Fig. 6-4), and there is a decreased recruitment pattern (see following discussion).*

**Comment:** *This patient has the particularly rapid form of motor neuron disease known as amyotrophic lateral sclerosis (ALS) or Lou Gehrig's disease, after the famous baseball star whose career was ended by the disease. In motor neuron disease (actually a host of different disorders), α-motoneurons become diseased and die, for reasons as yet unclear. In the ALS form, patients typically die from disseminated weakness of muscles throughout the body as well as of the tongue, muscles of swallowing, and muscles of respiration. One of the tasks of the neurologist, early in the disease course, is to determine whether the neurologic manifestations are relatively focal (and therefore might be caused by other disorders) or whether they are generalized.*

*Several of the patient's symptoms and signs deserve commentary. He has wasting of intrinsic hand muscles, reflecting loss of the trophic influence of α-motoneurons on muscle fibers (see Case 6-1). He has muscle twitches, known as fasciculations. These reflect the spontaneous depolarization of axons or α-motoneurons whose membranes have been rendered unstable as a result of disease. He also has cramps, which reflect a tendency for α-motoneurons engaged in a voluntary muscle contraction to continue firing at high rates even after voluntary effort has ceased, again because of membrane instability wrought from the loss of homeostatic functions subserved by the α-motoneuron cell bodies.*

*Electromyography detects the fasciculations, even when they are not visible on examination. In addition, as diseased α-motoneurons die, the axons of still-healthy neighbors sprout to supply new innervation to*

*Continued*

The Motor System

## Case 6-2—cont'd

the denervated muscle fibers (reinnervation). As a result, the average surviving α-motoneuron now supplies a much larger number of muscle fibers. Thus, the amplitude of MUPs is increased (Fig. 6-4). Furthermore, because new axon sprouts are often longer than normal, it takes longer for action potentials to travel to their terminal boutons than it does for action potentials traveling down the original axon branches. Thus, the time period over which all the muscle fibers belonging to a single α-motoneuron are depolarized is increased. For this reason, the duration of MUPs is increased as well (Fig. 6-4).

When the patient is asked to contract the muscle being studied, the smallest remaining α-motoneurons are recruited, as in a normal muscle. When more force is demanded, these small neurons fire faster. Normally, additional, slightly larger α-motoneurons would then be recruited. However, many of these are now dead. Thus, we are left with a situation in which a couple of motor units in the immediate vicinity of the needle tip are firing very rapidly (e.g., 50 Hz), unaccompanied by other MUPs firing at 40, 30, 20, or 10 Hz. This pattern, referred to as decreased recruitment, is indicative of loss of functioning axons, whether because of loss of α-motoneurons (as in ALS) or of axons (as in radiculopathy or neuropathy). The lower trace in Figure 6-4 reflects decreased recruitment.

In this way, electromyography is able to provide a detailed picture of the states of motor units that may not be evident from history and neurologic examination alone. In this particular patient, the electromyographic signs of denervation and renervation (decreased recruitment, increased MUP amplitude and duration, respectively) were found in multiple proximal and distal muscles of all limbs, providing strong support for the diagnosis of motor neuron disease, and eliminating the need to pursue a number of other diagnostic studies.

Normal

Reinnervation

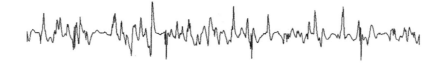

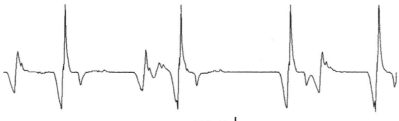

500 μV

10 ms

**Figure 6-4** Normal motor unit potentials (*top*) and motor unit potentials of increased amplitude and duration seen with denervation/reinnervation (*bottom*).

# Sensory Feedback and Segmental Reflexes

## Objectives

1. Be able to draw the reflex arc composed of an α-motoneuron, its axon, and group Ia sensory afferent projections.

2. Be able to explain the function of this reflex arc.

3. Be able to explain and give examples of the utility of abnormalities of myotatic reflex arcs in neurologic localization.

4. Be able to describe and explain the clinical differences between upper motor neuron and lower motor neuron lesions.

5. Be able to define the Jacksonian principle.

6. Be able to describe the two major roles of Golgi tendon organs and the type Ib afferent fibers innervating them.

In the beginning of this chapter we introduced the concept of the motor system as a hierarchical system. This hierarchy incorporates progressively more sophisticated levels of function as we ascend it. In addition, as the neurologist Hughlings Jackson proposed at the beginning of the 20th century, each level of the hierarchy has a certain degree of autonomy, and this autonomy is partially constrained by higher levels of the motor system. The level of the motor unit is no exception. The motor unit receives several modalities of sensory feedback. These sensory-motor connections, in turn, provide the basis for segmental reflexes: a primitive form of autonomous behavior. Later in the chapter, we will see how this behavior is constrained by higher levels of the motor system, and the consequences of loss of these constraints.

The α-motoneuron receives sensory feedback on the *length* of the muscle it innervates, the *rate of lengthening* of the muscle, and the *tension* the muscle exerts on the muscle tendon. These inputs also provide the basis for joint position sense (see Chapter 7).

## A. LENGTH FEEDBACK AND THE MUSCLE SPINDLE APPARATUS SYSTEM

Length feedback derives from a specialized organ within the muscle, the *muscle spindle apparatus* (Fig. 6-5). The muscle spindle apparatus consists of a highly elastic nuclear region, a deformable but not so elastic intermediate region, and polar regions composed of tiny striated (*intrafusal*) muscle fibers. The entire apparatus is enclosed in a membranous sac and the terminal portions of the polar regions, at either end of the sac, are attached to the *extrafusal* muscle fibers. Although this apparatus does contain muscle fibers, it is far too diminutive to induce joint movement. Rather, the nuclear and intermediate regions stretch or shorten as the extrafusal muscle stretches or shortens.

The Motor System

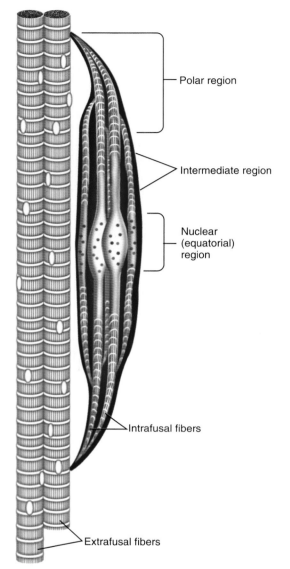

Polar region

Intermediate region

Nuclear (equatorial) region

Intrafusal fibers

Extrafusal fibers

**Figure 6-5** Muscle spindles (intrafusal fibers) are connected in parallel with striated muscle fibers (extrafusal fibers). (Modification of drawing by J. J. Warner.)

Stretching is detected by sensory nerve endings attached to the middle portion of the apparatus. There are two types of sensory nerves innervating this region: *group Ia* afferents (the largest of sensory nerves—see Table 6-1), which terminate in annulospiral endings wrapped around the nuclear region and are sensitive to the *rate* of muscle stretch, and the slightly smaller *group II* afferents, which terminate in "flower spray"

endings on the intermediate region and are sensitive to muscle *length* (Fig. 6-6).

The sensory neurons supplying the group Ia and group II endings (the cell bodies of which lie in the dorsal root ganglion) have axons that branch within the spinal cord. One branch sends information rostrally, via synapses on neurons supplying ascending sensory tracts, to the cerebral cortex, brainstem, and cerebellum. The other branch enters the ventral horn of the spinal cord, where it forms excitatory synapses on 50 to 80 percent of the α-motoneurons innervating muscle fibers within the parent (homonymous), extrafusal, muscle. When the muscle is stretched, these sensory nerves are stimulated. They then provide excitatory input to the α-motoneuron, inducing it to fire more rapidly, resisting the stretching force and preventing further muscle lengthening. The closed loop formed by the efferent axon of the α-motoneuron and the group Ia afferent fiber composes the *myotatic reflex arc* (Fig. 6-7). It provides the physiologic basis for *deep tendon reflexes* (a measure of phasic or *dynamic* muscle tone). The closed loop formed by the efferent axon of the α-motoneuron and the group II afferent composes another reflex arc (unnamed) that provides a physiologic basis for tonic (static) muscle tone.[2] For several reasons, both types of tone (but particularly dynamic tone) are among the most useful components of the entire neurologic examination: (1) they are readily assessed clinically; (2) both are highly localizing, as they are determined on a segmental basis (i.e., at one level of the spinal cord) (see Table 6-2); and (3) these reflexes are extremely resistant to influence by confounding factors (e.g., pain, lack of effort, psychiatric disease). Some of these attributes are illustrated in Case 6-3.

## Case 6-3

### Damage to S1 Nerve Root During Lumbar Disk Surgery

*A 50-year-old woman slips on an icy sidewalk and lands on her buttocks. For a couple of weeks she experiences aching low back pain. A year later, as she turns to get out of her car, she suddenly develops severe sharp pain in the left upper buttock radiating down the back of her left leg. This pain tends to*

[2]Unlike the myotatic reflex arc, this is not a monosynaptic reflex, as it incorporates one or more interneurons, and it probably involves γ- as well as α-motoneurons (see Box 6-1, The γ-Motoneuron System).

## Case 6-3—cont'd

fluctuate a great deal. It is aggravated by coughing, sneezing, lifting, the Valsalva maneuver (exhaling forcefully against a closed glottis), and tortional movements of the body. The pain does not subside, despite a week of bedrest. Diagnostic evaluation demonstrates a large L5–S1 herniated disk occupying the entire lateral recess of the bony spinal canal on the left side (see Case 1-3). She undergoes surgical resection of the disk. A year later, during a routine physical examination, her physician notices that her left "ankle jerk" (the deep tendon reflex elicited by striking the Achilles tendon with a reflex hammer) is absent. The remainder of her reflexes are graded 2 (on a scale of 1 to 5) and are normal (Table 6-3). In addition, there is less resistance to dorsiflexion of the left foot than of the right foot. Strength is normal throughout.

**Comment:** Tapping on the Achilles tendon transmits a brief pulse of vibration to the muscle spindles of the gastrocnemius and soleus ("gastroc-soleus") muscles. This elicits a burst of firing in the group Ia afferent

fibers that in turn leads to a burst of firing in the α-motoneuron—the jerk. Dorsiflexing the foot increases the firing rate in the group II afferent fibers and should, via a more modest increase in the firing rate of α-motoneurons, lead to modest resistance to dorsiflexion. Neither was found in this case. In the course of this patient's surgery, there was significant trauma to the S1 nerve root on the left (recall that the spinal cord ends at the L1–L2 level and that below this level, the bony spinal canal contains only nerve roots—the cauda equina). Although the S1 root exits through the S1–S2 neural foramen in the fused mass of sacral vertebral bodies known as the sacrum, it passes the L5–S1 disk far in the lateral recess of the bony spinal canal and is thus vulnerable to trauma, whether from the disk herniation itself or the surgery to remove the herniated fragment. It is quite common to find a missing deep tendon reflex after such surgery, reflecting damage to group Ia afferents. It is less common to encounter loss of static tone, reflecting damage to group II afferents.

## TABLE 6-1 Afferent Fiber Classes (Listed in Order of Declining Size)

| Conduction Velocity (m/sec) | Muscle Afferent | Cutaneous Afferent |
|---|---|---|
| 70–120 (myelinated) | Ia Primary muscle spindle (sensitive to velocity of muscle stretch) Ib Golgi tendon organ (sensitive to muscle tension) | |
| 25–75 (myelinated) | II Secondary muscle spindle (sensitive to muscle length) | Aβ Cutaneous receptors (sensitive to touch) |
| 10–30 (lightly myelinated) | III Muscle and visceral receptors (sensitive to pressure and pain) | Aδ Cutaneous receptors sensitive to touch, pressure, and pain |
| 0.5–2 (unmyelinated) | IV deep receptors (sensitive to pain) | C Cutaneous receptors (sensitive to temperature and pain) |

The Motor System

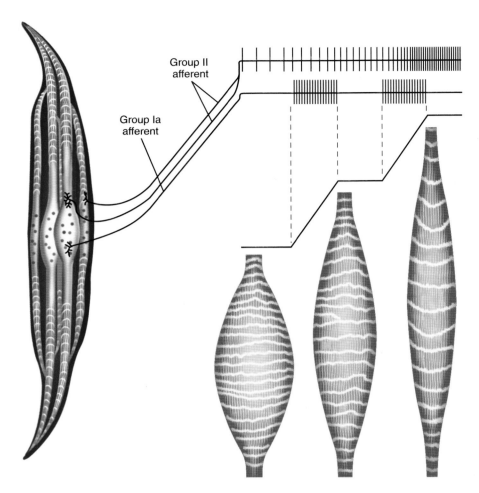

**Figure 6-6** Afferent innervation of the spindle fibers. Group Ia fibers fire transiently during the initial part of the stretch, that is, in relation to the rate of length change—the velocity—of stretch. Group II fibers fire in proportion to the length of the muscle. (Modification of drawing by J. J. Warner.)

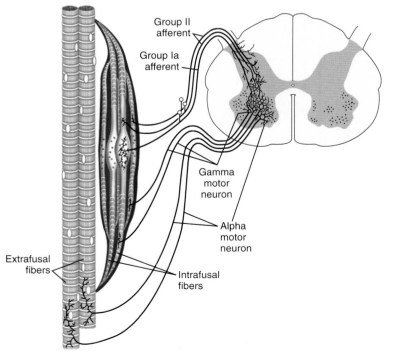

**Figure 6-7** Composite drawing of the entire extrafusal-intrafusal muscle apparatus, illustrating the axon of the α-motoneuron innervating the extrafusal fibers, and the group Ia (myotatic) and group II reflex arcs. Also illustrated are γ-motoneurons innervating the intrafusal muscle fibers (see Box 6.1). (Modification of drawing by J. J. Warner.)

**BOX 6-1**

*The γ-Motoneuron System*

In Figure 6-7, you will notice another efferent system stemming from small ventral horn motoneurons, the γ-motoneurons. The axons of these neurons synapse on the intrafusal muscle fibers of the spindle apparatus. When γ-motoneurons fire and contract the intrafusal muscle fibers, they stretch the intermediate and nuclear regions of the spindle apparatus and elicit firing of group Ia and II afferent fibers, which increases the firing rates of α-motoneurons supplying the extrafusal muscle fibers. In parallel with the functions of group Ia and II afferent fibers, there are static and dynamic γ-motoneurons.

The functions of γ-motoneurons cannot be differentially assessed in the course of the neurologic examination. However, γ-motoneurons clearly serve a crucial role. For example, given the peculiar arrangement of the group Ia and II reflex arcs, it is readily apparent that, as α-motoneuron firing begins to shorten a muscle, the muscle spindles will shorten as well, group Ia and II excitatory input to the α-motoneuron will drop, and the α-motoneuron will tend to stop firing. If this were the actual situation in the nervous system, any contractions that succeeded in shortening the muscle would cease almost as soon as they had begun. It appears that compensatory firing of

γ-motoneurons prevents this from occurring. They thus ensure that sensory feedback is available to the CNS throughout a movement. They provide a means by which the CNS can adjust the amplification of length- and velocity-dependent afferent feedback (i.e., the dynamic range of spindle afferent transmission). They make it possible to sustain continuous muscle shortening. In animal studies, spindle afferent firing remains nearly constant during muscle shortening. Because sustained complex movement involves continual lengthening and shortening of muscles, γ-motoneurons are generally just as active as α-motoneurons.

Gamma-motoneurons may be important in setting the equilibrium length for isometric muscle contraction. When they fire, they induce an increase in group Ia and II activity, in turn eliciting a higher firing rate in α-motoneurons. This shortens the extrafusal muscle until the inhibitory effect of shortening of the muscle spindle apparatus on group Ia and II activity is exactly counterbalanced by the excitatory effect of γ-motoneuron-induced stretching of the nuclear and intermediate zone of the muscle spindle. An increase in γ-motoneuron firing rate will reset the equilibrium at a state of greater muscle shortening.

**TABLE 6-2** Location of Myotatic Reflex Arcs Accessible to the Neurologic Examination

| Central Nervous System Level | Muscle Tested |
|---|---|
| CN V | Muscles of mastication ("jaw jerk") |
| CN VII | Muscles of facial expression |
| C5, C6 | Biceps, brachioradialis |
| C7 | Triceps |
| C8 | Finger flexors |
| L2, L3, L4 | Quadriceps femoris ("knee jerk") |
| S1 | Gastrocnemius-soleus ("ankle jerk") |

In principle, any lesion that damages the muscle stretch reflex arcs should cause hyporeflexia, regardless of whether it affects the α-motoneuron, its axon, the neuromuscular junction, the muscle, or the sensory afferent. The lesion might be peripheral, affecting a nerve root, peripheral nerve, or dorsal root ganglion, or it might be at the segmental level within the spinal cord, affecting the α-motoneuron, the proximal portion of its axon, or the portions of the axons from sensory neurons in the dorsal root ganglion that lie within the spinal cord. In practice, however, lesions of the sensory afferent fibers have the greatest impact, whereas lesions of the α-motoneurons, motoneuron axons, or muscle have variable and less dramatic effects. The impact of neuromuscular junction disease on deep tendon reflexes depends on the nature of that disease: it can be profound in Eaton-Lambert syndrome (Case

*The Motor System*

**TABLE 6-3** Grading of Deep Tendon Reflexes

| Grade | Rating | Significance |
|---|---|---|
| 0 | Absent | Usually pathologic |
| 1 | Just elicitable | Normal* |
| 2 | Easily elicitable | Normal* |
| 3 | Brisk | Normal* |
| 4 | Very brisk; associated with one or more reduplications (clonus) | Usually pathologic |
| 5 | Very brisk and associated with reduplications that continue as long as tension is maintained (sustained clonus) | Almost always pathologic |

*As we will show later in this chapter, all individual reflexes may fall in the normal range, whereas the pattern of reflexes may nevertheless suggest a pathologic condition.

4-1), and nonexistent in myasthenia gravis (Cases 4-16 and 5-1). This effect reflects the amount of neurotransmitter (acetylcholine) released at the first depolarizations of the terminal bouton of the $\alpha$-motoneuron in the two diseases (very small in Eaton-Lambert syndrome, normal in myasthenia gravis).

In the foregoing paragraphs, we discussed the importance of the group Ia afferent based myotatic reflex arcs and the group II afferent based reflex arcs in the localization of lesions of either peripheral portions of the nervous system or of spinal cord segments. The value of these reflexes is further enhanced by the fact that they are also modulated by cerebral and brainstem systems, and thus, central lesions will induce abnormalities in reflex tone as well. Neurons in brainstem centers (in part modulated by cerebral systems) send axons down the spinal cord that ultimately terminate on one or more interposed interneurons, which synapse on group Ia and II afferent endings in the spinal cord. In this way, they produce *presynaptic inhibition* of the excitatory effect of these sensory afferents on $\alpha$-motoneurons, resulting in reduced sensory input to the $\alpha$-motoneurons. With lesions of the cerebrum, brainstem, or the long connecting spinal cord pathways, this presynaptic inhibition is lost and the local reflex arcs are "released" from central control. The result is hyperactive deep tendon reflexes (increased dynamic tone) and augmented length-dependent resistance (increased static tone), a combination commonly referred to as *spasticity*. This phenomenon provides a cardinal example of the *Jacksonian principle that higher centers not only bring greater sophistication to neuronal processing but they also tonically inhibit lower centers*. The effect of CNS lesions on local dynamic and static stretch reflexes is illustrated in Case 6-4.

## Case 6-4

### Multiple Sclerosis

*A 35-year-old woman with multiple sclerosis is evaluated in clinic during a routine follow-up visit. She is generally doing well. She is known to have several spinal cord lesions and a number of cerebral lesions caused by this demyelinating disease. Examination is essentially normal but for the presence of abnormally brisk deep tendon reflexes everywhere (heightened dynamic tone) and increased resistance to passive limb movement (heightened static tone).*

**Comment:** *Because of the cerebral and spinal cord lesions, there has been loss of presynaptic inhibition to group Ia and group II terminals on $\alpha$-motoneurons, leading to abnormally high excitatory input from group Ia and group II neurons to $\alpha$-motoneurons at all levels. Thus, whereas hypoactive deep tendon reflexes are indicative of peripheral lesions or segmental spinal cord lesions (i.e., "lower motor neuron disease"), hyperactive deep tendon reflexes are indicative of CNS lesions (i.e., "upper motor neuron disease"). Peripheral lesions break myotatic reflex arcs whereas CNS lesions disinhibit or release myotatic reflex arcs. Whereas reduced resistance to slow muscle stretch is indicative of a peripheral lesion or a segmental spinal cord lesion, increased resistance to slow muscle stretch is indicative of a CNS lesion. Peripheral lesions break length-dependent reflex arcs, whereas CNS lesions disinhibit or release length-dependent reflex arcs (see Table 6-4).*

**TABLE 6-4** Summary: Effects of Lesions of the Motor System

|  | Peripheral | Central |
|---|---|---|
| Locus of lesion | Spinal cord segment, α-motoneuron, nerve root, or peripheral nerve | Rostral to α-motoneuron |
| Common terminology | "Lower motor neuron lesion" | "Upper motor neuron lesion" |
| Clinical features |  |  |
|   Atrophy | + | – |
|   Fasciculations | + | – |
|   Resistance to passive muscle stretch | Normal or decreased | Normal or increased |
|   Deep tendon reflexes | Usually decreased, especially with disease of sensory afferents | Increased |
| Distribution of impairment | Myotome, peripheral nerve, or disseminated | Hemibody (stroke, hemicord [Brown-Sequard] syndrome), or bilateral (myelopathy) |

## B. TENSION FEEDBACK AND THE GOLGI TENDON ORGAN SYSTEM

The Golgi tendon organ consists of a spray of specialized endings enveloped in a delicate capsule investing the muscle fascicle insertion point (Fig. 6-8). There is a Golgi tendon organ for each of the many muscle fascicles within a given muscle inserting on a tendon. The sensory neuron supplying each tendon organ projects via a Ib afferent fiber to an inhibitory interneuron between it and its α-motoneurons.

A Golgi tendon organ and its Ib afferent projections subserve two major roles. First, it provides feedback to an α-motoneuron regarding the tension exerted by its muscle fascicle on the muscle tendon. The greater the muscle fiber tension, the greater the inhibitory input to the α-motoneuron. In this way, the Golgi tendon organs appear to be the neuromechanical links that ultimately enable the equalization of the tension produced by the multiple α-motoneurons and their respective muscle fascicles on a tendon.

Second, the Golgi tendon organ provides information to the CNS regarding muscle tension that is used in the modification of muscle contraction pursuant to movement. The Ib afferent projections inhibit motoneurons supplying both homonymous and heteronymous (synergistic) muscles and they provide excitatory input to neurons supplying antagonist muscles. Through such circuitry, they may be useful in regulating the force of movement, particularly crucial when grasping a delicate object.

Afferent input from Golgi tendon organs as well as other tension-sensitive sensory neurons may also be important in preventing muscle overload.

## PRACTICE 6-3

**A.** A 68-year-old woman with a 5-year history of insulin-dependent diabetes mellitus (IDDM) presents to a neurologist because of a 1-year history of burning feet (a symptom of damage to peripheral sensory nerves). Examination reveals altered sensation for simple touch (the touch of the examiner's hands on her feet) in the distal lower extremities, extending halfway up the legs. The extensor digitorum brevis (EDB), on the dorsolateral surface of the feet, can no longer be palpated. Her deep tendon reflexes are 2 throughout (easily eli-

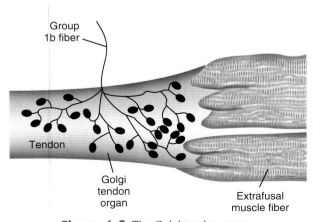

Group 1b fiber

Tendon

Golgi tendon organ

Extrafusal muscle fiber

**Figure 6-8** The Golgi tendon organ.

The Motor System

citable), with the exception of the ankle jerks, which are missing. It is known that diabetes results in damage to nerves, most likely because of associated disease of the vasa nervorum, the tiny blood vessels that supply the nerves. The longest nerves in the body are the most exposed to this pathologic process and, hence, are the most likely to be damaged. Explain the wasting of the EDBs and the missing ankle jerks.

**B.** A 25-year-old man is involved in an automobile accident. Evaluation in the emergency room reveals no evidence of serious injury. However, he has persistent neck pain, worse on the left side. He is evaluated by a physician who finds completely normal strength and opines that the patient is malingering in order to enhance the insurance settlement. You examine the patient and also find that his strength is normal, but in addition you find that his left triceps deep tendon reflex is unobtainable, whereas the remainder of his reflexes are normal. Can you localize the lesion?

**C.** A 45-year-old diabetic patient develops pain in his left thigh and weakness in his left leg. Examination reveals moderate weakness in the left iliopsoas (hip flexor) and quadriceps femoris. The patient is just able to walk. Deep tendon reflexes are 2 and symmetric in the upper extremities. The right knee jerk is 2, the left is absent, and both ankle jerks are absent. Localize all the lesions.

**D.** A 35-year-old woman presents with the chief complaint of numbness that has developed over the outer aspect of both thighs over the last month. The sensory loss is confirmed on examination. Deep tendon reflexes in the upper extremities are 2, and in the knees and ankles 4. The examination is otherwise normal. Localize the lesion.

**E.** A 50-year-old woman presents with difficulty walking that has developed insidiously over the last 6 months. On examination her gait is spastic and she has mild weakness of her iliopsoas bilaterally. Deep tendon reflexes are 3 to 4 throughout. The emergency room physician proposes getting a magnetic resonance image (MRI) of her lumbosacral spine, because she has proximal lower extremity weakness. What do you suggest? Why?

**F.** From a clinical point of view, Table 6-4 contains the most essential information in this entire chapter. If there is any aspect of this table that you do no understand or cannot readily explain, you should review this cycle.

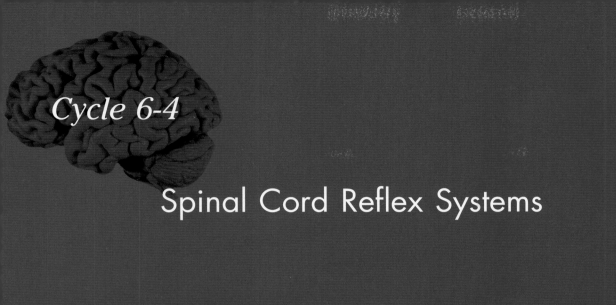

*Cycle 6-4*

## Objectives

1. Be able to describe the neural circuitry underlying spinal agonist-antagonist circuits, and list the three major types of input to the ventral horn that incorporate agonist-antagonist circuits.

2. Be able to describe the Babinski sign and triple flexion responses and explain how they occur.

3. Be able to explain the mechanisms underlying the spastic catch.

4. Be able to explain why signs of concurrent damage to descending and segmental motor systems have so much localizing value.

Up to this point, we have discussed only reflex systems based directly upon the afferent input to the α-motoneuron from the periphery. In this cycle, we will consider some reflex systems based upon simple circuits within the spinal cord. These circuits include agonist-antagonist circuits, circuits supporting withdrawal from noxious stimuli, and circuits supporting autogenic inhibition of muscle contraction (contraction-induced relaxation of a muscle).

## A. AGONIST-ANTAGONIST CIRCUITS

Group Ia afferents form excitatory synapses directly upon the α-motoneurons of their respective muscles (*homonymous* muscles) (e.g., the biceps). They also branch to form excitatory connections on the α-motoneurons of other *agonist* (synergistic) muscles (e.g., the brachioradialis) as well as on inhibitory interneurons that synapse on α-motoneurons supplying *antagonist* muscles (e.g., the triceps) (Fig. 6-9). Thus, the stretch of a muscle elicits contraction of that muscle and all other agonist muscles acting on its joint, while it inhibits all antagonist muscles, thus resisting further change in the angle of the joint. Activating group Ia afferents with a sudden vibratory pulse, as when eliciting deep tendon reflexes, achieves the same effect. This effect is also achieved when α- and γ-motoneurons are coactivated by motor centers in the cerebrum or brainstem: agonist muscles are co-contracted while antagonist muscles are concurrently inhibited. There is evidence of similar circuitry involving group II afferent fibers.

## B. WITHDRAWAL FROM NOXIOUS STIMULI

Group III and IV fibers from muscles and Aδ and unmyelinated C fibers from skin that are sensitive to nociceptive stimulation provide excitatory input to flexor α-motoneurons and inhibitory input to extensor α-motoneurons (via multisynaptic routes). For this reason, these are referred to as *nociceptive flexion reflex afferent fibers*. This circuitry provides the

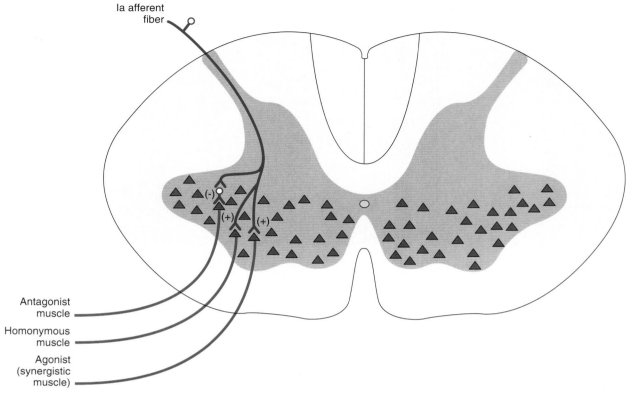

la afferent
fiber

(-)

(+)    (+)

Antagonist
muscle

Homonymous
muscle

Agonist
(synergistic
muscle)

**Figure 6-9** Agonist-antagonist circuits.

mechanism for very rapid withdrawal of a limb from a noxious stimulus. For example, these reflexes are responsible for the almost instantaneous withdrawal that occurs when one accidentally touches a hot stove. In the lower extremities in bipedal animals such as humans, and in all four extremities in quadrupedal animals, nociceptive flexor reflex afferents also provide excitatory input to extensor muscle groups of the other extremities (the crossed extensor response) (Fig. 6-10). This helps support the person or animal when sudden flexion of a limb is precipitated. However, the existence of a crossed extensor response (which in any event is difficult to demonstrate in humans) will not prevent falls when nociceptive flexion occurs as weight is being shifted to the affected leg. Fortunately, this nociceptive flexion reflex is normally inhibited by cerebral and brainstem systems (the medullary reticulospinal system, see later discussion). However, lesions of the cerebrum, the brainstem, or spinal cord pathways will interfere with this inhibition of the nociceptive flexion reflex, leading to uncontrolled action of this segmental reflex. This phenomenon, often referred to as *release*

of the reflex, is a classic example of the Jacksonian hierarchical principle. When the degree of release is relatively minimal, the result is the *Babinski sign*. When it is more nearly complete, the result is the *triple flexion response*. These responses are illustrated in Cases 6-5 and 6-6.

## Case 6-5

### Lacunar Infarct of the Posterior Limb of the Internal Capsule

*A 70-year-old man suddenly develops right-sided weakness, greater in his arm than his leg, due to a stroke involving the posterior limb of the left internal capsule (see Fig. 2-21). On examination, he has lost all useful function in the right hand and is profoundly weak in the right arm. He also exhibits weakness in the right leg but he is able to walk. When the outer portion of the sole of his left foot is scraped with the wooden end of a Q-tip, the great toe curls down*

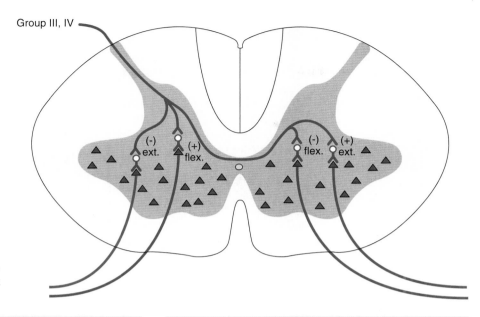

**Figure 6-10** Nociceptive flexion and crossed extension reflex pathways.

## Case 6-5—cont'd

*(flexes), a normal response. When the right foot is stimulated in similar fashion, the great toe goes up (extends)—a Babinski sign (also known as an extensor plantar response).*

**Comment:** *The nociceptive flexion reflex on the right has been partially released, or disinhibited, because of the damage to pathways between the cerebral cortex and regions of the medullary reticular formation that normally inhibit this reflex (to be discussed further).*

## Case 6-6

### Multiple Sclerosis
*The 35-year-old woman with multiple sclerosis introduced in Case 6-4 complains of repeatedly falling. The physician examining her has difficulty accounting for her complaint because her legs seem strong and her balance is only mildly impaired. However, when he scratches the bottom of either foot with the wooden end of a Q-tip, not only does he elicit a Babinski sign—he elicits a full triple flexion response: flexion at the ankle, knee, and hip.[3]*

---

[3]It may seem confusing that the terms "extensor plantar response" and "triple flexion response" are used to refer to the same fundamental physiologic process. The explanation is that the pathologic reflex involves withdrawal of four limb components from a noxious plantar stimulus: the great toe (extension), the foot (ankle dorsiflexion), the leg (knee flexion), and the thigh (hip flexion).

## Case 6-6—cont'd

**Comment:** *This patient is repeatedly falling because very minor stimuli to her feet, incurred in the course of routine standing and walking, elicit unilateral or bilateral triple flexion responses. This fullest expression of the released nociceptive flexion response may be further potentiated by excessively sensitive Golgi tendon organs systems (see the next section, Autogenic Inhibition of Muscle Contraction). Each time this happens, she falls. Fortunately, this symptom can almost always be treated with baclofen, a GABA$_B$ receptor agonist that potentiates potassium conductance, and thus inhibits the neuronal firing involved in the nociceptive flexion reflex.*

## C. AUTOGENIC INHIBITION OF MUSCLE CONTRACTION

The function of Golgi tendon organs and other, less well-defined systems sensitive to muscle tension, are normally inapparent to us. However, it is clear that these systems, like the nociceptive flexion reflexes, are subject to inhibition from higher centers in the cerebrum and brainstem and therefore susceptible to "release" with damage to these centers or their long connections to the various levels of the spinal cord. This release engenders the *spastic catch*, sometimes referred to as the "clasped knife reflex," as illustrated in Case 6-7.

The various reflexes we have discussed so far are summarized in Table 6-5.

**The Motor System**

## Case 6-7

### Multiple Sclerosis

*Further examination of the 35-year-old woman with multiple sclerosis introduced in Cases 6-4 and 6-6 reveals not only the hyperactive deep tendon reflexes and triple flexion plantar responses already described, but also spastic catches in her quadriceps femoris bilaterally. The examiner has her lie on her back on the examining table. As he asks her to relax as completely as possible, he lifts one leg and rapidly flexes the knee. Group Ia and group II, velocity- and length-dependent, afferent input rapidly increases, amplified by excessive γ-motoneuron activity. This maneuver leads to an abrupt catch as it induces a sudden dramatic increase in α-motoneuron firing. This catch is instantly followed by an abrupt release as force-sensitive afferents, possibly including Ib afferents from Golgi tendon organs, suddenly strongly inhibit α-motoneuron firing to the quadriceps femoris, thereby producing muscle relaxation, and briefly excite α-motoneurons supplying antagonist muscles.*

**Comment:** *Similar responses can often be elicited in other lower and upper extremity musculature, albeit less reliably. Spastic catches constitute a particularly important clinical sign because they are always abnormal, whereas even extremely brisk deep tendon reflexes may occasionally be normal.*

**TABLE 6-5** Summary of Reflex Systems

| | Reflex | Peripheral/Spinal Segmental | | Central | |
|---|---|---|---|---|---|
| **Response** | **Neural Basis** | **Physiologic Consequence** | **Behavioral Consequence** | **Physiologic Consequence** | **Behavioral Consequence** |
| **Muscle stretch reflex** | Group II—α-motoneuron | Loss of excitatory group II input to α-motoneuron | Flaccid tone | Loss of presynaptic inhibition of group II input to α-motoneuron | Excessive static tone |
| **Deep tendon reflex** | Group Ia—α-motoneuron | Loss of excitatory group Ia input to α-motoneuron | Reduced or absent deep tendon reflex | Loss of presynaptic inhibition of group Ia input to α-motoneuron | Hyperactive deep tendon reflex |
| **Babinski sign/triple flexion response** | Nociceptive flexion reflex circuits | NA | NA | Loss of central inhibition of reflex | Disinhibition of lower extremity flexion responses to noxious stimulation |
| **Spastic catch** | Group II/Ia—group Ib/other tension related afferent input to α-motoneuron | NA | NA | Loss of presynaptic inhibition of group II & Ia afferents followed by release of Ib mediated inhibition of α-motoneuron | Catch (II & Ia mediated) followed by release (Ib mediated) |

# D. THE INTERSECTION OF SEGMENTAL AND DESCENDING MOTOR SYSTEMS—KEY TO NEUROLOGIC LOCALIZATION

Focal lesions within the brainstem and spinal cord almost invariably disrupt both local, segmental systems and descending motor pathways. This phenomenon is of inestimable value in neurologic localization. For example, a patient who is normal but for a missing left triceps deep tendon reflex could have a lesion interrupting Ia afferent fibers anywhere between the muscle spindles of the triceps and the dorsal root entry zone at the C7 level of the spinal cord. We can guess as to the localization of this lesion based upon what we know about the prevalence of the various disorders that might be causing the problem (this would lead us to suspect a lesion at the root level due to a herniated disk or bony spurs). However, there is nothing about this patient's examination that enables us to pinpoint the lesion with certainty. By the same token, a patient who exhibits hyperactive reflexes and a spastic catch in the left leg together with a Babinski sign could, in principle, have a lesion affecting descending motor pathways anywhere above L2. Again, only the patterns of the most prevalent disorders producing such a pattern would help us in predicting the likely location of the lesion. However, the presence of both segmental and descending motor tract signs serves to pinpoint the lesion with certainty, as illustrated in Case 6-8.

## Case 6-8

### Herniated Cervical Disk with Cord Compression

*A 50-year-old man "ruptures" the C4-C5 disk as he is unloading some fertilizer. He experiences right-sided neck pain for 2 weeks. However, because of the break in the fibrous ring of the disk (the annulus fibrosis), and continued wear and tear on his neck, over time more and more of the disk material protrudes into the spinal canal. Eventually, it causes significant compression of the spinal cord at the C5 level and of the C5 nerve root on the right side (Fig. 6-11).*

**Comments:** *The spinal cord compression at C5 damages the gray matter of the cord at this level. This, in conjunction with damage to the right C5 nerve root, results in loss of the C5-C6 deep tendon reflexes (biceps, brachioradialis), weakness, and*

## Case 6-8—cont'd

*possibly some atrophy of C5 innervated muscles. It also damages descending motor pathways, leading to hyperactivity of all deep tendon reflexes represented below the lesion (triceps [C7], knee jerks [L2-L4], and ankle jerks [S1]), spastic catches in muscles innervated by α-motoneurons below the lesion, and bilateral Babinski signs (in aggregate, "long tract signs"). Because the entire cord is at least somewhat compressed, both lower motor neuron and upper motor neuron signs are bilateral, although more prominent on the right side.*

As we shall see in the chapter on cranial nerves, the combination of segmental and long tract signs provides an equally valuable index to localization within the brainstem—the major difference being that segmental damage within the brainstem produces cranial nerve abnormalities rather than lower motor neuron signs in the arms and legs.

## PRACTICE 6-4

**A.** A 70-year-old man with carcinoma of the prostate develops compression of the spinal cord at the T8 level as a result of a metastasis to a vertebral body. Predict his neurologic findings, including changes in the reflexes discussed so far in this chapter. Explain your predictions.

**B.** A 19-year-old college student develops Guillain-Barré syndrome 10 days after experiencing a gastrointestinal illness. This disorder is thought to be mediated by antibodies to antigenic sites shared by a myelin protein and certain infectious organisms, including viruses and some bacteria. The patient exhibits generalized weakness and loss of all deep tendon reflexes. Localize the lesions. Explain your localization. Do you think he would have Babinski signs? Why or why not?

**C.** A 70-year-old man with a lifelong history of heavy smoking has known small cell carcinoma of the lung. This highly malignant neoplasm has a strong propensity for widespread metastasis. He presents with bilateral leg weakness, absent deep tendon reflexes in the legs, and bilateral Babinski signs. His arms are normal. Localize the lesion.

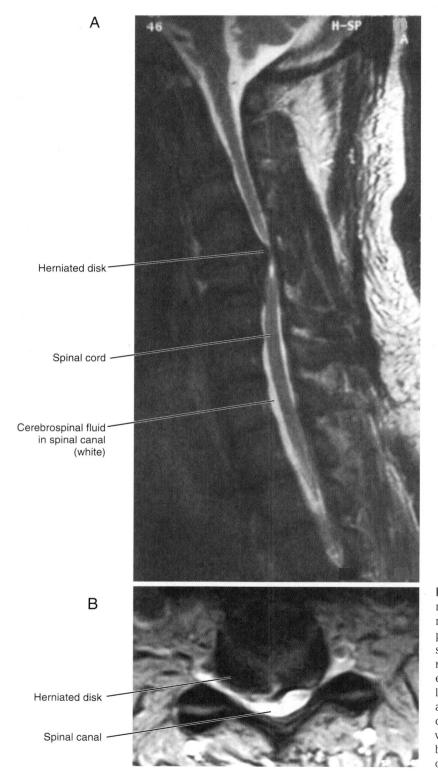

**A**

Herniated disk

Spinal cord

Cerebrospinal fluid
in spinal canal
(white)

**B**

Herniated disk

Spinal canal

**Figure 6-11** Cervical magnetic resonance image (MRI) in patient with a herniated C4–C5 disk with cord compression, predominantly on the right side. *A,* Sagittal slice. *B,* Coronal slice. So much disk material has been extruded in this case that it extends between the posterior longitudinal ligament and the posterior margins of C4 and C5 both above and below the C4–C5 disk level. The spinal cord is not visible within the spinal canal in the coronal slice because the MRI parameters were set to optimally demonstrate the spinal canal.

**D.** A 78-year-old woman slips and falls in her bathroom and breaks her left wrist. Two months later, when the cast is removed, she seems to have some difficulty using her hand. She also complains that she is having difficulty walking, tending to drag her left leg. She has a long history of arthritis affecting the left hip. Her physician concludes that her problems are related simply to disuse of the left hand and a flare-up of her arthritis. He prescribes an arthritis medication and sends her to physical therapy. You examine her and find that her entire left arm is weak, she has no reflexes in the left arm (those in the right arm are all 2), she has hyperactive reflexes in the left leg, and she demonstrates a left Babinski sign. Localize the lesion. Another physician evaluates the patient and finds both the left arm and leg weakness and concludes that she has had a cerebral hemispheric stroke. Is he right or wrong? How do you know?

# Cycle 6-5

# Spinal Cord Movement Systems

## Objectives

1. Be able to describe the concept of distributed representation as it applies to the motor system.
2. Be able to describe the advantages of this mode of motor system organization with respect to responses to injurious stimuli, loss of balance, and walking.
3. Be able to describe the major functions of Renshaw cells.

## A. DISTRIBUTED REPRESENTATION OF MOTOR FUNCTION

Up to this point, we have conceived of the spinal cord as a great stack of local segments, each comprising a slice of central gray matter (which includes α- and γ-motoneurons) and a dorsal root ganglion. Each segment supports local reflexes at the same time that its neurons are driven or inhibited from above by long tracts descending from the cerebral cortex and the brainstem. Unfortunately, this "executive-laborer" model does not do justice to the evolution of the CNS, and most seriously, it will not provide a satisfactory account for the patterns of clinical deficits we see with lesions of higher components of the motor system. These clinical patterns reflect the combined effect of

damage to higher systems, released functions at segmental levels, and preserved movement functions in lower systems. In no movement is this more evident than in walking.

Walking in both bipeds and quadrupeds requires coordinated, reciprocating movements incorporating muscles on both sides of the body innervated from the C4 through the S2 segments (arm swinging in bipeds helps to maintain balance). These movements are generated entirely within the spinal cord utilizing intersegmental connections known as propriospinal pathways. The earliest form of such multisegment-mediated coordinated movement was swimming. It is well developed in the most primitive of vertebrates, such as lampreys. Walking incorporates analogous reciprocating operations. However, it also requires balance and the maintenance of antigravity muscle tone, both of which are subserved by brainstem nuclei (to be discussed), and it also requires substrates for several different movement variations (e.g., strolling, walking, trotting, running, sprinting). The capacity of these ancient systems for executing the complex process of walking is no more dramatically illustrated than in experiments in cats in which the brainstem has been separated from the cerebrum by a cut at the junction between the thalamus and the midbrain. These decerebrate cats can be induced to walk on a treadmill by appropriate stimulation at a region of the midbrain known as the mesencephalic locomotor region. Such experiments have never been done in higher primates, but there is good evidence that the capacity of brainstem and spinal mechanisms for support of walking as well as a variety of other complex movements, such as those required to maintain balance or correct gait after tripping (postural reflexes), are preserved in more advanced organisms. These capacities are now being deliberately engaged in the rehabilitation of patients with spinal cord injury, as illustrated in Case 6-9.

---

### Case 6-9

#### Spinal Cord Injury

*A 45-year-old man is shot in the midthoracic spine during a robbery, rendering him acutely paraplegic. The spinal cord is severely contused (bruised) by bone fragments. A year later, following extensive rehabilitation, with great effort he is able to ambulate very short distances about his home using crutches. He then enters an investigational rehabilitation program in which he is suspended over a treadmill such that his feet contact the moving mat. Over the course of treatment, he eventually gains the ability to walk over 100 feet using a simple cane.*

**Comment:** *This rehabilitation technique engages the reciprocating spinal cord pattern generators responsible for walking movements and remodels their patterns of neural connectivity (with the strenuous efforts of the patient) so that the pattern generators are able to operate in the context of the dramatically altered pattern of descending input created by the cord lesion.*

---

These brainstem and spinal mechanisms support a *distributed representation of motor function*. That is, rather than movement being produced from the top down by an executive system, movement is the emergent product of the interaction of multiple systems—cortical, brainstem, spinal, and segmental—each with its own special expertise, each assuming a more or less dominant role automatically (without central directive), depending on the circumstances. In the decerebrate cat, walking could be induced by stimulation of the mesencephalic locomotor region. This walking depended on the action of reciprocating spinal cord pattern generator circuits, modified by vestibulospinal input (input from the inner ear critical to balance—to be discussed further), segmental sensory input, and segmental reflexes. In the normal animal or human, the relative contributions of these systems changes from moment to moment with changes in gait, perturbations of balance, changes in terrain, and encounters with objects to be stepped over or around. In Case 6-9, the capabilities conferred by the distributed representation of motor function had been lost, not only because of interruption of descending motor control, but also because of pathologic patterns of activity in spinal cord neuronal networks resulting from the injury. The rehabilitation program, by altering patterns of neural connectivity, succeeded in releasing spinal cord pattern generator circuits from their dominance by this pathologic activity, enabling them to operate effectively in the new environment.

A distributed representation is important for at least three major reasons. First, although the cerebrum, as we shall see, is capable of enormous precision as well as great speed in the production of internally initiated movements, it is very slow in producing reactive movements. Cerebral reaction times are on the order of hundreds of milliseconds. These delays are intolerable when urgent reaction is called for, such as withdrawing a hand from a hot stove, or avoiding falling when one loses balance. The brainstem and spinal mechanisms we have been discussing provide a far more optimal solution to these problems because of their capability for great speed (tens of milliseconds). Second, the cerebrum is generally ill equipped for maintaining two movement programs simultaneously. The relatively autonomous execution of sitting, standing, and walking by the brainstem and spinal cord enables us to carry out other activities, such as thinking, talking, or doing things with our hands, as we move about. Finally, in nearly all patients with cerebral injury, whatever the location or cause, there is a strong tendency for arm movements to be more affected than leg movements. This reflects the degree to which lower extremity functions are subserved by brainstem and spinal cord mechanisms that are spared by cerebral lesions.

## B. RENSHAW CELLS

Our discussion so far has focused exclusively on specific motor mechanisms to the exclusion of the general problems of information processing in the motor system. We will focus now on *Renshaw cells*. They have a salient role in the regulation of information processing in motor systems of the spinal cord. The manner in which these cell populations function provides a good illustration of a common approach that

*The Motor System*

has evolved in neural systems to deal with some inherent problems of information processing.

Renshaw cells are glycinergic inhibitory interneurons within the spinal cord that receive collateral projections from $\alpha$-motoneurons. They then synapse on these same $\alpha$-motoneurons as well as on homonymous and heteronymous (synergistic) $\alpha$-motoneurons. Renshaw cells serve to focus neural activity and to dampen excessive neural activity not precisely related to sensory stimulation or motor action (neural noise).

The problem of focus is nicely illustrated by the biathlon event in the Olympics, in which athletes alternate cross-country skiing with precision rifle shooting. Cross-country skiing requires generally high muscle tone, whereas precision marksmanship requires nearly complete relaxation of all muscles except those few directly involved in the task. To the extent that there is lack of focus, marksmanship suffers.

The diffuse connectivity of neurons and the prevalence of excitatory neurons provides a recipe for spreading and amplifying noise, yet Renshaw cells are so effective at dampening noise that we are rarely aware of the problem. The most dramatic demonstrations of the impact of these cells are seen in patients intoxicated with substances that seriously interfere with Renshaw cell function, such as tetanus toxin (see Case 4-7) and strychnine. In these patients, the slightest stimulation leads to sudden generalized muscular contraction. This reflects complete loss of focus and maximum noise in motoneuron populations.

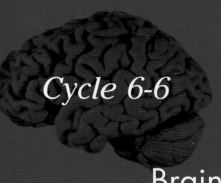

# Cycle 6-6

# Brainstem Centers: Tone, Posture, and Movement

## Objectives

1. Be able to distinguish the ventromedial and lateral tract groups in terms of their spatial relationship to motor neurons subserving different portions of the body, their role in tone, posture and precision movement, and their predominant effects on flexor and extensor (antigravity) muscle tone.

2. Be able to describe the effects on balance of lesions involving the vestibular labyrinths, the vestibular nuclei, or the vestibulospinal tracts.

3. Be able to characterize and explain the two major types of posturing (decorticate and decerebrate) observed in patients with lesions of the pons and lesions above the pons.

4. Be able to explain why the presence of upper extremity pronation drift and impairment in fine finger movements are such important neurologic signs.

5. Be able to distinguish the clinical manifestations of spinal shock from those of chronic spinal cord lesions.

Examination of a cross section of the spinal cord reveals five major descending motor tracts: the *vestibulospinal tracts*, the *pontine reticulospinal tract*, the *medullary reticulospinal tract*, the *lateral corticospinal tract*, and the *tectoreticulospinal tract* (Table 6-6) (Fig. 6-12*A*, *B*). A sixth set of tracts, the rubrospinal tracts, originate in the red nuclei of the midbrain. They have similar organization and share many functions with the lateral corticospinal tracts, and the effects of lesions of these tracts can rarely be distinguished clinically.

There are three major principles implicit in Table 6-6, which summarizes descending motor tracts:

1. All of the ventromedial tracts travel in close proximity to the medial aspect of the ventral horn of the spinal gray matter, which contains neurons innervating axial and limb girdle musculature, and all are primarily involved in actions involving axial and proximal muscle groups and in the regulation of posture and tone.

2. The major lateral tract, the lateral corticospinal tract, travels in close proximity to the lateral aspect of the ventral horn of the spinal gray matter, which contains neurons innervating distal musculature, and it is involved principally in precision movements of the distal extremities, especially the hands.

3. Ventromedial tracts, with the exception of the tectoreticulospinal tract, strongly favor extensor (antigravity) tone. The dominant lateral tract, the lateral corticospinal tract, has minimal effects on tone.

Almost all the axons within the descending motor tracts terminate on interneurons within the spinal cord

255

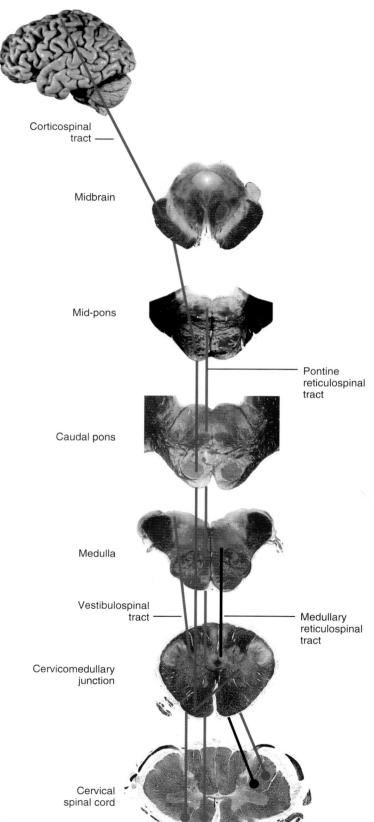

Corticospinal tract

Midbrain

Mid-pons

Pontine reticulospinal tract

Caudal pons

Medulla

Vestibulospinal tract

Medullary reticulospinal tract

Cervicomedullary junction

Cervical spinal cord

**Figure 6-12** The major descending motor tracts of the spinal cord.

A
256

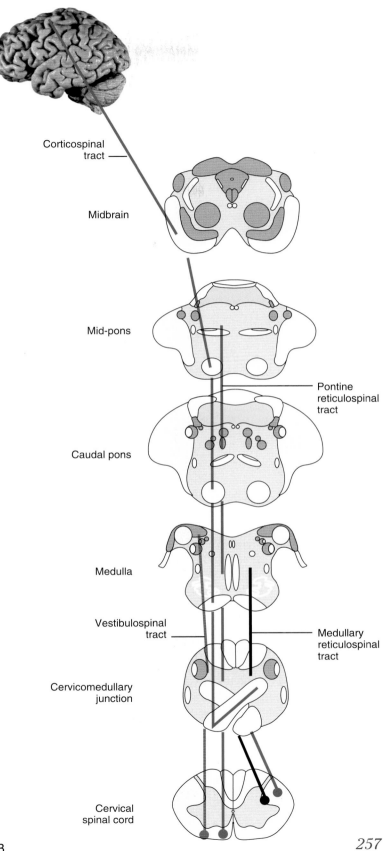

Corticospinal tract

Midbrain

Mid-pons

Pontine reticulospinal tract

Caudal pons

Medulla

Vestibulospinal tract

Medullary reticulospinal tract

Cervicomedullary junction

Cervical spinal cord

**Figure 6-12**, cont'd

B

**TABLE 6-6** Descending Motor Pathways

| Tract | Source | Spinal Cord Location | Flexor/Extensor Bias | Principal Targeted Musculature | Function |
|-------|--------|---------------------|---------------------|-------------------------------|----------|
| Lateral and medial vestibulospinal | Lateral and medial vestibular nucleus in the dorsolateral medulla | Ventromedial | Extensor | Axial/proximal | Posture, axial movement, muscle tone, and balance |
| Pontine reticulospinal | Nucleus reticularis pontis | Ventromedial | Extensor | Axial/proximal | Posture, axial movement and muscle tone |
| Medullary reticulospinal | Nucleus reticularis gigantocellularis | Lateral | Flexor | Axial/proximal | Posture, axial movement and muscle tone |
| Lateral corticospinal | Cerebral cortex | Lateral | Minimal | Distal | Distal, precision movement |
| Tectoreticulospinal | Deep layers of superior colliculus | Ventromedial | None | Axial | Head movements required for orienting reactions |

gray matter, either within the ventral horn or in the junctional zone between the dorsal and ventral horns. The interneurons, in turn, project to α- and γ-motoneurons as well as to group Ia and group II terminals (providing the basis for presynaptic inhibition of segmental reflexes). The major exception to this indirect projection pattern is certain lateral corticospinal tract fibers, particularly those linked to arm and hand movement, which synapse directly on α- and γ-motoneurons. This linkage provides the basis for the extremely rapid and highly focused activation of α-motoneurons necessary for quick, precise hand movements.

For all the descending tracts, with the single exception of the lateral corticospinal tract, the termination is predominantly ipsilateral to the point of origin. The lateral corticospinal tract, of course, originates in the contralateral cerebral cortex, and 90 percent of its fibers cross in the decussation of the medullary pyramids (Fig. 6-13); the remaining 10 percent travel without crossing within the ventromedial portion of the cord.

## A. THE VESTIBULOSPINAL TRACTS

The *vestibulospinal system* plays a dominant role in the maintenance of the antigravity tone necessary for us to sit, stand, and maintain any posture other than horizontal. It also produces the corrective movements necessary to keep us from falling when, in the course of routine movements, our center of gravity is no longer directly over our feet. The consequences of damage to this system are illustrated in Case 6-10.

### Case 6-10

**Parkinson's Disease**

*A 66-year-old man with a 15-year history of Parkinson's disease complained of repeatedly falling. His neurologist was at first puzzled by the complaint because the patient's anti-Parkinsonian medications had been very carefully titrated and the patient moved extraordinarily well. When asked, he promptly got out of his chair without evidence of any tendency*

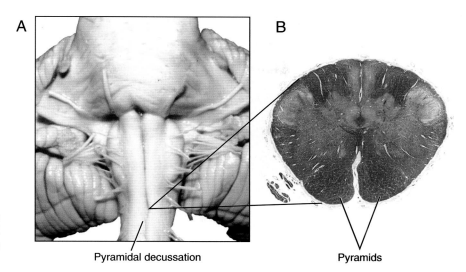

**Figure 6-13** Decussation of the medullary pyramids. *A,* Ventral view of the brainstem. *B,* Cross section of the medulla.

Pyramidal decussation     Pyramids

---

## Case 6-10—cont'd

*to go backward (retropulsion) and without pushing off with his hands. He easily initiated walking, his walking movements were fluid, and he made nearly normal turns. His stride was normal. The neurologist then asked the patient to stand with his feet together and his eyes closed. The patient did so without difficulty. Finally, as the patient was still standing with eyes closed, the neurologist suddenly grabbed him by the shoulders and forcibly yanked him backward. The patient failed utterly to make any corrective movements and would have fallen and experienced injury had the neurologist not caught him.*

**Comment:** *Although Parkinson's disease principally involves the dopaminergic neurons in the midbrain that modulate basal ganglia function (to be discussed), the disease eventually affects other neural systems, including vestibulospinal systems. As a result, patients eventually lose their postural reflexes, as in this case. Unfortunately, because this is not a dopaminergic system, the deficit cannot be corrected with the dopaminergic medication that so dramatically improves other motor deficits in these patients.*

Physiologic perturbation of the vestibular system by changes in the orientation of the head with respect to the gravitational field, or the induction of angular momentum in the head, lead to compensatory alterations in muscle tone and compensatory movements that precisely anticipate the consequences of the perturbations and thereby prevent falls. This principle can

be illustrated quite convincingly by inducing a non-physiologic perturbation by injecting cold water in one ear (cold calorics). Cold water injected in the right ear reduces the signal from the right labyrinth to the vestibular nuclei. This signal makes the brainstem "think" that there is a left body tilt, and it will compensate by inducing right body tilt. If you perform this experiment yourself, you will discover that, when walking, it requires some mental effort to avoid constantly drifting to the right and bumping into things. (Caution: restrict caloric stimulation to 30 mL of water chilled to 10°C injected over 30 seconds; larger amounts of colder water may induce frank vertigo, nausea, and vomiting.)

## B. THE MEDULLARY AND PONTINE RETICULOSPINAL TRACTS

The *medullary* and *pontine reticulospinal tracts* originate in the medulla and pons, respectively, and travel down the brainstem and spinal cord to terminate at the various segmental levels (Fig. 6-14). They are also involved in the maintenance of flexor and extensor muscle tone necessary to sustain posture and gait. In addition, they serve to immobilize the proximal portions of our extremities in order to provide a platform for distal extremity use. For example, when one types at a computer keyboard, the arms must be maintained in a semiflexed posture in such a way that the hands are suspended at the correct position over the keyboard. This positioning makes it possible for the fingers to make correct keystrokes through appropriate fine

*The Motor System*

**Pontine Reticular Formation**

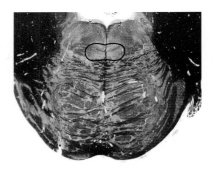

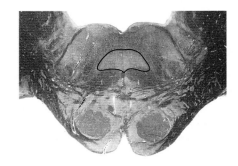

**Medullary Reticular Formation**

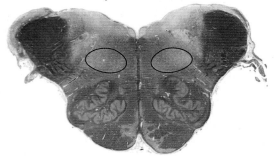

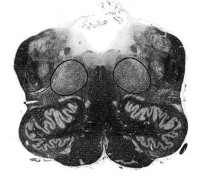

**Figure 6-14** The pontine and medullary reticular formations.

movements of finger flexor muscles and intrinsic hand muscles.

The medullary and pontine reticulospinal systems receive extensive input from the cerebral cortex, the cerebellum, and the spinal cord. The pontine reticulospinal system also receives major input from the vestibular nuclei. We believe that these systems operate according to the Jacksonian principle—that is, they add movement capability to that which is latent in lower systems within the spinal cord at the same time that they are regulated (predominantly inhibited) by higher systems. In Section E, we will discuss some of the consequences of disinhibition of the brainstem by more rostral lesions.

## C. THE TECTORETICULOSPINAL TRACT

The *tectoreticulospinal tract* derives from deep layers of the superior colliculus and projects to α- and γ-motoneuron pools in the cervical spinal cord. The deep layers of the superior colliculus receive visual, auditory, and somatosensory input. The superior colliculus, superficial and deep, is responsible for reactive orienting movements of the eyes and head. Reactive orienting movements are triggered when we encounter a salient sensory stimulus, such as a bright flash of light, a movement in our peripheral visual fields, a loud noise, or a painful somatosensory stimulus. Reactive orienting movements can be contrasted with intentional orienting movements, which are driven by the frontal eye fields.

Superficial layers of the superior colliculus provide the substrate for defining the targets of intended saccadic eye movements and are linked to eye movement control mechanisms. However, orienting responses also require, to one degree or another, movements of the head. Reactive orienting head movements are generated by the tectoreticulospinal tract.

## D. THE LATERAL CORTICOSPINAL TRACT

The *lateral corticospinal tract* derives from the pyramidal cells of area 4 of the cerebral cortex. These cells, their processes, and their projection targets compose the *pyramidal system*. The system will be our major focus in Cycle 6-8. The pyramidal system has minimal direct effects on muscle tone and is primarily involved in the execution of precise movements. It is most highly developed and operates with the least interaction with other motor systems in the control of the distal extremities, particularly the hands.

## E. CLINICAL EVIDENCE OF THE JACKSONIAN PRINCIPLE IN BRAINSTEM AND SPINAL CORD MOTOR SYSTEMS

In this section, we will consider the effects of lesions at various points in the motor system hierarchy that we have discussed. We have already reviewed the effects of spinal cord lesions that interfere with descending inhibitory influences on muscle stretch reflexes and local spinal cord reflexes. Both group Ia afferent fiber mediated reflexes (involving the myotatic reflex arc and dynamic tone) and group II afferent fiber mediated reflexes (involving static tone) are subject to tonic presynaptic inhibition at the site of afferent terminations on α-motoneurons. When this inhibition is lost, the result is hyperactive deep tendon reflexes (excessive dynamic tone), hyperactive stretch reflexes (excessive static tone)—the two in combination causing spasticity—and spastic catches, reflecting the combination of hyperactive stretch reflexes and disinhibited group Ib afferent input from Golgi tendon organs. Spinal cord lesions sever medullary reticulospinal projections that normally inhibit nociceptive flexion reflex systems, leading to the Babinski sign (the abbreviated response) and the triple flexion response (the full response). Because the medullary reticulospinal system is, in part, driven by corticobulbar projections,[4] lesions of either the cerebral cortex or of its projections to the medulla will also lead to a Babinski sign. The Babinski sign is commonly misinterpreted as a sign of corticospinal tract damage—a "pyramidal sign." This misconception is due to the company the corticospinal tract keeps—corticobulbar pathways projecting to the medullary reticular formation in the cerebrum and brainstem, and medullary reticulospinal pathways traveling in the lateral tract group in the spinal cord. Thus, lesions of the corticospinal tract will almost invariably

be associated with damage to adjacent tracts regulating nociceptive flexion reflexes.

At this point we need to add a very important caveat. The effects reviewed in the foregoing paragraph and discussed at greater length earlier in the chapter are seen only with subacute or chronic lesions. Acute lesions produce a phenomenon referred to as *spinal cord shock*, characterized by flaccid muscle tone, absent deep tendon reflexes, and no plantar responses. Although we do not fully understand the mechanisms underlying this syndrome, it appears that the sudden, complete loss of input to motoneurons from all descending motor tracts profoundly reduces the excitability of these neurons. This may reflect both a loss of excitatory input and the trans-synaptic effects of acute degeneration of the tracts.

Chronic lesions of motor systems in the brainstem, motor pathways within the cerebral hemispheres, or the cerebral cortex are associated with hyperactive muscle stretch reflexes, increased deep tendon reflexes, and extensor plantar responses. These reactions occur either because the brainstem centers that normally inhibit these responses have been damaged, or because the inhibitory effects of these centers are reliant on corticobulbar input. With lesions at or above the brainstem, we also see evidence of a new phenomenon—*posturing*. Posturing represents the most direct evidence we have for the role of brainstem motor systems in maintaining posture and, hence, axial tone. Lesions at the level of the pons produce *decerebrate posturing*, which is presumably mediated by disinhibition of the vestibulospinal and caudal portions of the pontine reticulospinal systems. It is characterized by profound extensor tone in all extremities (see Case 6-11, which follows, for explanation of mechanism). Lesions at or above the level of the midbrain produce *decorticate posturing*, which is presumably mediated by disinhibition or loss of cortical drive to the entire complex of brainstem motor systems. It is characterized by flexion and pronation of the upper extremity and extension of the lower extremity (see Case 6-12 ).

*The Motor System*

---

[4]The term corticobulbar is a generic designation applying to all projections from the cerebral cortex to the brainstem. In this chapter, we use it to describe projections from the cerebral cortex to brainstem centers involved in motor function. In subsequent chapters, we will also use it to refer to cortical projections to cranial nerve nuclei in the brainstem.

## Case 6-11

### Pontine Hemorrhage

*A 70-year-old woman with a long history of hypertension, poorly controlled largely due to poor compliance with medications, is admitted to the hospital in coma. She is observed lying quietly on her*

## Case 6-11—cont'd

back. Deep tendon reflexes are 1 to 2 and symmetric throughout and she has bilateral Babinski signs. Forceful sternal rub (a painful stimulus) promptly elicits extension of her neck and all extremities. A computed tomographic (CT) scan reveals a 1.5-cm diameter hematoma centered in the basis pontis.

**Comment:** The basis pontis is one of the common sites of CNS hemorrhage related to microvascular damage caused by sustained hypertension. This presentation is typical of pontine hemorrhage. Some of these patients will exhibit spontaneous posturing, often misinterpreted by inexperienced clinicians as epileptic seizures (and

therefore leading them to suspect a cortical lesion). However, more commonly, as in this case, noxious sensory input is necessary to elicit the response. Presumably the predominance of extensor tone in all extremities reflects the evolutionary age of the vestibulospinal system and the fact that it evolved primarily to maintain the antigravity tone needed to support posture and ambulation in quadrupeds. The likelihood that this patient will survive this hemorrhage is low, but if she does survive, her prognosis for long-term return of function is surprisingly good.

## Case 6-12

### Left Middle Cerebral Artery Distribution Stroke

A 65-year-old man with a long history of hypertension, diabetes, hypercholesterolemia, and heavy smoking awakes with severe right-sided weakness and inability to talk. On admission to the hospital, he is mute, can comprehend only the simplest of instructions, and has flaccid plegia of the right arm and proximal right leg with some spared ability to move the right foot. Deep tendon reflexes are absent on the right, but there is a right Babinski sign. Over the next 3 months, in the course of rehabilitation, he regains the ability to walk, but there is no return of useful function in the right arm and hand. At this point, he is hyper-reflexic on the right. He tends to hold the right arm across his chest in a flexed, internally rotated and pronated position and the right hand is contracted almost into a fist. It is very difficult for the examiner to straighten the right arm at the elbow or to open the patient's hand. In contrast, it is difficult for the examiner to flex the right leg at the knee. When the patient walks, he tends to circumduct the leg: that is, as he starts to step, he swings the leg wide because of hypertonus in the gluteus medius, and as he completes the step, he tends to excessively adduct the leg because of hypertonus in the adductor muscle group.

**Comment:** This patient has experienced a large left hemisphere stroke involving much of the middle cerebral artery territory. This stroke could have been caused by embolism from or propagation of clot from an

atheromatous lesion of the left internal carotid artery, or embolism from the heart, perhaps as a result of chronic atrial fibrillation. Acutely, the patient demonstrates some features—flaccidity, areflexia—which are reminiscent of spinal cord shock. In most stroke patients, this shock picture resolves considerably faster than the shock syndrome associated with spinal cord lesions. Ultimately, the patient develops the characteristic features of an "upper motor neuron" syndrome: hyper-reflexia and increased resistance to passive stretch. He also develops excessive flexion and pronation tone in the upper extremity and excessive extensor tone in the lower extremity. This finding may reflect the fact that all three major brainstem tone centers have been released and that the effects of the flexor bias of the medullary reticulospinal system are dominant in the arm, whereas the effects of the extensor bias of the pontine reticulospinal and vestibulospinal systems are dominant in the leg. It may reflect the release of antigravity mechanisms. Because the lesion is more rostral in the nervous system than that in Case 6-11, the pattern of antigravity tone may reflect the arboreal existence of our immediate evolutionary forebears—lower primates. In these animals, antigravity tone in the upper extremities involves flexion and pronation. The relative preservation of function in the right leg reflects the degree to which lower extremity functions, particularly standing and walking, are represented in the brainstem and spinal cord.

In Case 6-12, we observed decorticate posturing in the context of a devastating lesion. However, the development of excessive flexion and pronation tone in the arm turns out to be a very sensitive sign of a lesion of corticobulbar systems, as illustrated in Case 6-13.

## Case 6-13

### Left Frontal Brain Tumor

*A 45-year-old attorney presents with chief complaint of a 2-month history of headaches. On examination, when he closes his eyes and extends his arms in front of him (i.e., in sustention), with the palms up, he exhibits a very slight tendency to pronate the right arm, flex the fingers, and flex the arm at the elbow. The remainder of the neurologic examination is normal. The neurologist is not particularly alarmed by the headaches but the presence of this subtle sign leads her to obtain an MRI scan. This reveals a 3-cm diameter tumor of the left frontal lobe, which on subsequent biopsy proves to be a glioblastoma multiforme, a highly malignant tumor of glial origin.*

**Comment:** *Even though this tumor is centered in the frontal lobe, it is having some impact on corticobulbar motor pathways, either because it is infiltrating these pathways or because of pressure on these pathways from edema associated with the tumor. In this case, "pronation drift" was the only abnormality observed on examination. It can reasonably be viewed as a very abbreviated form of decorticate posturing. Because of the high sensitivity of this sign, a test for drift is considered one of the most important parts of the neurologic examination of the motor system. The presence of an abnormal sign confined to the arm, sparing the leg and the face, reflects not so much the localization of the tumor within the brain as the special role of cerebral motor systems in arm and hand function (see Cycle 6-8).*

## F. BRAINSTEM AND SPINAL MOTOR SYSTEMS IN PERSPECTIVE

At this point, although we have characterized the properties of the lateral and ventromedial brainstem and spinal motor systems and described some clinical consequences of naturally occurring lesions, a clear picture of the respective functions of these systems has probably not emerged. Now and again, an experiment is performed that suddenly brings extraordinary clarity to a complex scientific problem. Lawrence and Kuypers performed such an experiment in 1968 and it remains a landmark study to this day.

Lawrence and Kuypers made strategic lesions in the major motor systems at various points in the brainstem and spinal cords of rhesus monkeys, and they supported the monkeys through the often-difficult postoperative period so that they had the opportunity to observe the chronic effects of the lesions. Monkeys with lesions of the medullary pyramids (the point at which the corticospinal tract is most segregated from other pathways) appeared to function normally in every respect except that they could not independently move their fingers, insert a thumb and finger into a narrow well to retrieve food, or release food once they had grasped it (reflecting differential loss of finger extensor function). Monkeys with lesions of the lateral tract group in the cervical spinal cord (where the corticospinal tract has been joined by the medullary reticulospinal tract), while able to run around and grasp cage bars to climb, were generally unable to flex their hands to grasp food. In some cases, the grasping movement could be accomplished as part of a flexion movement involving the entire arm. In contrast, animals with lesions of the ventromedial system exhibited dramatic changes in posture, sitting with head slumped and limbs flexed and adducted, often falling to one side. Walking was unsteady and marked by frequent falls. When they jumped for overhead bars, they often missed. In reaching for food, there was severe slowing, inaccuracy and instability of proximal limb movements. However, dexterity in the hands was perfectly normal, and they could remove food from the smallest of food wells.

It is worth remembering that the pontine and medullary reticulospinal systems do not operate autonomously—they receive extensive corticobulbar fibers from the cerebral cortex as well as cerebellar projections. Cerebral hemispheric lesions, such as that described in Case 6-12, damage not just corticospinal but also corticopontine reticulospinal projections and corticomedullary reticulospinal projections. Consequently, the effects of such lesions are greater than those observed with the selective lesions made by Lawrence and Kuypers.

The results of the experiment in which the medullary pyramids were cut demonstrate the crucial importance of the pyramidal system, from motor cortex (area 4) to the lateral corticospinal tracts in the spinal cord, in the production of independent finger movements. *Because the capacity for independent finger movements is a sensitive and specific index of pyramidal system function, tests of this movement constitute one of the most important components of the neurologic motor examination.*

## PRACTICE 6-6

**A.** A 75-year-old man develops diverticulitis (infection and inflammation of small, age-related outpouchings of the colon) that is eventually complicated by the development of a pericolic abscess (accumulation of puss in the peritoneal cavity along the colon). During surgery, a portion of his colon is resected and the abscess is drained. During a long and stormy hospital course, he is treated with a number of antibiotics, including aminoglycosides, which are effective in the treatment of infections by Enterobacteriaceae (a major component of normal bowel flora). These drugs may be toxic to the hair cells in the vestibular labyrinths. Hearing, for reasons that are poorly understood, tends to be relatively spared. Predict the clinical consequences of such toxicity.

**B.** A 19-year-old man involved in a gang fight receives a stab wound to the spine that causes an immediate right hemiparesis. Localize the lesion. Will he have hyperactive or absent deep tendon reflexes on the right? Why?

**C.** A 65-year-old diabetic woman presents to the emergency room with the chief complaint of a 2-day history of difficulty walking. Past medical history is otherwise noteworthy for carcinoma of the right breast for which she underwent partial mastectomy and radiation therapy 3 years ago. On examination, she is barely able to stand. Cerebral and brainstem functions are normal. Deep tendon reflexes are 1 to 2 and symmetric in the arms, 3 at the knees, and 1 at the ankles (i.e., within normal limits). She has bilateral Babinski signs. Touch and vibratory sensation in the feet are impaired. Localize the lesions. Hint: what is the pattern of neural injury produced by diabetes? Is the reflex pattern really normal? Where do the Babinski signs suggest the lesion is? Would the combined effect of the lesion producing Babinski signs and the neural lesion caused by diabetes explain the reflex pattern observed?

**D.** Return to Case 6-13. It was said that, other than for the presence of pronation drift, the neurologic examination was normal. Considering that his lesion was impinging on projections from motor cortex (area 4), what other neurologic deficit would you predict?

**E.** Return to Practice 1-4B. Imagine that the year is 1899 and that you first see this patient relatively early in his course, when he first develops symptoms of the right hemispheric tumor. You then follow him as the herniation syndrome progresses until he ultimately dies. Because of the limitations of medical technology, your role is limited to explaining to the patient and his family what is likely to be going on, estimating prognosis, and providing emotional support and guidance. Describe the pattern and lateralization of weakness and posturing that are likely to occur as the tumor grows and the herniation process advances step by step.

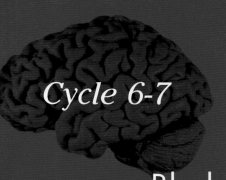

# Cycle 6-7

# Bladder and Bowel Control

### *Objective*

Be able to describe the neural mechanisms underlying bladder function and explain the basis for upper and lower motor neuron bladder syndromes and a lower motor neuron bowel syndrome.

The bladder and bowel are innervated by the autonomic nervous system. However, both have external sphincters that are under voluntary control, and even more important in the context of this chapter, their function quite precisely parallels that of the motor systems we have discussed.

Bladder function depends upon two major muscles: the detrusor, a dome-shaped muscle that is responsible for emptying the bladder, and the internal sphincter muscle, which restricts passage of urine through the bladder neck (Table 6-7). The detrusor is under parasympathetic control (supplied by fibers exiting the spinal cord with sacral nerve roots), and the sphincter is under sympathetic control (supplied by a splanchnic nerve [the hypogastric nerve] derived from paravertebral ganglia supplied by cells in the intermediate zone of the spinal cord at the T10–T12 levels). Generally, the detrusor is influenced to a greater degree by neurologic disease than the sphincter, for poorly understood reasons. Lesions of the neuronal cell bodies within the spinal cord responsible for bladder control (located at the S2–S4 cord levels), their axonal processes in the sacral parasympathetic outflow, or of

| Feature | Detrusor | Sphincter |
|---|---|---|
| **Function** | Empties bladder | Resists passage of urine through bladder neck |
| **Type of innervation** | Parasympathetic | Sympathetic |
| **Lower motor neuron syndrome** | Large, flaccid bladder, poor emptying | Overflow incontinence during increased abdominal pressure due to reduced tone |
| **Upper motor neuron syndrome** | Small capacity, "spastic" bladder | Difficulty initiating stream and emptying bladder; urgency incontinence when detrusor force exceeds sphincter resistance |

**TABLE 6-7** Summary of Bladder Control

265

the associated paravertebral ganglia and their projections will produce a "lower motor neuron bladder." A lower motor neuron bladder is large, commonly containing up to a liter or more, and flaccid, and it empties poorly. Catheterizing affected patients after they have "emptied" the bladder may yield several hundred milliliters of urine (normal is less than 30 mL). To the extent that the sphincter is affected also, there may be "overflow incontinence"—involuntary release of modest amounts of urine in the course of transient elevations in intra-abdominal pressure.

Chronic lesions of the spinal cord above the nerves innervating the detrusor lead to an "upper motor neuron bladder," yet another demonstration of the Jacksonian principle. The pathways inhibiting the detrusor originate in the pontine reticular formation and travel with the pontine reticulospinal tract in the ventromedial portion of the cord. With damage to these pathways, detrusor neurons become disinhibited, yielding a bladder that is small and hypertonic. Uncontrollable spasms of the detrusor occur at very small bladder volumes and produce a sudden sense of urinary urgency, often with incontinence as the patient is trying to get to the bathroom. Loss of urinary control may be a far more disabling symptom than weakness or spasticity in some patients with CNS lesions, such as the patent with multiple sclerosis discussed in Cases 6-4, 6-6, and 6-7.

In the same way that an acute spinal cord lesion producing spinal shock is associated with flaccid muscle tone and loss of all reflexes, it is associated with loss of detrusor tone and urinary retention. For this reason, it is always important to remember to catheterize such patients immediately (e.g., the patient in Practice 6-6C).

Bowel function is considerably less sensitive to neurologic dysfunction. The most common problem is a "lower motor neuron" bowel associated with a flaccid anal sphincter, most often caused by cancer invading the pelvic floor.

## PRACTICE 6-7

**A.** Tolterodine is a muscarinic acetylcholine receptor blocker that is relatively specific for cholinergic receptors on the detrusor. Discuss the pros and cons of using this drug in patients with upper and lower motor neuron bladders.

**B.** Return to Practice 6-3A, D, and E; 6-4A, B, C, and D; and 6-6C and determine whether these patients are likely to have an upper or lower motor neuron bladder.

# Cycle 6-8

# The Corticospinal System

## Objectives

1. Be able to list the major components of cerebral motor systems (areas 4, 6, supplementary motor cortex, primary sensory cortex, the basal ganglia and cerebellum), and be able to describe briefly their interrelationships.

2. Be able to describe the entire trajectory of the corticospinal tract and locate it on cross sections of the cerebrum, brainstem, and spinal cord.

3. Be able to list the major brainstem and spinal cord recipients of corticospinal projections.

4. Be able to describe the somatotopic organization of the corticospinal system throughout its course.

5. Be able to explain why most cerebral lesions affecting motor systems produce greater paresis in the arm and describe the major exception.

6. On the basis of discussions in Cycles 6-6F and 6-8C, be able to describe the definitive features of movements produced by the corticospinal system.

7. Be able to describe the microscopic representation of movements in area 4 and explain how and under what circumstances this provides the basis for the acquisition of new combinations of muscle contractions.

8. Be able to compare and contrast the roles of the supplementary motor area and dorsolateral premotor cortices in movement.

9. Be able to describe the localizing significance of all the major motor signs reviewed in Cycles 6-1 through 6-8.

The Motor System

This chapter so far has been devoted entirely to brainstem and spinal motor systems. We have repeatedly emphasized the great capabilities of these systems, as well as their crucial role in the distributed representation of motor function. However, it is cortical motor mechanisms that make possible the astonishing range, complexity, and precision of movements of which higher primates, particularly humans, are capable. Brief consideration of the range of human motor accomplishments gives one a full appreciation of the feats of which this system is capable: a 20-ft basketball shot, made under duress, that sinks the ball touching nothing but the net; a dive from a 10-m board including $2\frac{1}{2}$ somersaults and a full twist that culminates in little more than a ripple; a Bach partita for solo violin that to the ear is surely two violinists playing, not only executed to perfection but with the soaring intellect and depth of feeling that is inimitable Bach; 10 sutures placed by a neurovascular surgeon to secure an end-to-side anastomosis of two 2-mm arteries. Even in the untrained, the system defies the imagination. As Porter and Lemon noted,[5] first-year medical students have little difficulty using their unaided fingers to center a single red blood cell, 7 μ in diameter, within the field of view of a microscope. Even in a casual conversation between two friends, there is evidence of incomprehensible motor virtuosity in the rapidity and complexity of oropharyngeal movements required for speech. The versatility, complexity, and precision of movements of which the corticospinal system is capable reflect several factors: the large expanse of cerebral cortex and billions of neurons devoted to motor function; the presence of equally sophisticated sensory systems, particularly visual and somatosensory, that project heavily to motor cortices and provide data of sufficient detail and complexity to support complex movement programs; the close links between motor cortices and the prefrontal cortex, which is involved in developing appropriate behavioral responses to novel situations; and last but certainly not least, the enormous plasticity of this system.

In the first section of this cycle, we will review the macroanatomy of this system, the aspect we consider most directly in assessing motor deficits in patients. In the second section, we will consider the microanatomy and the physiology of this system. In the third section, we will introduce recent data that give us a sense of how discrete movements might logically combine into sequential movement programs. In the final section, we will consider the division of labor within cortical motor regions.

## A. THE MACROANATOMY OF THE CORTICOSPINAL SYSTEM

### Origin and Projections of the Corticospinal System

The major source of projections to the corticospinal tract is pyramidal neurons in layer V of the precentral gyrus, Brodmann's area 4 (Fig. 6-15). There are lesser projections from premotor cortex (area 6 over the frontal convexity) and the supplementary motor area (SMA), the portion of area 6 buried within the interhemispheric fissure. The corticospinal tract also con-

tains efferent fibers from the postcentral gyrus (areas 3, 1, 2), which terminate in sensory relay nuclei in the brainstem and in the dorsal horn of the spinal cord. These projections, about which we will have more to say in the next chapter, serve to regulate ascending sensory transmission.

The major afferent projections to area 4 are from premotor cortex and the supplementary motor area. These projections are predominantly ipsilateral, but there are substantial bilateral projections as well. Area 4 can be usefully viewed as subsidiary to area 6 in the cerebral hierarchy of motor function, that is, area 4 represents simple muscle contraction combinations, and these are engaged by projections from area 6 that help to combine these simple combinations into more complex movements. Area 4 also receives heavy afferent input from primary sensory cortex, which together with area 4, receives input from muscle spindles. Finally, areas 4 and 6 receive input from the ventral lateral nucleus of the thalamus, anterior parts of which relay projections from the putamen (a part of the basal ganglia) and posterior portions of which relay projections from the dorsal column (sensory) nuclei and the cerebellum. The basal ganglia and cerebellum function as "consultants" to cerebral cortical systems. We will review them in greater detail in Cycles 6-9 and 6-10.

Projections from area 4 descend through the corona radiata in the posterior third of the periventricular white matter. From the corona radiata, they coalesce into a compact bundle of fibers forming the genu and posterior limb of the internal capsule. Projections from area 4 supplying cranial nerve nuclei (corticobulbar fibers) travel through the genu of the internal capsule, while projections to limb musculature travel in the posterior limb of the internal capsule (Fig. 6-16). Corticospinal and corticobulbar fibers then continue caudally and ipsilaterally through the midportion of the cerebral peduncles (Fig. 6-17). Corticobulbar fibers terminate on interneurons in the vicinity of cranial nerve motor nuclei from the midbrain to the medulla, as well as on neurons of brainstem motor centers (e.g., the red nuclei, the pontine and medullary reticulospinal centers) (Fig. 6-18). Corticospinal fibers continue down into the basis pontis where they separate into several longitudinal bundles within the gray matter of the ventral pons (Fig. 6-19). At the pontomedullary junction, corticospinal fibers recoalesce to form the *medullary pyramids* (Fig. 6-13). At the cervicomedullary junction, 90 percent of the pyramidal fibers cross, in the *decussation of the pyramids*, from their ventral, midline location into the dorsolateral region of

---

[5]Porter R, Lemon R. Corticospinal Function and Voluntary Movement. Oxford, Clarendon, 1993.

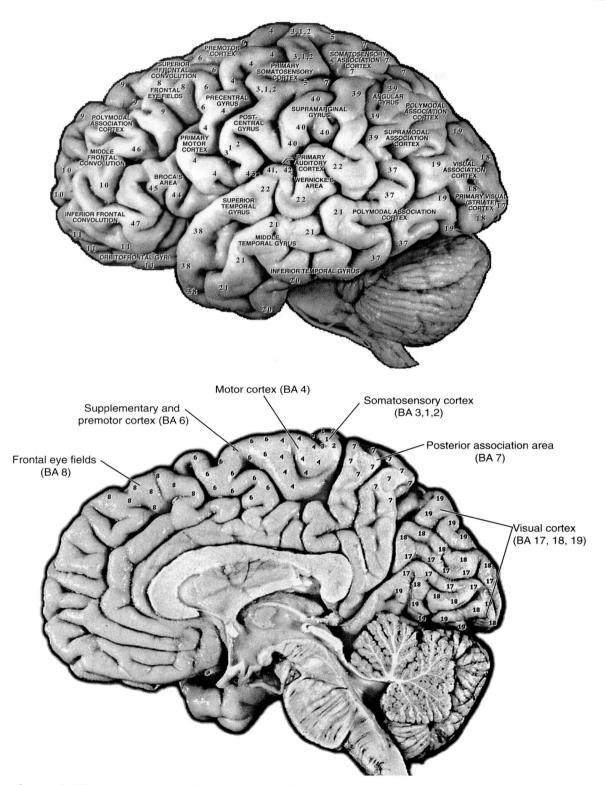

**Figure 6-15** Location of motor (area 4), premotor (convexity area 6), and supplementary motor areas (interhemispheric area 6). BA = Brodmann's area. (Modified from Warner JJ, Atlas of Neuroanatomy. Boston, Butterworth Heinemann, 2001, with permission from Elsevier Science.)

The Motor System

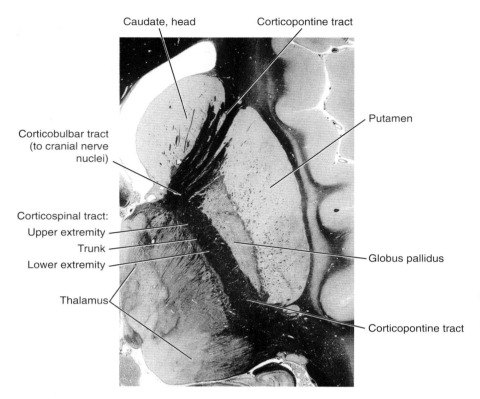

Caudate, head    Corticopontine tract

Putamen

Corticobulbar tract
(to cranial nerve
nuclei)

Corticospinal tract:
Upper extremity
Trunk
Lower extremity

Globus pallidus

Thalamus

Corticopontine tract

**Figure 6-16** Horizontal section showing organization of corticofugal tracts in the internal capsule.

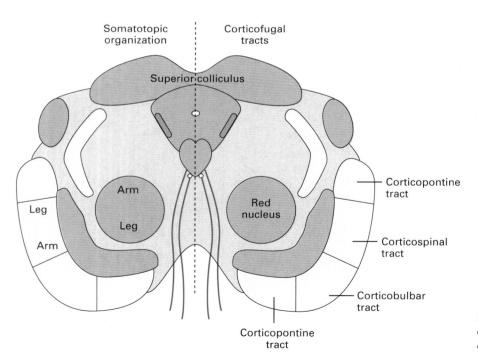

Somatotopic
organization    Corticofugal
tracts

Superior colliculus

Arm

Leg    Red
nucleus
Leg

Arm

Corticopontine
tract

Corticospinal
tract

Corticobulbar
tract

Corticopontine
tract

**Figure 6-17** Organization of corticofugal tracts in the mesencephalon.

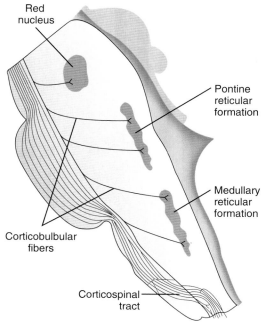

Red nucleus

Pontine reticular formation

Medullary reticular formation

Corticobulbular fibers

Corticospinal tract

**Figure 6-18** Corticobulbar connections in the brainstem (sagittal section).

the contralateral spinal cord. Ten percent continue ipsilaterally in the ventromedial portion of the spinal cord. The decussation of the pyramids is readily evident on gross inspection of the ventral aspect of the medulla (Fig. 6-13). Area 4 projections continue down the cord as the corticospinal tract until they exit at various levels to synapse, either on interneurons or directly on α-motoneurons in the ventral horn of the cord. *Central nervous system lesions above the pyramidal decussation produce weakness and incoordination contralateral to the lesion, whereas lesions below the decussation produce weakness and incoordination ipsilateral to the lesion.*

## Somatotopic Organization of the Corticospinal System

*The entire corticospinal system is somatotopically organized.* In area 4, neurons subserving movement of the face and tongue (including those implicated in speech) are located in the lateral, ventral portions of the precentral gyrus (abutting the sylvian fissure ventrally), those subserving arm movement are more dorsal, and neurons subserving the lower extremities are located in the parasagittal regions and the interhemispheric

portions of area 4 (i.e., legs medial, arms/face lateral). Replications of the somatotopic organization in area 4 can be seen in area 6 on the dorsolateral surface of the frontal lobe and in the supplementary motor area. As area 4 projections arc down through the corona radiata into the posterior limb of the internal capsule, this medial/lateral organization is reversed from the internal capsule all the way down to and including the corticospinal tract in the brainstem and spinal cord: face fibers are located medially and leg fibers are located laterally, with arm fibers in between.

The proportion of area 4 and the number of fibers within the corticospinal/corticobulbar tract devoted to movement of various regions of the body reflect the relative role of the cerebral cortex in the movement of these regions. Thus, there is extensive representation of the face and upper extremities (particularly distal portions) and relatively less representation of the lower extremities. The somatotopic organization of area 4 and the disproportionate representation of the body regions are captured in the homunculus depicted in Figure 6-20.

## The Reason for Greater Involvement of Arm and Hand with Most Cerebral Lesions

With rare exceptions, cerebral injuries produce contralateral motor impairment that affects the arm much more than the leg. We got a hint of this in Case 6-12. The traditional explanation for this phenomenon is that by far the most common cerebral lesion is an infarction in the middle cerebral artery distribution. This explanation seems quite logical as the middle cerebral artery supplies the face and arm regions of the motor homunculus, whereas the anterior cerebral artery supplies the leg regions. That is, there is a correspondence between the vascular anatomy and the neuroanatomy. However, an arm > leg hemiparesis is seen even when infarctions in the middle cerebral artery distribution largely spare the cerebral cortex as a result of large cortical collaterals (see Chapter 2). As it turns out, hemiparesis resulting from middle cerebral artery distribution strokes most often results from damage to corticospinal and corticobulbar fibers traveling down through the corona radiata in the periventricular region. In the periventricular region, unlike in the cerebral cortex, there is no correspondence between the somatotopic organization of corticobulbar/corticospinal fibers and the anatomic organization of

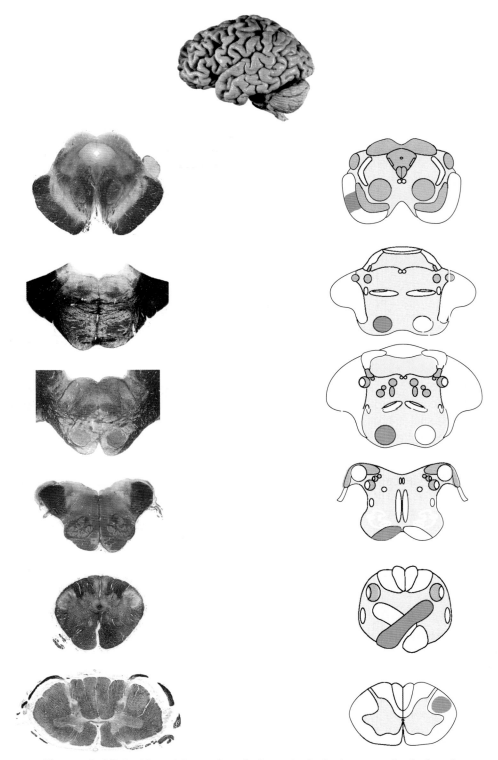

**Figure 6-19** Position of the corticospinal tract in the brainstem and spinal cord.

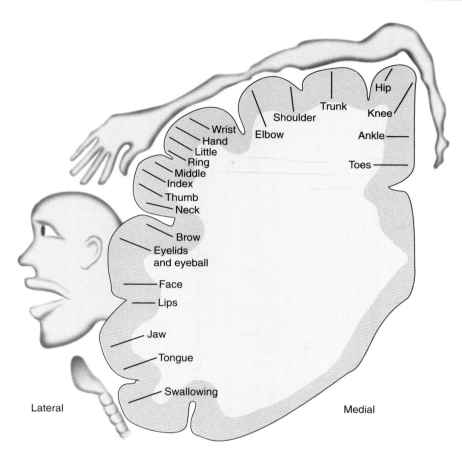

**Figure 6-20** The human motor homunculus.

the vascular supply, and hence no reason for upper extremity projections to be preferentially affected. Arm > leg hemipareses are also seen with lacunar infarctions of the posterior limb of the internal capsule, with proximal posterior cerebral artery occlusion, which may interrupt the vascular supply to the cerebral peduncle, and with brain tumors infiltrating the white matter of the hemisphere. Thus, in all these cases, we must look to a principle other than the relationship between the geography of the vascular supply and the somatotopic organization of the corticospinal system to explain the arm > leg hemiparesis.

The fundamental principle underlying the arm > leg hemiparesis phenomenon is that the corticospinal system is primarily involved in the function of the arm and hand, whereas leg movement, particularly in the realms of standing and walking, primarily falls within the purview of brainstem and spinal cord mechanisms. Furthermore, arm and hand movement is a minimally distributed function, substantially reliant on corticospinal systems, whereas leg movement is an exten-

sively distributed function, with contributions by corticospinal, brainstem, and spinal cord systems. Only with strokes characterized by unusual and extreme geographic distribution, such as anterior cerebral artery distribution infarcts, does the somatotopic organization of the corticospinal system become the dominant factor, resulting in violation of this principle. Patients with anterior cerebral artery distribution infarcts have predominantly lower extremity weakness.

## B. MICROANATOMY AND PHYSIOLOGY OF THE CORTICOSPINAL SYSTEM

Corticobulbar and corticospinal fibers ultimately terminate on interneurons in the vicinity of motor cranial nerve nuclei or the ventral horn of the spinal cord, respectively, or directly on α-motoneurons in these regions. However, on the way down, these pyramidal fibers, particularly those destined for the spinal cord,

The Motor System

send collateral projections to deep layers of the superior colliculus (origin of the tectospinal tract), to the red nuclei (origin of the rubrospinal tracts), and to regions of the pontine and medullary reticular formation from which the reticulospinal tracts originate. Thus, the corticospinal system is positioned to act as a supervisory system to all these subsidiary motor centers. This role is clearly necessary for the corticospinal system to be able to suppress background muscle tone produced by these systems in order to superimpose precisely composed movements. However, recall that we spoke earlier of a distributed representation of motor function, such that subcomponents of the motor system optimally suited to handle certain aspects of movement or certain types of movement automatically assume command of motor function without being directed to do so by a supervisory system. Neural network systems are intrinsically suited to precisely this kind of automatic shifting of labor, provided that they are extensively interconnected. Thus, the automatic and flexible shifting of responsibility for motor function from one portion of the motor system to another, depending upon the particular circumstances, would not be possible were there not extensive connections from the corticospinal system to the other motor centers, reciprocated by indirect projections from these other centers to area 4.

How does this corticospinal projection with its enormous complex of collaterals actually function in the execution of movement? In cerebral microstimulation studies, a tiny microelectrode inserted into the cortex stimulates a sufficient number of afferents in the immediate vicinity of a layer V corticospinal neuron to fire it at high frequency. These studies have shown that the latency to generate firing of an upper extremity α-motoneuron in the spinal cord that receives direct corticospinal projections is on the order of 7 ms. However, if we record from this same layer V neuron in the course of natural movement, we discover that, on average, 100 ms elapses between the first firing of this neuron and the onset of firing of the α-motoneuron. The intervening 93 ms provides time for other pyramidal neurons projecting to the same α-motoneuron to interact with each other and to generate EPSPs in the α-motoneuron. It also provides time for the layer V neuron and its cortical cohorts to influence the various brainstem motor systems that project indirectly to the α-motoneuron, and to be influenced by afferent input from these systems, ascending sensory information, and activity in the basal ganglia and the cerebellum that was elicited by the firing of the pyramidal cell. The α-motoneuron ultimately fires as the spatial and tempo-

ral summation of excitatory inputs succeeds in depolarizing it beyond threshold. In this way, the onset of firing of a pyramidal cell initiates a physiologic process that modifies tone and superimposes the targeted movement in a form that is appropriately modified to fit the particular constraints provided by the current state of the CNS and the environment. The principles governing the spatial and temporal shaping of neuronal activity during this 93 ms and the subsequent movement, largely unknown, constitute a major focus of motor systems research today.

The ultimate targets of corticospinal projections reflect the specialization of cerebral motor systems and the peculiar demands of that specialization. The primary focus of cortical motor systems is the upper extremity, particularly the hand. The famous turn-of-the-century British neuroscientist, Charles Sherrington, widely regarded as the father of motor system neurophysiology, likened the corticospinal representation of the hand to the fovea of the eye. The fovea, crammed with more neurons than the entire remainder of the retina, is entirely responsible for the exquisite visual acuity that enables us to see to perform precision tasks and to read. As we noted in describing the monkey experiment of Lawrence and Kuypers (Cycle 6-6), it is the corticospinal system that conveys the capacity for independent finger movement. In the monkey, this capacity is substantially facilitated by the existence of extensive projections from layer V pyramidal cells in area 4 that synapse directly upon α-motoneurons subserving hand muscles (without one or more intervening interneurons). This makes possible the extremely rapid neural transmission necessary to support rapid precision movements. At the same time, there are minimal projections from muscle spindles to these α-motoneurons, making them relatively free of reflex mechanisms and maximally available to the precise control exerted by corticospinal projections. In humans, the further evolutionary "corticalization" of motor systems is reflected in direct corticospinal projections to α-motoneurons subserving upper extremity muscles as proximal as the deltoids. Thus, a human with a lesion of a medullary pyramid would exhibit considerably more extensive and more severe motor deficits than did the monkeys of Lawrence and Kuypers.

Each corticospinal fiber projecting directly to α-motoneurons synapses on most or all of the α-motoneurons subserving the principal target muscle, most α-motoneurons subserving up to four synergistic (agonist) muscles, and some inhibitory neurons synapsing on α-motoneurons subserving antagonist muscles. Each of these α-motoneurons in turn receives direct projections from very large numbers of cortical pyramidal cells. At first glance, this appears to represent massive overcontrol of spinal motoneurons by the corticospinal system. As we will see in the next section, the purpose of this seemingly redundant connectivity is movement versatility. This enormous projection enables the contraction of agonist muscles to be combined in infinite graded combinations to achieve every conceivable nuance of a given movement or movement combination. The fact that a given α-motoneuron receives projections from so many cortical neurons means that the activity of α-motoneurons can be very finely adjusted relative to one another. Furthermore, some pyramidal cells exhibit large modulations of activity at very low force levels (force generated being proportional to firing rate), providing a further basis for precision grip—grip precisely modulated to the requirements of delicate tasks.

## C. THE ARCHITECTURE OF MOVEMENT

In Section A, we introduced the concept of somatotopic organization of the corticospinal/corticobulbar system. In fact, our description represented somewhat of an oversimplification. Area 4 neurons projecting to a given α-motoneuron are actually scattered over an area of the precentral gyrus spanning many square millimeters. Moreover, neurons subserving one muscle are admixed with neurons subserving a variety of other muscles. At first glance, this seems like a terribly disorganized arrangement. However, its ineffable logic becomes apparent when an experimental monkey is trained in a particular movement. For example, in one experiment, Randolph Nudo and his colleagues trained a monkey to retrieve food morsels from the bottom of a narrow well. The retrieval process required the monkey to insert its preferred fingers into the well and then flex the fingers at the metacarpophalangeal joints at the same time that it extended its wrist in a smooth, combined motion that resulted in dragging the morsel up the back side of the well until it emerged from the top of the well and could be grasped and eaten. These investigators mapped the monkey's motor cortex before and after the monkey was trained on this task. They discovered that with training, the monkey developed a number of columns of cells scattered through the forearm and hand area of the motor cortex, the microstimulation of

which elicited combined finger flexion and wrist extension. These and the findings of many other investigators suggest that the seemingly haphazard mixing of neurons subserving different muscles over a substantial cortical area exists in order to provide an enormous potential "vocabulary" of muscle contraction combinations. Each "word" in this vocabulary is defined by a particular combination of muscles that contract with a particular force/acceleration pattern in a particular temporal sequence, presumably modified in a flexible fashion by sensory input and interaction with subcortical and brainstem components of the motor system. The experiments of Nudo and his colleagues suggest that the cortical admixture of neurons subserving different muscle contractions provides only the "letter" and "syllable" substrate for the vocabulary and that the actual "words" are only created in the course of repeatedly performed movements. These movements spur the development of neural connections that bind neurons subserving different muscles to each other to achieve the optimal contraction combinations and force ratios and contraction sequences to meet the current spectrum of environmental demands. A change in the spectrum of environmental demands leads to the development of new vocabulary. Thus, when monkeys were extensively trained on a task that required a movement much like inserting a key into a lock and turning, finger flexion-wrist extension dual response representations failed to emerge, because this combined movement was not utilized in this task.

Training of monkeys in Nudo's food-well retrieval experiment also induced an increase in the extent of cortex from which finger movements could be elicited by cortical microstimulation and a decrease in areas from which wrist and forearm movements could be evoked. Training on the "key-turning" task induced changes in the opposite direction. These findings indicate that not only does training generate new task-specific motor "vocabulary," but it also expands the supply of particular motor "letters" and "syllables" in a way that will increase the resources brought to bear on the unique demands of the task.

Our focus on individual cortical neurons and columns in the preceding paragraphs may have obscured the fact that hundreds or thousands of cortical pyramidal cells may project to a given α-motoneuron. A particular muscle contraction in a particular context (e.g., contraction of the extensor carpi radialis during wrist extension versus contraction during wrist stabilization during a power grip) is defined by a particular pattern of activity of large numbers of cortical neurons (population coding of movement). The direction of particular movements is also defined by the pattern of activity of all the area 4 neurons linked to the relevant muscles, because direction is defined by the particular motor vocabulary involved in that movement.

An additional interesting finding of the experiments by Nudo and colleagues was that in the motor cortex contralateral to the preferred hand of the monkeys, the hand-forearm area of the motor cortex was larger, but a smaller number of columns was devoted to any particular movement. The finding of a greater area of cortex devoted to driving the preferred hand suggests that this cortex had the greater resources needed for the development of a larger variety of movement combinations. The finding of smaller numbers of columns devoted to any particular movement suggests that in addition, this cortex had achieved sufficiently greater refinement of neural connectivity to enable production of a given movement with a smaller number of cortical columns. There is evidence of a similar pattern in humans, corresponding to an aspect of handedness referred to as deftness—the greater skill and precision exhibited by the preferred hand. Handedness is determined by a number of factors, of which deftness is but one.

## D. SPECIALIZATION WITHIN CORTICAL MOTOR REGIONS

Area 4 provides the final common cortical pathway for all movements and, as we have seen, at least simple movement combinations. Area 4 is the recipient of extensive projections from convexity portions of area 6 (premotor cortex) and from parasagittal portions of area 6 (supplementary motor area). To invoke the metaphor employed in the previous section, if area 4 is viewed as defining operational motor "vocabulary," premotor and supplementary motor areas appear to be involved in generating motor "phrases" and "sentences." However, they appear to have substantially different and complementary roles in the development of movement programs. Premotor cortex appears to have a particular role in the development of movement sequences in response to the particular constraints imposed by the environment. It is well suited to do so by virtue of the extensive projections its receives from visual and somatosensory cortices. In contrast, the supplementary motor area appears to be primarily involved in the generation of heavily practiced movement sequences that, in principle, can be carried out in the abstract, without reference to specific environmental features.

The relative roles of areas 4 and 6 are best delineated in the course of motor learning. Both functional imaging studies (PET, fMRI) in humans and neurophysiologic studies in animals show that premotor cortex is most active during the early, learning phases of a movement sequence, and that as the sequences become practiced, the role of premotor cortex declines in parallel with increased engagement of the supplementary motor area. However, these two areas must also work in concert in the execution of practiced sequences. Much of what we do involves well-learned and rehearsed movement sequences that we initiate repeatedly to accomplish the myriad familiar tasks of daily life (a supplementary motor area specialty), but any given iteration of such a sequence must be modified to fit the particular requirements of the moment (a premotor cortex specialty).

The general theme of the division of labor between supplementary motor area and premotor cortex can perhaps be captured by considering handwriting. Handwriting represents internally developed movement sequences that have a distinctive and consistent personal character, no matter what the precise context of the movements—whether we are writing a minute margin note employing slight movements of three fingers, writing large at arm's length on a blackboard, writing with our nonpreferred hand, or writing clumsily but recognizably with a pen grasped between two toes. In all these situations, the handwriting remains inimitably our own. Handwriting style would thus appear to be primarily the province of the supplementary motor area. However, any physical alterations in the handwriting process required by the circumstances of the movement—writing with fingers, left or right hand, or foot; fitting the size and arrangements of written material to the space on the page—would appear to be more the province of the premotor cortex, which is privy to visual and somatosensory feedback and connected to engage the muscle spectrum required for the particular writing variation. Unfortunately, in large part because of the rarity of lesions confined to the supplementary motor cortex, there has not yet been clinical validation of this concept.

## PRACTICE 6-8

**A.** For each of the following neurologic manifestations, indicate the responsible locus of pathology: impaired independent finger movement ("fine motor move-ment"), Babinski sign, absent deep tendon reflex, pronation drift, muscle wasting (atrophy), hyperactive deep tendon reflexes, spastic catch, fasciculations, decorticate rigidity, decerebrate rigidity, flaccid tone.

**B.** Refer back to Practice 6-4D (cervical syrinx). Provide two reasons why the patient's arm was affected more than her leg.

**C.** A 30-year-old man presents with the chief complaint of imbalance. He has a spastic gait, hyperactive lower extremity reflexes, and bilateral Babinski signs. List all possible locations of a lesion that might explain his findings.

**D.** A 65-year-old man experiences a lacunar infarct of the posterior limb of the left internal capsule. Predict all his neurologic manifestations a month later.

The Motor System

# Cycle 6-9

# The Basal Ganglia

## A. ANATOMY

The basal ganglia consist of a group of large gray matter masses located deep within the cerebral hemispheres: the *caudate nucleus* and the *putamen* (collectively, the *striatum*), the *globus pallidus*, a portion of the substantia nigra, the *substantia nigra pars reticulata (SN$_{PR}$)*, the *subthalamic nucleus (STN)*, and an ancillary structure, the *substantia nigra pars compacta (SN$_{PC}$)* (the darkly pigmented portion of the substantia nigra) (Fig. 6-21). Return to Chapter 1 if you need to refamiliarize yourself with the gross anatomic features of these structures.

Although there is an enormous range of function subserved by these structures, they have a common structural organization (Fig. 6-22). Two basic functional routes have been delineated, the direct and the indirect. The direct route is defined by projections from most of the cerebral cortex to the striatum, which in turn projects to the globus pallidus interna (GP$_i$) and the SN$_{PR}$. The GP$_i$ and the SN$_{PR}$ are separated by the internal capsule, but functionally and structurally they are highly similar and for our purposes, can be considered as composing a unitary structure. The indirect route is defined by projections from the cerebral cortex (mainly areas 4, 6, and 8) to the STN, which in turn projects to GP$_i$/SN$_{PR}$. GP$_i$/SN$_{PR}$, the major output structure of the basal ganglia, projects to two major locations: (1) anterior portions of the ventral lateral nucleus (VL$_O$), the ventral anterior (VA) nucleus and the mediodorsal (MD; same as dorsomedial) nucleus of the thalamus, and (2) the superior colliculus (SC) and a region of the midbrain known as the pedunculopontine area (PPA). VL$_O$, VA, and MD then project to the frontal lobes. The PPA projects to the reticulospinal motor systems of the brainstem. The external portion of the globus pallidus (GP$_e$) is linked to both the direct and indirect basal ganglia routes. Because this nucleus appears only to refine the processing carried out via the direct and indirect routes, we will not consider it any further. For the remainder of this section, our focus will be exclusively on the core of the two functional routes: cortex → striatum → GP$_i$/SN$_{PR}$ → thalamus → cortex (direct), and cortex → STN → GP$_i$/SN$_{PR}$ → thalamus → cortex (indirect).

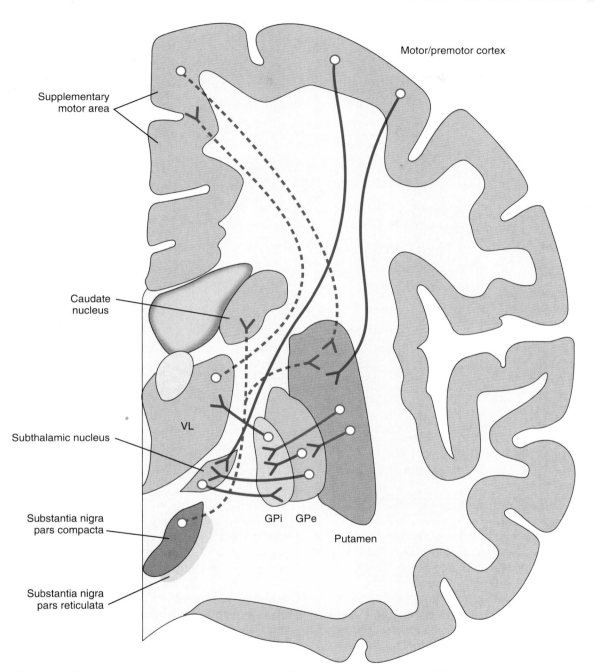

**Figure 6-21** Major components of the basal ganglia. VL = ventral lateral nucleus, GP$_i$ = globus pallidus interna, GP$_e$ = globus pallidus externa.

Information processing in the basal ganglia, as elsewhere in the cerebrum, is mediated primarily via the neurotransmitters glutamate and GABA. Neurons in the cortex projecting to the striatum and the STN, the neurons of the STN, and the neurons of the thalamic nuclei relaying basal ganglia output back to the cortex are all glutamatergic and excitatory. Neurons of the striatum and GP$_i$/SN$_{PR}$ are GABA-ergic and inhibitory.

The Motor System

32

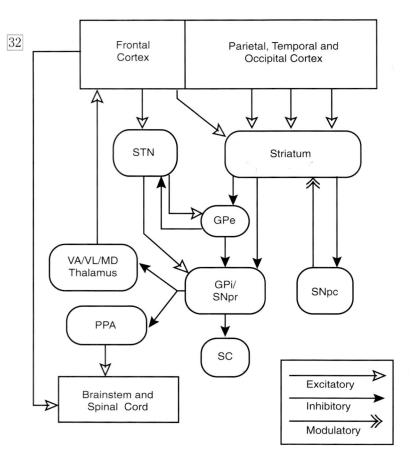

**Figure 6-22** Simplified schematic diagram of basal ganglia circuitry. See text for explanation. (Modified from Mink JW. Basal ganglia dysfunction in Tourette's syndrome: A new hypothesis. Pediatr Neurol 25:190–198, 2001, with permission from Elsevier Science.)

The function of the striatum is critically dependent upon modulation by the dopaminergic projection from the SN$_{PC}$. The activity of the dopaminergic neurons in the SN$_{PC}$ is remarkably constant under most circumstances, but it does increase in association with movements that will likely lead to reward.

Like nearly everything else in the nervous system, the basal ganglia demonstrate an exquisite somatotopic organization. The organization of the cortical projections to the striatum along its anteroposterior axis reflects the anteroposterior organization of cerebral cortical systems. Thus, particular portions of the head of the caudate nucleus receive projections from specific regions of the prefrontal cortex or the frontal eye fields and in turn project to discrete portions of the globus pallidus and the SN$_{PR}$. Therefore, different portions of the head of the caudate nucleus are implicated by their connectivity in higher neural functions and eye movements, respectively. In contrast, the putamen receives its major projections from areas 4 and 6, and the por-

tions of the thalamus to which the putamenal system ultimately projects send their efferent fibers predominantly to the supplementary motor area and convexity portions of areas 4 and 6. The putamen is therefore a component of the motor system.

The basal ganglia are somatotopically organized along the dorsoventral axis as well. Thus, portions of area 4 representing the leg project to the dorsal putamen, whereas portions representing the face project to the ventral putamen.

## B. FUNCTION

The basal ganglia provide a generic "consultant" service to cerebral cortical systems. That is, the nature of the neural processing performed appears to be the same, even though the actual neural information being processed differs widely from region to region, reflecting the somatotopic organization of corticostriatal and cortical-STN connections. The term "consultant" conveys the sense that the cerebral cortex obtains information from the basal ganglia before initiating an action. Thus, one might expect that if the putamen were a motor consultant, then neural activity in the putamen would precede the onset of neural activity in area 4. However, activity in the putamen actually parallels activity in area 4. Does this mean that the putamen does not act as a motor consultant? Probably not. Neural systems do not function by sending packets of information from one place to another. Rather, information exists only so long as the neural system that generated it persists in its particular firing pattern. Thus, a neural consultant system must function by modifying ongoing firing patterns, rather than modifying a packet of information before it is sent. Recall from Cycle 6-8B that nearly 100 ms elapse between the time when an area 4 neuron begins to fire and the time when one of its target $\alpha$-motoneurons begins to fire. It is during this 100 ms, as well as during actual muscle contraction, that the putamenal system has its opportunity to modify movement by influencing the evolution of the ultimate area 4 neuronal firing patterns that shape the movement.

Despite 30 years of intensive investigation, defining the essential neurologic principles of basal ganglia function continues to pose a major challenge to neuroscientific research. Some clinical observations encourage one to believe that the basal ganglia constitute an ancient, phylogenetically outmoded structure that does little that is positive and wreaks havoc when it malfunctions owing to disease. The basal ganglia first appeared on the evolutionary horizon with the development of amphibians. A case in point is Parkinson's disease. Parkinson's disease is a predominantly motor disorder caused by severe dopamine deficiency in the striatum as a result of neuronal dropout in the $SN_{PC}$. Patients with advanced disease may be treated with radiofrequency (microwave)-induced ablation of a portion of $GP_i$, in effect decommissioning the entire putamenal circuit (see Box 6-2). A few of these patients experience essentially complete recovery, seemingly doing well without any basal ganglia input to motor cortices. Another example is provided by patients with small strokes (lacunar infarcts) of the putamen, who are commonly asymptomatic.

However, it is hard to believe that the enormous mass of neural tissue composing the basal ganglia serves no useful function. Furthermore, pallidotomy patients have not undergone sufficient study to define all aspects of their neurologic function, most particularly their motor versatility and their capacity for motor system plasticity. Because pallidotomy is uniformly done in patients with very advanced disease, who have accumulated damage to a number of regions of the brain, including the cerebral cortex, such studies are extremely difficult to carry out and we will continue to rely on animal experiments to supplement human investigation in our efforts to solve this puzzle.

The currently most widely accepted theory of basal ganglia motor function has been most explicitly laid out by Jonathan Mink. He has proposed that the basal ganglia act to facilitate a single target movement while broadly inhibiting, in space and time, competing motor mechanisms that otherwise might interfere with the target movement. The principal mechanism underlying this function appears to reside in the peculiar nature of striatal and STN terminations on the neurons of $GP_i$ (most of the putamen projects to $GP_i$) (Fig. 6-23). Striatal projections for the most part terminate in a very dense contact with a single $GP_i$ neuron; that is, they are highly focused. In contrast, STN terminations ensheath many $GP_i$ neurons—they are more diffuse. Cortical-STN-$GP_i$-thalamic input is rapidly conducted and provides the basis for the early establishment of a broad inhibitory background. Through this, with some delay, the cortical-striatal-$GP_i$-thalamic input provides the basis for a subsequent, highly focused excitatory core that, projected back to the cerebral cortex, facilitates the target movement (Fig 6-24).

The precise nature of the potentially competing motor background that is apparently inhibited has not been defined precisely. It could include neural activity associated with preceding and following movements. It could include the background tone that must be inhibited in order for the target movement to take place.

The most serious failing of the Mink theory is that it is predicated on the tonic activity of basal ganglia neurons, whereas the invidious impact of basal ganglia lesions on neurologic function appears to be related in substantial part to pathologic alterations in the temporal firing pattern of basal ganglia neurons. Nevertheless, the Mink model does provide logical explanations for much of what we see clinically. Thus, in Parkinson's disease, the indirect route appears to be relatively overactive, resulting in excessive inhibition (insufficient facilitation) of all movements, even target movements. Furthermore, movements performed in close temporal sequence interfere with each other. Beneke and Marsden found that when normal subjects perform a simple two-movement sequence—flex the elbow and

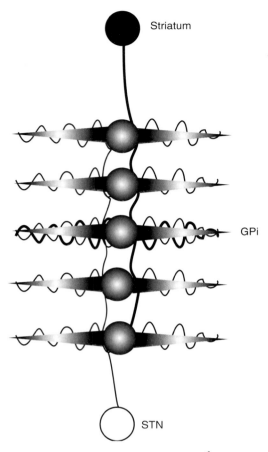

**Figure 6-23** Divergent excitatory projection from the subthalamic nucleus (STN)) and focused inhibitory projection from the striatum to globus pallidus interna (GP$_i$). (Modified from Mink JW. The basal ganglia: Focused selection and inhibition of competing motor programs. Prog Neurobiol 50:381–425, 1996, with permission from Elsevier Science.)

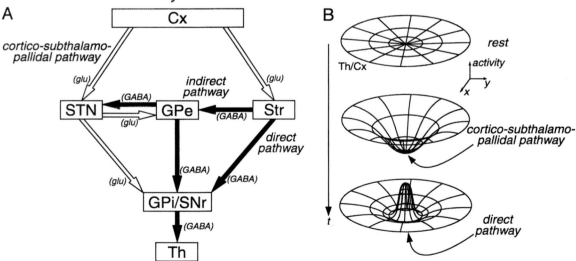

**Figure 6-24** A schematic diagram of the temporally evolving pattern of activity in the thalamus (Th) and cortex (Cx) as a result of the interacting input from the indirect and direct basal ganglia routes. From the state of rest *(top)*, the indirect pathway induces a broadly distributed inhibition of ongoing activity *(middle)* against which the direct route subsequently induces a sharply focused excitation *(bottom)*. Str = Striatum, glu = glutamate, STN = subthalamic nucleus, SNr = substantia nigra pars reticulata. (From Nambu A, Tokuno H, Hamada I et al. Excitatory cortical inputs to pallidal neurons via the subthalamic nucleus in the monkey. J Neurophysiol 84:289–300, 2000. Reproduced with permission of the American Physiological Society.)

**TABLE 6-8** Summary of Major Movements Disorders Stemming from Lesions of the Basal Ganglia

| Movement Disorder | Characteristics | Structure Implicated | Diseases Responsible |
|---|---|---|---|
| Akinesia | Difficulty initiating movement | Head of caudate (dopamine deficiency) | Parkinson's disease |
| Bradykinesia | Slowness of movement | | |
| Hypokinesia, rigidity, pill-rolling tremor | Small movements | Putamen (dopamine deficiency) | Parkinson's disease |
| Chorea | Small, quick, involuntary movements of fingers, hands, occasionally head, arms and legs. Lilting, dance-like gait | Putamen (intrinsic pathology) | Huntington's disease |
| Athetosis | Nearly constant, slow, sinuous, writhing movements | Putamen, globus pallidus (intrinsic pathology) | Hypoxia, carbon monoxide poisoning, Wilson's disease (an autosomal recessive disease causing tissue copper deposition) |
| Ballism | Violent, flinging movements, usually involving an entire arm | Subthalamic nucleus | Stroke |

then execute a pincer movement with the thumb and first finger—there is an approximately 200-ms delay between the termination of the first movement and the onset of the second. In parkinsonian patients, this inter-movement delay averaged 550 ms. These abnormally prolonged intermovement latencies provide a logical explanation for the slowing of movement sequences (bradykinesia) that is the hallmark of Parkinson's disease. Thus, many of the cardinal features of Parkinson's disease can be explained on the basis of insufficient facilitation of the target movement or excess inhibition of acceptable spatially or temporally proximate movements. In contrast, many of the pathologic movements associated with basal ganglia disease (e.g., chorea, ballismus: see next section) can be explained on the basis of dysfunction in the indirect basal ganglia route, with failure to inhibit potentially competing movements, or dysfunction in the direct route, with excess focal excitation in the striatum generating uninhibitible competing movements. By either mechanism, the direct striatal route manages to "punch holes" in the inhibitory background provided by the indirect route, leading to pathologic excitation of thalamocortical neurons and pathologic movements.

## C. MANIFESTATIONS OF BASAL GANGLIA DYSFUNCTION

Our best intuitions about the function of the basal ganglia derive from our observations of patients with basal ganglia disease.[6] The following cases exemplify the spectrum of impairment (see also Table 6-8).

### Case 6-14

**Parkinson's Disease**
*A 68-year-old woman with an 8-year history of Parkinson's disease consults a neurologist in hopes of better management of her disease. On examination, she exhibits very little facial expression (hypomimia or masking of faces). As she sits with her arms at rest,*

*Continued*

[6]Basal ganglia disease is still often referred to clinically as extrapyramidal disease, clearly a very misleading misnomer born of an early misconception that the pallidum projected exclusively to the brainstem. Thus, the basal ganglia appeared to constitute a second system, operating in parallel to the pyramidal system.

## Case 6-14—cont'd

she exhibits a 6-Hz rotatory tremor of the right forearm and hand (referred to as a "pill-rolling" tremor as it emulates the movement pharmacists once used to align pills in the hand preparatory to pouring them into a small bottle). Slow flexion and extension of one of her arms at the elbow by the neurologist reveals increased resistance that is constant throughout all phases of the movement ("plastic" or "lead-pipe" rigidity). When asked what diagnosis she has been given, she responds in a very quiet voice (hypophonia), "P-p-p-arkins-s-s-ons dis-s-sease." This peculiar form of stuttering is known as palilalia. She is generally slow to respond to questions (slowness of thinking or bradyphrenia) and to execute commands (bradykinesia). She tends to sit, silent and immobile, unless pressed to move by the examiner (akinesia). When asked to repeatedly oppose the thumb and index finger of one hand, she exhibits a normal capacity for individual finger movement (i.e., intact pyramidal function), but her movements are very small (hypokinesia). When asked to stand, she makes several attempts, repeatedly falling backward into the chair (retropulsion) and ultimately she requires the examiner's assistance to get up. She is very slow to begin to walk and when she finally does walk, her stride is shortened. She almost comes to a complete stop as she is about to pass through the door to the examining room ("freezing"). When she walks, she holds her entire body very stiffly and her arms are absolutely immobile. When she turns, rather than making a graceful, fluid movement that is integrated into her walking, she stops and makes half a dozen short steps in order to pivot her rigid body 180 degrees (pedestal turn). As she approaches her chair in the examining room, her steps suddenly get much shorter and more rapid as she begins to fall forward ("festination").

**Comment:** This patient exhibits all the classic features of Parkinson's disease. These features reflect the particular pattern of striatal (primarily putamenal) dysfunction that follows from loss of the normal supply of dopamine, as the darkly pigmented cells in the substantia nigra pars compacta that normally supply dopamine prematurely die. As a result, the balance between the direct and indirect basal ganglia routes is tipped toward the indirect route. There is insufficient facilitation of target movements or excess inhibition of

## Case 6-14—cont'd

acceptable spatially or temporally proximate movements. An analogous pathologic process appears to affect basal ganglia circuits involving the prefrontal cortex, hence the akinesia and bradyphrenia. With the provision of appropriate doses of dopaminergic medications (both the dopamine precursor, levodopa, and direct dopamine receptor agonist drugs), this patient should be able to achieve nearly normal function. However, the disease is relentlessly progressive, and the day will eventually come when, despite optimal medical therapy, she will be substantially disabled.

## Case 6-15

### Huntington's Disease

A 35-year-old man is brought in by his family because of a 1-year history of inappropriate behavior and abnormal movements. Because of irresponsibility, he lost a job he had held for 10 years. He is inappropriately familiar with strangers and is wont to launch into discussion of personal body functions after barely an introduction. His relationship with his wife has become shallow and impersonal and he has not exhibited any sexual interest in some time. He was recently apprehended by police after pocketing some candy bars in a grocery store. As the neurologist enters the room, his jovial demeanor belies the seriousness of the occasion. He immediately addresses her by her first name and continues to do so throughout the examination. As he sits, he appears very restless. He exhibits frequent quick, involuntary movements of his fingers, hands, and arms, and occasional quick turning movements of his head, and he repeatedly crosses and uncrosses his legs. When asked to walk, his stride is frequently interrupted by brief lilting movements.

**Comment:** This patient has Huntington's disease, which is a neurodegenerative disease affecting the cerebral cortex, particularly the frontal lobes, and the basal ganglia, particularly the caudate nucleus. It is inherited in autosomal dominant fashion. It first came to widespread public attention in this country when the folk singer Woody Guthrie was afflicted. The pattern of inappropriate behavior displayed by this patient is

## Case 6-15—cont'd

typical and reflects disease of the prefrontal cortex, particularly its orbitofrontal portions (to be reviewed in greater detail in Chapter 12). The movements he exhibits are referred to as chorea, a term actually inspired by the peculiar lilting gait of these patients, which is reminiscent of dancing. Even though the caudate nucleus is far more severely affected in this disease than the putamen, it is likely that chorea derives from putamenal dysfunction, because the putamen is the motor component of the striatum. The movements are completely different from those observed in Parkinson's disease because they reflect the loss of the principal neurons of the striatum, rather than simply loss of dopaminergic supply. As a result, the balance between the direct and indirect basal ganglia routes is tipped toward the direct route. There is a lack of inhibition of inappropriate movements that presumably represent fragments of the repertoire of movements that normally compete with the target movement. The choreiform movements of Huntington's disease can be curbed using dopamine receptor blockers, such as haloperidol. However, it is a relentlessly progressive disease that ultimately culminates in severe dementia, and there is no effective treatment for the disorder of higher neural function.

## Case 6-16

### Carbon Monoxide Poisoning

A 25-year-old man is found in his home, unconscious but still alive, a victim of carbon monoxide poisoning due to a malfunctioning heater. He is promptly treated with hyperbaric oxygen but makes a very slow recovery. When seen by a neurologist a year later, he exhibits modest generalized impairment in cognitive function. He also demonstrates nearly constant, sinuous, writhing movements of his arms and hands and, to a lesser extent, his head and legs (choreoathetosis). He also exhibits dramatic chorea when he walks.

**Comment:** Although this patient exhibits effects of a generalized hypoxic insult to the brain, his choreoathetosis reflects the particular susceptibility of the globus pallidus to the effects of carbon monoxide poisoning (Fig. 6-25). The reasons for this effect are not known. As in Huntington's disease, the balance

## Case 6-16—cont'd

between the direct and indirect basal ganglia routes is tipped toward the direct route, resulting in the appearance of uncontrollable inappropriate movements. The different character of the movements in these two disorders reflects the peculiar nature of the two different pathologies.

## Case 6-17

### Subthalamic Stroke

A 75-year-old woman suddenly develops repeated, violent, flinging movements of her right arm. These movements wax and wane, tend to worsen when she becomes anxious, and subside when she sleeps.

**Comment:** This patient exhibits hemiballismus. It is caused by a small stroke (a lacunar infarct) involving the left subthalamic nucleus. The neurons of the subthalamic nucleus project to the internal segment of the globus pallidus. They are glutamatergic (excitatory) and normally fire more or less steadily at a high rate. It appears that the loss of this more or less tonic excitatory input from the STN to the cells of $GP_i$ frees VLo of the inhibitory influence of $GP_i$ and results in the paroxysmal surges of neural activity in area 4 that are responsible for these violent movements. The essentially complete loss of the indirect basal ganglia pathway results in unfettered activity by the direct route. These patients will benefit substantially from treatment with dopamine receptor blockers such as haloperidol. Furthermore, the disorder gradually abates, reflecting plasticity in the affected motor systems.

The Motor System

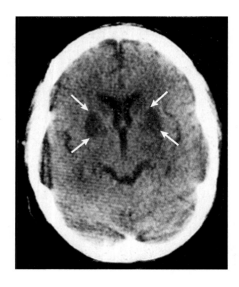

**Figure 6-25** Computed tomographic (CT) scan of a patient who experienced severe carbon monoxide poisoning, demonstrating bilateral necrosis of the globus pallidus.

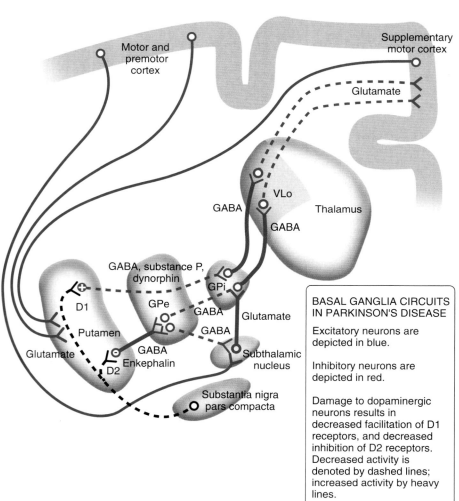

**BASAL GANGLIA CIRCUITS IN PARKINSON'S DISEASE**

Excitatory neurons are depicted in blue.

Inhibitory neurons are depicted in red.

Damage to dopaminergic neurons results in decreased facilitation of D1 receptors, and decreased inhibition of D2 receptors. Decreased activity is denoted by dashed lines; increased activity by heavy lines.

**Figure 6-26** Neural connectivity in the putamenal subsystem of the basal ganglia. See Box 6-2 for explanation.

## BOX 6-2

*The Convergence of Basal Ganglia Science and a Bold Operation for Parkinson's Disease*

In 1960, Oleh Hornykiewicz discovered that the pigmented cells of the substantia nigra pars compacta, long known to be depleted in Parkinson's disease, were dopaminergic. Seven years later, George Cotzias reported the successful treatment of Parkinson's disease with levodopa. This now-standard therapy, although not entirely satisfactory (particularly in late stages of the disease), has nevertheless so transformed the clinical picture of the average afflicted patient that most neurologists have only a remote sense of the desperate nature of the untreated disease. Before levodopa, this severe disability motivated many valiant attempts to deal with the disease surgically. The earliest operations, dating back to Victor Horsley in 1905, were often arcane procedures such as extirpation of the entire premotor cortex. In the late 1930s, Russell Meyers introduced an operation in which the output pathways of the globus pallidus were sectioned via an open craniotomy with a transventricular approach. Although the results of these procedures were often dismal, there was enough information in his reports to encourage trials of stereotactic ablation of these pathways or the pallidum itself after Spiegel introduced stereotactic neurosurgery in 1947. Pallidotomy became a popular procedure in the 1950s. However, for reasons unclear, an anterodorsal site became the favored lesion locus. Between 1952 and 1960, Lars Leksell in Lund, Sweden, systematically explored pallidotomy lesions sites, and in his paper in 1960, he reported a 95 percent success rate with posteroventral pallidotomy. Unfortunately, in the meantime, the world had moved on. The unpredictable and generally less than salutary results of anterodorsal pallidotomy led to disenchantment with the procedure in general. This surgery, which was uncomfortably close to the posterior limb of the internal capsule and the optic tract, was often fraught with complications. A different operation, cryoablation of the ventral lateral nucleus of the thalamus, introduced by Hassler and Reichert in 1954, had a dramatic impact on tremor and achieved widespread favor. Leksell gave up on his operation.

However, in 1985, Leksell encouraged a junior colleague, Lauri Laitinen, to retry the procedure. In 1992, Laitinen and his colleagues reported substantial success with the operation in 92 percent of their patients. This time around, the operation has achieved widespread acceptance, despite success rates considerably less than those reported by Laitinen, in part because of the availability of superior surgical techniques (e.g., CT-guided stereotactic localization), in part because of the unfolding neuroscience of the basal ganglia, which has enhanced the theoretical rationale for the procedure. That neuroscientific knowledge, still incomplete, is as follows:

Parkinson's disease is due to premature death of dopaminergic neurons in the substantia nigra pars compacta. As a result, dopamine levels in the putamen are eventually reduced by as much as 99 percent. Dopaminergic neurons project to all the median spiny neurons (MSNs), which compose 95 percent of the neurons in the putamen and also constitute the major source of output of the putamen. The two populations of MSNs in the putamen define two subsystems (see Fig. 6-26). One population expresses $D_1$ dopamine receptors, upon which dopamine has an excitatory effect. The second population expresses $D_2$ receptors, upon which dopamine has an inhibitory effect. All MSNs are GABAergic and therefore inhibitory. However, the $D_1$ receptor-bearing MSNs project to the globus pallidus interna ($GP_i$), whereas the $D_2$ receptor-bearing MSNs project to the globus pallidus externa ($GP_e$), which projects in turn to a portion of the $GP_i$. and to the STN (subthalamic nucleus). Whereas $GP_e$ input to $GP_i$ is GABAergic and inhibitory, STN input to $GP_i$ is glutamatergic and excitatory.

The depletion of dopamine in Parkinson's disease, and the opposite effects of dopamine on the two putamenal subpopulations, provide the key to the current hypothesis regarding the physiologic mechanism of Parkinson's disease, originally proposed by Mahlon DeLong and his colleagues and since further elaborated by Jonathan Mink. Because of the differential effect of dopamine on the two basal ganglia routes, dopamine deficiency results in a pathologic shift of the balance between the two routes in favor of the indirect route (Fig. 6-26). The loss of the excitatory effect of dopamine on putamenal neurons bearing $D_1$ receptors results in diminished inhibition of the projection targets of these neurons in $GP_i$ (the direct route). The loss of the inhibitory effect of dopamine on putamenal neurons bearing $D_2$ receptors results in excess inhibition of projection targets in $GP_e$. Target $GP_e$ neurons thus fail to inhibit $GP_i$. Target neurons in $GP_e$ also fail to inhibit STN, which then excessively

*Continued*

**BOX 6-2—cont'd**

excites neurons in $GP_i$ (the indirect route). Thus, as a result of dopamine deficiency, neurons of $GP_i$ are inadequately inhibited by the direct route and excessively excited by the indirect route. The excessive activity of these neurons pathologically inhibits neurons in $VL_O$, and $VL_O$ thus fails to provide adequate excitation of cortical neurons in areas 4 and 6.

It can now be seen that the effect of Leksell's ablative operation on the $GP_i$ is to destroy the pathologically inhibitory input to $VL_O$ from $GP_i$. As we noted in the main text, the results of this operation occasionally border on the miraculous—patients brought to the operating room frozen and unable to walk literally climb off the operating room table and stroll out of the room. Unfortunately, such dramatic results are rare, for unclear reasons. However, about a third of patients experience some benefit, and equally important, 80 percent enjoy substantial relief of dopamine-induced dyskinesias (at times violent writhing movements of the head and extremities that become a severe problem in advanced Parkinson's disease). This makes it possible for their physicians to give them higher doses of dopaminergic medications. Leksell's operation, reborn in the 1990s, has thus gained a major place in the therapeutic armamentarium of advanced Parkinson's disease.

Extensive trials are also taking place employing stimulation of the $GP_i$ or STN via stereotactically placed indwelling electrodes, which deliver constant high-frequency stimulation, which achieves a "physiologic ablation." The particular value of physiologic ablation is that the extent of the affected region of the brain can be adjusted after the operation simply by adjusting the stimulation current.

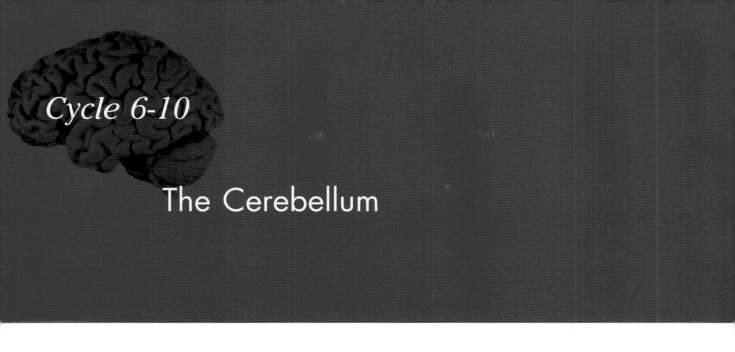

## *Objectives*

1. Be able to list the four major cerebellar subsystems, briefly describe their major afferent and efferent projections, and summarize the basic function of each.
2. Be able to describe the clinical consequences of lesions of the cerebellar vermis, hemispheres, and flocculonodular lobe, and of lesions involving the gray matter of the basis pontis.

## A. ANATOMY AND FUNCTION

Like the basal ganglia, the cerebellum acts as a consultant to the cerebral cortex in motor behavior. Unlike the basal ganglia, it also acts as a consultant to the brainstem and spinal motor systems we reviewed in earlier cycles of this chapter.

The gross architecture of the cerebellum is relatively simple (Fig. 6-27). When viewing the cerebellum from its ventral aspect, one can see the two large cerebellar hemispheres and a small caudal appendage composed of the central nodulus and the lateral flocculi. The cerebellar cortex is deeply folded into folia (long, thin, fronds; folium means "leaf of fern"). These folia are aligned in the coronal plane, transverse to the long axis of the brainstem. The foliation of the cerebellar cortex serves to accommodate a vast surface area within a small space, in a fashion similar to, though considerably more dramatic than, that observed with the gyrification of the cerebral cortex. Like the cerebrum, the gray matter of the cerebellum is located near its surface, and the deep portions of the cerebellum are composed predominantly of the white matter pathways traveling to and from the cerebellar cortex.

Four major regions can be delineated within the cerebellar cortex: the midline *vermis*, the paramedian *intermediate zone*, the lateral *hemispheres*, and the *flocculonodular lobe*. Each of these four regions comprises a cerebellar subsystem with a distinctive pattern of connections and a specific function, and each is linked to a specific cerebellar nucleus located deep within the cerebellar white matter or in the brainstem (Table 6-9). The vermis is linked to the fastigial nucleus, the intermediate zone to the interpositus nucleus, the lateral hemispheres to the dentate nucleus, and the flocculonodular lobe to the vestibular nuclei (Fig. 6-28).

The pattern of neural connections within each of these subsystems is the same. The cerebellar cortex consists of three layers: a thick, superficial, molecular layer consisting largely of the neuronal processes of the cells in the layers beneath and containing most of the connections supporting cerebellar circuitry; a thick deep layer composed predominantly of cerebellar granule cells, and in between, a one-cell layer of Purkinje cells (Fig. 6-29). Approximately 50 billion granule

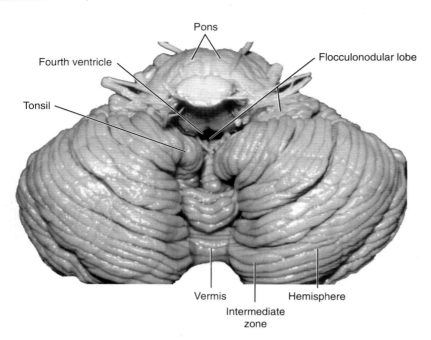

Pons

Fourth ventricle

Flocculonodular lobe

Tonsil

Vermis

Intermediate
zone

Hemisphere

**Figure 6-27** Major functional regions of the cerebellum.

cells are in the cerebellum, and the granule cells make up 50 percent of all neurons in the CNS. Afferent fibers to the cerebellum generally terminate in two branches, one synapsing on neurons of one of the deep cerebellar nuclei, and one synapsing on a number of granule cells (Fig. 6-30). Each granule cell gives rise to an axon that rises to the molecular layer and bifurcates, sending each branch (a "parallel fiber") 5 to 10 mm along the long axis of a cerebellar folium. Each parallel fiber contacts the large, fan-shaped dendritic arborizations of up to several thousand Purkinje cells, which also project up into the molecular layer. Each Purkinje cell receives contacts from up to 80,000 parallel fibers and sends its axon to terminate on the neurons of its respective deep cerebellar nucleus. The cells of the deep cerebellar nuclei are tonically active, and the Purkinje cells are inhibitory. Thus, the Purkinje cells act to shape the activity of the neurons in the deep cerebellar nuclei over time. These deep nuclear neurons then project their now-modified activity pattern to the motor systems in the cerebrum, brainstem, and spinal cord that are both the sources of cerebellar afferents and the recipients of cerebellar "consulting expertise." The connections and functions of the four cerebellar subsystems are outlined in Table 6-9.

Most spinal cord afferents enter the cerebellum via the inferior cerebellar peduncle, located in the dorsolateral regions of the medulla. Afferent projections from the cerebrum, relayed by the gray matter islands in the basis pontis, enter via the middle cerebellar peduncles (Figs. 6-31, 6-32). Cerebellar projections to the cerebrum exit via the superior cerebellar peduncle, which forms the lateral aspects of the fourth ventricle in the rostral pons.

Cerebellar systems are all located ipsilateral to the muscles whose activity they modulate. Thus, the major cerebral projections to the cerebellum descend via the frontopontocerebellar and occipitopontocerebellar pathways in the anterior and posterior limbs of the internal capsule (see Fig. 6-16) and the most medial and lateral portions of the cerebral peduncles to synapse (see Fig. 6-17), without crossing, on gray matter within the basis pontis (see Fig. 6-32). Neurons composing this gray matter then send their axons across the pons (as the pontine transverse fibers), through the middle cerebellar peduncle, to synapse on their target dyads in the cerebellum. In turn, cerebellar output projections from the deep cerebellar nuclei destined for the cerebrum exit the cerebellum via the superior cerebellar peduncles, cross in the decussation of the brachium conjunctivum, variably send collaterals into the contralateral red nucleus, and eventually terminate on the caudal region of the contralateral ventral lateral nucleus of the thalamus ($VL_C$).[7] Neurons in

---

[7]Recall that projections of the putamenal system project, via $GP_i$ and $SN_{PR}$, to VL pars oralis ($VL_o$). Thus, cerebellar and basal ganglia projection pathways do not overlap except in the cerebral cortex.

**TABLE 6-9** Anatomy and Function of Cerebellar Subsystems

| | Vermis | Intermediate Zone | Lateral Hemispheres | Flocculonodular Lobe |
|---|---|---|---|---|
| **Deep Nucleus** | *Fastigial* | *Interpositus* | *Dentate* | *Vestibular* |
| Major sources of afferent connections | Vestibular nuclei, spinocerebellar pathways originating in the intermediate zone of the spinal gray matter (between dorsal and ventral horns) at all levels, proprioceptive, muscle and joint, and skin receptors | Spinocerebellar pathways; cerebral area 4 via frontopontocerebellar pathway | Cerebral areas 4, 6 (premotor and supplementary motor cortex), somatosensory and visual association cortices via frontopontocerebellar and occipitopontocerebellar pathways (Figs. 6-16, 6-17) | Vestibular apparatus |
| Major targets | Vestibular and pontine reticulospinal systems (ventromedial descending motor tracts) | Red nucleus (source of the rubrospinal tract), motor and premotor cortex via $VL_C$ nucleus of thalamus | Red nucleus, motor and premotor cortex via $VL_C$ nucleus of thalamus | Vestibular nucleus (with subsequent projections to head and eye movement systems), fastigial nucleus |
| Effects of ablation of cortex or deep nucleus in animals and inferences regarding function | Imbalance during sitting, standing, and walking | *Tremor:* impaired balance of agonist-antagonist activity during movement; instability of stretch reflexes due to impaired adjustment of sensitivity and gait; *impaired compensation for perturbations of maintained postures or movement execution.* | *Particularly profound impairment in movements involving multiple joints, e.g. reaching (irregular trajectory, inaccuracy in meeting target).* Presumably reflects impaired correction for interaction torques (the interacting clockwise and counter-clockwise angular momentum of two bones linked at a joint) generated during multijoint movements; both formulation and execution of multijoint movement are impaired | |
| Clinical features of dysfunction in humans | Poor balance during sitting and standing, broad-based, unsteady gait, tendency to fling legs while walking | Oscillatory tremor (ataxia), irregular trajectory and fluctuating velocity during reaching movements (dyssynergia); inaccuracy of reaching (dysmetria); exaggerated movement when resistance to a movement is suddenly eliminated (Holmes' sign) | | Saccadic breakdown of ocular smooth pursuit, hypo- or more often, hypermetric ocular saccades, nystagmus |

**The Motor System**

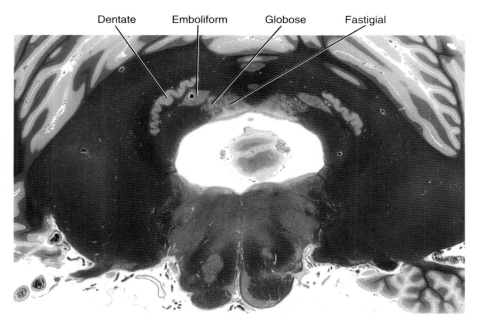

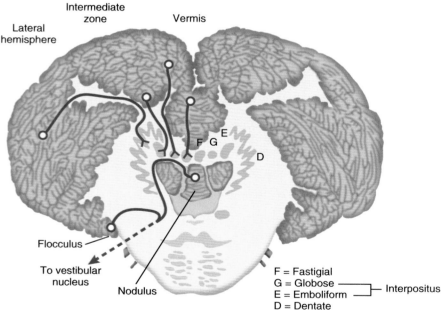

**Figure 6-28** Relationship between cerebellar cortex and the deep cerebellar nuclei. (Top picture modified from Warner JJ. Atlas of Neuroanatomy. Boston, Butterworth Heinemann, 2001, with permission from Elsevier Science. Bottom drawing modified from J.J. Warner.)

$VL_C$ then send their projections to target regions in motor and premotor cortex. Cerebral lesions produce contralateral motor signs because corticobulbar/ corticospinal projections cross only once, whereas cerebellar lesions produce ipsilateral motor signs because corticocerebellar-cortical pathways cross twice.

Despite intensive investigation spanning much of the 20th century, the essential neurophysiologic princi-

ples of cerebellar function remain a subject of intensive investigation, and our intuitions about cerebellar function, like those regarding basal ganglia function, are substantially guided by the nature of the neurologic manifestations of disease (see Section B). The cytoarchitecture of the cerebellar folia incorporates long parallel fibers linking Purkinje cells subserving multiple muscles and potentially crossing system boundaries

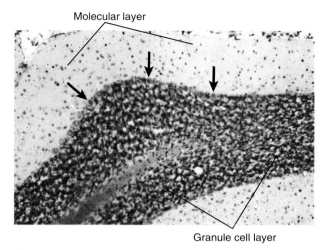

**Figure 6-29** Histologic features of the cerebellum. Arrows point to Purkinje cell layer.

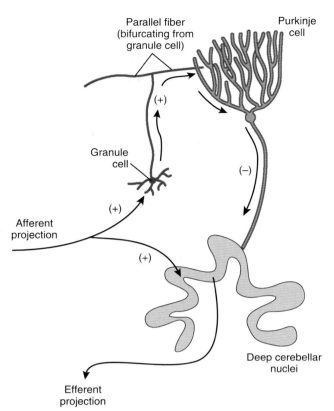

**Figure 6-30** The prototypical cerebellar "circuit."

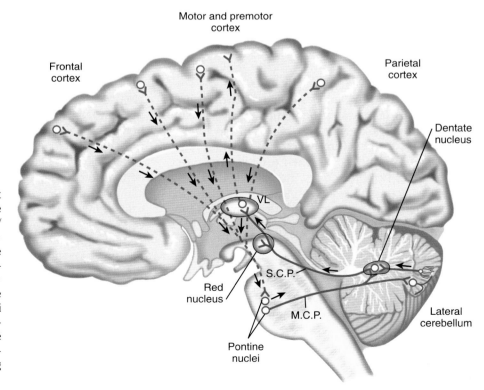

**Figure 6-31** Major afferent and efferent pathways of the lateral cerebellar hemisphere/ dentate subsystem. S.C.P. = superior cerebellar peduncle (fibers decussate to contralateral hemisphere). M.C.P. = middle cerebellar peduncle (fibers from pontine nuclei project across midline to contralateral cerebellar hemisphere via the middle cerebellar peduncles). (Modification of drawing by J.J. Warner.)

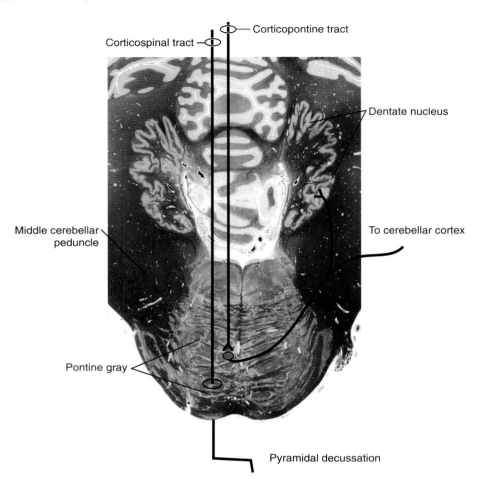

Corticopontine tract

Corticospinal tract

Dentate nucleus

Middle cerebellar
peduncle

To cerebellar cortex

Pontine gray

Pyramidal decussation

**Figure 6-32** The corticopontocerebellar pathways to the lateral cerebellar hemispheres and the dentate nucleus. (Modified from Warner JJ. Atlas of Neuroanatomy. Boston, Butterworth Heinemann, 2001, with permission from Elsevier Science.)

(e.g., between the two sides of the body, and between the intermediate zone and the lateral cerebellar hemisphere). Thus, it appears to be set up to coordinate the activity of multiple muscles involving multiple joints. It also appears to be set up to reconcile motor system conflicts, which may arise when a movement developed by the cerebral cortex (ramified through the cerebellar hemisphere/dentate system) is perturbed by something in the environment (as conveyed to the CNS by ascending sensory and spinocerebellar pathways and ramified through the intermediate zone/interpositus system).

Not only do the long parallel fibers provide the mechanism for coordinating the activity of multiple muscles, but they may provide the neurophysiologic basis for regulating the relative timing of muscle contractions. Because these fibers are small, they have relatively slow conduction velocities. It takes time for impulses to travel down these tiny fibers, and the fibers travel varying distances between Purkinje cell synapses.

This variance provides the basis for different and precisely defined delays between Purkinje cell excitations, possibly forming the basis for the precise delay needed between sequential muscle contractions in a multimuscle, multijoint movement. The multiplicity of parallel fibers makes feasible a multiplicity of muscle contraction combinations and timing relationships.

As in the case of the basal ganglia and Renshaw cells in the spinal cord, inhibitory interneurons in the cerebellum serve to focus neural activity and suppress competing but somewhat less active muscle contraction combinations and sequences. As is the case with the basal ganglia, much of the cerebellar influence is exerted during the roughly 100 ms that elapse between onset of pyramidal cell firing in the cortex and the onset of $\alpha$-motoneuron firing in the spinal cord, and during the subsequent course of $\alpha$-motoneuronal firing during the movement. Unlike the basal ganglia, the cerebellum, particularly the lateral hemisphere/dentate system, via its links with premotor cortex and supplementary motor cortex, is significantly involved in motor planning. Both the cerebellum and the basal ganglia have been implicated in motor learning.

As with the basal ganglia, a question arises as to what degree the functions of the cerebellum have been or can be subsumed by the cerebral cortex. The cerebellum is an ancient structure, already evident in the most primitive vertebrates. This question has some clinical significance. Patients who experience cerebellar strokes generally exhibit substantial recovery, and surgery to remove cerebellar tumors or evacuate cerebellar hemorrhages is remarkably well tolerated. On the other hand, under certain circumstances, the cerebellum is capable of considerable mischief. Degenerative cerebellar disease is typically associated with profound disability, as indicated in the following section.

## B. MANIFESTATIONS OF CEREBELLAR DYSFUNCTION

Our best clues to the essential functions of the cerebellum derive from observations of cerebellar disease in humans, as Cases 6-18 to 6-20 illustrate.

### Case 6-18

#### Alcoholic Cerebellar Vermal Degeneration
*A 65-year-old man, a lifelong alcoholic, is admitted to the hospital because of seizures resulting from abrupt cessation of alcohol consumption. His seizures are immediately brought under control with phenytoin and nervousness and agitation related to alcohol withdrawal are well controlled with lorazepam (a GABA$_A$ receptor agonist). Three days later, he is anxious to go home. However, he can barely walk. His gait is extremely wide-based, and with each step he tends to roughly fling the foot and leg forward. He is dangerously unstable when attempting to walk and repeatedly has to be caught by one of his physicians. When asked to lightly slide one heel down the length of the shin (heel-to-shin maneuver), he cannot keep the foot from swinging wildly from side to side, and he only intermittently contacts his shin. In contrast, when asked to alternately touch the examiner's finger and his own nose with the same hand (finger-to-nose maneuver), he performs nearly normally.*

**Comment:** *This patient has degeneration of the cerebellar vermis due to the chronic toxic effects of*

### Case 6-18—cont'd

*alcohol (Fig. 6-33). The reasons for the peculiar susceptibility of the vermis to the effects of alcohol are not known. Typically such patients will improve significantly during the weeks following the alcohol binge.*

### Case 6-19

#### Paraneoplastic Cerebellar Degeneration
*A 38-year-old woman develops a flulike illness. As she remains bed-bound over the next 3 weeks, she discovers that she can no longer control the use of her hands, stand, or walk. On examination, there is severe saccadic breakdown of ocular smooth pursuit (normal smooth following movements of the eyes have been replaced by a series of small, quick, saccadic jerks). When asked to alternate gaze between the examiner's nose and the examiner's raised hand, her eyes consistently shoot past the target, following which she has to saccade back (hypermetric saccades). Her speech has a singsong intonation in which vowel sounds are frequently abnormally prolonged (scanning speech). When asked to perform a finger-to-nose maneuver, her hand and arm irregularly accelerate and decelerate and the hand follows a ragged trajectory (dyssynergia). She tends to swing her hand back and forth as she tries to zero in on the target (ataxia/cerebellar tremor) and she typically misses the target by several centimeters (dysmetria). On the heel-to-shin maneuver, she is also very ataxic and dysmetric. As she sits on the side of the bed, she totters from side to side (truncal titubation). Her balance is so bad that she is completely unable to stand. Her strength is completely normal.*

**Comment:** *This patient has paraneoplastic cerebellar degeneration, a rare disorder in which Purkinje cells throughout the cerebellum are destroyed. There is evidence of severe dysfunction of all four major cerebellar systems. This syndrome is caused by antibodies to a tumor antigen (usually breast or ovarian carcinoma in women) that also react with a Purkinje cell antigen. A correct diagnosis may lead to early detection and resection of the tumor, potentially saving the patient's life. Unfortunately, the neurologic disorder typically progresses so rapidly that even rapid excision of the tumor will not reverse the cerebellar damage.*

The Motor System

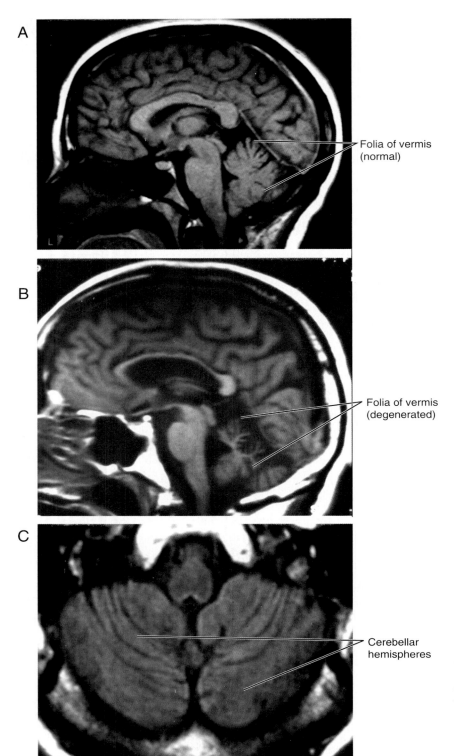

A

Folia of vermis
(normal)

B

Folia of vermis
(degenerated)

C

Cerebellar
hemispheres

**Figure 6-33** Magnetic resonance image (MRI) of the cerebellum of a chronic alcoholic with cerebellar vermal degeneration. *A*, Normal cerebellar vermis. *B*, Severe atrophy of the folia of the vermis. *C*, Note the relative sparing of the cerebellar hemispheres in this patient.

## Case 6-20

### Friedreich's Ataxia

*A 16-year-old girl is brought to the neurology clinic because of clumsiness. It seems she has always been clumsy, but her parents think that the problem may be progressive. On examination, there is mild saccadic breakdown (eyes advance by small jerks when she visually follows slow-moving objects) of ocular smooth pursuit. The finger-to-nose maneuver is moderately dyssynergic and slightly dysmetric. She exhibits mild truncal titubation while sitting on the examining table, and her gait is somewhat wide-based and unsteady. She is barely able to walk at all with her eyes closed and nearly falls in the attempt. Deep tendon reflexes are 1 and symmetric in the arms and absent in the legs. She has severe impairment of position sense in the great toes (ability to detect passive flexion or extension of the great toes). Her 10-year-old brother, who came along for the adventure, looks a bit ungainly as he runs down the hall. He has no ankle jerks.*

**Comment:** *This patient has Friedreich's ataxia, an autosomal recessive disorder characterized by degeneration of neurons in the dorsal root ganglia and of cells in the intermediate zone of the spinal cord gray matter projecting to the cerebellum. Her cerebellum is perfectly normal. She has cerebellar signs because of loss of sensory input to the cerebellum (joints, muscle spindles). The disease of the dorsal root ganglia also breaks the myotatic reflex arcs; hence the loss of deep tendon reflexes. Her impairment of walking is worse with her eyes closed because she is then forced to rely exclusively on her defective somatosensory function and impaired vestibulocerebellar function to maintain her balance. The disease is slowly progressive and patients are usually wheelchair-bound by age 40. They often also have scoliosis (curvature of the spine) and typically develop cardiac disease that may cause early death. The disease is not treatable. However, the gene has recently been located, providing the potential foundation for treatment in the future. Her little brother probably also has the disease.*

## PRACTICE 6-10

**A.** A 67-year-old man with a long history of hypertension, hypercholesterolemia, and smoking suddenly develops right-sided weakness and incoordination. On examination he has mild to moderate weakness of the right arm, proximally and distally, slight weakness of the proximal right lower extremity, severe impairment of independent finger movement in the right hand, a right pronation drift, and severe ataxia, dysmetria, and dyssynergia of the right arm during finger-to-nose maneuver (see Table 6-9). Despite nearly normal strength in the right leg, he tilts severely to the right while attempting to walk, and it is all his examiner can do to support him. He has a right Babinski sign. Locate this patient's stroke (hint: several loci are possible).

**B.** An 80-year-old woman with a history of hypertension and a heart attack suddenly develops severe dizziness, nausea, vomiting, and a tendency to fall to her left. Examination reveals ataxia, dyssynergia, and dysmetria of the left arm during finger-to-nose maneuver. She is unable to even stand because of her tendency to fall to the left. An MRI angiogram reveals distal occlusion of the left vertebral artery. Locate her lesion and explain why she has cerebellar signs on the left (hint: refer to Cycle 2-3).

**C.** Return to Practice 6-6A. If there were no history of aminoglycoside use, how would you determine whether this man had disease of the vestibular labyrinths or disease of the cerebellar vermis?

**The Motor System**

# Summary: Central Nervous System Motor Function

## A. A SYSTEMS PERSPECTIVE

All movements, to one degree or another, represent a combination of articulated muscle activity, selective manipulation of background muscle stiffness or tone, and reflex activity. The neural substrate for each of these three components is distributed differently within the CNS.

The neural substrate for the various types of articulated muscle activity depends upon several interrelated factors: the need for rapidity and precision, the need for custom design of movement, and the relative recency of the evolution of a particular capacity. The corticospinal system provides capacities for high precision and speed, is eminently capable of providing novel movements tailored to every situation, and has evolved most recently. Although the function of the corticospinal system is manifest in precision movements involving every part of the body, the singular marker of dysfunction in this system is loss of the capacity for independent finger movement. At the other extreme are neural systems of ancient origin subserving what might be viewed as automatic movements. The best example of this is the system underlying walking. As we have seen, spinal cord pattern generators produce the reciprocating limb movements of walking, and brainstem systems, most importantly the vestibulospinal system, provide the basis for the corrective movements during walking that are needed for balance. The corticospinal contribution to walking is modest: initiation, change of direction, and customizing steps to fit the demands of the terrain.

Muscle tone is necessary for us to maintain posture while we are upright, whether sitting, standing, or moving (i.e., antigravity tone). Muscle tone in proximal muscles also provides the platform upon which we can produce precision movements with the distal extremities, particularly the hands. The distribution of neural systems that control muscle tone parallels, both anatomically and functionally, that of systems underlying articulated muscle activity. Anatomically, precision movements are largely mediated via the lateral corticospinal tract of the spinal cord, whereas tone is maintained by the descending ventromedial tracts. Functionally, enhancement of proximal limb tone preparatory to precision movement of distal extremities is substantially driven by corticobulbar connections to brainstem motor centers. In contrast, antigravity tone is maintained primarily by the pontine and medullary reticular formations and the vestibulospinal system and must be selectively suppressed by the corticobulbar/corticospinal system to allow articulated muscle activity. Cerebral lesions lead to increases in extensor tone (spasticity) in the lower extremities and increases in pronation and flexion tone in the upper extremities (e.g., pronation drift, decorticate posturing), in a sense the recapitulation of a pattern of tone that had some functional value in our arboreal ancestors. Lesions in the pons lead to excessive extensor tone in all extremities (decerebrate rigidity), in a sense causing the reca-pitulation of a pattern of tone that had some functional value in our even more ancient quadrupedal forebears.

Neural systems underlying reflexes are the most phylogenetically primitive of all components of the motor system. They are located exclusively in the brainstem and spinal cord. They serve functions as various as resisting muscle lengthening during load bearing (myotatic reflex arcs), equalizing the force applied by muscle fascicles to tendons and protecting against tendon overload (Golgi tendon organs), withdrawal from noxious stimuli (nociceptive flexion reflexes), and correction of postural deviation to prevent falls (postural reflexes). The distribution of these systems is substantially complementary to that of the corticospinal system. Thus, in the hands, where the corticospinal system reigns supreme, there are relatively fewer muscle spindles. Like tone systems, reflex systems are bound by the Jacksonian principle. Thus, lesions of corticospinal or brainstem motor systems, or lesions of their projections in the spinal cord, lead to disinhibition of myotatic reflexes (hyper-reflexia), Golgi tendon organ systems (together with disinhibited myotatic reflexes resulting in spastic catches), and nociceptive flexion reflexes (Babinski signs, triple flexion responses).

The basal ganglia and cerebellum act as consultants to the corticospinal system in the production of articulated muscle activity, and the basal ganglia contribute to the regulation of tone. The consequences of basal ganglia disease depend on locus and type of lesion. Thus, dopamine depletion of the putamen in Parkinson's disease leads to excessively small movements (hypokinesia), suppression of simultaneous but mutually compatible movements, prolongation of the interval between mutually compatible sequential movements (bradykinesia), and increased tone (plastic rigidity). A number of different lesions of the basal ganglia result in the generation of inappropriate movements: chorea with degeneration of the caudate nucleus and putamen in Huntington's disease, choreoathetosis with hypoxic injury to the pallidum, and hemiballismus with infarcts of the subthalamic nucleus.

The consequences of cerebellar disease reflect the broad spectrum of motor activity influenced by the cerebellum: balance by the vermis, eye movements by the flocculonodular lobes, and articulated limb movement by the cerebellar hemispheres. The essential manifestation of cerebellar disease can be characterized as decomposition of movement—over or under computation of the duration and magnitude of muscle activity needed to move to a target (hypo- and hypermetric ocular saccades, limb dysmetria), and impaired coordination of the contraction of the multiple muscles involved in a movement subsuming multiple bones and joints, manifested as ataxia (oscillation) and dyssynergia (jerky, wandering movements).

# B. A NEUROLOGIST'S PERSPECTIVE

An alternative way of gaining some perspective on the roles of the various components of the motor system is to view this system as a neurologist does: observing abnormalities of the neurologic examination and reasoning backward to infer the neural systems in which function must be impaired. Neurologists effectively utilize an axial movement/appendicular movement dichotomy that corresponds quite well to the roles of the motor systems reviewed in Section A.

## Midline Neuraxis

Lesions of the midline neuraxis produce disorders of posture, balance, muscle tone, gait, and predominantly lower extremity movement. The type of disorder depends on the locus of the lesion. Because the spinal cord is a small structure in cross section, lesions generally affect both midline and appendicular systems, and the pattern of neurologic dysfunction is chiefly defined by the level of the lesion in the spinal cord. Lesions of the spinal cord may produce muscle weakness, wasting, and fasciculations in segments directly involved in the lesion by directly destroying the final common pathway for movement—$\alpha$- and $\gamma$-motoneurons. They also produce weakness by disrupting the descending motor pathways that influence $\alpha$- and $\gamma$-motoneurons to produce movement—principally the corticospinal, ponto-, and medullary reticulospinal tracts and the vestibulospinal tracts. After weeks to months, they may lead to abnormalities of muscle tone so great that they directly suppress movement (because of muscle stiffness), and they render dysfunctional spinal cord movement systems that are still intact, such as the spinal cord pattern generators responsible for walking movements. Finally, they release potentially dysfunctional reflexes, such as nociceptive flexion reflexes, resulting in some cases in spontaneous triple flexion reflexes.

The Motor System

Lesions of the brainstem lead to weakness and abnormalities of muscle tone that are similar in many ways to those seen with spinal cord lesions. Lesions of the brainstem may also produce impairment in balance, even in the absence of significant weakness or dystonia, due largely to impairment in vestibulospinal function. Brainstem lesions lead to the patterned abnormalities of tone referred to as posturing: decerebrate with lesions of the pons, and decorticate with lesions at the level of the midbrain.

Lesions of the midline cerebellum do not affect strength but wreak havoc with the coordination of motor systems implicated in balance and lower extremity movement. Patients with vermal lesions are very unsteady on their feet; their gait is wide-based, sloppy, and unsteady (ataxic); they tend to clumsily fling their legs forward as they walk; and they are unable to precisely control the movements of their legs, as in the heel-to-shin maneuver, which is characterized by oscillation (ataxia), inaccuracy (dysmetria), and lack of smoothness (dyssynergia). Gait abnormalities due to midline cerebellar and vestibular lesions often look nearly identical. The most effective way to distinguish between them is the heel-to-shin maneuver, which is severely impaired with cerebellar lesions, but normal with vestibular lesions.

Lesions of the basal ganglia often lead to increased stiffness of all muscles (e.g., plastic or cogwheel rigidity in Parkinson's disease), but axial muscles are often the most affected. Axial and appendicular movements tend to be equally affected in basal ganglia disease— both steps during walking and hand movements are too small (hypokinetic) in Parkinson's disease, and choreiform movements are evident in both hands (brief, inadvertent, irregular jerks) and feet (the lilting gait that inspired the term "chorea") in Huntington's disease. Basal ganglia lesions do not affect strength.

Disorders of the midline cerebrum chiefly affect midline motor functions and leg movement. They engender impairment in those aspects of gait that are deliberate as opposed to automatic, for example, the characteristic pattern of difficulty initiating walking, ceasing walking, making turns, and fitting steps to irregularities in the terrain known as gait apraxia. They also lead to degradation of rapid, precise movements of the feet (e.g., slow, irregular foot tapping). Because of heavy corticobulbar projections regulating tone, midline cerebral lesions lead to tone abnormalities that in many ways resemble those seen with brainstem and spinal cord lesions. Finally, like brainstem and spinal cord lesions, they may lead to release of primitive spinal cord mediated reflexes, e.g., Babinski signs.

## Lateral Neuraxis

Lesions of the lateral cerebellum—the cerebellar hemispheres—lead to inaccurate (dysmetria), oscillatory (ataxia/intention tremor), and irregular movements (dyssynergia) of the arms and hands, without weakness.

Basal ganglia disease, as we have noted, tends to affect axial and appendicular movements equally. However, in practical terms, the impact on axial function may be greater because, for example, parkinsonian patients can still perform most activities of daily living with small hand and finger movements (albeit more slowly), but the ability to get around is profoundly affected by difficulty getting out of chairs, leg stiffness, and tiny stepping movements, despite normal strength.

Lateral cerebral lesions have profound effects on arm and hand function—largely because, when compared with axial functions, there are far fewer alternative systems to subsume arm and hand function in the face of cerebral lesions. Thus, lateral cerebral lesions lead to severe impairment of skilled movements in the contralateral hand and marked weakness that is maximal in distal upper extremity muscles, attributable to damage to the corticospinal system, and abnormalities in tone (spasticity, pronation drift, decorticate posturing) that reflect damage to corticobulbar systems.

## CYCLE 6-3

**A.** Diabetics experience neural damage throughout the body. Because of the particularly severe damage to the axons of α-motoneurons supplying the EDB, one of the most distal muscles in the body, the trophic influence of the α-motoneurons on the muscle fibers has been lost. Because the pathologic process has outpaced renervation, the muscles have atrophied. The diffuse nerve damage has also affected group Ia afferents supplying muscle spindles in the gastrocnemius-soleus bilaterally; hence the loss of ankle jerks. Loss or attenuation of ankle jerks is generally a very sensitive sign of disseminated neuropathy (polyneuropathy).

**B.** C7 nerve root. This scenario is fairly typical for a herniated cervical disk. This patient is likely to benefit from surgical resection of the disk.

**C.** The proximal left lower extremity weakness and missing left knee jerk could be due to lesions of the α-motoneurons or nerve roots at the L2, L3, and L4 levels or of the peripheral nerves deriving therefrom (i.e., the femoral nerve). In this case, the disease is actually a peculiar inflammatory neuritis, not uncommonly seen in diabetics, that affects nerve roots and peripheral nerves, almost invariably in the legs (a radiculoneuropathy). Prognosis for spontaneous recovery is quite good. The missing ankle jerks, of course, reflect the more garden-variety diabetic polyneuropathy, which breaks the S1 myotatic reflex arcs.

**D.** The lesion must be below C8 (finger jerks are normal) and above L2 (knee jerks are hyperactive). In fact, this is an unusual disk herniation at the T11–T12 vertebral level, which compresses the cord at the L2 level, producing the peculiar pattern of sensory loss (remember the mismatch between spinal cord and vertebral body levels [see Chapter 1]). From what you learn in the next chapter, you will be able to explain the pattern of sensory loss.

**E.** Hopefully you suggested a cervical MRI. This patient's diffuse hyper-reflexia, including very brisk biceps and brachioradialis deep tendon reflexes, suggests a lesion above the C5–C6 level. In fact, this patient has a meningioma (a benign tumor) at the C2 level. She will do well with surgical resection of the tumor.

## CYCLE 6-4

**A.** There would be increased deep tendon reflexes and increased resistance to passive movement of the lower extremities due to loss of presynaptic inhibition of group Ia and group II afferents, respectively; spastic catches in the legs as a result of this same disinhibition combined with release of group Ib mediated inhibition of α-motoneuron activity; and bilateral Babinski signs due to loss of inhibition of nociceptive flexion reflexes. He would also have significant weakness of his legs, the basis for which will be discussed in subsequent sections. His arms will, of course, be completely normal.

**B.** The lesions affect exclusively peripheral nerves and nerve roots. Demyelination often completely blocks all neural transmission in a nerve (i.e., conduction block). Alternatively, it may variably slow the conduction velocity of axons within a nerve. Thus, a brief pulse of excitation generated at one end of such a nerve will no longer be transmitted down the nerve as a brief wave of depolarization. Instead, it will be spread out over considerable time (dispersed) and the peak amplitude will be reduced. Conduction block and dispersion particularly impair group Ia and II afferent transmission, thus breaking myotatic reflex arcs and passive stretch reflex arcs throughout the body, hence the absence of deep tendon reflexes.

We would not expect Babinski signs. In some circumstances, as we shall see, peripheral lesions can mask some of the effects of central lesions. However, unless we posit a completely hidden central lesion, there is nothing in the clinical presentation to suggest CNS disease. In actual fact, patients with Guillain-Barré syndrome do not have CNS disease and do not exhibit Babinski signs.

**C.** The tumor has metastasized to the lumbosacral region of the spinal cord, where it has broken the myotatic reflex arcs underlying the knee jerks (L2–L4) and ankle jerks (S1) at the same time that it has damaged descending pathways inhibiting nociceptive flexion reflexes, hence the bilateral Babinski signs. The presence of Babinski signs is the most important clue because it tells you the lesion is central. Once you know this, it is just a question of figuring out the location of the segmental lesion(s) that would break the appropriate myotatic reflex arcs.

**D.** This patient has segmental ("lower motor neuron") signs at the C5, C6, and C7 levels on the left, and long tract ("upper motor neuron") signs in the left leg. These findings pinpoint the lesion to the C5, C6, and C7 levels of the cord. If she had had a hemispheric stroke, she would have had upper motor neurons signs in both the arm and the leg.

This patient evidently bruised her spinal cord during the fall (in part because of narrowing of the spinal canal due to degenerative disease). This impact produced a small hemorrhage into the cord substance (hematomyelia). Subsequently, as the hematoma was cleared, the hematoma cavity continued to expand, forming a long cavity or syrinx (Fig. 6-34). The mechanisms for this expansion are controversial.

The syrinx, largely confined to the left half of the cord, has damaged the gray matter over many levels, most particularly C5, C6, and C7, and it has damaged descending motor pathways at these same levels, hence the "upper motor neuron signs" in the left leg.

## CYCLE 6-6

**A.** Patients like this, who experience aminoglycoside-mediated vestibulotoxic effects, acutely have severely impaired balance. They walk with a wide-based gait, are quite unstable, and are at considerable risk of falling. Eventually, they characteristically demonstrate some recovery. Without adequate vestibular input, the vestibulospinal system cannot produce appropriate corrective movements to maintain an upright body posture.

**B.** The lesion must be on the right side at or above the C5 level. The lateral corticospinal tract decussates in the medulla, so below the medullary level, clinical features of tract damage will be ipsilateral to the lesion. The other descending motor pathways are uncrossed throughout their extent, so clinical manifestations will always be ipsilateral to the lesion. The arm is innervated by the C5 through T1 levels, so if the entire arm is paralyzed, the lesion must be at or above C5. Right-sided deep tendon reflexes will be absent because of spinal shock. The somatosensory and motor manifestations of spinal cord hemisection are referred to as the Brown-Sequard syndrome, to be discussed further in Chapter 7 (Somesthesis).

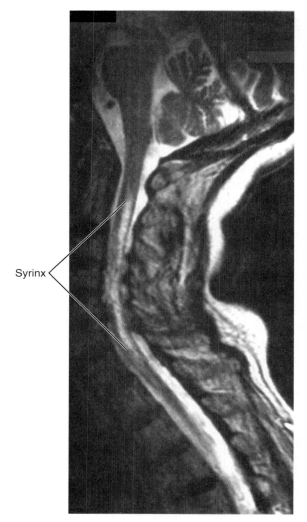

**Figure 6-34** See Feedback for Cycle 6-4D. Magnetic resonance image (MRI) of syrinx.

Syrinx

**C.** This patient presents with a relatively common problem that is often misdiagnosed, with tragic results. The most important localizing clue (other than a high index of suspicion born of clinical experience) is the presence of Babinski signs, indicating the presence of a central lesion. These lead, in turn, to a reanalysis of the deep tendon reflexes. Diabetic polyneuropathy normally breaks the afferent limb of the myotatic reflex arc underlying the ankle jerks (because the nerve fibers involved are among the longest in the body and therefore are most exposed to diabetic pathologic change). The fact that this patient has ankle jerks indicates that reflexes are actually so brisk that, even with the periph-

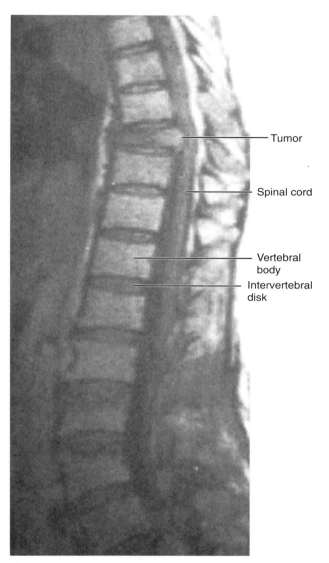

— Tumor

— Spinal cord

— Vertebral body
Intervertebral disk

**Figure 6-35** Magnetic resonance image (MRI) of thoracic spine of patient in Practice 6-6C.

single day of delay, she may be rendered permanently paraplegic.

**D.** Because the lesion is impinging upon the pyramidal system, the patient is likely to have impairment of independent finger movements in the right hand.

**E.** As the tumor first becomes symptomatic, there will be pronation drift of the left arm during sustention (holding the arms extended in front of the body), weakness on the left side (greater in the arm), and impairment of fine motor movement in the left hand. These deficits reflect damage to the corticospinal tract (fine motor movement) and damage to corticobulbar fibers leading to release of all brainstem tone centers and incipient development of decorticate posturing on the left. As the mass grows, weakness becomes worse and the patient develops frank decorticate posturing on the left, much as in Case 6-10. As the tumor grows further, it shifts the brainstem down (central herniation) and to the left (uncal herniation), eventually compressing the left midbrain against the margin of the tentorium and thereby crushing the left corticospinal and corticobulbar tracts in the cerebral peduncle against the margin of the tentorium. This produces weakness and decorticate posturing on the right side. As the herniation process continues to progress, it begins to impact the pons (bilaterally) and the patient develops bilateral decerebrate posturing. In practice, once the herniation process begins, it tends to advance very rapidly, leading to the patient's demise within 1 to 3 days, hence the need for urgent surgical intervention.

## CYCLE 6-7

**A.** In an upper motor neuron bladder, there is hypertonicity of the detrusor, small capacity, and an excessive propensity for spontaneous contractions and resultant urinary frequency, urgency, and urgency incontinence. Tolterodine is highly effective in mitigating the impact of disinhibited detrusor neurons and reducing bladder hypertonicity, and it is a very beneficial drug for patients with this problem.

In a lower motor neuron bladder, there is reduced bladder tone, increased capacity, and increased residual volume after urination (known as postvoid residual, or PVR). The increased PVR heightens the risk of infection because bacteria are no longer efficiently cleared from the bladder. Tolterodine will aggravate these problems by further reducing detrusor tone.

eral nerve lesion, they are still detectable. Thus, there is masked hyper-reflexia. The 3 level knee jerks and the 2 level upper extremity reflexes suggest that the lesion may be somewhere along the thoracic spinal cord (although a higher lesion is possible). In this case, the cord compression could be due to breast cancer metastatic to a vertebral body, now extending into the spinal canal (Fig. 6-35). If this patient gets radiation therapy on the day of her emergency room visit, her ability to walk can probably be preserved. With even a

**TABLE 6-10** Summary of Neurologic Signs in Relationship to Lesion Localization

| Sign | Localization |
|---|---|
| Impaired independent finger movement | Lesion of corticospinal tract |
| Babinski sign | Lesion of medullary reticulospinal tract or cortical projections thereto |
| Absent deep tendon reflex | Segmental lesion breaking myotatic reflex arc, most likely, lesion of group Ia afferents |
| Pronation drift | Lesion of corticobulbar fibers releases flexion and pronation tone in the upper extremity generated by pontine and medullary reticulospinal systems. In effect, an extremely abbreviated form of decorticate rigidity |
| Muscle wasting | Lesion of α-motoneuron or its axon with resultant loss of trophic effect on muscle |
| Hyperactive deep tendon reflexes | Lesion of corticobulbar or reticulospinal or vestibulospinal pathways, resulting in disinhibition of myotatic reflex arcs |
| Spastic catch | Lesion of corticobulbar, reticulospinal or vestibulospinal pathways, resulting in both disinhibition of myotatic reflex arcs and autogenic inhibitory, Ib/Golgi tendon organ-based circuits |
| Fasciculations | Lesion of α-motoneuron or its axon, leading to propensity for spontaneous depolarizations |
| Decorticate rigidity | Lesion of corticobulbar fibers releasing medullary and pontine reticulospinal systems |
| Decerebrate rigidity | Lesion of pons releasing extensor tone in all extremities generated by the vestibulospinal tract and vestibular input to the pontine reticulospinal tract |
| Flaccid tone | Usually, lesion of group Ia and II afferent pathways. May be seen with very acute lesions of the cord, causing spinal shock, or of the cerebral hemispheres. |

Many patients with upper motor neuron bladders (i.e., those with lesions above T10) have both a spastic sphincter and a spastic detrusor. Therefore, whether the bladder in these patients is very small or very large depends on which muscle "wins," the detrusor or the sphincter. The moral of the story is, before you give anyone tolterodine (or any comparable drug), you should check a PVR.

**B.**

| | |
|---|---|
| 6-3A | Diabetic polyneuropathy: LMN |
| 6-3D | T11–T12 level disk with L2 level myelopathy: UMN |
| 6-3E | High cervical meningioma with myelopathy: UMN |
| 6-4A | T8 level myelopathy due to metastatic prostate cancer: UMN |
| 6-4B | Guillain-Barré syndrome (polyradiculoneuropathy): LMN |
| 6-4C | Metastasis to the conus medullaris—could be UMN if lesion is predominantly above S2–S4 or LMN if it substantially invades S2–S4 levels of the cord |
| 6-4D | Cervical syrinx: UMN |
| 6-6C | Diabetic with myelopathy: LMN due to diabetic polyneuropathy or UMN due to |

cord lesion from metastasis. The actual clinical situation will depend on which lesion has the greatest effect.

# CYCLE 6-8

**A.** Table 6-10

**B.** Corticospinal fibers to the leg travel more laterally and thus, are more likely to by spared by the lesion. Ventromedial fibers (pontine reticulospinal and vestibulospinal), which play a relatively greater role in lower extremity function, tend to be spared by the lesion because of their ventral location.

**C.** Parasagittal cerebral cortex, such as falcine meningioma, affecting leg region of the motor homunculus. Periventricular white matter carrying fibers from parasagittal cortex around the bodies of the lateral ventricles down to the spinal cord, for example, due to pressure induced demyelination from hydrocephalus, inflammatory demyelination, as in multiple sclerosis, or ischemic demyelination. Thoracic spinal cord. The lesion could conceivably be in the brainstem, but because of the somatotopic organization of corticospinal and corticobulbar pathways (arms medial, legs lateral), one would also expect prominent upper extremity involvement. Finally, the lesion could be in the cervical spinal cord and associated with only very subtle lower motor neuron manifestations in the upper extremities (see Case 6-8). Many patients with cervical spondylotic myelopathy do not complain about their arms, and it is only the presence of reflex alterations in the arms that provides the clue to the cervical location of the lesion.

**D.** Arm > leg hemiparesis, right upper motor neuron facial palsy, right pronation drift, impaired independent finger movement on the right, right-sided hyper-reflexia, increased resting tone on the right, reduced right arm swing while walking, spastic gait on the right, right Babinski sign.

## CYCLE 6-10

**A.** This patient has what is commonly referred to as ataxic hemiparesis—pyramidal and cerebellar signs on the same side of the body. The question is, where do pyramidal and cerebellar pathways subserving the right side of the body pass sufficiently close to each other to be susceptible to damage by the same small stroke?

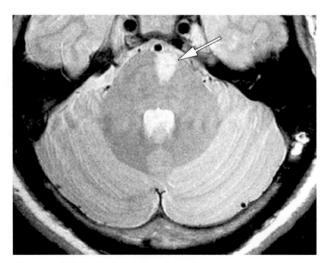

**Figure 6-36** Median infarction of the basis pontis caused by occlusion of single penetrating vessel from the basilar artery, producing ataxic hemiparesis.

The most common location is the left side of the basis pontis (see Practice 2-3B and Feedback, Fig. 6-32 and Fig. 6-36). This stroke, cause by thrombotic occlusion of a single small vessel supplying the left median portions of the basis pontis, damages corticospinal fibers destined for the right arm, still on the left side because they have not yet decussated. It also damages gray matter in the basis pontis that receives frontopontine corticobulbar fibers and projects, via the middle cerebellar peduncle, to the contralateral (right) cerebellar hemisphere, hence the right-sided cerebellar signs. There are at least a couple of other locations where a single small stroke might simultaneously damage both pyramidal and cerebellar pathways supplying the same side of the body. One is in the midbrain, where the stroke could damage the cerebral peduncle and the slightly more dorsal cerebellorubrothalamic fibers that have just crossed in the decussation of the brachium conjunctivum. For unclear reasons, this is an extraordinarily rare event. Another location is in the posterior corona radiata, where a single small lesion could simultaneously damage descending pyramidal fibers destined for the posterior limb of the internal capsule and ascending fibers from $VL_C$ in the thalamus destined for motor and premotor cortex. This location is second only to the basis pontis in frequency.

**B.** The vertebral artery thrombosis occludes the orifice of the posterior inferior cerebellar artery (PICA), which supplies the dorsolateral medulla on its way to the inferior portions of the cerebellar hemisphere (see Practice 2-3C and Feedback and Figs. 8-31, 8-32). The inferior cerebellar peduncle, located in the dorsolateral medulla, is severely damaged, thus depriving the cerebellum of most of its afferent input from the spinal cord. This damage is probably the major contributor to the patient's cerebellar signs and symptoms. Damage to the inferior cerebellar hemisphere could also account for some of her manifestations. The severe dizziness, nausea, and vomiting are caused by damage to the vestibular nuclei, which are located in the same region. This patient has a lateral medullary or Wallenberg infarction, about which we will have more to say in subsequent chapters. Her prognosis for recovery is quite good.

**C.** Have him perform a heel-to-shin maneuver. If he has vestibular disease, it will be normal.

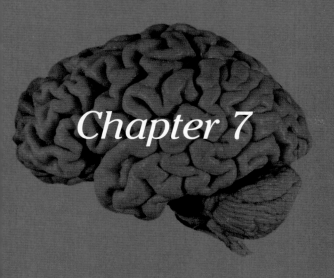

*Chapter 7*

# SOMESTHESIS

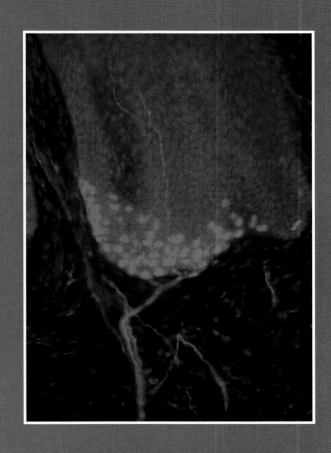

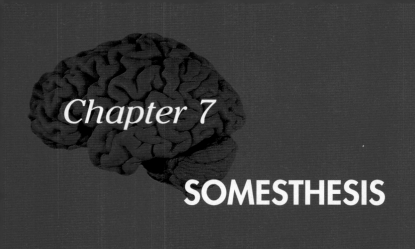

# Chapter 7

# SOMESTHESIS

# Introduction

The term "somesthesis" subsumes all the sensory systems that bring information to the brain and spinal cord regarding direct stimulation of the face and body. It includes sensations of touch, vibration, joint position, limb movement, temperature, and pain as well as visceral sensation—the different modalities of somatic sensation. As we shall see, different somesthetic systems incorporate sensitivity to several different dimensions of somatosensory information, including intensity, timing (onset and offset of the sensory stimulus), velocity, direction, and spatial configuration. They also incorporate signal-sharpening facilities that may evolve rapidly over time, potentially optimizing our capability for detecting the most critical features of a particular stimulus. The brain's capacity for receiving and processing somatosensory information in multiple modalities and dimensions is achieved through the linkage of a variety of highly specialized peripheral receptors to specific ascending neural pathways that maintain substantial segregation of different classes of sensation all the way to the cerebral cortex.

From a clinical point of view, understanding somesthetic systems is important for two reasons. First, although the sensory examination, because of its substantial subjective component, is less useful than the motor examination in identifying and localizing dysfunction within the nervous system, it can still help us in addressing specific hypotheses about localization generated by the history and the motor examination. Division I of this chapter will be devoted to delineating the principles that enable us to use the somatosensory examination as a means of interrogation of the nervous system.

Second, one component of somatosensory systems, that subserving nociception (pain sensation), is the substrate for one of the most common and distressing human experiences. No physician can escape the obligation to alleviate pain and the suffering that it entails. Division II of this chapter will focus on nociceptive systems and the principles underlying the means we have for manipulating these systems to the patient's benefit.

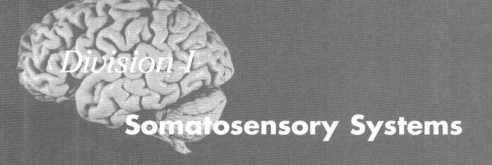

# Division I

# Somatosensory Systems

Meissners + Pacinian Corpuscles = Fast Adapting

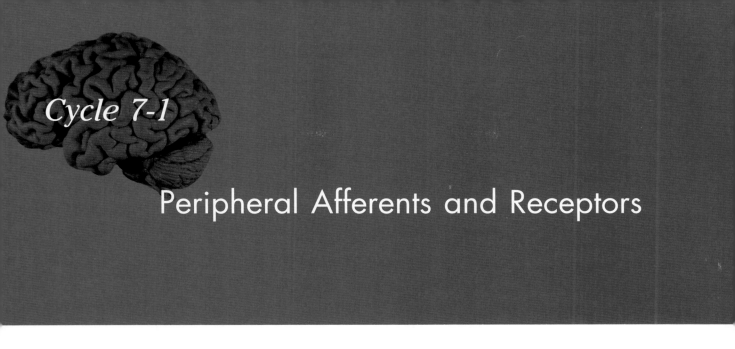

# Peripheral Afferents and Receptors

## Objective

Be able to describe the major somatosensory special receptors, the neural fiber sizes with which they are associated, and the types of sensation for which they are particularly important.

As for motor systems, it is convenient to begin our review of somatosensory systems at the bottom, in the periphery, and proceed centrally through the hierarchical organization. Table 7-1 summarizes the major peripheral somatosensory fiber systems.

## A. PROPRIOCEPTION

Proprioception is the physical sense of the position and movement of limbs in relation to each other and the body. Together with visual and vestibular input, proprioception provides the basis for our knowledge of the position of our bodies in space. Proprioception is provided primarily by the group Ia and II afferent fibers from muscles that play a major role in motor function. These systems achieve an extraordinary degree of precision, being able to detect changes in proximal joint angles of as little as 0.2 degree. In the chapter on motor systems, we noted that group Ia and II afferent input to reflex arcs plays a major role in proximal limb movement, but a much lesser role in distal limb and hand movements, which are almost exclusively the domain of the pyramidal system. There is evidence of a parallel organization of proprioceptive systems. Whereas group Ia and II afferent systems subserve proprioception in the proximal extremities, in the distal extremities, particularly the hands, this input is supplemented by input from Ruffini endings, which are bound to collagen fibrils in the skin and are responsive to skin stretch.

## B. MECHANORECEPTION

Mechanoreceptor systems underlie our various capacities for touch (Fig. 7-1). The specificity of each system for particular aspects of touch is conveyed by the mechanical properties of its respective receptors.

Two types of mechanoreceptors are located in the superficial dermis—Merkel disks and Meissner's corpuscles. Both respond to skin deformation in a tiny region in their immediate vicinity, and the density of both is particularly high in the fingers. Merkel disks are slowly adapting receptors (they tend to continue firing so long as a stimulus is applied). They are therefore well adapted to the sustained detection of skin deformation. This ability enables us not only to detect and precisely localize touch (and regions of maximal stimulation, such as edges of objects) but also to appreciate form and texture (Fig. 7-2). Meissner's corpuscles, in contrast, are rapidly adapting, responding briefly at the onset and offset of stimuli (Fig. 7-3). As a result, they

**TABLE 7-1** Major Peripheral Somatosensory Fiber Systems

| Sensory Modality | Receptor Type | Receptor | Fiber Size | Conduction Velocity (m/sec) | Functional Submodality |
|---|---|---|---|---|---|
| Proprioception | Muscle spindles | Type Ia | Aα | 70–120 | Velocity of muscle stretch |
| | Muscle spindles | Type II | Aβ | 40–70 | Muscle length |
| | Type II slowly adapting | Ruffini endings (deep and cutaneous) | Aβ | 40–70 | Joint angle in hands and feet |
| Mechanoreception | Type I slowly adapting | Merkel disk (cutaneous) | Aβ | 40–70 | Detection of skin pressure; sensation of form, texture |
| | Rapidly adapting | Meissner's corpuscles (cutaneous) | Aβ | 40–70 | Detection of flutter, motion, slippage |
| | Type II slowly adapting | Ruffini endings (cutaneous) | Aβ | 40–70 | Skin stretch |
| | Rapidly adapting | Pacinian corpuscle (deep) | Aβ | 40–70 | Vibration |
| Thermoreception | Warm | Bare nerve endings | C | 0.5–1 | Warmth |
| | Cold | Bare nerve endings | Aδ, C | 0.5–35 | Cold |
| Nociception | Mechanical, thermal | Bare nerve endings | Aδ | 10–35 | Sharp pain |
| | Polymodal | Bare nerve endings | C | 0.5–1 | Burning pain |

are particularly sensitive to dynamic aspects of skin stimuli. They appear to be responsible for the perception of stimulus movement along the skin. This sensibility assumes particular importance when it involves slippage of an object being gripped. We are acutely sensitive to slippage, and the sensation immediately and automatically elicits the increase in grip force needed to prevent further slippage.

Two types of mechanoreceptors are located in the deep dermis—Ruffini endings and Pacinian corpuscles. Both respond to tactile events involving large areas of the body surface. Ruffini endings, which are slowly adapting, are important in detecting skin stretch. They thereby contribute to sensation of objects moving across the skin that deform the skin, and to movements of fingers and toes that stretch the skin. They thus make a major contribution to proprioception in the hands and feet. Pacinian corpuscles are rapidly adapting (Fig. 7-4). They are exquisitely sensitive to even the faintest of vibratory stimuli.

Hairs are innervated by several specialized mechanoreceptors. Movements of individual hairs can be sensed.

## C. THERMORECEPTION

Our sensation of temperature is provided by two separate systems, one sensitive to a broad range of temperatures between 0° and 40°C, the other sensitive to a somewhat narrower range of temperatures between 30° and 50°C (Fig. 7-5). If these two systems produced an indefinitely sustained discharge in response to a given stimulus, they would together provide the basis for an ability to determine absolute temperatures within the range of 30° to 48°C. However, they adapt to maintained stimulation. For this reason, they endow considerable capacity for determining relative temperature and temperature changes, but very modest capability for determining absolute temperature. You will note in Figure 7-5

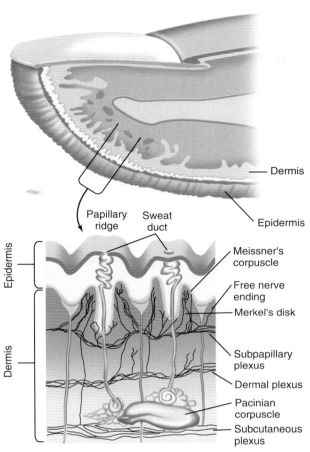

**Figure 7-1** Drawing of a transverse section of skin illustrating the positions of the various mechanoreceptors.

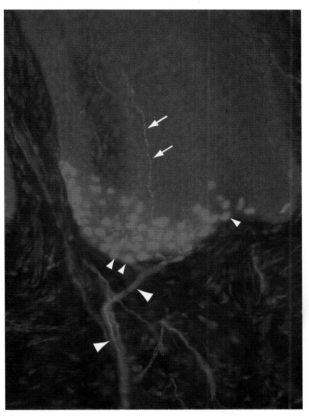

**Figure 7-2** A high magnification micrograph of human gum tissue, providing a closeup view of Merkel disks (*small arrowheads*), the large axon innervating these disks (*large arrowheads*), and an intraepithelial C fiber (*arrows*).

that the two curves cross at 37°C, body temperature, thus maximizing our capability for determining changes in temperature to higher or lower than body temperature. These basic properties can be demonstrated through a very simple experiment: if one submerges one hand in a bucket of ice water and the other in a bucket of hot water, and then subsequently plunges both hands into a bucket of lukewarm water, the tepid water will feel hot to the hand that was in ice water and cold to the hand that was in hot water.

## D. NOCICEPTION

### Two Peripheral Pain Systems

There are two general cutaneous and muscular peripheral pain systems:

1. Mechanical/thermal nociceptors respond to high-intensity stimuli, and rapidly transmit highly localized pain sensations to the central nervous system via lightly myelinated Aδ fibers.

2. Polymodal nociceptors respond to high-intensity mechanical stimuli, exogenous chemical stimuli, endogenous chemical stimuli (e.g., bradykinin, histamine), and thermal stimuli. They slowly transmit poorly localized pain sensations to the central nervous system via C (unmyelinated) fibers.

We all have had direct experience with the relative contribution of these two systems to pain. When we inadvertently cut ourselves, we immediately feel a highly localized, sharp pain, transmitted via the mechanical/thermal Aδ nociceptive system. As this sharp pain rapidly subsides, it is replaced by a long-lasting burning pain, transmitted via the polymodal C fiber nociceptive system.

*Somesthesis*

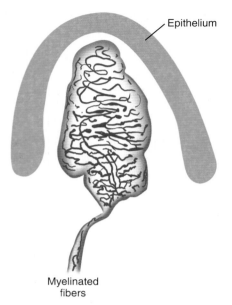

Epithelium

Myelinated
fibers

**Figure 7-3** A Meissner's corpuscle.

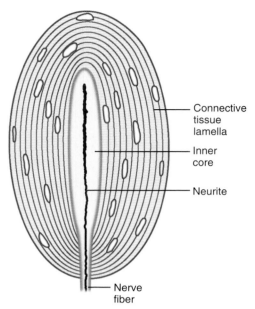

Connective
tissue
lamella

Inner
core

Neurite

Nerve
fiber

**Figure 7-4** A Pacinian corpuscle. The neurite, or nerve ending, is encased in a multilayered capsule of supporting cells and fluid. Because of the connective tissue lamellae, constant or low-frequency stimuli do not perturb the nerve ending within the inner core of the Pacinian corpuscle—they are damped. Only rapid vibration is transmitted. Thus, the connective tissue lamellae act as a high pass filter.

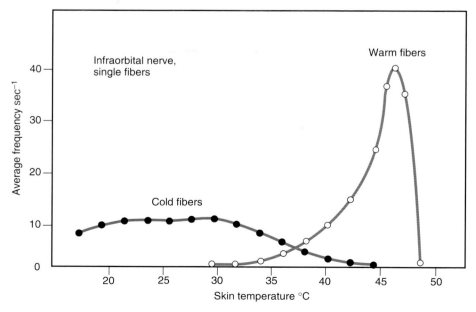

**Figure 7-5** Average responses of cold and warm fibers to different, sustained skin temperatures.

A third pain system subserves the viscera. These fibers are responsive to stretch or distention of the viscera, and to various chemical stimuli. For example, the abdominal pain associated with gastrointestinal infections is related to intestinal distention, and the chest pain associated with myocardial ischemia (angina) is related to the drop in pH in the heart muscle consequent to lactate production by anaerobic metabolism. Visceral nociception is transmitted to the central nervous system by both segmental dorsal root ganglion neurons and by the vagus nerve (CN X). Thus, patients with severe spinal cord damage are still capable of experiencing visceral pain.

## Referred Pain

Pain from any deep source may be referred to a distant location. For example, patients experiencing a heart attack often describe pain in the left arm. This mislocalization of pain reflects the convergence of visceral and somatic afferents onto the same dorsal horn neurons in the spinal cord[1] and the fact that "twigs" from a single nerve root may supply disparate regions of the body, as illustrated in Case 7-1.

---

[1]Convergence of different dorsal root ganglion neuronal projections onto a single dorsal horn neuron is the most common basis for referred pain. However, another mechanism sometimes accounts for referred pain of visceral origin. The nociceptive afferent fibers supplying viscera often have a second branch, which terminates in a somatic dermatome. This was demonstrated in a remarkably simple and elegant experiment in which uterine pain was induced in female rats after they were injected with Evan's blue dye. Evan's blue dye extravasates into areas of enhanced vascular permeability. Active polymodal nociceptive terminals release vasoactive substances such as substance P and calcitonin gene-related peptide (CGRP). In association with pain of uterine origin, Evan's blue dye was noted in the skin and muscle of the pelvis and thighs, clearly demonstrating activity of the somatic branch of the nociceptive fibers concurrent with the activation of the visceral branches.

### Case 7-1

**Referred Pain**

*A 65-year-old man presents with a history of several years of severe, aching low back pain radiating into both hips and down both legs. The pain in both the back and the legs is constant and unremitting. If the patient engages in any sustained exertion, he will suffer increased pain for hours. He denies any numbness or tingling in his legs. A magnetic resonance image (MRI) scan of the lumbar spine demonstrates extensive degenerative disease of the bones and joints but no significant disk herniation and no evidence of nerve root compression.*

**Comment:** *This patient stands in sharp contrast to the patient in Case 1-3, who experienced intermittent sharp, shooting pain, often in association with tingling and burning in one leg, in response to any activity that increased the pressure of a herniated disk fragment on a nerve root (coughing, sneezing, lifting). Case 1-3 described pain of neurogenic origin. The pain in this patient stems from degenerative disease (osteoarthritis) in spinal facet joints. Even though these facet joints are located immediately adjacent to the spinal canal, they are innervated by twigs of nerve roots that pass by them to portions of the legs. Nerve fibers supplying the legs and nerve fibers supplying the facet joints project to the same neurons in the spinal cord. Thus, facet joint pain is experienced as leg pain because it is referred to the legs. The fact that the pain tends to be sustained and that it is not associated with tingling or burning sensations helps to distinguish it from pain due to nerve root compression.*

Somesthesis

# Central Nervous System Somatosensory Pathways

1. Be able to list the sensory modalities subserved by the protopathic and epicritic systems, the properties of peripheral afferent fibers and central neural pathways required for transmission within these systems, and the types of neural fibers involved.

2. Know the functions of the dorsal root ganglia, their spatial relationship to the spinal canal and segmental levels of the spinal cord, and the neural basis for dermatomes.

3. Be able to describe the spinal segmental neural systems and the spinal cord and brainstem pathways subserving protopathic and epicritic sensation.

## A. TWO SENSORY SYSTEMS

The peripheral somatosensory modalities that we have discussed fall naturally into two major systems: (1) the *protopathic* system, which is critical to the well-being of the organism, and can suffice with poor spatial and temporal resolution, and (2) the *epicritic* system, which involves high spatial or temporal resolution, often both (see Table 7-2). The protopathic system, phylogenetically the oldest, involves the modalities of temperature and pain. The epicritic system involves the modalities of proprioception, discriminative touch, and vibration. Both systems are capable of determining the presence or absence of touch. The protopathic system can function with small, slowly conducting fibers that actually perform a service through their propensity for spatial and temporal dispersion, which acts to increase the

**TABLE 7-2** Protopathic and Epicritic Systems

| Feature | Protopathic | Epicritic |
|---|---|---|
| Sensory modalities | Temperature, pain, touch | Form, texture, touch, pressure, slippage, vibration, position |
| Spatial and temporal resolution | Low | High |
| Fiber type | Small, slowly conducting, lightly myelinated and unmyelinated | Large, rapidly conducting, myelinated |
| Ascending tract | Lateral spinothalamic tract | Dorsal and dorsolateral columns |

impact of peripheral input. The epicritic system requires large myelinated fibers capable of supporting the high spatial resolution needed for sensory precision and the high temporal resolution necessary for precise timing. Within the spinal cord, protopathic sensation is carried by the lateral spinothalamic tract, whereas epicritic sensation is carried by the dorsal and dorsolateral columns (to be discussed further).

Fibers subserving the epicritic and protopathic systems are blended within peripheral nerves and nerve roots. Despite this blending, the distinctive functional properties of these two systems can be put to good use, as illustrated in Case 7-2.

Peripheral protopathic and epicritic systems are also differentially affected by disease, as Cases 7-3 and 7-4 illustrate.

*Damage to protopathic*

## Case 7-2

### Local Anesthetics

*Local anesthetic drugs such as lidocaine (Xylocaine) and bupivicaine (Marcaine) are used routinely to achieve local anesthesia in dental procedures (see Case 5-5). They pass into axons via open voltage-sensitive sodium channels and bind preferentially to the inactivated conformation of these sodium channel proteins, thereby preventing the inward flow of sodium necessary for propagation of action potentials. Because the action potentials traveling along the smaller axons of neurons subserving protopathic modalities have a relatively longer duration (relative to those traveling along the larger fibers subserving epicritic modalities), more local anesthetic flows into these axons. Thus, although the degree of sensory loss (anesthesia) achieved with dental anesthesia is somewhat variable, blockade of transmission along protopathic axons (producing analgesia) is more easily and reliably achieved than the loss of epicritic sensations.*

*This principle is used to even greater advantage in treating postoperative pain. Patients who have undergone chest operations (thoracotomy) are at high risk for developing pneumonia, in part because their chest pain inhibits them from coughing. It is now relatively routine in these patients to administer a constant, slow infusion of local anesthetic into the upper thoracic spinal epidural space. Small nerve fibers in the nerve roots traversing this space are rendered completely dysfunctional, producing excellent analgesia. Large fibers continue to function relatively normally, interfering with sensation only to the extent of producing a light tingly feeling. Movement in the limbs is preserved, in part because of preservation of large fiber function, in part because cervical and lumbosacral roots are exposed to a lower concentration of anesthetic than are the thoracic roots.*

*Damage to epicritic*

## Case 7-3

### Vincristine Neurotoxicity

*A 35-year-old woman with Hodgkin's disease (a cancer involving lymphocytes) receives a multi-drug chemotherapy regimen that includes vincristine, a neurotoxic drug that interferes with microtubule function important for both axonal transport and maintenance of axonal structural integrity. It predominantly affects large peripheral nerve fibers subserving epicritic modalities. Her cancer goes into remission. However, she subsequently notes loss of feeling in her feet. Examination reveals altered sensation to the touch of the examiner's hands, extending halfway up the patient's legs and maximal loss of sensation in her feet. Vibratory sensation is absent in the great toes and reduced at the medial malleoli of the ankles. Position sense is markedly reduced in the great toes. Sensation of pinprick (pain) and temperature is relatively preserved, and her feet look normal. Ankle jerks are absent. Intrinsic foot musculature is atrophic.*

**Comment:** *Selective damage to large axons has permanently affected sensory fibers supporting epicritic modalities. Group Ia fibers are also damaged, hence the absent ankle jerks. Axons of α-motoneurons are damaged; hence, the atrophic foot musculature. Because longer axons make greater demands on their supporting neurons than do shorter axons, they are relatively more vulnerable to the effects of any toxin; hence the maximal involvement of the feet. Because unmyelinated fibers have relatively fewer microtubules and are relatively less dependent on microtubule function, they are spared, and protopathic sensory modalities remain substantially intact.*

**Somesthesis**

## Case 7-4

### Diabetic Polyneuropathy

*A 60-year-old man with a 15-year history of diabetes, now insulin-dependent, complains of burning sensations in his feet. On examination, there is loss of sensation for all sensory modalities in his feet and distal legs with gradual normalization of sensation as one moves proximally. His feet are red, there is no hair on them, and the skin is thin and atrophic. The skin blanches with sustained pressure, but it takes several seconds for the red color to return.*

**Comment:** *Diabetes causes damage to nerve fibers of all sizes. Thus, both* <u>epicritic and protopathic</u> *sensory modalities are involved. Therefore, in contrast to the patient in Case 7-3, this patient also has impairment of pain and temperature sensation in the feet. The pathology involves small, unmyelinated fibers of all types, including efferent autonomic fibers—hence, the loss of hair, thinning of the skin, and slowed capillary refill in the feet. In Division II in this chapter, we will consider the mechanisms underlying the burning pain in this patient's feet.*

*[handwritten margin note: Both epicritic and protopathic]*

## B. SENSORY ORGANIZATION AT THE SPINAL SEGMENTAL LEVEL

### The Dorsal Root Ganglion

All peripheral somatosensory fibers derive from cells in the dorsal root ganglia. The dorsal root ganglia are nestled in the fat within the bony neural foramina of the vertebral column (see Fig. 1-54, Case 1-3). Because spinal cord levels are progressively more rostral than vertebral levels as one descends the vertebral column (the spinal cord ends at about the L1 vertebral level) (see Fig. 1-49), there may be a considerable distance between a dorsal root ganglion and the point at which its projection actually enters the spinal cord. This is particularly the case in lumbosacral regions, where all the sensory fibers within the cauda equina are proximal to their respective dorsal root ganglia. Because the cell body of a neuron supplying a sensory axon within a peripheral nerve lies within the dorsal root ganglion, lesions of the nerve root or nerve distal to the dorsal root ganglion will interfere with the support provided by the cell body to the peripheral portion of the axon. Lesions proximal to the dorsal root ganglion will not

have this effect on the peripheral portion of the axon. This principle can be used to advantage in localizing injury within the peripheral nervous system, as illustrated in Case 7-5.

Neurons within the dorsal root ganglia have no dendrites. Rather, they produce an axon that bifurcates, sending one branch distally to end in one or more sensory receptors, and one branch proximally, to

## Case 7-5

### Lumbosacral Radiculopathy versus Plexopathy

*A 30-year-old man who has undergone orchiectomy and chemotherapy for testicular carcinoma develops pain radiating down his left leg in association with fluctuating paresthesias over the outer aspect of his left leg and the dorsum of his left foot. Examination reveals sensory impairment involving all modalities over the dorsum of the left foot. The patient's urologist is concerned that the patient may have metastatic cancer spreading along the lymph nodes of the lumbosacral retroperitoneum and invading the lumbosacral plexus. A neurologist performs a nerve conduction study of the superficial peroneal nerves, which are almost purely sensory nerves supplying the dorsum of the feet. The amplitude of the potential generated by peripheral electrical stimulation of the nerve is the same on the left as on the right. This finding indicates that the entire pathway from the left superficial peroneal nerve to its supporting dorsal root ganglion (including the portion passing through the lumbosacral plexus) must be intact. The neurologist suggests that the lesion must therefore be proximal to the dorsal root ganglion, possibly caused by a herniated disk, and not by infiltration of the lumbosacral plexus. He counsels a brief period of bed rest followed by a more prolonged period of restricted activity in which the patient refrains from anything that would increase vertical pressure on the spinal column. With this treatment, the patient's symptoms resolve.*

**Comment:** *Cancer infiltrating a nerve plexus is often very difficult to document, even with the best of imaging studies. Electrophysiologic studies can therefore be of great value. In this case, the administration of further courses of chemotherapy, with all their side effects, hinged on the diagnostic outcome.*

synapse in the spinal cord. The distal branch supplies a region of the body that is defined as the *receptive field* of that neuron. The receptive fields of individual, low-threshold, large-diameter, epicritic fibers are generally quite small, particularly in the hands. The receptive fields of individual, high-threshold, small-diameter, protopathic fibers are generally quite large. The receptive fields from all the neurons in one dorsal root ganglion define a *dermatome*, a region of the skin surface supplied by the neurons in that ganglion. The various dermatomes are illustrated in Figure 1-48. There is significant overlap between dermatomes, so that the extent of sensory loss produced by damage to a single nerve root or dorsal root ganglion will be considerably more circumscribed than the extent defined in dermatomal maps. For example, a patient with L5 root damage cause by a herniated disk or surgery to evacu-ate such a disk may have sensory loss limited to a patch on the upper, outer aspect of the leg and the dorsolateral margin of the foot, where there is relatively little overlap with innervation provided by the neighboring L4 and S1 nerve roots.

Sensory fibers in the cervical and lumbosacral regions, after emerging from the spinal canal as nerve roots, may coalesce, separate, and coalesce repeatedly with fibers from neighboring roots in their course through the brachial and lumbosacral plexuses, ultimately emerging in mixed nerves that include fibers destined for multiple dermatomes. Thus, the geographic areas supplied by sensory fibers in peripheral nerves in the arms and legs generally have very little correspondence to those supplied by nerve roots (dermatomes). This distinction may be important for localization and differential diagnosis, as seen in Case 7-6.

## Case 7-6

### C8 Radiculopathy versus Ulnar Neuropathy

*A 62-year-old man undergoes coronary artery bypass surgery in which the internal mammillary arteries, traveling beneath the anterior rib cage, are grafted to coronary vessels distal to sites of stenosis. When he awakes from surgery, he complains of weakness in his left hand and numbness of the medial portion of the hand (fourth and fifth fingers and hypothenar surface) and the medial left forearm. A neurologist examines the patient and suspects inadvertent intraoperative compression of the ulnar nerve in the ulnar groove at the elbow. Given today's operative standards, this would represent malpractice. However, she is bothered by the presence of numbness in the medial forearm, weakness in the flexors of the fourth and fifth fingers, and weakness of both wrist flexion and extension when the hand is adducted at the wrist (i.e., displaced medially as the patient lies on his back with his arm at his side, palm up). After some research, the neurologist concludes that there was no malpractice.*

**Comment:** *Damage to the ulnar nerve in the ulnar groove produces sensory loss and motor impairment in a peripheral nerve distribution. The sensory loss includes the fifth finger, the medial aspect of the fourth finger, and the medial portion of the hand extending to the wrist and not beyond. Weakness includes the interossei (the finger spreaders), the adductor pollicis (the muscle in the webspace of the thumb that adducts the thumb) and occasionally, the flexor carpi ulnaris, which flexes the wrist when the wrist is in the adducted position. The patient described has considerably more extensive sensory and motor impairment, which is incompatible with an ulnar nerve lesion at the elbow. The answer to this conundrum lies in the fact that internal mammillary to coronary artery grafts require particularly wide spreading of the rib cage during thoracotomy. Sometimes, unavoidably, the first rib dislocates at its articulation with the lateral vertebral process. The proximal, dislocated end of the rib may then press against the C8 nerve root, producing a C8 radiculopathy. The result is that the patient has sensory loss involving the C8 dermatome, which includes both the medial hand and the medial forearm. He also has weakness of all C8-innervated muscles in the upper extremity, including those supplied by the ulnar nerve (interossei, adductor pollicis, flexor carpi ulnaris, and ulnar portion of the flexor digitorum profundus, which flexes the distal phalanx of the fourth and fifth fingers) and those supplied by the radial nerve (extensor carpi ulnaris, which extends the adducted wrist). Thus, in this case, the clinical distinction between a root and a peripheral nerve injury was a crucial one.*

Somesthesis

## The Spinal Cord Segment

As soon as somatosensory fibers enter the spinal cord, protopathic and epicritic systems become, to a large degree, spatially segregated.

*Protopathic sensory fibers* terminate primarily on neurons within the most dorsal, superficial regions of the dorsal horn, often referred to as Rexed's lamina I and II (Fig. 7-6A). Within this region, innumerable suc-

cessive and parallel synapses occur in a complex neural network. Segmental networks within lamina I and II are linked to networks in adjacent spinal cord segments via propriospinal fibers (short ascending and descending pathways within the spinal cord) located in Lissauer's tract at the dorsal-most margin of the dorsal horn. Neural impulses entering the dorsal horn along the lightly myelinated (Aδ) and unmyelinated (C) peripheral fibers of the protopathic system encounter further

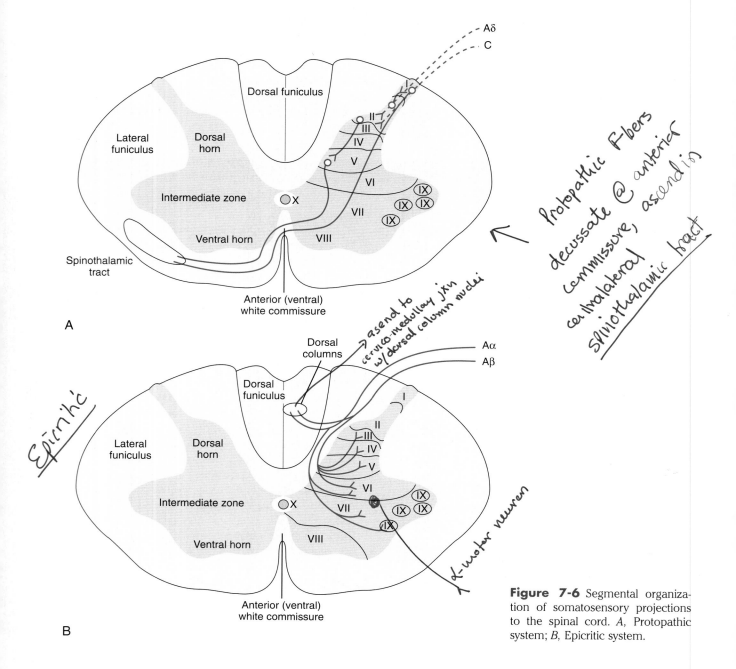

Figure 7-6 Segmental organization of somatosensory projections to the spinal cord. *A,* Protopathic system; *B,* Epicritic system.

transmission delays as they travel through the networks of the dorsal horn. Eventually, activation of neurons in lamina I and deeper lamina of the dorsal horn generates impulses in axons that cross the spinal cord in the *anterior commissure* near the central canal (not to be confused with the anterior commissure of the cerebrum) to the contralateral ventrolateral region of the white matter of the spinal cord. These axons ascend all the way to the brainstem and thalamus as the *lateral spinothalamic tract*. This anatomic organization, in which protopathic fiber pathways cross the spinal cord within one or two spinal levels of the point of entry of peripheral input, renders them particularly vulnerable to certain types of injury, as Case 7-7 illustrates.

## Case 7-7

### Lumbar Central Cord Syndrome

*A 35-year-old woman presents with the chief complaint of numbness that has developed over the outer aspects of her thighs over the past month. On examination, she has sensory loss confined to an L2 distribution over the outer aspect of each thigh that maximally involves pain and temperature sensation (see Fig. 1-48A). She also has mild weakness of hip flexors, hyperactive knee and ankle jerks, and bilateral Babinski signs.*

**Comment:** *The fact that this patient has bilateral, symmetric sensory loss in the absence of polyneuropathy suggests a spinal cord lesion. This impression is confirmed by the presence of signs of damage to descending spinal cord motor pathways. She actually has a highly unusual central disk herniation at the T11-T12 level (most low back disk herniations occur at the L4-L5 and L5-S1 levels). This herniated disk compresses the spinal cord at the L2 level (recall the mismatch between spinal cord and vertebral body levels—[Fig. 1-49]). At some time, perhaps the occasion of the disk herniation, the trauma to the cord produced a small hemorrhage within the center of the cord (hematomyelia). As the hemorrhage resolved, a small cavity or syrinx was left in its place. This cavity, over time, has enlarged, something observed quite commonly in this situation. With enlargement, the cavity has particularly damaged the fibers of the protopathic system crossing in the anterior commissure of the cord. This damage produces abnormalities of pain and temperature sensation confined to the dermatomes corresponding*

## Case 7-7—cont'd

*to cord segments actually involved by the cavity. Cord segments below this level are spared because the ascending sensory tracts are spared. The cord compression or the syrinx has also produced subtle damage of descending lateral and ventral motor pathways, hence the hyper-reflexia and Babinski signs, and the mild proximal lower extremity weakness.*

All *epicritic sensory fibers* enter the ipsilateral dorsal column of the spinal cord (Fig. 7-6B). From there, they follow one of two major trajectories. Some immediately enter the dorsal horn, send collaterals into ventral regions of the dorsal horn (subserving segmental proprioception), and ultimately terminate on or in the vicinity of α-motoneurons in the ventral horn (subserving motor functions). Others, with or without immediate collateral projections to the dorsal horn, travel rostrally in the ipsilateral dorsal column all the way to the dorsal column nuclei at the cervicomedullary junction. In addition, there are neurons within the dorsal horn itself that receive epicritic fiber synapses and project via the ipsilateral dorsolateral column to the dorsal column nuclei. *Note that within the spinal cord, fibers of the protopathic system are crossed (travel contralateral to the side of the body they represent), whereas those of the epicritic system are uncrossed.*

## C. ASCENDING SOMATOSENSORY SYSTEMS

In the protopathic system, axons course rostrally in the lateral spinothalamic tract and eventually terminate in one of three locations: (1) the *medullary, pontine, and midbrain reticular formations*, (2) the *periaqueductal gray matter*, and (3) the *ventral posterolateral nucleus* (VPL) of the thalamus. Projections to the brainstem reticular formation account for the arousing effect of painful stimuli and for the impact of pain on muscle tone. Projections to the periaqueductal gray provide, in part, the basis for central nervous system regulation of ascending nociceptive transmission (see Division II, Pain). Projections to the ventral posterolateral nucleus of the thalamus and thence to the cortex subserve localization of pain and qualitative and quantitative analysis of protopathic information.

Somesthesis

Spinal fibers representing the epicritic system travel rostrally within the dorsal columns all the way to the cervicomedullary junction, where they synapse on neurons within one of the dorsal column nuclei. Fibers derived from cord segments below spinal cord level T6 travel in the medial portion of the dorsal columns, in the *gracile fasciculus* (Fig. 7-7), and terminate on the medially located *nucleus gracilis* (Fig. 7-8). Fibers derived from upper thoracic levels and the cervical regions travel in the adjacent, more lateral *cuneate fasciculus*, and terminate on the *nucleus cuneatus*. The somatotopic representation of the body in the dorsal columns—arms lateral, legs medial—is peculiar and characterizes only three other structures within the central nervous system, the cerebral motor and primary sensory homunculi in the pre- and postcentral gyri, respectively, and the cerebellar hemispheres. In all other nuclear and tract systems, the legs are represented laterally and the arms medially.

Neurons within the nucleus gracilis and nucleus cuneatus send their axons across the caudal brainstem in the sensory decussation to the contralateral *medial lemniscus* (Fig. 7-9). Thus, above the sensory decussation, both epicritic and protopathic pathways represent the contralateral side of the body. Epicritic fibers ascend in the medial lemniscus, eventually to terminate in the *ventral posterolateral nucleus* (VPL) of the thalamus. Within the most caudal portions of the medial lemniscus, leg fibers travel ventrally and arm fibers dorsally. As the medial lemniscus moves laterally and simultaneously rotates into a mediolateral orientation in the caudal pons, the leg fibers assume a lateral position (the typical somatotopic organization for nuclei and fiber tracts).

Focal lesions of the peripheral nerves produce patterns of sensory loss corresponding to the somatic distribution of the nerves injured. Focal lesions of ascending spinal cord pathways produce sensory loss extending to all portions of the body from some level below the injury. The finding of a sensory level strongly suggests the presence of a spinal cord lesion (Case 7-8).

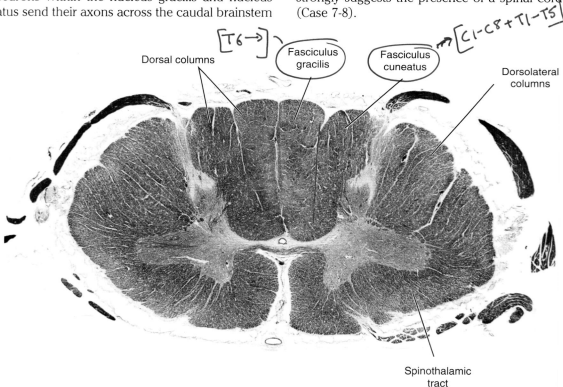

**Figure 7-7** Transverse section of the cervical spinal cord, illustrating the fasciculus gracilis, the fasciculus cuneatus, the dorsolateral columns, and the lateral spinothalamic tract.

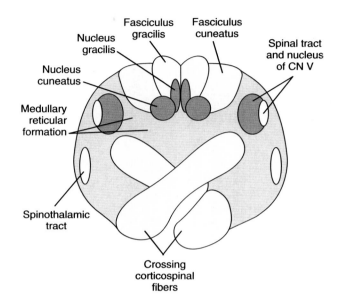

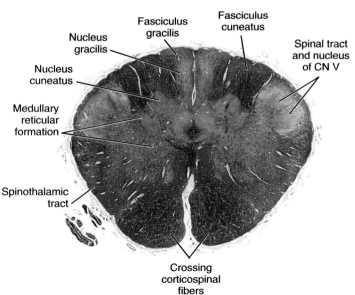

**Figure 7-8** Transverse section of the spinal cord at the cervicomedullary junction (the level of the pyramidal decussation), illustrating the nucleus gracilis, the nucleus cuneatus, and the lateral spinothalamic tract.

Somesthesis

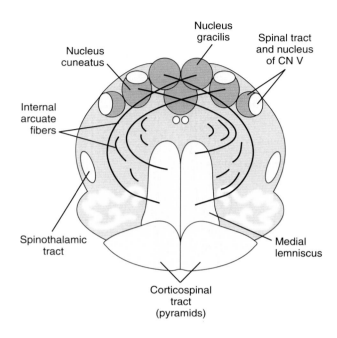

Nucleus
gracilis

Nucleus
cuneatus

Spinal tract
and nucleus
of CN V

Internal
arcuate
fibers

Spinothalamic
tract

Medial
lemniscus

Corticospinal
tract
(pyramids)

*Sensory Fibers ~~which~~ (Epicritic) terminate in N. gracilis and N. cuneatus.*

*Then decussate in medial lemniscus*

*[Protopathic fibers cross in the s.c. itself]*

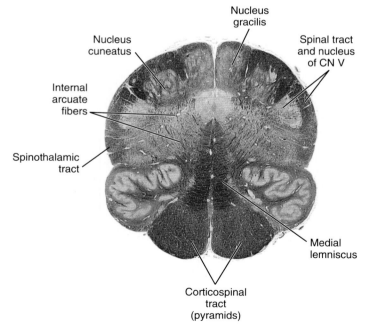

Nucleus
cuneatus

Nucleus
gracilis

Internal
arcuate
fibers

Spinal tract
and nucleus
of CN V

Spinothalamic
tract

Medial
lemniscus

Corticospinal
tract
(pyramids)

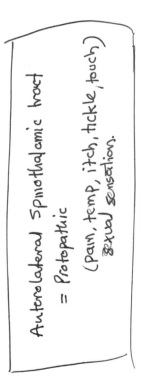

*Anterolateral Spinothalamic tract = Protopathic (pain, temp, itch, tickle, touch) Sexual sensation.*

**Figure 7-9** Transverse section of the brainstem illustrating the sensory decussation.

## Case 7-8

### Cervical Myelopathy and Sensory Level

*A 40-year-old policeman presents with the chief complaint of progressive difficulty walking and urinary urgency. On examination, he has mild weakness of his hip flexors. Biceps and brachioradialis reflexes cannot be elicited, but triceps and finger flexor reflexes, knee jerks, and ankle jerks are 3 to 4. He has bilateral Babinski signs. His gait is narrow-based and spastic. He has diminished pain and temperature sensation bilaterally below the L1 dermatomal level.*

**Comment:** *The reflex abnormalities clearly point to a spinal cord lesion at the C5–C6 level (loss of C5–C6 reflexes, hyperactive C7, C8, L2, L3, L4, and S1 deep tendon reflexes). Both the sensory level and the Babinski signs also point to a spinal cord lesion. This patient has a congenitally narrow cervical spinal canal compounded by a centrally herniated C5–C6 disk. The disk herniation in the context of a narrow canal results in significant cord compression.*

*In this case, the motor signs were so clear-cut that they left little doubt about the presence of a spinal cord lesion (myelopathy), and the precise localization of the lesion. The presence of the sensory level was thus of little clinical value. However, in some patients the motor signs are confusing and the presence of a sensory level is crucial in identifying a spinal cord lesion. Consider,*

*for example, if the patient were diabetic and had generalized hyporeflexia due to polyneuropathy, and furthermore, his plantar reflexes were either equivocal or unobtainable (because of weakness of the extensor hallucis longus due to polyneuropathy). In such a case, a sensory level might be the only clue to the existence of a cord lesion.*

*You may be curious as to why the patient in this case had an L1 sensory level in the presence of a C6 cord lesion. This phenomenon reflects a general rule of sensory levels—they indicate only that a lesion exists somewhere higher in the cord, not the precise level of the lesion. Presumably, this reflects the fact that vascular injury is responsible for a significant portion of the damage produced by spinal cord compression. Spinal cord compression in the anteroposterior direction particularly compresses transverse branches of the anterior spinal artery. This compression results in infarction in the territory of branches of the anterior spinal artery supplying the core of the spinal cord (Fig. 7-10). If this damage implicates the entire spinothalamic tract, then the sensory level will be at the level of the lesion. If this damage spares the most medial portions of the spinothalamic tract (subserving upper extremities and thoracic levels in Case 7-8), then the sensory level may be lower, perhaps at L1.*

---

## BOX 7-1 The Epicritic/Protopathic Distinction

The epicritic/protopathic distinction we have drawn in this chapter, a conceptualization that originated with the British neurologist Henry Head early in the 20th century, represents somewhat of an oversimplification, albeit a clinically useful one. The ways in which this simplification breaks down provide a topic of considerable interest. It is clear that the senses of touch and limb movement are conveyed by both epicritic and protopathic pathways, and will not be eliminated by lesions of just one type of pathway. The fact that most patients who have undergone surgical destruction of the lateral spinothalamic tract to eliminate chronic pain eventually redevelop pain raises the possibility of alternative pain transmission pathways. For example, nociceptive and possibly other afferents from the viscera have been shown to travel in

the ventral portions of the dorsal columns. This finding explains the analgesic effectiveness of an old operation, midline myelotomy (cutting the medial portions of the dorsal columns), once used in patients with intractable visceral pain (e.g., due to cancer).

It has been discovered relatively recently that both the dorsal and the dorsolateral columns support vibratory and position sense and two-point discrimination, but only the dorsal columns have the very large fibers and secure synapses necessary for the temporal precision and high resolution necessary to support precise hand movements and tactile directional sensitivity. Indeed, the neurologic deficits seen with pure dorsal column lesions resemble those seen with pyramidal tract lesions.

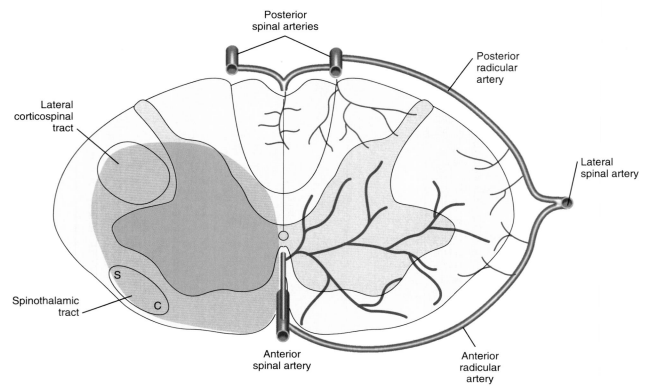

**Figure 7-10** Cross section of the spinal cord at the C5 level. The branches of the anterior spinal artery supplying the core of the spinal cord are illustrated on the right. Repeated anterior-posterior compression of the cord compresses these branches, resulting in the pattern of infarction shown on the left. The somatotopic organization of the lateral spinothalamic tract is also indicated on the left (S, sacral; C, cervical).

Figure 7-11*A* through *D* demonstrates the ascending somatosensory systems through their entire extent.

Thalamocortical relay neurons in the ventral posterolateral nucleus of the thalamus project, via the posterior limb of the internal capsule and the corona radiata, to Brodmann's *areas 3, 1, and 2 in the postcentral gyrus of the cerebral cortex* (in aggregate, SI), and to the secondary somatosensory area, SII (Fig. 7-13). Although protopathic and epicritic systems travel to common destinations within the thalamus and the cerebral cortex, they remain locally segregated, as do representations of the different somatosensory modalities within these systems. This preserves the capability for cerebral responses that are specific to information in a given sensory modality. As the output of thalamocortical neurons is a linear function of their input, and there is modest convergence and divergence of input to thalamocortical neurons, these neurons reliably relay their input to the cerebral cortex with minimal change. Recall from Chapter 1, Cycle 1-8, that this relay is gated by nucleus reticularis, the envelope-like layer of cells

surrounding the thalamus. Nucleus reticularis is, in turn, regulated by the midbrain reticular formation, ascending noradrenergic and serotonergic pathways, the prefrontal cortex, and overlying temporoparietal cortices. Nucleus reticularis, by regulating thalamocortical transmission, provides one of many mechanisms by which portions of the cerebral cortex are selectively engaged in a particular task (see Chapter 12). When the nucleus reticularis gates selected sensory information to the cerebral cortex, it defines the particular source of sensory input that the brain focuses on, so it provides a mechanism for focusing attention. In humans, unlike more primitive mammals, this particular mechanism has little impact on visual attention and only some impact on auditory attention; however, it still appears to have a substantial impact on somatosensory attention.

A precise somatotopic organization is preserved throughout sensory systems. Within the cerebral cortex, as in motor systems, the cortical extent devoted to specific body regions reflects the relative functional

*Text continued on p. 332*

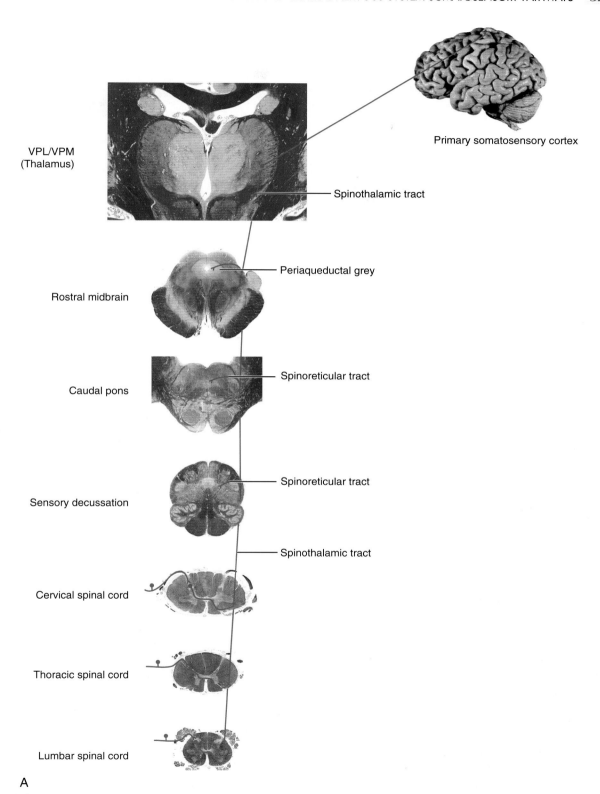

Primary somatosensory cortex

VPL/VPM
(Thalamus)

Spinothalamic tract

Rostral midbrain

Periaqueductal grey

Caudal pons

Spinoreticular tract

Sensory decussation

Spinoreticular tract

Spinothalamic tract

Cervical spinal cord

Thoracic spinal cord

Lumbar spinal cord

A

**Figure 7-11** *A* and *B,* Ascending protopathic system. VPL, ventral posterolateral nucleus; VPM, ventral posteromedial nucleus. *C* and *D,* Ascending epicritic system. The stick figures in *C* and *D* illustrate the somatotopic organization of the epicritic system.                                                       *Continued*

**Somesthesis**

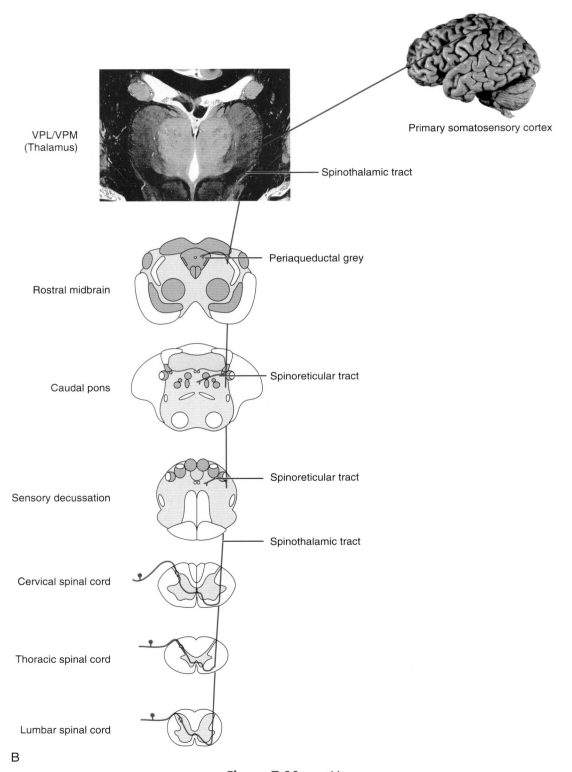

VPL/VPM
(Thalamus)

Primary somatosensory cortex

Spinothalamic tract

Rostral midbrain

Periaqueductal grey

Caudal pons

Spinoreticular tract

Sensory decussation

Spinoreticular tract

Spinothalamic tract

Cervical spinal cord

Thoracic spinal cord

Lumbar spinal cord

B

**Figure 7-11**, cont'd

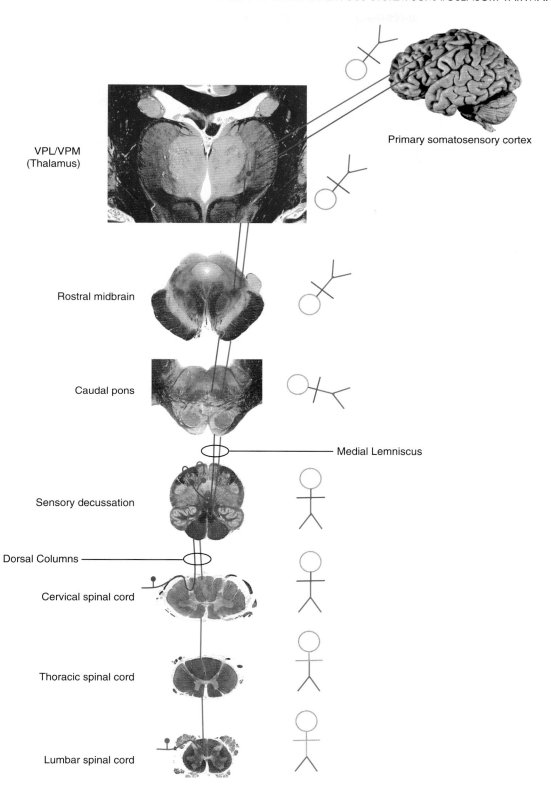

Primary somatosensory cortex

VPL/VPM
(Thalamus)

Rostral midbrain

Caudal pons

Medial Lemniscus

Sensory decussation

Dorsal Columns

Cervical spinal cord

Thoracic spinal cord

Lumbar spinal cord

**Figure 7-11**, cont'd

Somesthesis

Continued

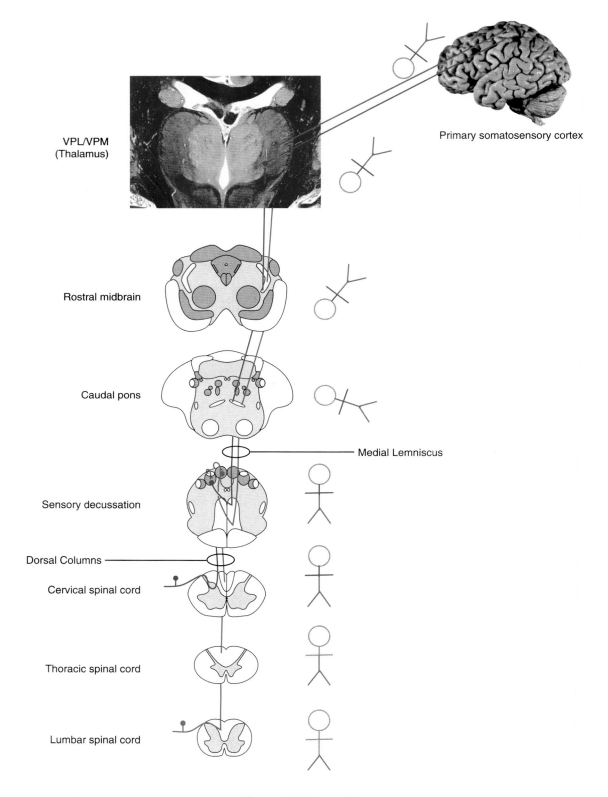

VPL/VPM
(Thalamus)

Primary somatosensory cortex

Rostral midbrain

Caudal pons

Medial Lemniscus

Sensory decussation

Dorsal Columns

Cervical spinal cord

Thoracic spinal cord

Lumbar spinal cord

**Figure 7-11**, cont'd

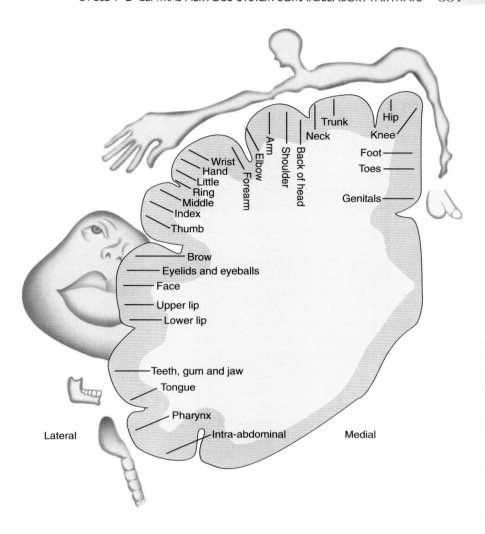

**Figure 7-12** The sensory homunculus.

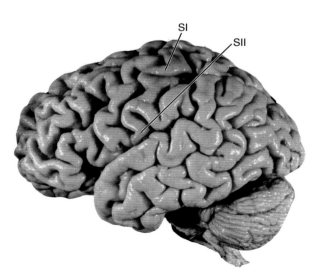

**Figure 7-13** First (SI) and second (SII) somatosensory areas of the cerebral cortex.

Somesthesis

importance of these regions; thus, the sensory homunculus is every bit as distorted as the motor homunculus (Fig. 7-12).

## PRACTICE 7-2

**A.** Return to Practice 6-4D (Spinal Cord Syrinx). Predict the pattern of sensory loss.

**B.** Return to Practice 6-6B. Assume that the knife injury has completely transected the right half of the spinal cord. Predict the pattern of sensory loss one would find.

**C.** A 40-year-old man has pernicious anemia caused by an inherited defect in the synthesis of intrinsic factor in the stomach. Intrinsic factor is needed for adequate absorption of vitamin $B_{12}$. Vitamin $B_{12}$ deficiency causes anemia as well as demyelination in both the central and peripheral nervous systems. The central nervous system demyelination predominantly involves the dorsal columns and the lateral motor tracts. Predict the neurologic abnormalities one would find on examination.

**D.** A 70-year-old woman with longstanding hypertension, diabetes, and a lifelong history of smoking one pack per day suddenly develops sensory loss over the entire right side of her body. All sensory modalities are affected. Arm and leg are equally involved. Her examination is noteworthy for the absence of all the follow-ing: weakness, impairment in fine motor movement in her right hand, upper extremity drift, language impairment, reflex asymmetry, and Babinski signs. Localize the lesion.

**E.** An 80-year-old man with a long history of hypertension, hypercholesterolemia, and heavy smoking suddenly develops paraparesis. On examination, he has no motor function in his legs. Vibratory and position senses are normal, but pain and temperature sensations are severely impaired from the T6 level down. His bladder is severely distended. Localize the lesion. The sudden onset of the neurologic deficit suggests a vascular event. What blood vessel is implicated?

**F.** Indicate whether impairment in each of the following sensory functions assessed in the sensory neurologic examination is seen with lesions of the protopathic system, the epicritic system, neither, or both.

Ability to distinguish cutaneous stimulation at one
    point from stimulation at two points (two-point
    discrimination)
Pain sensation ("pinprick")
Temperature
Vibration
Limb position
Simple touch:
    Detection
    Alteration of subjective experience

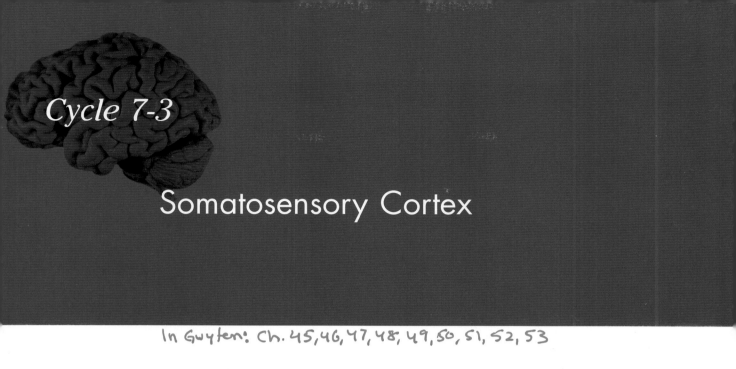

# Cycle 7-3

# Somatosensory Cortex

*In Guyton: Ch. 45, 46, 47, 48, 49, 50, 51, 52, 53*

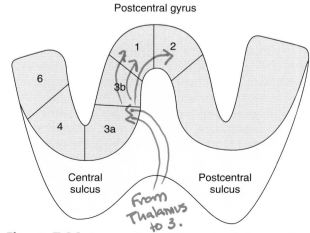

## Objectives

1. Be able to identify the primary somatosensory cortex and related somatosensory association cortex.

2. Be aware of the specialization of different subregions of primary somatosensory cortex.

3. Be able to describe and give two examples of what is meant by plasticity of somatosensory cortices.

4. Be able to define graphesthesia and explain its localizing importance.

The somatosensory cortex includes two separate regions that receive input from the somatosensory thalamus. One, SI, occupies nearly all the postcentral gyrus. The second, SII, occupies a small area abutting the sylvian fissure and adjacent to the most ventral portion of the postcentral gyrus (Fig. 7-13).

## FIRST SOMATOSENSORY AREA  57

The first somatosensory area (SI) is further divided into cytoarchitectonically distinct regions, each of which is engaged in processing specific types of somatosensory information (Fig. 7-14). Thus, the broad spectrum of somatosensory information that was captured in the periphery through various specially adapted receptors,

and temporarily obscured in the ascending somatosensory pathways and the thalamus, is again manifested in its fully differentiated form in the postcentral gyrus (Table 7-3).

Brodmann's area 3 can be viewed as the cortical receiving area for thalamic projections, 3a for muscle and nociceptive afferents, and 3b for non-nociceptive cutaneous afferents. The subdivisions of area 3 then project to Brodmann's areas 1 and 2, which subserve further specialization of function.

Within area 3b, the cortex is further subdivided into a mosaic of tiny abutting patches of cortex, some

Postcentral gyrus

**Figure 7-14** Cross section of the postcentral gyrus illustrating the cytoarchitectonic organization.

333

**TABLE 7-3** Cytoarchitectonic and Functional Subdivisions of the First Somatosensory Area (SI)

| Brodmann's Area | Sensory Afferents | Function |
|---|---|---|
| 3a | Muscle and nociceptive (cutaneous and possibly visceral) afferents via the thalamus | Proprioception<br>Pain |
| 3b | Slowly and rapidly adapting cutaneous input via the thalamus | Tactile perception (shape, size, texture)<br>Vibratory sensation<br>Thermal sensation |
| 1 | Slowly and rapidly adapting cutaneous input from area 3b | Texture perception |
| 2 | Cutaneous input from area 3b and nociceptive and muscle input from area 3a | Position and edge detection, size perception, 3-dimensional shape perception (stereognosis)<br>Pain |

specialized for vibratory sensation, others for touch, still others for thermal discrimination. These areas are remarkably fluid, showing rapid changes in extent and topography according to the demands of tasks in which the individual is routinely engaged.

The neuronal systems of the postcentral gyrus also display considerable fluidity in their somatotopic organization. This is reflected in two ways: the skin of the fingers is normally divided into dozens of tiny cortical receptive fields, each a few millimeters across, each subserved by a column of cells in somatosensory cortex. Normally the receptive fields of fingers are dominated by input from a single digit, reflecting the substantially independent sensations the fingers experience in their independent movements. However, if two fingers are experimentally bound together, so that they move as one, new receptive fields soon appear that are dominated by input from both fingers, showing that somatosensory cortex now treats the two fingers as one.

Until the 1980s, it was thought that the sensory homunculus in an adult is largely immutable. However, experiments performed by a number of investigators have proved otherwise. In one such experiment, all the cervical dorsal roots were severed on one side in adult monkeys. According to the old way of thinking, this would have left the enormous extent of the postcentral gyrus representing the hand and arm deafferented and silent. However, to everyone's surprise, cortex originally devoted to hand and arm evolved to represent the lower face. Thus, eventually, the entire postcentral gyrus was once again actively engaged in somatosensory processing. From this and other experiments, it appears that somatosensory cortex is just as plastic as

motor cortex in its ability to adapt to environmental and behavioral demands and constraints.

# SECOND SOMATOSENSORY AREA

The second somatosensory area, SII, receives direct projections from the thalamus and has extensive reciprocal connections with all portions of SI. It appears to be primarily involved in shape and texture discrimination. Unlike SI, the two SIIs are heavily linked to each other by transcallosal connections. This link potentially provides the basis for bimanual coordination, bihemispheric transmission of unilateral sensory input, and rapid transfer of acquired tactile skills, such as tactile discrimination, from one hand to the other. It also provides the basis for a unified somatosensory representation of the entire body surface. Finally, it may provide, in part, the substrate for graphesthesia, the ability to identify numbers traced on the body surface. Because the afferent input underlying graphesthesia ascends to the brain via the dorsal columns, graphesthesia could be viewed as a test of dorsal column function. However, the ability to translate this information into number representations is a uniquely cortical function. Therefore, testing of graphesthesia is most often clinically useful as a means of detecting cortical lesions, as Case 7-9 illustrates.

Both Brodmann's areas 5 and 7 receive somatosensory projections from area 2, and caudal portions of area 7 (7a) receive projections from visual association cortices (see Fig. 6-15). Both area 5 and rostral area 7 (7b) project heavily to precentral motor areas, providing a basis for sensorimotor integration. For this reason,

## Case 7-9

### Middle Cerebral Artery Distribution Stroke

*A 68-year-old left-handed woman suddenly develops moderate weakness and incoordination of the right hand. Her language is completely normal. However, graphesthesia is impaired in the right palm relative to the left. A magnetic resonance imaging (MRI) study of the brain is normal. A magnetic resonance angiogram (MRA) reveals 80 percent stenosis of the left internal carotid artery. The patient is referred for carotid endarterectomy.*

**Comment:** *In patients with stroke, it is crucial to distinguish between large vessel and small vessel (lacunar) infarcts. Large vessel infarcts are caused by embolism or propagation of clot from unstable atheromatous lesions (e.g., in the proximal internal carotid artery) or the heart. Lacunar infarcts are caused by intrinsic disease of small brain vessels. Large vessel infarcts usually damage the cerebral cortex and therefore are associated with deficits in neural functions uniquely subserved by the cortex. Language, graphesthesia, and stereognosis (the ability to identify objects from the tactile experience of their three-dimensional shape) are three such uniquely cortical functions. In the patient described,*

*the absence of language impairment is of uncertain significance because she is left-handed, and therefore may have substantial right hemisphere language function. That is, the absence of language impairment does not rule out a cortical injury. Stereognosis requires the motor function necessary to manually explore the object—a function that this patient has lost. The MRI scan was normal, as it is in many patients with stroke, particularly those with modest deficits. Thus, the impairment in graphesthesia was the only sign that the patient had a cortical lesion. The impairment in graphesthesia suggested that the left internal carotid artery stenosis was probably symptomatic, and that the patient's likelihood of having another, perhaps even larger stroke, was greater than 40 percent. Thus, carotid endarterectomy to remove the necrotic, thrombotic atheromatous lesion in the neck was strongly indicated. The precise cerebral substrate for graphesthesia is uncertain. It could include areas SII and Brodmann's area 5, because these regions are commonly involved by middle cerebral artery distribution strokes.*

parietal lesions (whether of the postcentral gyrus, area 5, or both is uncertain) may so disrupt sensorimotor integration as to produce disorders resembling those stemming from motor system lesions (Case 7-10).

As we shall see in Chapter 12, on higher neural functions, area 7 appears to provide the basis for aligning our body-centered spatial coordinate system with the environmentally defined spatial coordinate system, on the basis of somatosensory and visual inputs, which converge on this cortical area.

Somesthesis

*[handwritten annotation:]* Graphesthesia → test for dorsal columns, but mainly cortical lesions

*[handwritten diagram:]* → Thalamus → Area 3a, 3b → Area 1, Area 2 → { Visual Association cortices } → Area 5, Area 7 ← → Motor Cortex (∴ sensorimotor coordination)

## Case 7-10

### Middle Cerebral Artery Distribution Stroke

*A 72-year-old man suddenly develops incoordination of the right arm and some difficulty speaking as a result of a left middle cerebral artery distribution stroke. Strength in his right arm is normal. When asked to close his eyes and extend his arms in front of him in a supinated position, the right arm tends to slowly drift up—a "parietal drift." He also exhibits nearly continuous, uncontrollable, wormlike movements of the fingers, a phenomenon referred to as pseudoathetosis. When he is asked, while his arms are still extended and eyes closed, to touch his right index finger to his chin, he can barely get his hand to his face and his arm movements are very clumsy. When allowed to open his eyes (permitting visual guidance of the movement) he fairly accurately touches his chin with only modest incoordination.*

**Comment:** *The mechanism of parietal drift is uncertain. However, it is not the same as the mechanism underlying the much more commonly observed pronation drift, seen with lesions of motor pathways, which represents incipient decorticate posturing. The term "pseudoathetosis" derives from the fact that although the movements look very much like those seen with basal ganglia lesions (see Case 6-15), they actually reflect loss of cortical sensory input to motor cortices. He can perform a finger-to-chin maneuver reasonably well when he can rely on visual guidance, but when he has to depend on proprioceptive input alone, he is very inaccurate, and his movements very much resemble the ataxia that results from lesions of the cerebellar hemispheres. Disruption of parietopontocerebellar pathways may contribute to this "pseudoataxia."*

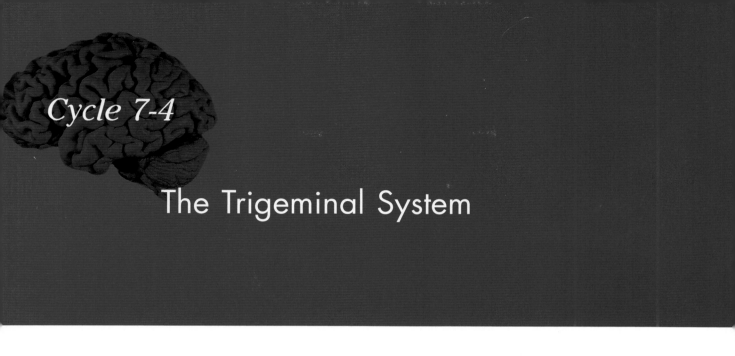

# Cycle 7-4

# The Trigeminal System

## Objectives

1. Be able to describe the peripheral trajectories and regions of the face and head supplied by the three trigeminal branches.

2. Be able to describe the three major brainstem trigeminal nuclei, locate them on axial sections, describe their major functions, and describe their projections to the thalamus.

3. Be able to explain the mechanism of headache in patients with intracranial structural or inflammatory processes.

The trigeminal nerves subserve somesthesis for the face. The various components of the trigeminal system almost exactly parallel somatosensory systems subserving the body.

The cell bodies of all three divisions of the trigeminal nerve are located in the floor of the cavernous sinus in the gasserian (trigeminal) ganglion, effectively the dorsal root ganglion of the trigeminal nerve. The first or ophthalmic division of the trigeminal nerve (V1) supplies the forehead from the eyebrows to well behind the hairline, and the eyes, including the corneas (Fig. 7-15). V1 fibers enter the cavernous sinus via the superior orbital fissure of the skull, immediately behind the orbits. The second or maxillary division of the trigeminal nerve (V2) supplies the central regions of the face, including the nose (inside and out), upper lip,

cheeks, and spatially adjacent regions inside the mouth. V2 enters the cranial vault via the foramen rotundum. The third or mandibular division of the trigeminal nerve (V3) supplies the chin, lower lip, the margin of the mandible, the floor of the mouth, and the tongue. It enters the cranial vault via the foramen ovale.

V1 and, to a much lesser extent, V2 also innervate the meninges and dura within the supratentorial compartment of the cranial vault. The headache component of migraine reflects events transpiring at trigeminal terminals in the meninges and their microvasculature. Pain due to destructive processes involving the meninges typically has a major component that is referred to the cranium, as Case 7-11 illustrates.

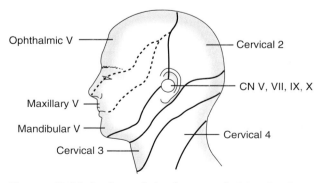

**Figure 7-15** Regions of the face supplied by the three divisions of CN V.

337

## Case 7-11

### Metastatic Cancer in Middle Cranial Fossa Causing Headache

*A 55-year-old man with a lifelong history of heavy smoking presents with a 2-week history of progressively more severe, steady, boring pain in his right forehead and temple. On examination, he is visibly in terrible pain. The neurologic examination is normal. An MRI scan reveals a 3-cm diameter contrast-enhancing plaque on the floor of the right middle cranial fossa encroaching on the cavernous sinus. A chest x-ray reveals a 4-cm diameter hilar mass.*

**Comment:** *This patient has carcinoma of the lung with metastasis to the dura of the middle cranial fossa, which is innervated by branches of V1. His pain is referred to the forehead and temple. Patients with diffuse inflammation of the meninges due to meningitis experience generalized headache via the same mechanism.*

Intermittent traction on the meninges also elicits cranial pain (Case 7-12).

## Case 7-12

### Brain Tumor Causing Headache

*A 60-year-old man presents with a 1-month history of waxing and waning, dull, generalized headache, worse on the right side. When asked what happens when he sneezes, he says it feels like the top of his head is going to blow off. The headache is also worsened by coughing, bending over, lifting, or straining when he moves his bowels. On examination, he exhibits a left pronation drift when his arms are extended in front of him in supination, he has some degradation of fine motor movement in his left hand, and he fails to swing his left arm when he walks. His deep tendon reflexes are slightly brisker on the left and he has a left Babinski sign. An MRI scan reveals a 6-cm diameter right temporoparietal mass associated with effacement of sulci over the right hemisphere, flattening of the right lateral ventricle, and nearly 1 cm right-to-left shift of midline cerebral structures. Biopsy of the mass reveals a malignant primary brain tumor, a glioblastoma multiforme.*

## Case 7-12—cont'd

**Comment:** *This patient's tumor is so large that it has eliminated all extra space in the right hemicranium and through subfalcine herniation, substantially reduced the space in the left hemicranium. Coughing, sneezing, Valsalva maneuver, and bending over transiently increase the intracranial pressure (mainly via pressure transmitted through the venous system), causing sudden traction of the meninges between the brain and the skull and a sudden explosion of pain.*

Trigeminal receptors and nerve fibers are identical to those in somatosensory nerves supplying the body. As in the body, they define protopathic and epicritic subsystems. As in the somatosensory system serving the body, these subsystems spatially segregate as soon as they enter the brainstem in the lateral pons (Fig. 7-16).

Fibers of the protopathic system descend in the spinal tract of V to synapse in the nucleus of the spinal tract of V, which extends from the caudal pons down to the C2 level of the spinal cord, where it merges imperceptibly with lamina I and II of the dorsal horn (Fig. 7-6). Thus, the spinal nucleus of V could be viewed as the trigeminal analog of spinal lamina I and II.

Neural transmission within the spinal nucleus of V follows a multisynaptic pathway ending in projections to neurons that send their axons across the brainstem. These coalesce along the length of the caudal brainstem into the trigeminothalamic tract, which ultimately travels just dorsal to the medial lemniscus. It sends terminals and collaterals into the brainstem reticular formation and the periaqueductal gray and eventually terminates in a portion of the ventral posterior nucleus of the thalamus, the *ventral posteromedial nucleus* (VPM). It is located ventromedial to the ventral posterolateral nucleus that receives sensory projections from the body (Fig. 7-17).

Most epicritic fibers within the trigeminal nerves synapse on the chief sensory nucleus of V, within the lateral pons just rostral to the spinal nucleus of V (adjacent to the CN V entry zone) (Fig. 7-18). However, there is one peculiar subset of fibers within the trigeminal nerve. These fibers supply muscle spindles within the muscles of mastication, innervated by the motor nucleus of CN V, and within the extraocular muscles. They are peculiar in that their cell bodies are located not in the gasserian ganglion but within the mesen-

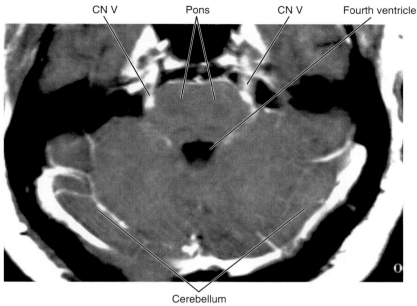

CN V          Pons          CN V          Fourth ventricle

Cerebellum

**Figure 7-16** Axial contrast-enhanced magnetic resonance image (MRI) of the brainstem, illustrating the pathway of the trigeminal nerves between the cavernous sinuses on either side of the sella turcica and the trigeminal entry zones in the lateral portions of the pons. Note that the brainstem portion of this slice corresponds quite precisely to an anterior-posterior inverted version of the slice depicted in Figure 7-18. The nerves are unusually conspicuous here because this patient had diffuse infiltration of the meninges by adenocarcinoma. The meninges investing the trigeminal nerves are heavily infiltrated as well. Because the blood-brain barrier is broken down by the cancer, gadolinium (the contrast agent used here), leaks into the tissue, where it appears white on this image.

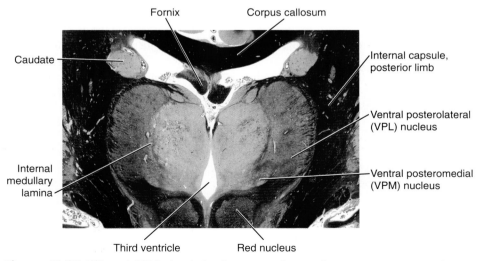

Fornix          Corpus callosum

Caudate

Internal capsule, posterior limb

Ventral posterolateral (VPL) nucleus

Internal medullary lamina

Ventral posteromedial (VPM) nucleus

Third ventricle          Red nucleus

**Figure 7-17** VPL and VPM, the thalamic targets of ascending somatosensory pathways. (Modified from Warner JJ. Atlas of Neuroanatomy. Boston, Butterworth Heinemann, 2001, with permission from Elsevier Science.)

Somesthesis

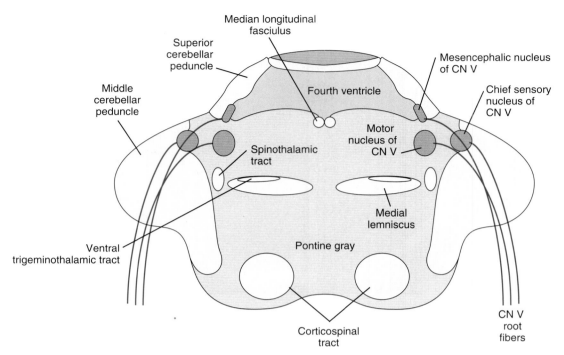

**Figure 7-18** The chief sensory and mesencephalic nuclei of CN V.

cephalic nucleus of V, which lies in the lateral midbrain, just rostral to the chief sensory nucleus. Thus, the mesencephalic nucleus of V is, in effect, a fifth cranial nerve dorsal root ganglion lying within the substance of the brainstem. The axons of cells in the mesencephalic nucleus synapse on cells in the motor nucleus of V bilaterally, providing the basis for jaw reflexes. Cells in the chief sensory nucleus of V project rostrally, via the trigeminothalamic tract, to terminate in the contralateral ventral posteromedial nucleus of the thalamus. As for the somatosensory system of the body, although targets of protopathic and epicritic trigeminal systems are admixed throughout the ventral posteromedial nucleus, they remain segregated in their connections. The trigeminal system is summarized in Figure 7-19.

Thalamocortical relay cells in the ventral posteromedial nucleus send their projections via the genu of the internal capsule and the corona radiata to lateral portions of the postcentral gyrus—the face portion of the sensory homunculus.

## PRACTICE 7-4

**A.** Return to Practice 2-3C (lateral medullary infarction). Predict the pattern of sensory loss this patient would exhibit.

**B.** A 72-year-old woman complains of a 2-week history of constant, boring pain in the right temporal region that has progressed steadily in intensity and is now excruciating. Three years ago she underwent partial mastectomy, radiation therapy, and chemotherapy for carcinoma of the breast. On examination, she has subjectively altered sensation to touch over the right forehead and upper cheek region. A cold tuning fork applied to these areas feels neither cold nor warm, whereas on the left side of the face it feels cold to her. The right corneal reflex (blink induced by touching the cornea with a wisp of cotton) is diminished compared to the left. The remainder of the neurologic examination is completely normal. Localize the lesion.

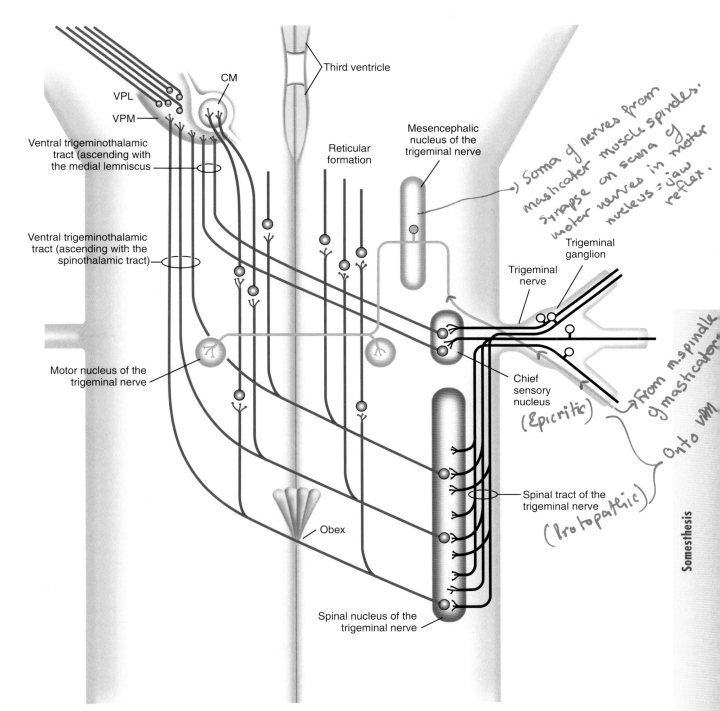

**Figure 7-19** The trigeminal nuclei and pathways. VPL, ventral posterolateral nucleus; VPM, ventral posteromedial nucleus; CM, central medial nucleus. (Modified from Warner JJ. Atlas of Neuroanatomy. Boston, Butterworth Heinemann, 2001, with permission from Elsevier Science.)

**TABLE 7-4** Summary of Protopathic and Epicritic Sensory Systems

| Features | Protopathic | Epicritic |
|---|---|---|
| Sensory modalities | Temperature, pain, touch | Form, texture, touch, pressure, slippage, vibration, position |
| Spatial and temporal resolution | Low | High |
| Site of major afferent neuron | Dorsal root ganglion at each, spinal segment | Dorsal root ganglion at each spinal segment |
| Fiber type | Small, slowly conducting, lightly myelinated and unmyelinated | Large, rapidly conducting, myelinated |
| Segmental organization | Complex polysynaptic route through dorsal horn involving intersegmental propriospinal fibers | Pauci-synaptic organization: all dorsal root fibers enter dorsal columns without synapse, some ascend to dorsal column nuclei with or without dorsal horn collaterals, and some enter and terminate in dorsal horn to subserve reflex functions |
| Ascending tract | Lateral spinothalamic tract | Dorsal (fasciculus gracilis and cuneatus) and dorsolateral columns |
| Laterality of ascending tract | Contralateral (fibers cross within 1–2 levels of dorsal root entry) | Ipsilateral (fibers do not cross until sensory decussation) |
| Somatotopic organization of ascending tracts | Typical (legs lateral and dorsal) | Atypical (arms lateral) |
| Targets of ascending tracts | Brainstem reticular formation and VPL (thalamus) | Ipsilateral nuclei cuneatus and gracilis at cervicomedullary junction; relay via medial lemniscus to contralateral VPL |
| Cortical target | Postcentral gyrus (particularly Brodmann's areas 3a and 2) (arm and leg portions of sensory homunculus) | Postcentral gyrus (Brodmann's areas 3a, 3b, 1, 2) (arm and leg portions of sensory homunculus) |
| Trigeminal equivalent | Spinal nucleus of V | Chief sensory and mesencephalic nuclei of V |
| Site of major trigeminal afferent neuron | Gasserian ganglion (floor of cavernous sinus) | Gasserian ganglion except proprioceptive fibers of mesencephalic nucleus of V |
| Trigeminal projection target | VPM (thalamus) | VPM (thalamus) |
| Trigeminal cortical projection target | Postcentral gyrus (areas 3a and 2) (face portion of sensory homunculus) | Postcentral gyrus (areas 3a, 3b, 1, 2) (face portion of sensory homunculus) |

*Key*: VPL, ventral posterolateral nucleus; VPM, ventral posteromedial nucleus.

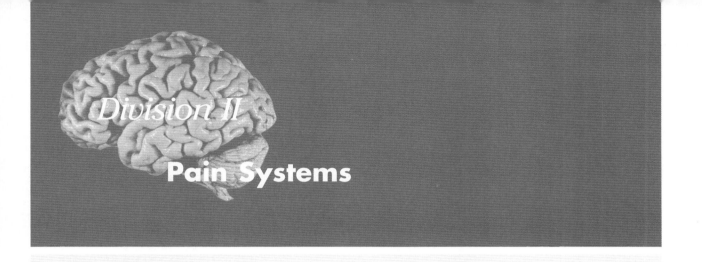

# Division II

# Pain Systems

Pain is an unpleasant sensory and emotional experience. Under most circumstances, acute pain is useful in that it informs us of actual or potential tissue damage. Causes of such damage include contact with hot objects, wasp stings, broken bones, and serious or life-threatening infections such as appendicitis or spinal epidural abscesses. Pain lasting days or weeks may also be useful to the extent that it encourages immobilization and protection of the injured area. However, most such pain rapidly outlives its usefulness, persisting long after the problem has been detected and effectively dealt with. Some types of acute pain, such as perioperative pain, migraine headache, and essentially all types of chronic pain, never serve any useful purpose, cause patients inordinate suffering, seriously interfere with the pursuit of normal life, and may even contribute to physical disease and death. Until very recently it was thought that the use of perioperative analgesics was not necessary in neonates because they were not sentient—that is, in some fundamental way, they were incapable of suffering. However, a controlled clinical study showed that the provision of analgesia markedly reduced the perioperative mortality rate.

Thus, there is an enormous impetus to treat pain effectively. The perception and experience of nearly all types of pain involves a complex central nervous system apparatus that includes the afferent nociceptive pathways we reviewed in Division I of this chapter, a number of efferent (descending) systems and pathways that serve to modulate afferent nociceptive transmission, and cerebral systems, most important being the limbic system, that instantiate the suffering that may be associated with pain. In order to take a logical, scientific approach to pain management, one needs to have some understanding of these systems. Some types of pain stem from peripheral neural injury. The mechanisms by which such injury leads to the generation of nociceptive input provide the basis for still other techniques of pain management. Finally, some chronic pain is perpetuated by central nervous system changes reflective of neural plasticity. Although these changes are complex and incompletely understood, having an awareness of their existence substantially alters the approaches we take to patients in chronic pain.

In this Division, we will begin with a review of central nervous system mechanisms that modulate nociceptive input (Cycle 7-5). We will then consider mechanisms of peripheral neurogenic pain (Cycle 7-6). Finally, we will consider central nervous system changes that may occur in response to chronic pain, and their implications for pain management (Cycle 7-7).

# Cycle 7-5

# Central Nervous System Pain Modulatory Mechanisms

### Objectives

1. Be able to describe the sites of origin and termination of the two major anti-nociceptive descending spinal cord systems, their neurotransmitters, and their mechanism of action.

2. Be able to describe the sites of action and potential mechanisms of analgesia for tricyclic antidepressants, opiates, and clonidine.

3. Be able to describe the essential principles of the gate control theory of pain modulation and give clinical examples that support its validity.

4. Be able to distinguish between pain perception and pain experience, describe the concept of suffering and its central nervous system substrate, and give examples of techniques to reduce suffering.

## A. BRAINSTEM, SPINAL CORD, AND SEGMENTAL MECHANISMS

In Cycle 7-1, we noted that nociceptive input is conveyed from the periphery by (1) mechanical/thermal nociceptors, which respond to high-intensity mechanical stimuli and transmit highly localized pain sensations via lightly myelinated $A\delta$ fibers; and (2) polymodal receptors, which respond to high-intensity mechanical stimuli, thermal stimuli, and chemical stimuli and transmit poorly localized pain sensations via unmyelinated C fibers. These polymodal receptors and their C-fiber afferents appear to provide the major substrate for the most distressing aspects of pain. We noted in our earlier review that these C fibers synapse in superficial layers of the dorsal horn (layers I and II) upon neural targets within a complex neural network that includes a neuron that sends its axon across the spinal cord in the anterior commissure to the ascending lateral spinothalamic tract.

### Serotonergic Systems

Within the complex dorsal horn neural network subserving nociceptive transmission lie several types of inhibitory interneurons that serve to suppress central transmission of nociceptive input (Fig. 7-20). Some inhibitory interneurons are enkephalinergic and synapse on primary afferent terminals of nociceptive C fibers, on excitatory interneurons in the multisynaptic relay of nociceptive transmission, and on cells giving rise to spinothalamic tract fibers. Some dorsal horn cells and the terminals of nociceptive C fibers express $\mu$–opioid and dynorphin (another endorphin) receptors. Enkephalin, $\mu$–opioid, and dynorphin receptors are activated by endogenous opioids and by exoge-

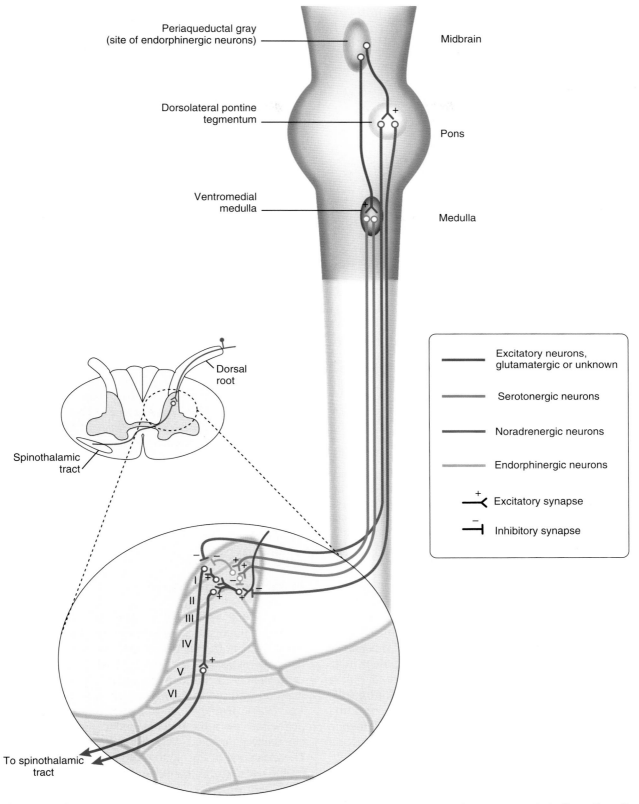

**Figure 7-20** Brainstem, spinal cord, and segmental pain modulatory mechanisms. Roman numerals indicate Rexed's laminae.

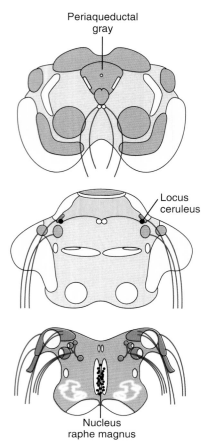

Periaqueductal
gray

Locus
ceruleus

Nucleus
raphe magnus

**Figure 7-21** Location of the periaqueductal gray in the midbrain (endorphinergic neurons), the locus ceruleus in the dorsolateral pontine tegmentum (noradrenergic neurons), and the nucleus raphe magnus in the ventromedial medulla (stippled area) (serotonergic neurons).

## Case 7-13

### Painful Diabetic Polyneuropathy

*A 55-year-old woman with a 10-year history of diabetes comes to clinic complaining of severe burning, searing pain in her feet and distal legs. The pain is constant but is at its worst after she has been on her feet for a while. It is becoming very difficult for her to work, and she cannot sleep at night because of the pain. On examination, there is reduced vibratory sensation in the feet. Light touch is experienced as irritating, as if her feet are being stroked with stinging nettles. She is given doxepin (Sinequan), a tricyclic antidepressant. Her symptoms improve dramatically, but she still experiences a rough period in the late afternoon after she gets off work. The pain at this time makes her irritable and she is unable to enjoy dinner with her family. Her physician prescribes a single dose of Percocet (acetaminophen + oxycodone, an opioid analgesic) at 4 p.m. With this addition, pain ceases to be a major problem for her.*

**Comment:** *This patient clearly has diabetic polyneuropathy. Doxepin and other tricyclic antidepressants inhibit the reuptake of both serotonin and norepinephrine by terminal boutons, thus increasing the concentration of these neurotransmitters in the synaptic cleft. They potentiate the action of the descending spinal cord serotonergic and noradrenergic pathways (see next section) involved in suppressing nociceptive input. Oxycodone acts in both the superficial layers of the dorsal horn and the periaqueductal gray to suppress the transmission of nociceptive input.*

nously administered opiates. The inhibitory enkephalinergic neurons receive excitatory input from serotonergic and nonserotonergic fibers that originate in the serotonergic nucleus raphe magnus and immediately adjacent portions of the ventromedial medulla (Fig. 7-21). These fibers descend in the dorsolateral region of the spinal cord. Neurons of the ventromedial medulla in turn receive excitatory input from the periaqueductal gray, a region rich in endorphinergic neurons of a number of different types. Thus, the neural circuitry in this descending, pain inhibitory system includes two points at which opiate drugs, and one point at which serotonergic drugs might act to alleviate pain. This system is commonly engaged to good effect in the treatment of patients, as Case 7-13 illustrates.

## Noradrenergic Systems

Spinothalamic tract neurons and the terminals of C fibers in the dorsal horn receive descending inhibitory input from noradrenergic fibers that originate in the dorsolateral pontine tegmentum (DLPT), in the immediate vicinity of the locus ceruleus. These fibers also descend in the dorsolateral region of the spinal cord. The DLPT, like the ventromedial medulla, receives projections from the periaqueductal gray. It is also reciprocally connected with the ventromedial medulla. The existence of this system provides a potential role for the use of drugs that potentiate noradrenergic activity in the treatment of pain. The targets of this pathway are $\alpha_2$-noradrenergic receptors that gate a potassium ionophore. These observations suggest that the $\alpha_2$-

agonist clonidine should be a particularly effective analgesic. Clonidine does indeed have some value in treating pain (see Case 7-16), but in general, systemic administration has at best very modest effects, probably because the doses that are effective in animal studies (up to 150 μg/kg/dose) are far greater than can be administered to humans (up to 10 μg/kg/day) without producing unacceptable sedation and hypotension. Sedation appears to be mediated through presynaptic inhibition of the locus ceruleus. Hypotension is apparently mediated by presynaptic inhibition of sympathetic cells in the intermediate zone of the spinal cord and of the baroreceptor complex in the rostral medulla, which includes the dorsal motor nucleus of the vagus and the nucleus of the solitary tract. The adverse effects of systemic administration of clonidine in humans can be circumvented through intrathecal or epidural administration of this drug.

## The Gate Control Theory of Pain Modulation

Some inhibitory neurons in the dorsal horn receive input from large, myelinated, peripheral nerves and synapse on neurons in the superficial layers of the dorsal horn relaying nociceptive transmission (Fig. 7-22). This circuitry provides the basis for the gate control theory of pain modulation, a highly influential concept derived from circumstantial clinical evidence and explicitly formulated by Melzack and Wall. The concept is that nociceptive C fiber transmission can be suppressed by enhancing myelinated fiber afferent transmission. This may be the basis for the frequency with which people who have experienced an acute painful injury will repeatedly shake the involved extremity or rub the areas of skin immediately adjacent to the site of injury. However, the strongest evidence of the

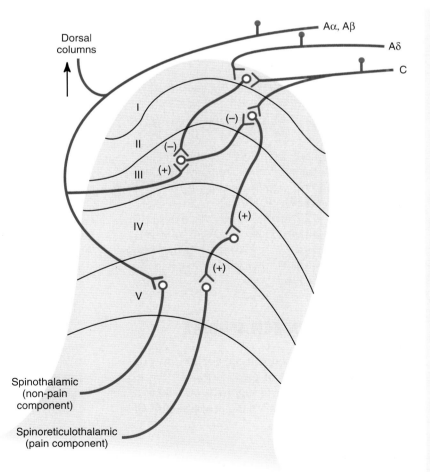

**Figure 7-22** A theoretical segmental neural substrate for the gate control theory of pain modulation.

validity of this theory lies in the effective use of nerve stimulators to treat pain, as illustrated in Case 7-14.

## Case 7-14

### Dorsal Column Stimulation for Treatment of Pain due to Neural Injury

*A 25-year-old man develops refractory nausea and vomiting due to a viral gastrointestinal illness. He visits a local emergency room where he is rehydrated and given an intramuscular dose of promethazine (Phenergan) in an effort to control the nausea and vomiting. Unfortunately, the drug is injected improperly, into the patient's right sciatic nerve. He immediately experiences excruciating pain shooting down the back of his leg. The pain eventually subsides, but over the ensuing weeks he develops severe, constant, burning pain involving his right foot and lateral side of his right leg. Aggressive treatment with a variety of drugs fails to bring adequate relief, and the patient remains incapacitated. An electrode is threaded through a needle into the epidural space immediately overlying the dorsal columns of the sacral spinal cord and connected to an implanted electrical stimulator. With high-frequency stimulation of the sacral cord, the patient experiences marked relief of his pain. He is still dependent on intensive drug therapy but is now able to return to work and resume a reasonable family life.*

**Comment:** *We presume that the stimulator acts by exciting low threshold, large, myelinated afferent fibers with collateral projections to inhibitory interneurons synapsing on nociceptive afferent pathways. A similar principle motivates the use of transcutaneous electrical nerve stimulators (TENS units), which involve the application of a stimulating electrode to the skin. Unfortunately, TENS units are only occasionally effective.*

## B. CEREBRAL MECHANISMS

The mechanisms discussed in Section A primarily involve the perception of pain. However, the experience of pain involves the component we refer to as suffering. Suffering derives from the processing of afferent nociceptive transmission by the cerebrum and, more particularly, by the limbic system. The limbic system provides the means by which we attach value to experience (see Chapter 12). Thus, happiness, sadness, elation, and misery each reflect particular patterns of neural activity in the limbic system. There is not a tight relationship between the intensity of afferent nociceptive activity and the degree of suffering instantiated by the limbic system. Thus, patients in intense pain may experience very little suffering, and patients with relatively modest pain may experience severe suffering. Experience with victims of wartime injury has provided the most dramatic demonstration of this principle. Soldiers pressed into action often seem to experience very little suffering despite terrible injuries. Only later, when divested of responsibility, do they experience suffering commensurate with their wounds. This principle has important ramifications for clinical practice. Patients suffering intensely are often dismissed in cavalier fashion because it does not seem likely that such a minor problem could cause so much suffering. On the other hand, physicians do not always take full advantage of our capability for controlling suffering by manipulating the patient's activity and mental state. Thus, in Case 7-13, doxepin was particularly useful because, in addition to suppressing ascending nociceptive transmission, it helped the patient to sleep, and it effectively treated depression (which also reflects an adverse limbic state). Few things are worse than enduring pain during a long sleepless night. Few things amplify suffering associated with pain to a greater degree than depression. In Case 7-14, the epidural stimulator directly suppressed nociceptive transmission. However, the ultimate benefits of this intervention were not completely realized until the patient returned to work, where the responsibility, reward for accomplishment, and social interaction served to alter limbic system activity in a positive way via the same mechanisms as in the wounded soldier pressed into combat. There is also evidence of opiate receptors in parts of the limbic system (amygdala, nucleus accumbens) that could directly mediate some of the salutary effects of opiate drugs on pain. It is not clear to what extent the benefits of manipulating cerebral responses to pain are due to altered patterns of neural activity in the limbic system, or to cerebral suppression of ascending nociceptive transmission.

# Cycle 7-6

# Peripheral Mechanisms Underlying Neurogenic Pain

## Objectives

1. Be able to describe ectopic impulse generation and the factors that predispose to it and provide two clinical examples.
2. Be able to describe the mechanism of drugs that suppress ectopic impulse generation.
3. Be able to describe the processes that occur in the dorsal root ganglion following nerve injury that lead to enhanced nociceptive transmission.

Neurogenic pain is caused by nerve injury. Nerve injury can produce pain via at least two mechanisms: (1) ectopic impulse generation and (2) changes in dorsal root ganglia that lead to enhanced nociceptive transmission to the dorsal horn of the spinal cord.

## ECTOPIC IMPULSE GENERATION

Ectopic impulse generation refers to the spontaneous generation of action potentials, usually at sites of axonal demyelination. Neurons appear to compensate for demyelination by producing an exceptionally high density of voltage-sensitive sodium channels in the demyelinated membrane. This substantially enhances the probability that action potentials will be transmitted through the demyelinated segment, despite the loss of

current due to membrane leakiness and the layering of large numbers of ions along the neural membrane (capacitance "current").[2] It also enhances the probability that action potentials will be spontaneously generated at the site of demyelination. Often mechanical pressure, to which nerves are normally relatively impervious, is sufficient to trigger such ectopic impulses.[3] This is particularly true of new axon sprouts, which are intrinsically mechanosensitive. The high density of voltage-sensitive sodium channels, coupled with very slow propagation of action potentials in a demyelinated segment, may lead to a situation in which membrane

---

[2] A substantial change in a type of voltage-gated sodium channel also occurs after injury. Many neurons insert sodium channels originally present only during development. These "regressive" channels are more likely to lead to spontaneous generation of action potentials.

[3] This is the basis for the Tinel's and Phalen's signs of peripheral nerve injury. Tinel's sign can be elicited by brisk tapping over the site of damage (the central crease of the palm just distal to the wrist in a patient with carpal tunnel syndrome). In this syndrome, damage to the median nerve is caused by excessive pressure where the nerve passes with the finger tendons into the hand beneath the flexor retinaculum of the wrist. A positive Tinel's sign is characterized by brief electrical sensations radiating distally, in this case, into the thumb and first two fingers. Phalen's sign can be elicited by application of prolonged pressure to a nerve. In the patient with carpal tunnel syndrome, this sign can be produced by gently pressing the wrist into marked flexion or extension for a minute or so. The sign is present if the patient experiences tingling in the median nerve innervated portions of the hand.

*349*

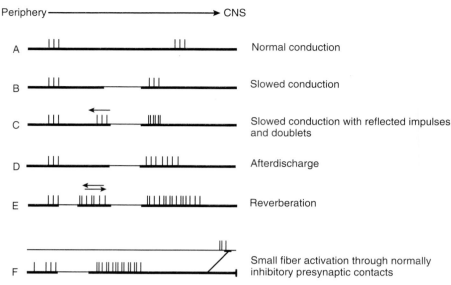

**Figure 7-23** Patterns of somatosensory afferent activity in ectopic impulse generation. In *A*, impulses are conducted toward the CNS in a normal fashion. In *B*, impulse transmission is slowed through an area of demyelination. In *C*, impulse transmission is slowed sufficiently for additional impulses to be generated in adjacent demyelinated membrane. The additional impulses are conducted to the CNS in the form of doublets (two impulses very close together), and back toward the periphery as reflected impulses. In *D*, conduction through a segment of demyelination produces after-discharge. In *E*, multiple sites of demyelination create reverberation of impulses between ectopic sites, and massive discharge towards the CNS. In *F*, transfer of activity from large to small afferents occurs through presynaptic mechanisms.

depolarization outlasts the refractory period of the nearby sodium channels. Action potentials can then be generated that travel antidromically (from proximal to distal) along the nerve—a reflected impulse. The same thing can happen at multiple demyelinated segments, leading to reverberating antidromic and orthodromic pulses between sites. Thus, one action potential generated by stimulation of a distal receptor can result in the generation of a large number of reflected pulses and a resultant barrage of action potentials at the sensory terminal in the dorsal horn (Fig. 7-23). Cases 7-15 and 7-16 illustrate these principles.

In some circumstances, for example, postherpetic neuralgia, either ectopic impulse generation or normal neural activity that is pathologically amplified by it can be ameliorated by topical application to involved dermatomes of another class of voltage-sensitive sodium channel agents, local anesthetics, such as lidocaine (Xylocaine). Postherpetic neuralgia is focal pain of neural origin in a dermatomal distribution that follows local reactivation of herpes zoster infection ("shingles").

It is not understood precisely why such high-frequency, ectopically generated or amplified impulses are perceived as painful. It is clear that high-frequency stimulation of Aδ fibers supplying mechanical or thermal receptors produces a sensation of pain. There is also reason to believe that rapid discharge of large fibers not normally implicated in nociception can be "transferred" to small-diameter fibers subserving nociception. One mechanism that might mediate this is primary afferent depolarization. Primary afferent depolarization reflects an interaction between large, myelinated fiber terminals and C fiber terminals in the dorsal horn. Some large-fiber terminals make collateral axoaxonic synapses on the terminal boutons of C fibers. When these large fibers fire at low or moderate rates, they partially depolarize the C fiber terminals. This depolarization has the effect of reducing the amount of neurotransmitter released when the C fibers actually fire—a form of presynaptic inhibition (an alternative substrate for the gate control mechanism of pain modulation). However, if a large myelinated fiber fires at a sufficiently high rate, it may generate an action potential in the C fiber terminal—primary afferent depolarization.

## Case 7-15

### Arsenic Polyneuropathy

*A middle-aged woman seeks retribution on her husband for suspected infidelity by lacing his food with arsenic. After several weeks, he presents to a local hospital with the chief complaint of progressive generalized weakness, severe burning in his feet and distal legs, and persistent gastrointestinal distress. The pain is almost more than he can stand when he is lying in bed, but it becomes excruciating and intolerable whenever he bears weight on his feet. Hospital staff marvel at the sweetness of the patient's wife, who brings him tasty treats every day. His neurologist suspects Guillain-Barré syndrome (acute postinfectious demyelinating polyradiculoneuropathy), but astutely collects a 24-hour urine sample to check for arsenic. Her suspicions are borne out by the discovery of high levels of arsenic in the urine and in the treats the patient's wife is bringing him. With incarceration of his wife, the administration of chelating agents to* reduce the tissue arsenic burden, and the administration of a drug that inhibits the opening of voltage-sensitive sodium channels (carbamazepine, Tegretol), the patient's strength steadily improves and his pain is substantially alleviated.

**Comment:** *Arsenic is a neurotoxin that primarily produces axonal injury. Painful neuropathies are usually associated with significant axonal involvement. However, axons and their investing myelin have sufficient interdependence that purely axonal or purely demyelinative lesions are never actually realized in practice. The extreme pain produced by the pressure of weight bearing on this patient's feet illustrates the pathologic pressure sensitivity that may develop in diseased nerves. The efficacy of carbamazepine is consistent with the role of voltage-sensitive sodium channels in the genesis of the reverberating ectopic impulses ultimately experienced as severe pain.*

## Case 7-16

### Trigeminal Neuralgia

*A 75-year-old woman presents to clinic with a 6-week history of excruciating facial pain. There is a constant background of dull ache in her left jaw and this is punctuated many times a day by bursts of piercing, electrical pain that radiate up her jaw along the V3 dermatome. This lancinating pain can be precipitated by lightly touching certain parts of the left lower face, chewing, or talking. As she talks to you, she constantly flinches and tears pour down her face. She cowers as you approach her face to examine her. Examination is normal. You confirm that touching a region around the left angle of the mouth will often precipitate a burst of pain. The patient eventually achieves almost complete relief of pain with an appropriate dose of phenytoin (Dilantin).*

**Comment:** *This patient has trigeminal neuralgia. It appears to reflect ectopic impulse generation in* proximal portions of the trigeminal nerve just outside the brainstem, or within the brainstem just beyond the trigeminal entry zone. In elderly patients, extra-axial segmental demyelination is often produced by pressure from an ectatic loop of artery, most often the superior cerebellar artery, pulsating against proximal portions of the nerve. In young patients with multiple sclerosis, inflammatory demyelination can occur within the neuraxis at the nerve entry zone. In either circumstance, afferent neural impulses generated by normal stimulation of certain tissue receptors ("trigger points") lead to the generation of reverberating impulses in the demyelinated zone, transforming low rates of neural firing into bursts of extremely high frequency activity. Phenytoin, like carbamazepine, binds preferentially to the inactivated state of voltage-sensitive sodium channels, thus inhibiting action potentials and ectopic impulse generation.*

Somesthesis

## DORSAL ROOT GANGLION AND RELATED DORSAL HORN CHANGES

Peripheral nerve injury leads to at least three important changes in affected dorsal root ganglia and peripheral axons: (1) increased density of voltage sensitive sodium channels in Aβ neurons (low threshold, fast conducting, non-nociceptive neurons), and enhancement of their conductivity; (2) increased production of growth factors by neurons, Schwann cells, and macrophages; (3) increased expression of α₁-noradrenergic receptors by polymodal nociceptive afferent neurons. The increased density of sodium channels in type A neurons increases the probability of action potential generation in these neurons, spontaneous firing, and pathologically sustained and high-frequency firing in response to peripheral stimuli. This could mediate pain by primary afferent depolarization in the dorsal horn (see previous discussion). The increased production of growth factors induces sympathetic neurons innervating the vasculature of the dorsal root ganglion to send sprouts into the ganglion itself (Fig. 7-24). Thus, when these sympathetic neurons fire and release norepinephrine, this leads to pathologic firing of polymodal nociceptive afferent neurons, which express abnormally large numbers of α₁-noradrenergic receptors on cell bodies,

at the site of injury in damaged axons, and at the terminals of intact axons. Because of upregulation of α₁-receptors, these neurons are particularly sensitive to norepinephrine, to the extent that firing may also be inducible by circulating norepinephrine of adrenal origin. These mechanisms are thought to be the basis for "sympathetically mediated" pain.

Parallel changes in the dorsal horn of the spinal cord following peripheral nerve injury are only beginning to be understood (see also Cycle 7-7). The increased production of growth factors (as well as many other neuroactive substances) induces collateral sprouting of low threshold, rapidly conducting, A fibers with the development of terminals in regions of the dorsal horn in which C fibers normally terminate. With sustained firing, C fibers synapsing in the dorsal horn may sprout and form additional synapses on preganglionic sympathetic neurons in the intermediate zone of the spinal cord. This in turn may generate excessive sympathetic activity in the areas of pain. The heightened activity of large fibers after nerve injury may lead to glutamate-mediated excitotoxic death of inhibitory neurons in superficial lamina of the dorsal horn; by producing disinhibition, this may facilitate pain transmission.

Case 7-17 illustrates the clinical consequences of some of these phenomena.

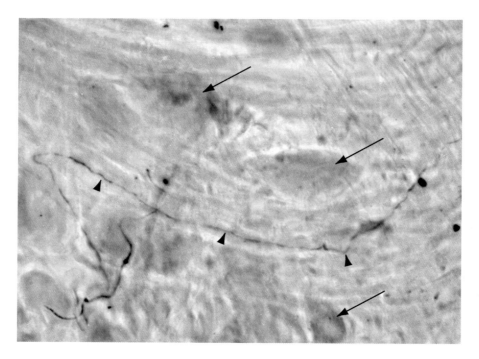

**Figure 7-24** Photomicrograph of a dorsal root ganglion following peripheral nerve injury, illustrating a sympathetic axon (*arrowheads*) that has extended well into the ganglion, far from its normal site of termination on a blood vessel. Dorsal root ganglion neurons (*arrows*).

## Case 7-17

### Sympathectomy for Treatment of Refractory Neural Pain

*A 22-year-old woman experiences a brachial plexus injury in a motor vehicle accident. Although she has only modest weakness in proximal muscles of the left arm (reflecting injury to upper portions of the plexus), she develops severe burning, searing pain maximal over the C5 and C6 dermatomes. Even the touch of light clothing is very painful, and the light brush of the examiner's hand across the involved region produces a surge of pain. Autonomic hyperactivity is readily evident: the limb is cold and cyanotic from vasoconstriction, and there is excessive sweating. A variety of medications, including tricyclic antidepressants, anticonvulsants, opiates, and clonidine are employed with only partial success. Ultimately, sympathectomy is performed via chemical ablation of the superior cervical ganglion. This procedure provides substantial relief of pain.*

**Comment:** *The traditional medical therapies employed in this patient sought to engage central pain suppression mechanisms (tricyclic antidepressants, opiates) and dampen ectopic impulse generation (anticonvulsants). Clonidine, an $\alpha_2$-agonist, reduces release of norepinephrine by postganglionic sympathetic endings by stimulating $\alpha_2$-receptors that inhibit opening of voltage-gated calcium channels. It also acts at spinal cord sites to directly suppress nociceptive transmission, as discussed earlier. However, in this case, only complete elimination of efferent autonomic activity in the limb was successful in treating the pain. Without such relief, not only do patients continue to suffer from severe pain, but the affected limb undergoes profound changes, including thinning of the skin, muscle atrophy, joint contractures, and osteoporosis. Ultimately, the limb becomes completely useless. Unfortunately, sympathectomy is frequently unsuccessful; it may bring only transient relief of pain, and in some cases, it may actually add a sympathetic component to the chronic pain syndrome, perhaps by contributing to upregulation of $\alpha$–adrenergic receptors on peripheral nociceptive afferent fibers.*

Somesthesis

# The Role of Central Nervous System Plasticity in the Generation of Chronic Pain States

### *Objectives*

1. Be able to describe the major processes involved in wind-up.
2. Be able to describe what is meant by the term "pathologic learning" and give three examples.

Learning consists of changes in the strengths of neural interconnections in the central nervous system. We tend to think of learning as conscious, intentional, and positive. However, a moment's reflection indicates that many things that we recognize as learning, for example, improving skills in a particular sport, are not conscious—they just happen. Learning is not always intentional: experiences teach us, whether we intend to learn or not. It is also clear that we can learn incorrect facts and develop "bad habits" in any sport we engage in. Finally, we tend to think of learning as the exclusive province of the cerebrum. In fact, learning may occur wherever there are interneural connections. In this section we consider some learning processes, some of which substantially involve the spinal cord and the brainstem, that are clearly bad in that they effectively constitute the process of learning to experience long-lasting, if not permanent, pain. They constitute one example of a group of central nervous system learning processes that might be referred to as *pathologic learning*.

## A. THE DORSAL HORN: WIND-UP

If nociceptive input is sufficiently sustained, changes occur in dorsal horn and dorsal root ganglion cells such that the impact of peripheral input on central pain transmission becomes steadily greater. Painful stimuli become even more painful and formerly nonpainful stimuli induce pain. This process is referred to as "*wind-up*," or "central sensitization." The initial perception of pain derives from release of glutamate by C fiber nociceptive afferent endings. However, these same afferent endings release other neurotransmitters, including substance P and calcitonin gene-related peptide (CGRP). The effects of glutamate at NMDA receptors, in the presence of substance P, if sustained and of sufficient magnitude, may lead to a strengthening of connections between nociceptive afferent fibers and dorsal horn neurons (see also Box 7-2). This increases the sensitivity of dorsal horn neurons to all inputs. The receptive fields of these neurons then may increase, as formerly subthreshold inputs now succeed in eliciting action potentials. Consequently, stimuli from a more extensive area of the body will cause them to fire. These processes underlying wind-up lead to the development of hypersensitivity to subsequent noxious stimuli (*hyperalgesia*), and to the experience of non-noxious stimuli, such as simple touch, as painful (*allodynia*). Hyperalgesia and allodynia reflect a normal learning process, strengthening of neural connections (known as long-term potentiation) that occurs throughout the nervous system. In the course of wind-up, this normal process yields a pathologic outcome—hypersensitivity of cells in the dorsal horn to input from both nociceptive C fibers and non-nociceptive terminals. Sustained nociceptive C fiber input causes these neurons to respond as strongly to non-nociceptive input as they originally did to nociceptive input. Similar mechanisms may underlie the pathologically low pain tolerance of patients with fibromyalgia and "psychosomatic" disorders.

## B. CENTRAL PAIN SYNDROMES

Return to Case 7-17 and consider an alternative scenario observed in many such patients. Suppose sympathectomy is not effective. The patient then undergoes multilevel cervical rhizotomy (cutting of the dorsal roots). This procedure provides relief of pain for about 6 months (as well as a numb arm), after which the pain returns with even greater severity. She then undergoes anterolateral tractotomy (cutting of the contralateral spinothalamic tract). This procedure, too, provides dramatic relief of pain, but again, for only 6 months. Consider another equally compelling situation. A patient undergoes above the knee amputation because of intractable ischemia of the leg related to peripheral vascular disease. The amputation site heals well and the patient is successfully fitted with a prosthesis so that he can walk again. However, the severe ischemic pain in his leg that he experienced before amputation persists in the now "phantom" limb.

How can such cases be explained? The answers are far from clear, but a number of clues are emerging, some of which we have already touched upon in this chapter.

First, extensive remodeling occurs at all levels of the central nervous system in response to loss of input from peripheral nerves, in response to sustained peripheral stimulation, or even in response to repetitive movement. Some aspects of this remodeling suggest that it is a positive adaptation through which measurable improvements in performance occur. For

---

### BOX 7-2 The Role of Inflammation and Glia in the Genesis of Chronic Pain: An Emerging Science

Evidence is rapidly emerging that suggests that inflammatory processes involving peripheral nerves, Schwann cells and macrophages in dorsal root ganglia (mentioned above), and astrocytes and microglia in the dorsal horn of the spinal cord may play a role in the genesis of chronic pain. There are not yet any clear clinical correlates of these discoveries, but they provide a potential basis for novel and far more effective treatments of pain.

Any type of peripheral nerve injury induces an inflammatory response. This initially involves neutrophils, and more chronically it involves macrophages. In animal experiments, interventions that reduce infiltration of sites of nerve injury by these inflammatory cells reduce hyperalgesia and allodynia. Neutrophils, and to a greater extent, macrophages, secrete a large variety of immunoreactive substances called cytokines, many of which act on neurons. Giving antibodies to tumor necrosis factor alpha (TNF-$\alpha$), one of these cytokines, prior to peripheral nerve injury, also reduces hyperalgesia and allodynia. So, too, does the administration of interleukin-10.

In the dorsal horn, peripheral nerve injury of almost any type results in swelling of astrocytes and increased production within these astrocytes of glial fibrillary acidic protein (a marker of astrocytic activation). It also results in an increased number of microglia bearing a characteristic marker (OX42) that indicates activation. Glial activation can be induced by substance P and glutamate released from C fiber terminals, and by nitric oxide and prostaglandins released by nociceptive neurons within the superficial lamina of the dorsal horn. Activated glia release nitric oxide, prostaglandins, and a number of cytokines, including interleukin-1, interleukin-6, and TNF-$\alpha$. Both glia and neurons express receptors for these substances. These substances mediate pain induced by peripheral nerve inflammation or injury. Inhibition of glial metabolic activity, interference with glial activation, or disruption of the action of glial products (interleukin-1, TNF-$\alpha$, and nerve growth factor) reduces hyperalgesia and allodynia following peripheral nerve injury, suggesting that glia are contributors to the genesis of these pain responses. The administration of nonsteroidal anti-inflammatory drugs in animals and humans, at least when done at the time of pain onset, can attenuate subsequent pain.

Somesthesis

example, as we noted in Cycle 7-3, when the nerves to a monkey's arm are cut, the arm regions of the sensory and motor homunculi in the cerebral cortex are "rewired" so that previously very weak synapses with projections from the face are markedly strengthened, effectively expanding the face representation. Monkeys required to make ever finer frequency discriminations during repetitive vibratory stimulation demonstrate marked expansion of neuronal fields representing the vibratory modality in sensory cortex. Monkeys and humans expand the extent of motor cortex involved in a complex skilled movement as they repeatedly practice the movement and become more skilled at carrying it out.

However, it is also clear that these normally adaptive and beneficial learning processes may run amok. Musicians, particularly violinists and pianists, who perform extremely large numbers of repetitive movements, are at risk for developing a repetitive movement dystonia, in which their hands will suddenly lock into a dystonic posture as they perform. Many careers have been ruined as a result. In a recent experiment, when monkeys were trained to repeat a stereotyped finger movement thousands of times over, they developed dystonia. Examination of their sensory cortices revealed extensive remodeling with marked expansion of the receptive fields and loss of specificity of the neurons. These results suggest that pathologic patterns of neural connectivity (i.e., pathologic learning) occurred as a result of the repetitive movement, even if it is difficult to explain why such abnormal connectivity in somatosensory cortex produces dystonia. Analogous experiments have not been carried out in animals experiencing chronic pain, but it is quite plausible that dysfunctional remodeling of sensory cortex occurs in these circumstances as well, such that the brain "learns to hurt" as a result of chronic input from nociceptors or central cells that contribute to ascending nociceptive transmission. Both repetitive movement dystonia and certain pain states appear to represent "pathologic learning."

Comparable remodeling occurs within the spinal cord, brainstem, and thalamus, in response to sustained nociceptive input. Thalamic cells that receive input from the spinothalamic tract are normally active only when an appropriate stimulus is applied to their peripheral receptive fields. This activity signals pain when it reaches a certain firing rate in a sufficient number of cells. After a lesion of the spinothalamic tract, these cells become active in the absence of peripheral stimulation, and the activity tends to involve

## Case 7-18

### Pain with Multiple Sclerosis

*Return to Case 5-6, which presents a patient with multiple sclerosis. During a follow-up visit, this patient complains of chronic discomfort in the right side of her body that is punctuated by sudden surges of burning/tearing pain. These episodes sometimes occur many times in a day, and may last up to 30 minutes at a time. Treatment with phenytoin (Dilantin), 400 mg per day, completely relieves the pain.*

**Comment:** *In the discussion of Case 5-6, we noted that in response to demyelination, axons in the central nervous system increase the density of voltage-sensitive sodium channels (just as in the periphery). This serves to increase the probability of successful transmission of an action potential. However, also as in the periphery, it increases the probability of ectopic impulse generation. It is thus quite logical that a drug that reduces the rate of opening of voltage-sensitive sodium channels should be effective in relieving pain generated in this way.*

high-frequency bursts. When this activity reaches a critical level in a population of cells that previously received nociceptive input, it is likely that spontaneous pain will be experienced. This may provide one explanation for the occasional success of antiepileptic medications in control of chronic central pain. However, the unstable bursting activity of deafferented neurons is highly resistant to tonic suppression.

Finally, evidence suggests that ectopic impulse generation (discussed in peripheral nerves in Cycle 7-6) also occurs in the central nervous system, either as a result of disease or as a result of surgical procedures performed to alleviate pain. This is probably the explanation for the symptoms observed in the patient in Case 7-18.

## PRACTICE 7-7

**A.** For each of the following drugs, identify the site of action and the probable mechanism of analgesic effect:

Doxepin (tricyclic antidepressant)
Morphine sulfate (opiate)
Carbamazepine, phenytoin
Clonidine

## CYCLE 7-2

**A.** Damage would be maximal to protopathic fiber pathways crossing at the C5, C6, and C7 levels of the cord. Because right-to-left and left-to-right fibers would be affected by the cavity within the cord, the patient would have bilateral loss of pain and temperature sensation in these dermatomes. This pattern of sensory loss is often referred to as a "cape" distribution.

**B.** One would find impairment in epicritic modalities (position and vibratory sense) ipsilateral to the lesion (i.e., over the right hemibody) because the epicritic system has not yet crossed. One would find impairment in protopathic modalities contralateral to the lesion, because fibers of the protopathic system cross within one or two segments of cord entry. Illustrating the principle of sensory levels seen with spinal cord lesions, the impairment in epicritic modalities would extend up to the lesion and the impairment in protopathic modalities would extend to 1 or 2 levels below the lesion. This pattern of sensory loss, in conjunction with the right hemiparesis, defines the Brown-Sequard syndrome.

**C.** There would be loss of epicritic sensation (vibratory and position sense), because of both damage to the dorsal columns and damage to large myelinated fibers in peripheral nerves. There would be weakness and bilateral Babinski signs due to damage to the lateral motor tracts. Ankle jerks would be absent because of damage to the longest group Ia sensory afferents (breaking the S1 myotatic reflex arcs).

**D.** This patient has a lacunar infarct involving the ventral posterolateral (VPL) nucleus of the thalamus caused by thrombosis of one of the thalamogeniculate arteries (twigs arising from the proximal posterior cerebral arteries) as a result of localized atheromatous disease. Because this lesion affects a point of confluence of epicritic and protopathic pathways, all sensory modalities are affected. The lesion spares the posterior limb of the internal capsule—hence the absence of motor signs.

If your answer is a postcentral gyrus lesion due to thromboembolic occlusion of a middle cerebral artery branch, give yourself full credit. The only thing wrong with this answer is that such events are extraordinarily rare, simply because damage associated with middle cerebral artery distribution infarcts is rarely confined to the postcentral gyrus.

**E.** See Case 2-5 and Figure 2-25.

**F.** Two-point discrimination

    E

Pain sensation ("pinprick")

    P

Temperature

    P

Vibration

    E

Limb position

    E

Simple touch:

   Detection

      Neither

   Alteration of subjective experience

      Both

## CYCLE 7-4

**A.** There would be ipsilateral loss of pain and temperature sensation in the face, due to involvement of the spinal nucleus and tract of CN V, and contralateral loss of pain and temperature sensation in the body, due to involvement of the lateral spinothalamic tract. This "crossed" pattern of neurologic abnormalities is a common marker of brainstem lesions, which combine damage to sensory or motor nuclei with damage to sensory or motor tracts that cross below the level of the injury.

**B.** Clearly she has evidence of impaired function in V1 and V2. The complete absence of any other neurologic abnormalities suggests that the lesion is outside the brainstem. The fact that both V1 and V2 are involved indicates that the lesion must be involving the trigeminal nerve in that portion of its course where these two divisions are juxtaposed, i.e., the subarachnoid or cavernous sinus portions of the nerve. The severe headache implicates the meninges and, thus, the cavernous sinus portion of the nerve. Direct neural damage does cause pain, but it is usually sharp, stabbing, burning, or searing in quality. Boring or aching pain points to meninges. The most likely cause in this case is metastatic cancer. It might or might not show up on an MRI scan at this early stage. However, the line of logic we have pursued here would lead to prompt and effective treatment with radiation therapy.

## CYCLE 7-7

**A.** See Table 7-5.

### TABLE 7-5

| Drug | Site/Mechanism of Action |
| --- | --- |
| Doxepin | Stimulates inhibitory interneurons in the dorsal horn by potentiating descending serotonergic and noradrenergic transmission from the ventromedial medulla and the DLPT, respectively. |
| | Promotes sleep, treats depression by potentiating cerebral serotonergic activity. |
| Morphine sulfate | Potentiates transmission from the periaqueductal gray to the ventromedial medulla. |
| | Emulates activity of inhibitory enkephalinergic neurons in the dorsal horn. |
| | Produces presynaptic inhibition of nociceptive C fiber terminals by binding to $\mu$-opioid and dynorphin receptors. |
| | Binds to opioid receptors in the limbic system (amygdala, nucleus accumbens), ameliorating suffering. |
| Carbamazepine | Reduces ectopic impulse generation at sites of injury in peripheral nerves and in the central nervous system by binding to the inactivated conformation of voltage-sensitive sodium channels. |
| Clonidine | Inhibits spinothalamic tract neurons in the dorsal horn. |
| | May produce presynaptic inhibition of nociceptive C fiber terminals by binding to $\alpha_2$ receptors. |
| | May benefit sympathetically mediated pain by binding to presynaptic $\alpha_2$ receptors and thereby reducing release of norepinephrine. |

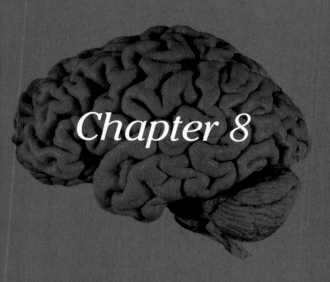

*Chapter 8*

# CRANIAL NERVES AND
# BRAINSTEM ORGANIZATION

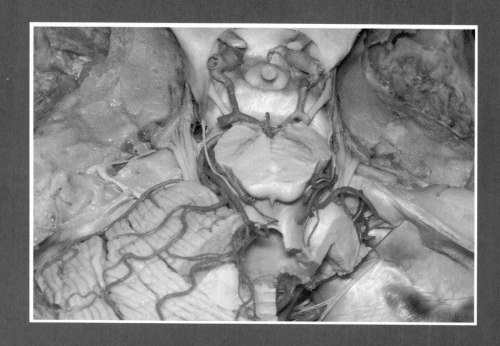

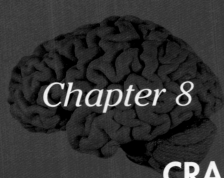

# Chapter 8

# CRANIAL NERVES AND BRAINSTEM ORGANIZATION

The importance of the functions of cranial nerves speaks for itself: vision, hearing, smell, the capacity to move our eyes at will and maintain stable vision during rapid body movement, feeling and pain in the face and head, chewing, the nuances of facial expression, speaking, swallowing, and head movement. For the neurologist and neurosurgeon, however, cranial nerve function takes on additional significance. Cranial nerves and their controlling pathways span the extent of the cerebrum and brainstem. For this reason, the pattern of cranial nerve dysfunction, in conjunction with the pattern of sensory and motor impairment, is invaluable in localizing lesions within the cranium. The cranial nerve examination provides a highly effective means for interrogating the brain and brainstem in order to localize lesions, and indirectly, draw conclusions about the nature of the pathologic processes causing them.

In Motor Systems (Chapter 6), we discussed the localizing value provided by a combination of lower motor neuron and upper motor neuron ("long tract") signs. For example, the presence of hyporeflexia in the right biceps and brachioradialis, evidence of a C5-C6 lower motor neuron lesion, and hyper-reflexia in the triceps, knee, and ankle deep tendon reflexes on the right, absolutely localizes the lesion to the right C5-C6 spinal cord region, just as certainly as designating the junction of two highways pinpoints an accident to a particular intersection. This principle applies equally to cranial nerves and, within the brainstem, is just as useful in pinpointing lesions. Thus, the presence of a facial palsy (cranial nerve [CN] VII) on the right side in conjunction with loss of pain and temperature sensation over the contralateral body absolutely pinpoints the lesion to the right dorsolateral pontomedullary junction.

As we shall see, even pure lower motor neuron or pure upper motor neuron cranial nerve deficits have considerable localizing value, because, unlike sensory and motor pathways in the spinal cord and peripheral nerves, both the supranuclear and infranuclear pathways of cranial nerves are relatively short. For example, inability to voluntarily direct the eyes to the right (a supranuclear eye movement disorder) in a person with a right hemiparesis tells us the lesion must be rostral to the pontomesencephalic junction. The presence of paralysis of one half of the face in the absence of any evidence of sensory or motor tract damage tells us the lesion must be between the cerebellopontine angle and the region within the parotid gland where the facial nerve fibers disperse to supply the muscles of facial expression.

In the course of this brief introduction, it should have become obvious that cranial nerve signs are best interpreted in the context of the clinicopathologic "company" they keep. This interpretation requires an understanding of the geography of the brainstem—the second major topic of this chapter.

In this chapter, we will review cranial nerves I, III, IV, V (motor component), VI, VII, IX, X, XI, and XII. The sensory components of cranial nerve V were discussed in Somesthesis (Chapter 7). Cranial nerves II and VIII will be considered in the following two chapters (Chapters 9 and 10).

**Cranial Nerves and Brainstem Organization**

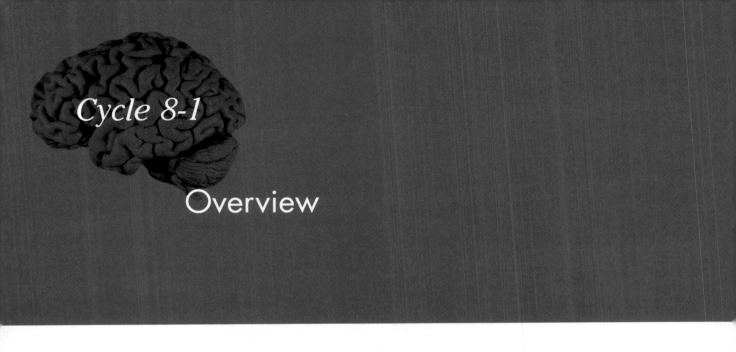

# Cycle 8-1

## Overview

**Objectives**

1. On a drawing of the ventral brainstem, be able to indicate the points of emergence of CN III and V through XII.

2. On axial sections of the brainstem, be able to identify the corticospinal tract, lateral spinothalamic tract, medial lemniscus, and the mesencephalic, chief sensory, and spinal nucleus and tract of CN V (trigeminal nerve).

3. By the end of the chapter, be able to draw from memory the three most representative and clinically most important axial sections of the brainstem—those of CN III, VI-VII, and VIII-IX.

One of our major goals in this chapter will be to enable you to develop a three-dimensional conceptualization of the cranial nerve nuclei, their relationship to ascending and descending tracts in the brainstem, and their peripheral trajectories. We begin with what is already familiar to you: the points of emergence of the cranial nerves in the brainstem (Fig. 8-1) and the points of egress of the cranial nerves in the base of the skull (Fig. 8-2). Figure 8-3 depicts the levels of axial sections to which we will refer repeatedly in this chapter in our exploration of the brainstem, and Figure 8-4 displays these axial sections. At this point, you can view these sections as the objectives of this chapter—what we hope you will understand thoroughly by the chapter's conclusion.

*Text continued on p. 370*

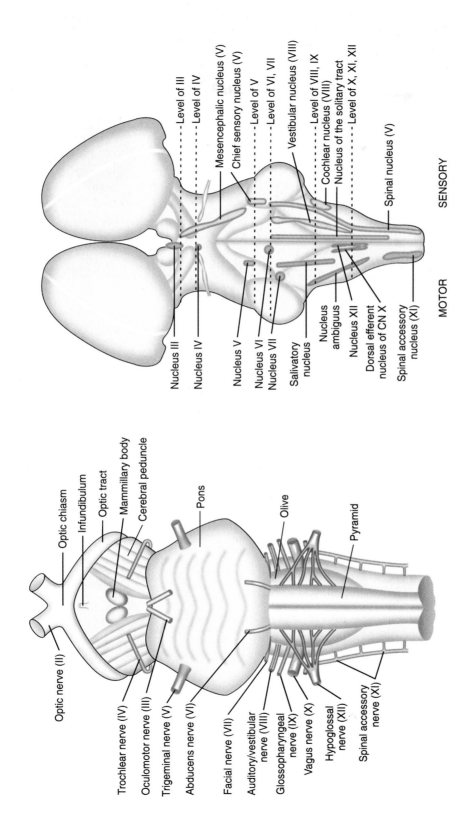

**Figure 8-1** Emergence of the cranial nerves from the brain (*left*), with the location of the nuclei in the brainstem (*right*).

Left figure labels:

Optic nerve (II)
Optic chiasm
Infundibulum
Optic tract
Mammillary body
Cerebral peduncle
Pons
Olive
Pyramid
Trochlear nerve (IV)
Oculomotor nerve (III)
Trigeminal nerve (V)
Abducens nerve (VI)
Facial nerve (VII)
Auditory/vestibular nerve (VIII)
Glossopharyngeal nerve (IX)
Vagus nerve (X)
Hypoglossal nerve (XII)
Spinal accessory nerve (XI)

Right figure labels:

Level of III
Level of IV
Mesencephalic nucleus (V)
Chief sensory nucleus (V)
Level of V
Level of VI, VII
Vestibular nucleus (VIII)
Level of VIII, IX
Cochlear nucleus (VIII)
Nucleus of the solitary tract
Level of X, XI, XII
Spinal nucleus (V)

Nucleus III
Nucleus IV
Nucleus V
Nucleus VI
Nucleus VII
Salivatory nucleus
Nucleus ambiguus
Nucleus XII
Dorsal efferent nucleus of CN X
Spinal accessory nucleus (XI)

MOTOR    SENSORY

**Cranial Nerves and Brainstem Organization**

363

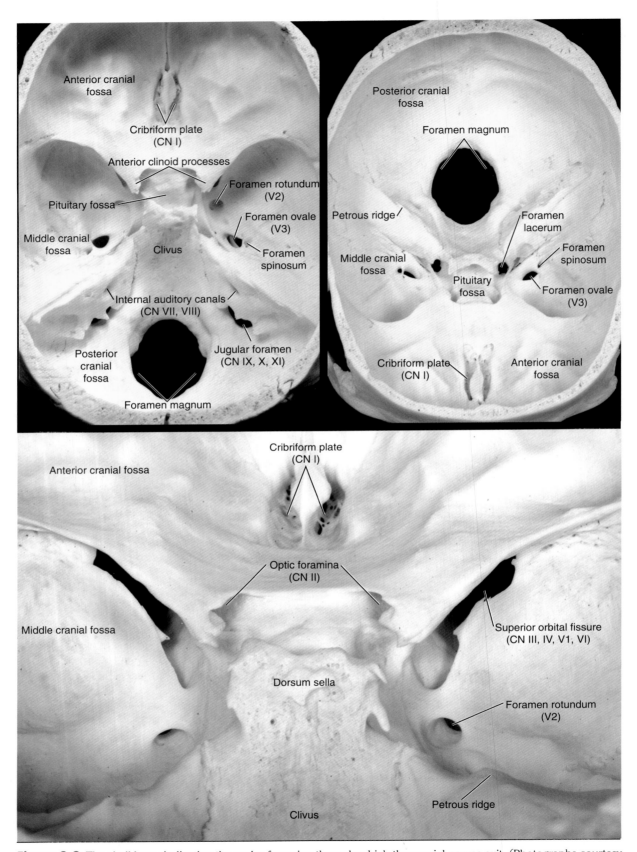

**Figure 8-2** The skull base, indicating the major foramina through which the cranial nerves exit. (Photographs courtesy of Greg Westlye.)

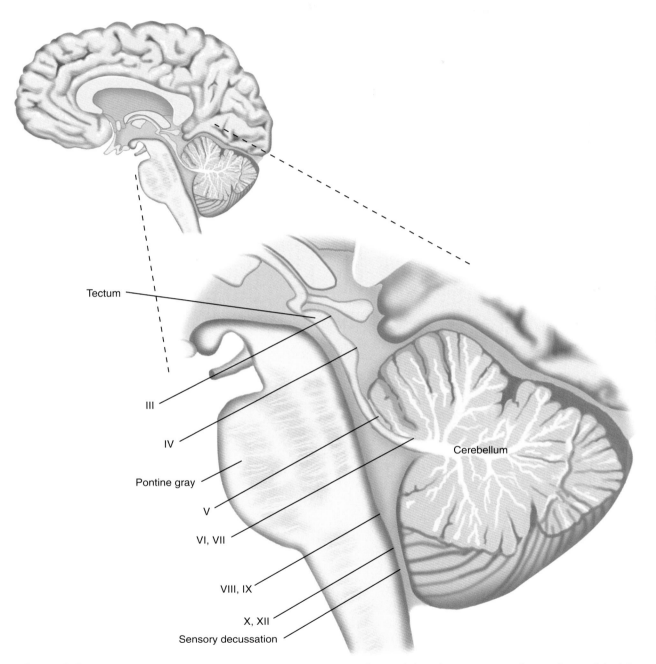

**Figure 8-3** Sagittal section of the brainstem, showing the levels of the axial sections corresponding to the nuclei of the cranial nerves (indicated by roman numerals).

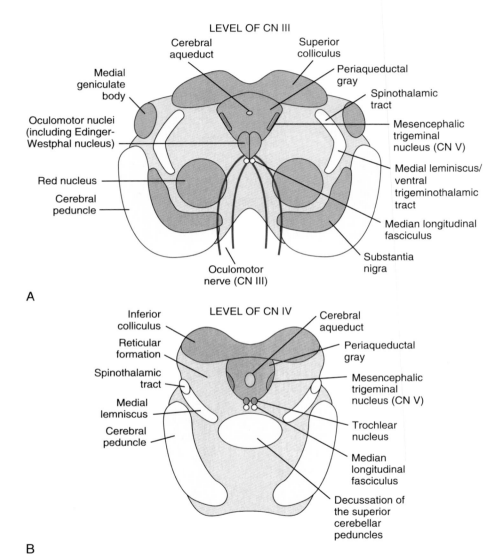

**Figure 8-4** Axial sections at the levels of the cranial nerve nuclei indicated in Figures 8-1 and 8-3. *A,* Level of CN III. *B,* Level of CN IV. *C,* Level of CN V. *D,* Level of CN VI-VII. *E,* Level of CN VIII-IX. *F,* Level of CN X-XI. *G,* Sensory decussation. *H,* Motor decussation.

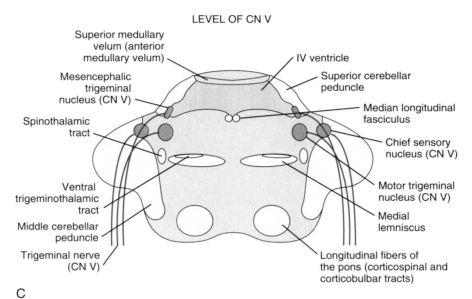

**LEVEL OF CN V**

Superior medullary velum (anterior medullary velum)

Mesencephalic trigeminal nucleus (CN V)

Spinothalamic tract

Ventral trigeminothalamic tract

Middle cerebellar peduncle

Trigeminal nerve (CN V)

IV ventricle

Superior cerebellar peduncle

Median longitudinal fasciculus

Chief sensory nucleus (CN V)

Motor trigeminal nucleus (CN V)

Medial lemniscus

Longitudinal fibers of the pons (corticospinal and corticobulbar tracts)

C

**LEVEL OF CN VI, VII**

Abducens nucleus (CN VI)

Superior cerebellar peduncle

Median longitudinal fasciculus

Nucleus solitarius

Salivatory nucleus

Motor nucleus (CN VII)

Ventral trigeminothalamic tract

Facial nerve (CN VII)

Longitudinal fibers of the pons (corticospinal and corticobulbar tracts)

IV ventricle

Facial colliculus

Vestibular nuclei (CN VIII)

Spinal trigeminal nucleus and tract (CN V)

Middle cerebellar peduncle

Spinothalamic tract

Medial lemniscus

Abducens nerve (CN VI)

D

**Figure 8-4**, cont'd

Cranial Nerves and Brainstem Organization

*Continued*

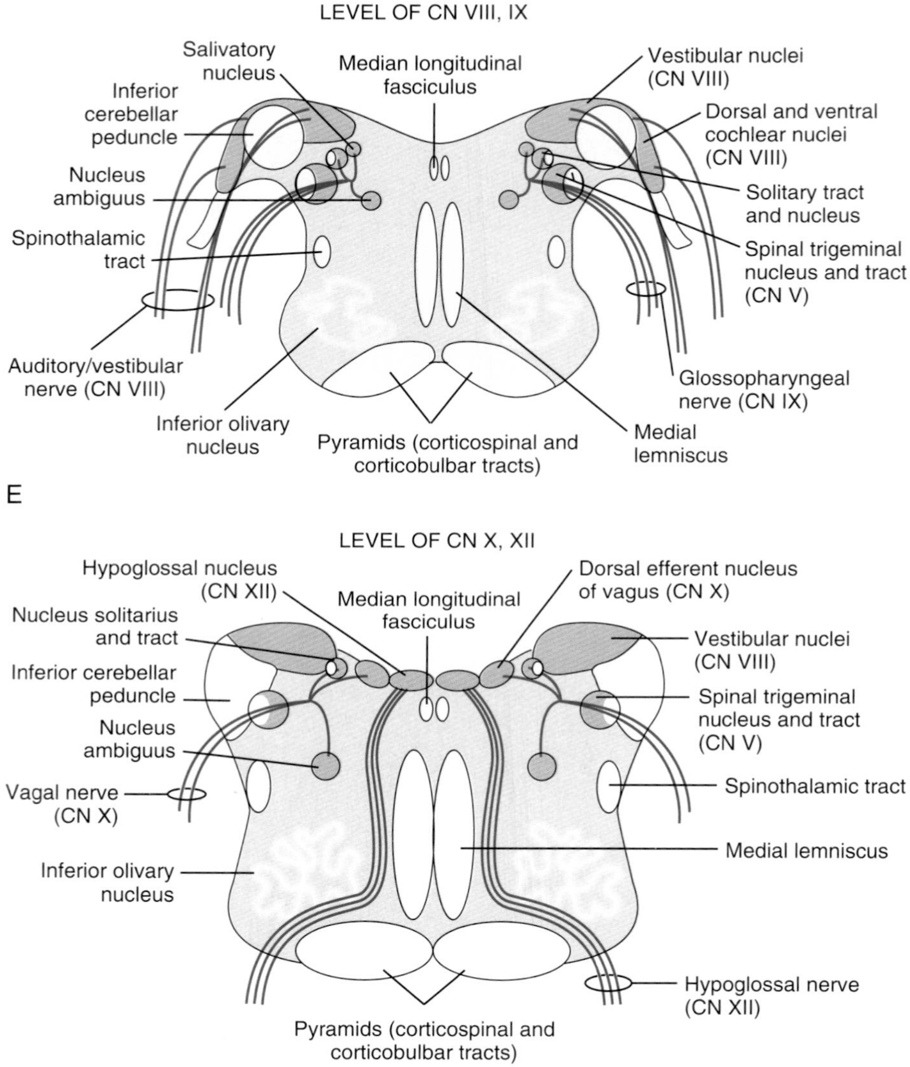

LEVEL OF CN VIII, IX

E

LEVEL OF CN X, XII

**Figure 8-4**, cont'd

SENSORY DECUSSATION

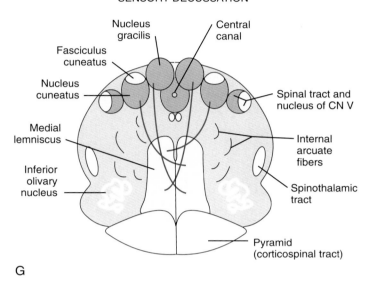

MOTOR DECUSSATION

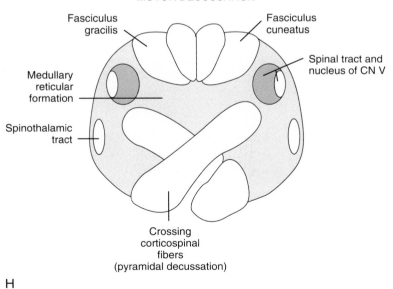

**Figure 8-4**, cont'd

## PRACTICE 8-1

On the following sections, identify the corticospinal tract, lateral spinothalamic tract, medial lemniscus, and the mesencephalic, chief sensory, and spinal nucleus and tract of CN V.

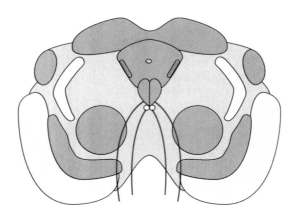
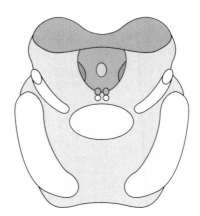
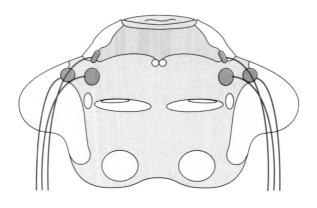
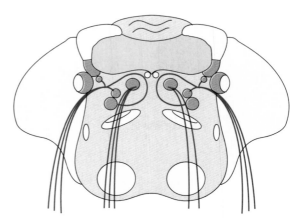

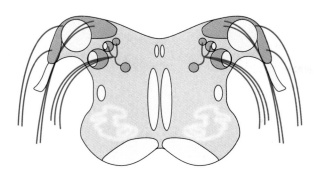

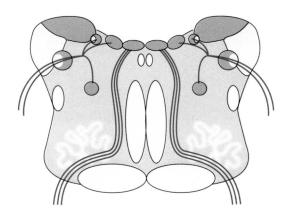

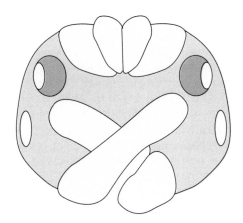

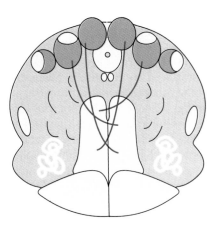

# Cycle 8-2

# Cranial Nerve I

### Objectives

1. Be able to describe the anatomy of the olfactory apparatus from its receptors to its projection targets in the cerebrum.

2. Be able to account for human limitations and proclivities in describing smells in terms of the sites of olfactory projections.

Cranial nerve I subserves the sense of smell. The olfactory receptor cells are located between the cribriform plate and the mucosa in the most rostral portion of the nasopharynx. Cilia on the mucosal end of these neurons extend into the mucosa. These cilia, in aggregate, contain an enormous variety of receptor proteins. Each receptor will generate an action potential when it comes in contact with any one of a broad but specific range of molecules. The particular pattern of firing of the entire population of olfactory epithelial cells (CN I, proper) defines one's olfactory experience at any given moment. The axons of olfactory epithelial cells extend through the cribriform plate and synapse within a complex neural network within the olfactory bulb known as an olfactory glomerulus. Neurons within the glomeruli project backward, along the olfactory tract (Fig. 8-5). Their axons terminate largely in the pyriform cortex overlying the amygdala, the amygdala itself, and portions of the entorhinal cortex overlying the adjacent hippocampus. There are also olfactory projections, via the thalamus, to orbitofrontal cortex, which is involved in defining our goals and plans for action according to our own, internally defined criteria (see Chapter 12).

Sense of smell is probably less important in humans than in any other species. Furthermore, since the advent of high-resolution computed tomographic (CT) and magnetic resonance imaging (MRI), testing of smell is rarely done as part of the neurologic examination. Nevertheless, two aspects of human olfaction are of particular interest. First is our overwhelming sense of smells as either "good" or "bad," a dichotomy that contrasts markedly with our experience of visual, auditory, or somatosensory sensation. The explanation for this phenomenon appears to be quite straightforward: not only are there no olfactory projections to association cortices, which provide the basis for the extraordinarily complex experience of vision, hearing, and touch, but nearly all olfactory projections are to the amygdala or periamygdaloid cortex. The amygdala is one of the most important components of the limbic system, which defines our sense of value (see Chapter 12). This unique direct link between olfactory and limbic systems may also account for the ability of some smells to evoke very vivid memories. The particularly prominent limbic component of memories that can be evoked by smell may provide the basis for the evocation of particularly detailed images via strong activation of sensory association cortices linked with the limbic system.

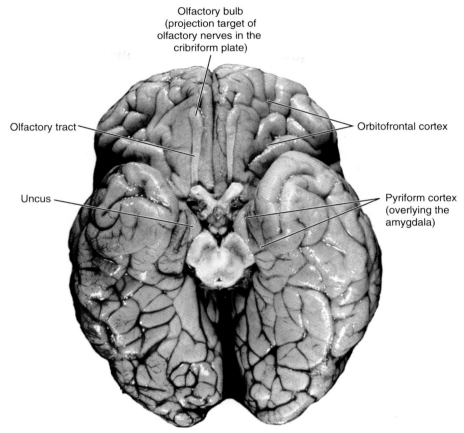

Olfactory bulb
(projection target of
olfactory nerves in the
cribriform plate)

Olfactory tract

Orbitofrontal cortex

Uncus

Pyriform cortex
(overlying the
amygdala)

**Figure 8-5** The olfactory bulb, the projection target of the olfactory nerve (which derives from olfactory epithelial cells in the mucosa of the nasopharynx), the olfactory tract, and its major cerebral sites of termination.

Second, we are remarkably inept at describing smells, resorting almost always to similes to other smells. This phenomenon also probably reflects the lack of olfactory projections to association cortices, projections that would indirectly link them to language cortex.

1. Be able to name and describe the actions of the six extraocular muscles and the levator palpebrae.

2. Be able to define the innervation of the extraocular muscles and levator palpebrae, locate the cranial nerve nuclei supplying them on axial sections of the brainstem, and describe the intra- and extra-axial pathways these nerves take and the consequences of lesions of these nerves.

3. Be able to explain the mechanisms of neural control of pupillary size and lens shape.

4. Be able to account for the particular neurologic importance of a unilateral dilated and unreactive pupil and explain the mechanisms by which this typically occurs.

5. Be able to define Horner's syndrome and explain the mechanism of the two most common lesions causing it.

Cranial nerves III, IV, and VI control the movements of the eyes. Because the function of these three sets of nerves is coordinated by supranuclear mechanisms and they act in tandem, we will consider them together. We will begin with a review of the extraocular muscles and their effects on eye movement. We will then consider the location of the nuclei of CN III, IV, and VI in the brainstem, the anatomic relationship of these nuclei to other brainstem structures, and the trajectory these cranial nerves take in their course to the orbits. Finally, we will review neural control of pupillary size and lens shape. The functions of CN III, IV, and VI are summarized in Table 8-1. We will consider supranuclear control of eye movements in Cycle 8-4.

## A. THE EXTRAOCULAR MUSCLES

Figure 8-6 depicts the location of the four rectus muscles in relation to the eye. The *superior rectus (SR)* elevates (supraducts) the eye when it contracts. The *inferior rectus (IR)* infraducts the eye. Both muscles pull at a slight angle (23 degrees) to the straight-ahead (primary) position of the eye, but for practical purposes, the function of these muscles can be viewed as simply raising and lowering the eye, respectively. The *medial rectus (MR)* rotates the eye medially to adduct the eye. The *lateral rectus (LR)* rotates the eye laterally to abduct. Clinicians often use the expressions "A-D-duct" and "A-B-duct" to make themselves clear.

There are two other muscles, the *superior oblique (SO)* and the *inferior oblique (IO)*, which have somewhat more complicated insertions and actions. The SO originates in the posterior portion of the orbit, like the rectus muscles. However, its tendon passes through a loop in the anterior, superior, medial portion of the orbit, the trochlea (Fig. 8-7), and then travels backward

**TABLE 8-1** Summary of Control of Ocular Movements

| Cranial Nerve | Common Nomenclature | Muscles Innervated | Action on Eye |
|---|---|---|---|
| III | Oculomotor | Superior rectus (SR) | Supraduction |
| | | Inferior rectus (IR) | Infraduction |
| | | Medial rectus (MR) | Adduction |
| | | Inferior oblique (IO) | Extortion |
| | | | Supraduction during extreme adduction |
| | | Levator palpebra | Elevation of upper eyelid |
| | | Pupillary sphincter | Pupillary constriction |
| IV | Trochlear | Superior oblique (SO) | Intortion |
| | | | Infraduction during extreme adduction |
| VI | Abducens | Lateral rectus (LR) | Abduction |

to insert on the posterior, superior portion of the eye. When the eye is looking at the trochlea (i.e., adducted 51 degrees), contraction of the SO pulls the top portion of the eye forward, causing the eye to infraduct (Fig. 8-8). When the eye is abducted 39 degrees, SO contraction produces only internal rotation (intortion) of the eye (Figs. 8-9, 8-10). The inferior oblique (IO), located beneath the eye, has exactly corresponding actions, even though its anatomy is slightly different. There is no trochlea for it to pass through. Instead, it simply originates at the anterior, inferior, medial portion of the orbit, where an inferior trochlea might be located, if there were one. It inserts posteriorly on the inferior, posterior aspect of the eye, in direct homology to the SO. When the eye is adducted 51 degrees, contraction of the IO pulls the inferior aspect of the eye forward, thus supraducting the eye. When the eye is abducted 39 degrees, contraction of the IO produces external rotation (extortion).

The tortional effects of the SO and IO might seem peculiar and unnecessary. However, as we will consider at greater length later in this chapter, the extraocular muscles function not just to direct our eyes where we want them, but also to produce reflexive movements of our eyes that will keep them stable, as if they were controlled by gyroscopes, despite head motions. Head motions include tilt. The tortional effects of the SO and IO serve to compensate for tilt.

One final muscle, the levator palpebra, lifts the upper eyelid. Although it is not an extraocular muscle, it is innervated by CN III, and drooping of the lid *(ptosis)* may be a useful localizing sign.

## B. THE NUCLEI AND TRAJECTORIES OF CRANIAL NERVES III, IV, AND VI

### Cranial Nerve III

Cranial nerve III, the oculomotor nerve, innervates the SR, IR, MR, IO, and the levator palpebra. Within each oculomotor nucleus, a separate subnucleus innervates each of the extraocular muscles. A single subnucleus, shared by the two oculomotor nuclear complexes, innervates both levator palpebrae. The third cranial nerve nuclear complex is located just ventral to the periaqueductal gray in the midbrain (Fig. 8-4, III). Nerve fibers emerge from the entire 1-cm rostrocaudal extent of the CN III nuclear complex and fan out laterally and ventrally through the midbrain tegmentum and the red nuclei, ultimately coursing medially to emerge as rootlets in the interpeduncular fossa. These rootlets immediately coalesce into the two third cranial nerves, which pass through the dura at the posterior roof of the cavernous sinus on either side of the sella turcica. Each third cranial nerve traverses the cavernous sinus and ultimately passes through the superior orbital fissure into the orbit to supply the various muscles.

The dispersion of CN III fibers in the brainstem means that midbrain lesions usually cause partial rather than complete palsies. The proximity of CN III nerve fibers to the cerebral peduncles means that lesions within the brainstem (intra-axial lesions) causing CN III palsies are commonly associated with contralateral hemiparesis. Both phenomena are exemplified in Case 8-1.

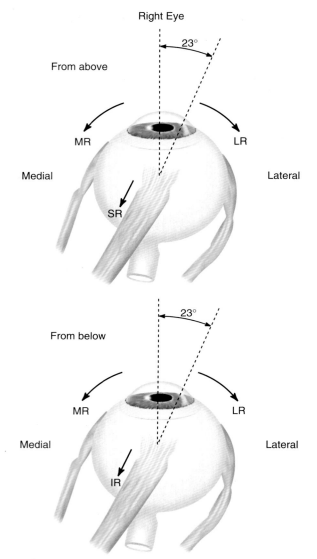

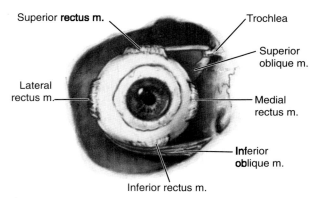

**Figure 8-7** Anterior view of the orbit showing the trochlea. (Modified from Poxanas MT, Anderson RL. Extraocular muscles. In: Clinical Orbital Anatomy. Baltimore, Williams & Wilkins, 1984. Reproduced with permission of Lippincott Williams and Wilkins.)

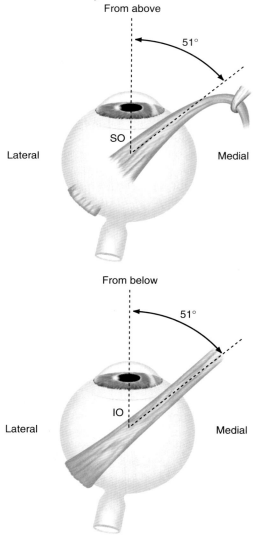

**Figure 8-6** Insertion of the rectus muscles on the right eye, viewed from above and below. The eyes in this figure are directed straight ahead (the primary position of gaze). The angles in this and subsequent figures refer to angular deviation from the primary position. MR, medial rectus; LR, lateral rectus; SR, superior rectus; IR, inferior rectus.

**Figure 8-8** Combined infraduction/intortion of the right eye by the superior oblique muscle (*top*) and supraduction/extortion of the eye by the inferior oblique muscle (*bottom*).

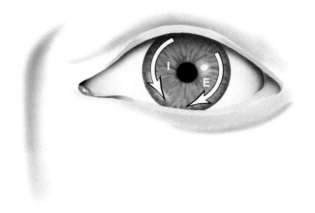

**Figure 8-9** An eye in the primary position of gaze, arrows illustrating intortion (I) and extortion (E).

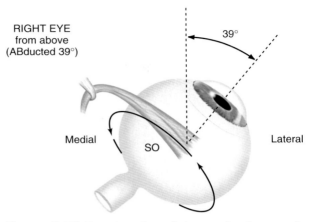

**Figure 8-10** Pure intortion of the eye by the superior oblique muscle.

## Case 8-1

### Carcinoma Metastatic to Midbrain

*A 65-year-old man with a lifelong history of heavy smoking presents with a 2-week history of progressive left-sided weakness and incoordination and double vision. On examination, there is severe ptosis on the right. Supraduction of the right eye is severely impaired, adduction is limited to approximately 10 degrees, and infraduction is nearly normal (Fig. 8-11). The pupils are equal and react symmetrically to light. He has mild to moderate left-sided weakness, worse in the arm, substantial loss of fine motor movement in the left hand, severe pronation drift on the left, left-sided hyper-reflexia, and a left Babinski sign. An MRI scan reveals a 1-cm diameter, contrast-enhancing mass involving the right midbrain tegmentum and cerebral peduncle (Fig. 8-12). A chest x-ray reveals a 6-cm diameter hilar mass in the left lung.*

**Comment:** *This unfortunate gentleman has carcinoma of the lung that has metastasized to the right midbrain, damaging some of the CN III fibers on their way to the interpeduncular fossa, as well as descending motor pathways in the right cerebral peduncle. The enhancement with contrast reflects the fact that in brain tumors in general and metastases in particular, there is breakdown of the blood-brain barrier, which allows the contrast material (gadolinium in an MRI) to leak into the brain parenchyma, where it appears white on the images. This man has what is known as Weber's syndrome, after the neurologist who first described this clinical picture at the turn of the twentieth century in a patient with a small hemorrhage into the cerebral peduncle.*

## Cranial Nerve IV

Cranial nerve IV supplies only the SO, and for this reason it is often referred to as the trochlear nerve. The nucleus of CN IV is also located at the ventral aspect of the periaqueductal gray, somewhat caudal to the third nerve nuclear complex (Fig. 8-4, IV). The fourth cranial nerves take an extraordinary course, passing dorsally from the nuclei, around the periaqueductal gray and through caudal margins of the inferior colliculi, where they cross to emerge on the dorsal aspect of the brainstem (the only cranial nerve to do so). They then travel around the midbrain, in the sulcus formed by the junction of the midbrain and the cerebellum, to enter the dura of the posterior aspect of the cavernous sinuses. These nerves pass through the cavernous sinuses and enter the orbits via the superior orbital fissures, like the third cranial nerves. For poorly understood reasons, perhaps the minuteness of the nerve, perhaps its long circuitous course, the fourth cranial nerve is particularly susceptible to damage by trauma (Case 8-2).

## Case 8-2

### Traumatic CN IV Palsy

*A 25-year-old woman was involved in an automobile accident. She was not wearing her seatbelt and in the course of the accident, her head smashed into the windshield. She lost consciousness but was awake and alert by the time she arrived at the emergency room. Although she complained of double vision, emergency room physicians were unable to find any neurologic abnormalities, and a CT scan of the head*

*Continued*

1    2

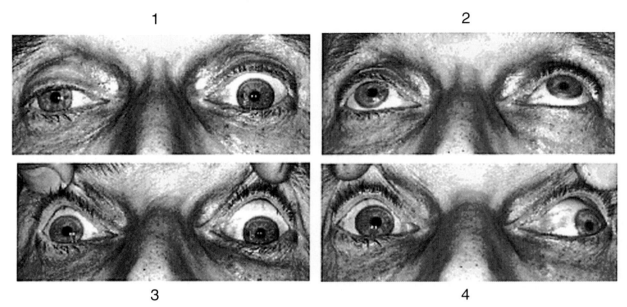

3    4

**Figure 8-11** Ocular examination in Case 8-1: (1) Primary position; (2) upgaze; (3) downgaze; and (4) left gaze. (From Warner JJ, Atlas of Neuroanatomy. Boston, Butterworth Heinemann, 2001, with permission from Elsevier Science.)

### Case 8-2—cont'd

was normal. She was discharged from the hospital after an overnight stay. When seen in a neurology clinic a month later, she felt she had completely recovered except for persistent, albeit fluctuating, double vision. The double vision was described as vertical, and it subsided if she covered one eye (i.e., it was "binocular"). On examination, she tends to sit with her head tilted to the right. When directed to visually follow the examiner's finger, all extraocular movements are normal except when she gazes to the right and down. In this position, there is defective infraduction of the left eye (Fig. 8-13). The remainder of her neurologic examination is normal.

**Comment:** This patient has a left fourth cranial nerve palsy. As she looks to the right, the left eye adducts into the position at which it is directed straight at the trochlea. In this position, the left CN IV, via the left SO, serves only to infraduct the eye. Thus, this is the position at which the left CN IV palsy becomes most evident. In the primary position, infraduction of the left eye can be accomplished by the left IR, innervated by CN III. Hence her otherwise normal extraocular movements. The left CN IV palsy also allows the left eye to extort (rotate counterclockwise from her perspective). She tilts her head to the right (rotates

### Case 8-2—cont'd

it clockwise) to compensate for this. The excessive clockwise rotation of the right eye produced by this head tilt is reflexively corrected by intortion of the right eye, achieved by supranuclear brainstem mechanisms that align the two eyes about their axes. The fact that the remainder of her neurologic

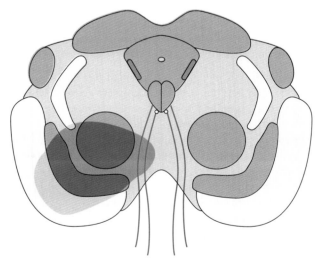

**Figure 8-12** Drawing of axial section through the midbrain, diagramming the lesion in Case 8-1.

## Case 8-2—cont'd

*examination is completely normal gives us some assurance that the lesion is outside the brainstem (i.e., extra-axial), involving the fourth cranial nerve in its peripheral course.*

## Cranial Nerve VI

CN VI innervates but a single muscle, the LR. Because the LR abducts the eye, CN VI is often referred to as the abducens nerve. The nuclei of CN VI are located near the midline in the caudal pontine tegmentum, just below the floor of the fourth ventricle. In a very peculiar arrangement, the fibers of the facial nerve (CN VII, the nucleus of which is located ventral and lateral to the nucleus of CN VI) (Fig. 8-4, VI, VII), loop over the nucleus of CN VI before coursing ventrolaterally to exit the brainstem. The masses of the abducens nuclei, in conjunction with the arching fibers of the facial nerve, produce the bumps on the floor of the fourth ventricle known as the facial colliculi. The sixth cranial nerves course ventrally, through the pontine tegmentum and the basis pontis, to exit near the midline at the pontomedullary junction (see Fig. 8-1). From here CN VI passes forward and slightly rostrally to enter the floor of the cavernous sinus via a passageway through the dura and abutting the apex of the petrous bone known as Dorello's canal. CN VI then pass through the cavernous sinus, with CN III, IV, and V1 (Fig. 8-14), to enter the superior orbital fissure.

Possibly because of the very short distance between the egress point of CN VI at the pontomedullary junction and its entry into Dorello's canal, it is particularly susceptible to the effects of increased intracranial pressure, which tends to push the entire brainstem caudally (central herniation), stretching this nerve (Case 8-3).

## Case 8-3

**Increased Intracranial Pressure due to Posterior Fossa Tumor with Hydrocephalus**

*A 9-year-old girl is brought to a pediatrician by her parents because of a several-month history of progressive clumsiness and imbalance and a 1-week history of diplopia. On examination, she is able to abduct either eye only partially, and as she attempts*

## Case 8-3—cont'd

*to look straight ahead, both eyes tend to deviate medially (Fig. 8-15). She also has evidence of papilledema (edema of the optic nerve heads due to increased intracranial pressure), some incoordination of the right arm, a slightly wide-based gait with a tendency to fall to the right, generalized hyper-reflexia, and bilateral Babinski signs. An MRI scan reveals a large, contrast-enhancing mass in the right cerebellar hemisphere that compresses the fourth ventricle to the extent that it interferes with the flow of cerebrospinal fluid, causing enlargement of the lateral and third ventricles (hydrocephalus). A neurosurgeon resects the tumor, which proves to be a pilocytic astrocytoma.*

**Comment:** *Obstruction of the flow of cerebrospinal fluid with secondary hydrocephalus is a common occurrence with posterior fossa tumors. In this case, the marked increase in the volume of supratentorial contents (brain and cerebrospinal fluid) produced downward pressure on the brainstem. This in turn produced traction on the sixth cranial nerves at their point of entry into Dorello's canals. The pressure of the expanded ventricles on descending corticobulbar pathways destined for the pontine and medullary reticulospinal systems caused hyper-reflexia and Babinski signs. Pressure on the descending corticospinal tracts caused lower extremity incoordination. The direct effects of the tumor mass on the right cerebellar hemisphere and the midline cerebellum were responsible for the incoordination of the right arm and contributed to the gait instability. Compression of the brainstem by the tumor may also have contributed to neurologic abnormalities in the legs. With expert surgery, the prognosis in a patient with this type of tumor is quite good.*

## C. NEURAL CONTROL OF PUPILLARY SIZE

Two muscles within the iris control the size of the pupil: the *pupillary sphincter* and the *pupillary dilator*. The pupillary sphincter is innervated by parasympathetic fibers and the pupillary dilator by sympathetic fibers.

### Parasympathetic Innervation

Parasympathetic fibers controlling the pupillary sphincter originate within a ventral subnucleus of the third

Right

Left

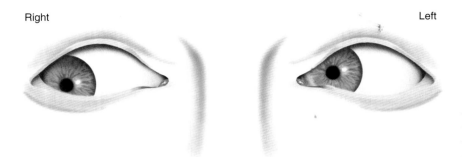

**Figure 8-13** Drawing of eye positions of patient in Case 8-2 during gaze to the right and down, demonstrating the impaired infraduction of the left eye.

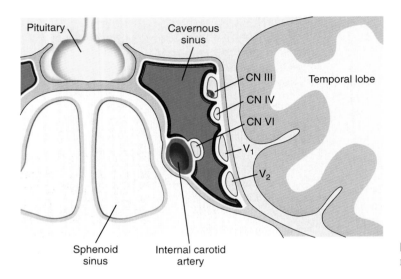

Pituitary

Cavernous sinus

CN III

CN IV

CN VI

V₁

V₂

Temporal lobe

Sphenoid sinus

Internal carotid artery

**Figure 8-14** Anteroposterior view of the cranial nerves passing through the cavernous sinus.

Right

Left

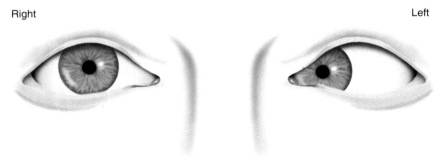

Right

Left

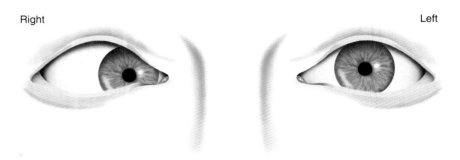

**Figure 8-15** Eye positions of patient in Case 8-3 during right gaze (*top*) and left gaze (*bottom*), demonstrating bilaterally impaired abduction.

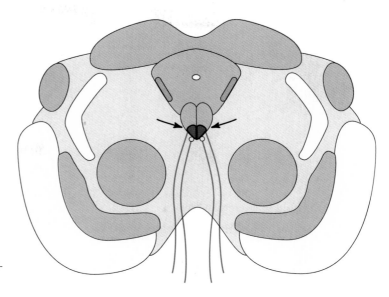

**Figure 8-16** Drawing of axial section of the mid-brain showing the Edinger-Westphal nuclei.

nerve nuclear complex, the preganglionic Edinger-Westphal nucleus (Fig. 8-16). Preganglionic fibers from the *Edinger-Westphal nucleus* coalesce with other CN III fibers in the interpeduncular fossa and follow CN III all the way into the orbit, where they synapse in the postganglionic ciliary ganglion. Postganglionic neurons in the ciliary ganglion then innervate the pupillary sphincter.

Lesions of the third cranial nerve that involve the fibers innervating the pupillary sphincter result in pupillary dilatation and impairment in pupillary constriction in response to a bright light or looking at near objects. The fibers from the Edinger-Westphal nucleus travel in the very outer margin of the third cranial nerve, in its dorsal, medial aspect. They are particularly vulnerable to compression in this location, as illustrated in Cases 8-4 and 8-5.

---

## Case 8-4

### Aneurysmal Subarachnoid Hemorrhage

*A 35-year-old man suddenly develops a very severe headache. He is brought by family members to the emergency room. Other than mild neck stiffness, his examination is most remarkable for a widely dilated right pupil that does not constrict when a bright light is shone in it (Fig. 8-17), and some impairment in supra-, infra-, and adduction of the right eye. An emergency CT scan reveals blood in the basal cisterns (Fig. 8-18). A cerebral angiogram demonstrates an intracranial aneurysm at the junction of the right internal carotid and posterior communicating arteries (Fig. 8-19).*

**Comment:** *Figure 8-20 illustrates the mechanism by which internal carotid—posterior communicating artery junction aneurysms cause third cranial nerve palsies as they suddenly expand in the course of rupture. Third cranial nerve compression may cause a complete palsy or a partial palsy with severe involvement of the pupil, as in this case. In any event, the pupil is consistently involved. Thus, pupillary dilatation of acute onset always suggests an internal carotid—posterior communicating artery junction aneurysm until proved otherwise. The very high case fatality rate associated with aneurysmal ruptures mandates immediate neurosurgical intervention in these cases.*

Cranial Nerves and Brainstem Organization

Right                                                                                              Left

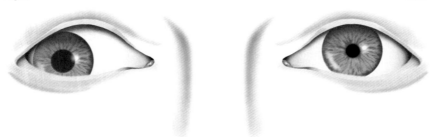

**Figure 8-17** Drawing of eyes of patient in Case 8-4, demonstrating dilatation (mydriasis) of the right eye and slight downward and outward deviation of the eye due to the unopposed action of the lateral rectus and superior oblique muscles.

Temporal lobe

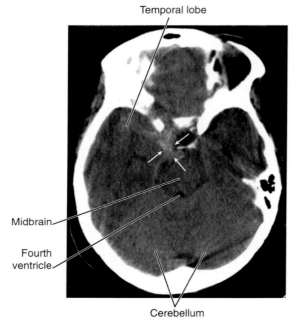

Midbrain

Fourth
ventricle

Cerebellum

**Figure 8-18** Computed tomographic (CT) scan of the head of patient in Case 8-4, revealing blood (*arrows*) in the basal cisterns (the cerebrospinal fluid filled spaces at the base of the brain). Extravascular blood reliably has high signal on CT scans, imaging as white.

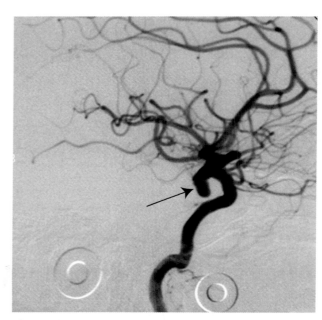

**Figure 8-19** Cerebral angiogram of patient in Case 8-4, revealing an aneurysm at the junction of the right internal carotid and posterior communicating arteries.

## Case 8-5

### Subdural Hematoma with Herniation

*A 55-year-old man, driving while intoxicated and not wearing a seat belt, is involved in a high-speed collision. He is comatose when he arrives at the emergency room. His left eye is deviated down and out and the pupil is widely dilated and poorly responsive to light. Painful sternal rub elicits decorticate posturing on the right. An emergency CT scan reveals a large, acute left subdural hematoma and both uncal and* central herniation (Fig. 8-21; also see Cycle 1-4, Practice B).

**Comment:** *Figure 8-22 illustrates the mechanism of the third cranial nerve palsy in this case. At this stage in the herniation process, death is imminent, and prognosis is guarded even with prompt evacuation of the hematoma. Cases 8-4 and 8-5 serve to illustrate the great diagnostic importance of acute, unilateral pupillary dilation.*

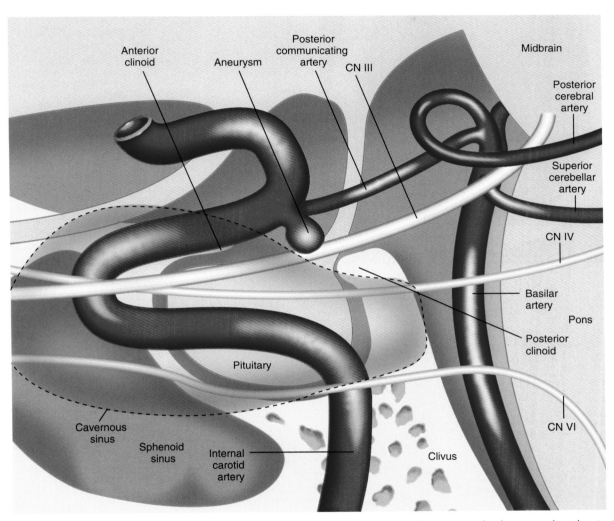

**Figure 8-20** Diagram of the anatomic relationship of the internal carotid—posterior communicating artery junction to the dorsum of the cavernous sinus. Aneurysms at this junction, as depicted here, typically extend downward such that, as they rapidly expand, the aneurysm apex compresses the third cranial nerve at the point where it enters the cavernous sinus and is immobilized. The dorsomedial position of the pupillary fibers renders them especially susceptible to this compressive force.

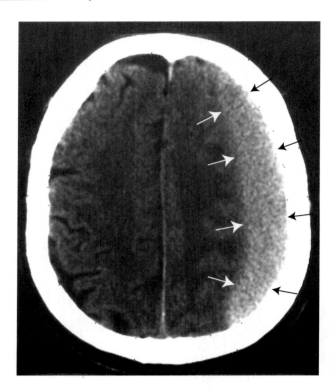

**Figure 8-21** Acute left-sided subdural hematoma (*arrows*) (Case 8-5). The subdural fluid collection appears white on this computed tomographic (CT) scan because of the high blood content. The great mass of the hematoma acts to push the left hemisphere down (central herniation) and to the contralateral side (incipient uncal herniation).

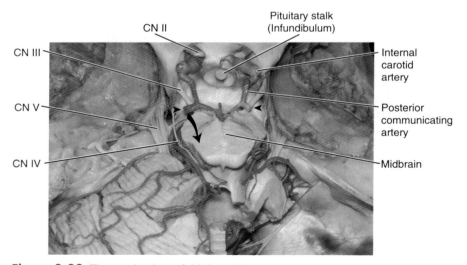

**Figure 8-22** The mechanism of third cranial nerve palsies in cerebral herniation syndromes. In this view from the upper occipital region of the skull, we are looking down at the floor of the middle cranial fossa, the sella turcica, the transected midbrain, and the dorsum of the cerebellum. Note that CN III passes immediately beneath the posterior cerebral artery (*arrowheads*). Herniation due to a large left hemisphere mass will push the brainstem down and tip the midbrain to the left (as indicated by the large arrow over the midbrain). Both proximal posterior cerebral arteries will be pulled down on the dorsal aspect of CN III (where the pupillary fibers pass). However, because of the midbrain tipping, pressure on the left CN III will be greater, and pupillary dilation will appear first on the left—the side of the lesion. (Dissection by Riusai Tanaka, M.D.)

## Sympathetic Innervation

Sympathetic pathways innervating the pupillary dilator take a very long and circuitous course through the brainstem and neck back up into the head and the eye (Fig. 8-23). They also innervate a small muscle in the upper lid, the tarsus, which elevates the upper eyelid, and they innervate sweat glands in a small patch of skin above the eyebrow.

The sympathetic pathway originates in the lateral hypothalamus. A multisynaptic pathway descends from the hypothalamus through the dorsolateral quadrant of the brainstem all the way down to the T1 level of the spinal cord. Here, descending sympathetic axons synapse on cells within the intermediate zone of the spinal cord. Preganglionic cells in the intermediate zone send their axons out the ventral root into the paravertebral chain ganglia. The axons ascend the chain, ultimately to synapse on cells in the superior cervical ganglion, high in the anterior triangle of the neck. The axons of neurons in the superior cervical ganglion then accompany the internal carotid artery all the way up into the cavernous sinus, where they then join V1 in its course into the orbit. There they variously innervate the pupillary dilator, the tarsus muscle, and sweat glands in the skin above the brow. This long, meandering pathway renders these sympathetic fibers vulnerable to damage at a number of locations. The most common and most serious is at the point where the intermediate zone preganglionic cell projections pass out with the ventral root at T1 and join the vertebral chain ganglia (Case 8-6).

---

### Case 8-6

#### Oculosympathetic Paresis due to Tumor of Lung Apex

*A 60-year-old man with a 45-year history of smoking three packs of cigarettes a day consults his physician because of a 50-pound weight loss over the prior 6 months. She notes a rather cachectic looking gentleman with moderate ptosis (drooping) of the right lid and mild constriction of the right pupil (miosis) that is most conspicuous in dim light. She immediately orders a chest x-ray, which reveals a 10-cm diameter mass in the right pulmonary apex.*

**Comment:** *This patient has lung cancer, which is damaging the sympathetic pathway to the orbit where it exits the T1 ventral root to enter the chain of*

---

### Case 8-6—cont'd

*paravertebral sympathetic ganglia. The combination of eyelid ptosis, pupillary miosis, and loss of sweating over the brow (anhydrosis) defines Horner's syndrome. The ptosis is much less severe than that seen with CN III lesions. The miosis is best seen in dim light because this elicits maximal sympathetic pupillary tone, thus maximizing the difference between the normal pupil and the denervated pupil. This case illustrates the potentially ominous significance of Horner's syndrome.*

## D. NEURAL CONTROL OF LENS SHAPE

Cells in the ciliary ganglion, supplied by parasympathetic fibers from the Edinger-Westphal nucleus, also innervate the ciliary muscle. Contraction of the ciliary muscle releases tension on the lens, allowing it to assume the more nearly spherical shape necessary to focus on near objects (*accommodate*). The administration of high doses of anticholinergic (antimuscarinic) drugs may compromise this function, as illustrated in Case 8-7.

---

### Case 8-7

#### Inability to Focus due to Anticholinergic Drugs

*A 23-year-old man is admitted to the psychiatry inpatient service because of the development of paranoid schizophrenia. He is treated with high doses of a neuroleptic drug, chlorpromazine (Thorazine), and an anticholinergic drug, trihexyphenidyl (Artane). As his acute psychosis subsides, he finds he is unable to read unless he holds printed material at arm's length. On examination, his pupils are 5 mm in diameter and sluggishly reactive. His visual acuity at 3 ft is normal but declines to 20/100 at 1 ft.*

**Comment:** *Chlorpromazine is a potent $D_2$-dopamine receptor blocker. Its therapeutic effects are mediated by blockade of transmission in the mesolimbic dopamine pathway (see Chapter 12). Unfortunately, its effects are not limited to this pathway, and it typically produces significant Parkinsonian symptoms by blocking dopaminergic transmission in nigrostriatal pathways. To combat these symptoms, patients given*

Continued

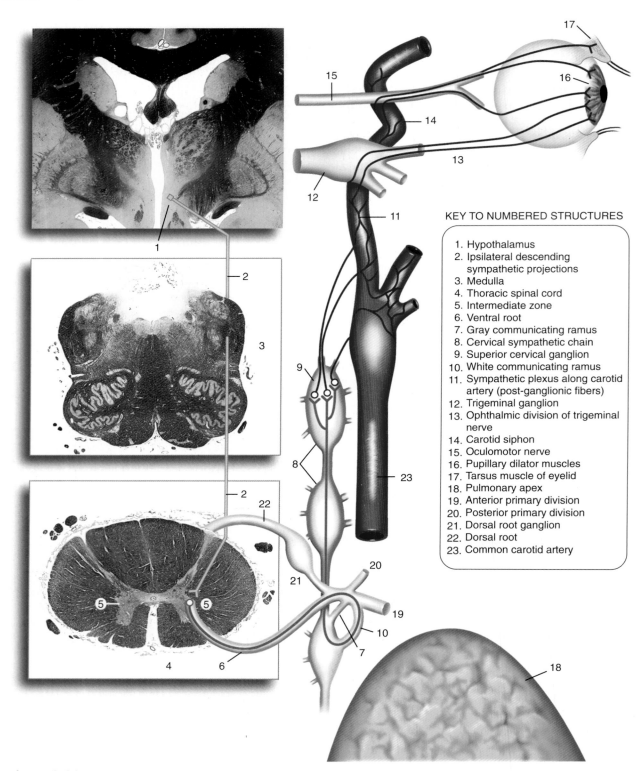

KEY TO NUMBERED STRUCTURES

1. Hypothalamus
2. Ipsilateral descending sympathetic projections
3. Medulla
4. Thoracic spinal cord
5. Intermediate zone
6. Ventral root
7. Gray communicating ramus
8. Cervical sympathetic chain
9. Superior cervical ganglion
10. White communicating ramus
11. Sympathetic plexus along carotid artery (post-ganglionic fibers)
12. Trigeminal ganglion
13. Ophthalmic division of trigeminal nerve
14. Carotid siphon
15. Oculomotor nerve
16. Pupillary dilator muscles
17. Tarsus muscle of eyelid
18. Pulmonary apex
19. Anterior primary division
20. Posterior primary division
21. Dorsal root ganglion
22. Dorsal root
23. Common carotid artery

**Figure 8-23** Pathway of sympathetic fibers to the pupillary dilator and adjacent structures. (Modified from Warner JJ, Atlas of Neuroanatomy. Boston, Butterworth Heinemann, 2001, with permission from Elsevier Science.)

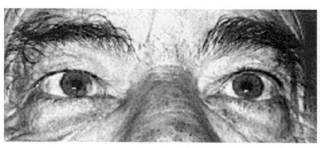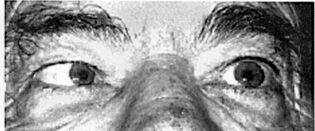

**Figure 8-24** Practice 8-3E. (From Warner JJ, Atlas of Neuroanatomy. Boston, Butterworth Heinemann, 2001, with permission from Elsevier Science.)

### Case 8-7—cont'd

*chlorpromazine and other similarly acting neuroleptic drugs are commonly also given anticholinergic drugs, such as trihexyphenidyl, which have modest anti-Parkinsonian effects—in fact, they were the mainstay of treatment of Parkinson's disease before levodopa became available in the late 1960s. Chlorpromazine is also a very potent anticholinergic drug. Thus, this patient is receiving high doses of two anticholinergic (antimuscarinic) medications. The result is impairment in both pupillary constriction and rounding up of the lens during near vision; hence his difficulty reading. More modern neuroleptic agents, such as risperidone and olanzepine, have minimal anticholinergic effects and very modest Parkinsonian effects.*

## PRACTICE 8-3

**A.** A 70-year-old woman with insulin-dependent diabetes develops otitis externa, an infection of the external auditory canal, in the right ear. Her family physician treats the infection with topical antibiotics instilled into the ear. The infection continues to fester and the patient increasingly complains of right-sided headache and generally feeling unwell. She subsequently develops severe boring pain maximal in the right maxillary and mandibular regions. When she develops double vision, her physician refers her to a neurologist. He notes complete inability to abduct the right eye and reduced sensation for all modalities in the right V2 and V3 distributions. The remainder of the neurologic examination is normal. Localize the lesion.

**B.** A 75-year-old man with a 20-year history of diabetes awakes one morning with diplopia. On examination, there is severe ptosis on the right and his right eye is tonically deviated down and out. He is unable to supra-, infra-, or adduct the eye. The pupils are equal in size and both constrict briskly in response to a bright light. The remainder of his examination is noteworthy only for loss of sensation for all modalities in his feet and distal legs and missing ankle jerks. Localize the lesion responsible for his ophthalmoplegia. Bonus: should this patient get a CT scan and a cerebral angiogram? Why or why not?

**C.** A 68-year-old woman with a history of hypertension awakes with severe dizziness, nausea, and vomiting. She has difficulty controlling her right hand and cannot walk, tending to fall to the right. On examination, she has moderate ptosis of the right eyelid, the right pupil is smaller than the left, and pain and temperature sensation is diminished over the right face and the left hemibody. She exhibits ataxia, dyssynergia, and dysmetria during a right finger-to-nose maneuver, and her gait is very ataxic with an overwhelming tendency to fall to the right. She has no weakness, reflexes are symmetric, and plantar responses are flexor (i.e., no Babinski signs). Localize the lesion.

**D.** A 65-year-old man suddenly develops diplopia and severe generalized headache maximal in the right frontal region. On examination, there is severe ptosis on the right. The right eye does not move at all. The pupil is slightly dilated and does not constrict when exposed to a bright light. There is no right corneal reflex (i.e., stroking the right cornea with a wisp of cotton fails to elicit a blink). The patient reports that a cold tuning fork applied to various regions of the face feels somewhat colder on the left than the right, and touch sensation is subjectively altered over the right side of the face. The remainder of the neurologic examination is completely normal. Identify the cranial nerve deficits and localize the lesion. Bonus: Can you explain why the pupil is only slightly dilated?

**E.** Which cranial nerve is affected in the patient shown in Figure 8-24?

# Cycle 8-4

# Supranuclear Control of Eye Movements

The fact that under nearly all normal circumstances the eyes move in perfect tandem (i.e., their movements are *conjugate*), despite the scattering of oculomotor control through a number of variously dispersed brainstem nuclei, clearly indicates the presence of an apparatus above the nuclei of CN III, IV, and VI in the hierarchy of eye movement control referred to as supranuclear. In this cycle, we will first consider in some detail the supranuclear apparatus that enables conjugate eye movements, and then briefly consider the supranuclear apparatus that controls the dysconjugate, inward turning of the eyes during focus on near objects, known as vergence. We will then consider the major means by which the brain manipulates the supranuclear conjugate gaze apparatus in order to achieve appropriate eye movements under various circumstances.

## A. MECHANISMS OF CONJUGATE EYE MOVEMENT

The key to conjugate movements of the eyes lies in the existence of neural yoking mechanisms that assure the cocontraction of different muscles in each of the two eyes as needed to move the eyes together in a given direction. The most important yoking mechanism from a clinical diagnostic point of view is that underlying horizontal eye movements. Each abducens nucleus actually contains two thoroughly admixed populations of cells. One population gives rise to the axons of the sixth cranial nerve and the other population gives rise to axons that cross the brainstem and course rostrally in the contralateral median longitudinal fasciculus (MLF), ultimately to synapse on neurons in the contralateral nucleus of the MR in the third cranial nerve nuclear complex (Fig. 8-25). In this way, any input to the right abducens nucleus that terminates equally on the two cell populations (as all inputs do) will elicit contraction of the right LR, rotating the right eye to the right, and contraction of the left MR, rotating the left eye to the right. The net result is that the eyes are conjugately rotated to the right. In analogous fashion, input to the left abducens nucleus achieves conjugate deviation of the eyes to the left.[1]

The relatively long distance that the fibers responsible for the adductive component of conjugate horizontal eye movement have to travel in the MLF renders them susceptible to damage, as demonstrated in Case 8-8.

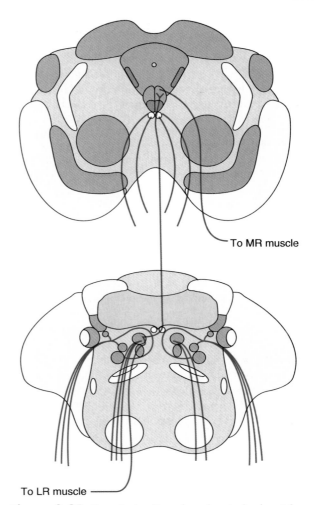

To MR muscle

To LR muscle

**Figure 8-25** Neural circuitry of conjugate horizontal eye movements. LR, lateral rectus; MR, medial rectus.

---

[1]All mechanisms controlling conjugate eye movements entail reciprocal excitation and inhibition of agonist and antagonist muscles (a discovery of Sherrington shortly after 1900). Thus, conjugate deviation of the eyes to the right entails excitation of cells in the right abducens nucleus projecting to the right LR and the left MR nucleus, but also inhibition of cells in the left abducens nucleus projecting to the right MR nucleus and the left LR muscle. Because it is not necessary to take these reciprocal innervation patterns into account in the neuro-ophthalmologic evaluation of patients, we will omit further reference to them for the sake of brevity.

### Case 8-8

**Multiple Sclerosis**

*An 18-year-old college sophomore presents to a neurology clinic complaining of a 1-week history of intermittent double vision (diplopia) in which the images are side by side. Further inquiry reveals a 1-year history of urinary urgency and urgency incontinence. She also concedes that despite a promising career as a gymnast in high school, her performance once she got to college has been very disappointing, to the extent that she has completely given up gymnastics. On examination, extraocular movements are normal except when she gazes to the*

*Continued*

## Case 8-8—cont'd

*right, in which case there is normal abduction of the right eye but very little adduction of the left eye. She also exhibits generalized hyper-reflexia and bilateral Babinski signs, and her gait is marked by mild spasticity.*

**Comment:** *This patient has evidence of damage to the fibers from the right abducens nucleus ascending in the left MLF to synapse in the left MR nucleus—a left internuclear ophthalmoplegia (INO) (Fig. 8-25). The term internuclear is used because the lesion is between oculomotor nuclei (the third and the sixth). She also has evidence of bilateral damage to descending motor pathways, either corticobulbar or the pontine and medullary reticulospinal tracts. Finally, she has evidence of damage to descending pathways mediating urinary bladder tone and sphincter control (see Chapter 6, The Motor System). Because the MLF is nowhere near the corticobulbar pathways (which travel in the cerebral peduncles and basis pontis), it is unlikely that a single lesion is responsible for all these deficits. Multifocal CNS disease occurring in a young person, especially in stepwise fashion as in this patient, overwhelmingly suggests multiple sclerosis (Fig. 8-26). Unilateral or bilateral INOs commonly develop in patients with multiple sclerosis. A unilateral INO may also develop in an older person as a result of a lacunar infarction of the brainstem involving the MLF.*

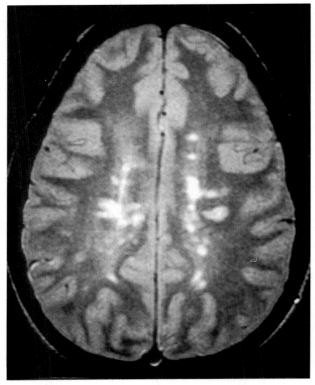

**Figure 8-26** Magnetic resonance image (MRI) of the head in patient with multiple sclerosis, demonstrating multifocal lesions within the deep cerebral white matter compatible with demyelination.

The yoking mechanism underlying conjugate horizontal eye movements is linked to supranuclear eye movement control systems subserving voluntary gaze, voluntary smooth pursuit (following a moving target with one's eyes), and eye movements induced by acceleration or rotation of the head. These systems will be discussed in some detail in succeeding sections.

An analogous yoking mechanism enables vertical (up or down) eye movements, effectively linking neurons in the oculomotor subnuclei for the SR, IR, and IO, and in the trochlear nuclei. Separate nuclear groups in the dorsal rostral midbrain constitute both links within this yoking mechanism and points of connection of the yoking mechanism with other brain and brainstem mechanisms (which subserve vertical voluntary gaze, vertical voluntary smooth pursuit, and vertical eye movements induced by acceleration or rotation of the head). Lesions that involve the general vicinity of the third cranial nerve nuclei, such as top of the basilar artery embolic stroke, may cause deficits in vertical eye movements. Masses in the vicinity of the aqueduct, such

as pineal tumors, may compress the various nuclear groups subserving vertical eye movements and their connections with the oculomotor and trochlear nuclei, leading to impairment in vertical eye movements, especially upgaze (Parinaud's syndrome) (Fig. 8-27).

## Vergence and the Near Triad

There is one natural eye movement in which ocular movement is dysconjugate, yet still coordinated, and that is when the eyes are both directed medially as one focuses on a near object, something known as *vergence*. Mechanisms underlying vergence are located in the dorsal midbrain reticular formation near the third nerve nuclear complex. Fibers from the vergence center project directly to the MR nuclei without passing through the MLF. Thus, the patient described in Case 8-8 would almost certainly have exhibited normal adduction of the left eye during vergence. In fact, it is crucial to have such a patient look at something very close in order to differentiate a lesion of the MLF from

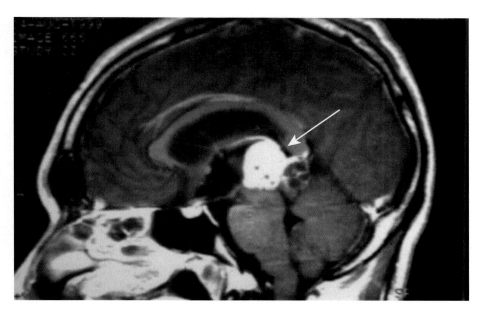

**Figure 8-27** Sagittal magnetic resonance image (MRI) of a patient with a pineal tumor (*arrow*) compressing the rostral dorsal midbrain and causing paralysis of upgaze. Such patients also commonly exhibit impairment of convergence and pupillary reactions (see text).

a selective lesion of the MR muscle (not uncommon), third nerve fibers supplying it, or the nucleus of the MR (exceedingly rare).

Ocular vergence is associated with rounding up of the lens (accommodation) and pupillary constriction. The combination of ocular vergence, accommodation and pupillary constriction is referred to as the *near reflex* or the *near triad*. Accommodation and pupillary constriction are produced by neurons in the Edinger-Westphal nuclei projecting to the ciliary ganglia in the orbits (Cycle 8-3). The circuitry underlying accommodation is located in the same region of the dorsal midbrain reticular formation that is involved in vergence (see preceding paragraph). The circuitry underlying pupillary constriction, whether during exposure to bright light or while focusing on near objects, is located in a region of the dorsal midbrain just rostral to the superior colliculi known as the pretectal area. The entire near triad involves projections from various portions of the cerebrum conveying responses to the amount of disparity between the images seen by the two eyes, the amount of blur, and possibly also reflecting the intention to focus on a near object. The retinal-pretectal mechanism underlying pupillary constriction to light will be discussed in Chapter 9 (Vision).

# B. CONTROL OF CONJUGATE EYE MOVEMENT

In Section A, we discussed the "wiring harness" that enables conjugate eye movement. In this section,

we will discuss the supranuclear mechanisms that link to this wiring harness to enable the control of conjugate eye movement needed to deal with environmental contingencies. The supranuclear control of conjugate eye movement can, for practical purposes, be divided into three domains: vestibular, gaze, and smooth pursuit.

## Vestibular Control of Conjugate Eye Movement: Reflex Ocular Stabilization

In the course of our nearly continual movements in pursuit of a day's activities, we move our heads countless times, sometimes very quickly, at times quite violently. If our eyes were fixed in the orbits except when we voluntarily chose to move them, they too would be constantly and sometimes violently moved with our heads. If there were no mechanism to compensate this—to, in effect, maintain gyroscopic control of the position of the eyes—we would be faced with repeated jarring and blurring of vision. Fortunately, this blurring is almost completely prevented by the *vestibulo-ocular reflex (VOR)*. To gain an appreciation for the power of the VOR, perform the following experiment. Hold your index finger upright at arm's length and move your arm and hand rapidly from side to side as you focus on your index finger. The image of the finger is reduced to a barely resolvable blur. Now hold your arm still while you rapidly rotate your head from side to side. In this condition, in which you are recruiting the assistance of your VOR, your index finger remains in nearly perfect focus.

The vestibular apparatus will be discussed in considerable detail in Chapter 10. It provides the mechanisms for stabilization of eye position in the course of all head movements involving acceleration. This includes rotation in any direction (which involves angular acceleration), linear acceleration in any direction, and any movement involving a change in the angular orientation of the head with respect to the gravitational field. We will confine our discussion to the impact of the vestibular apparatus on eye movement in the course of rotation of the head in the axial plane (i.e., horizontal eye movements), as this will suffice for understanding the most important clinical phenomena.

The vestibular component of the inner ear sends a constant signal to the medial vestibular nucleus. The medial vestibular nucleus, in turn, provides tonic input to the abducens nuclei and the midbrain vertical eye movement network. The tonic input from the medial vestibular nucleus to the ipsilateral abducens nucleus effectively serves to inhibit ipsilateral conjugate eye movement.[2] If that tonic vestibular input is reduced, by a head turn to the opposite side, a lesion of the vestibular apparatus or the vestibular nucleus, or cooling of the vestibular apparatus (through injection of cold water into the external auditory meatus), then the eyes will conjugately deviate to the side of reduced input. In the case of a head turn to the opposite side, this ipsilateral eye deviation serves to precisely compensate for the head movement so that the eyes remain pointed in exactly the same direction and there is no movement of the visual image across the retina as the head turns.

This marvelous compensatory mechanism also provides us with two maneuvers that are very useful in testing the integrity of vestibular systems and of the brainstem conjugate eye movement apparatus. These maneuvers are illustrated in Cases 8-9 and 8-10.

---

[2]Each medial vestibular nucleus actually sends inhibitory input to the ipsilateral abducens nucleus and excitatory input to the contralateral abducens nucleus. Furthermore, because both medial vestibular nuclei innervate both abducens nuclei, the net effect of vestibular input on horizontal eye movement reflects the balance of input from both vestibular nuclei. However, to simplify our discussion, we will focus exclusively on the ipsilateral inhibitory input from the medial vestibular nucleus.

## Case 8-9

### Multifactorial Dysequilibrium Syndrome

*An 80-year-old man presents to a neurology clinic with the chief complaint of insidiously progressive imbalance while walking. He has a 10-year history of mild hypertension. On neurologic examination, he has moderate to severe impairment in position sense in the great toes. He exhibits a moderate gait apraxia (particular problems with initiation of walking and making turns). His best-corrected visual acuity (using both eyes) is 20/30—he is able to see at 20 ft what a normal person would be able to see at 30 ft. When visual acuity is retested as he rotates his head back and forth, his visual acuity drops to 20/200. In fact, it becomes so bad that he repeatedly tries to momentarily freeze the movement of his head so that he can catch a glimpse of the test card. Finally, he is asked to stand with his feet together and his eyes closed. The examiner, standing behind him, suddenly and without warning, grabs his shoulders and jerks him backward. He falls with very little in the way of compensatory movement and is saved from injury only by the timely intercession of the examiner.*

**Comment:** *This patient has what is often referred to as a multifactorial dysequilibrium syndrome. That is, his imbalance is caused by several factors. First, he has impairment in proprioceptive input from his feet, presumably due to polyneuropathy. Second, he has difficulty modifying his walking to the specific requirements of the terrain or demands of the situation—gait apraxia. In this patient, this is most likely caused by damage to the descending white matter fibers traveling from the leg region of the cerebral motor homunculus to the brainstem and spinal cord as a result of multiple tiny strokes (ischemic demyelination). Finally, he has impairment in vestibular function, something that occurs quite commonly and for uncertain reasons in the elderly. This impairment is manifested in two ways. First, he has severe impairment in his VOR, revealed by the test of visual acuity during sinusoidal head movement. Second, he has severe impairment in vestibulospinal tract function, revealed in his loss of postural reflexes. In aggregate, these various deficits are sufficient to account for his gait instability.*

## Case 8-10

### Brain Death

A 17-year-old high school student is struck in the sternum with a baseball during practice. He immediately collapses in cardiac arrest. Extensive resuscitative efforts are unsuccessful until emergency medical technicians arrive and apply direct current cardioversion. A normal cardiac rhythm is reestablished and the patient is hospitalized. However, 3 days later, he remains comatose and there is no evidence of CNS function. The organ transplant team is anxious to harvest multiple organs before they are damaged in the course of the vicissitudes of a long intensive care unit stay, and the boy's parents agree that this is what their son would have wanted. Before organ harvest can occur, it must be established that the patient's brain is dead. This conclusion requires a complete inventory of cranial nerve function, a test for the existence of any residual respiratory function, and tests for the presence of brainstem motor system reflexes (decorticate or decerebrate posturing). As part of this testing, the patient's eyes are held open while his head is suddenly rotated from one side to the other (oculocephalic testing or the "Doll's eye" maneuver). The eyes move with the head, suggesting that alterations in the vestibular input to the abducens nuclei fail to elicit any compensatory eye movement (eye movement in the direction contralateral to the head rotation). In addition, 60 mL of ice water is injected in one ear, and 8 minutes later, into the other ear. This too fails to elicit any ocular movement. Failing these and all other tests for residual CNS function, the patient is deemed brain dead and is transferred to the surgical service. Ultimately, he is able to provide two kidneys, two lungs, a liver, a heart, and corneas to other patients.

**Comment:** Blunt trauma to the sternum is now a well-established, albeit rare cause of sudden ventricular fibrillation in susceptible individuals. In this patient, as in many patients experiencing out-of-hospital cardiac arrest, a normal cardiac rhythm and cerebral perfusion were not established soon enough to prevent severe CNS damage. In the late 1970s, physicians throughout the world agreed upon a set of strict criteria for defining brain death. These criteria are, in effect, criteria for brainstem death. In this patient, two maneuvers involving the vestibular apparatus and its connections to eye movement pathways were used to test the integrity of these systems. In the oculocephalic maneuver, a sudden head rotation to the right normally reduces the signal from the left vestibular apparatus to the left medial vestibular nucleus, resulting in increased firing in the left abducens nucleus and conjugate compensatory deviation of the eyes to the left (note that actually both vestibular apparatuses are potentially engaged in this maneuver, the left apparatus reducing its signal to the brainstem, the right increasing its signal). Proprioceptive input from the neck also contributes to the oculocephalic response. In this patient, there was no oculocephalic response with head movement to either side, suggesting severe brainstem damage. In the second test, injection of ice water in the right ear, a far more potent stimulus than that provided by the oculocephalic maneuver, should have reduced the input from the right vestibular apparatus to the brainstem and resulted in tonic conjugate deviation of the eyes to the right. The failure of this to occur provided further evidence of severe damage to the brainstem implicating the eye movement apparatus (CN III, IV, and VI, and the MLF) and the vestibular nuclei.

## Gaze Mechanisms: Voluntary and Reactive Control of Ocular Saccades

In addition to the reflexive control of eye movements provided by the vestibular apparatus and its connections to the oculomotor network, we have two systems that enable voluntary control of eye movements: gaze and smooth pursuit. *Gaze* movements consist of conjugate movements of the eyes known as *saccades* that enable us to center a particular visual target on the fovea, the point of maximal visual acuity in the retina ("foveation"). These movements can be very rapid, up to 450 degrees per second. *Smooth pursuit* movements are used to maintain foveation of a moving target. They are considerably slower, up to 60 degrees per second. Separate, albeit linked systems control these two classes of conjugate eye movements. As in the foregoing sections, we will limit our discussion to horizontal eye movements.

Cranial Nerves and Brainstem Organization

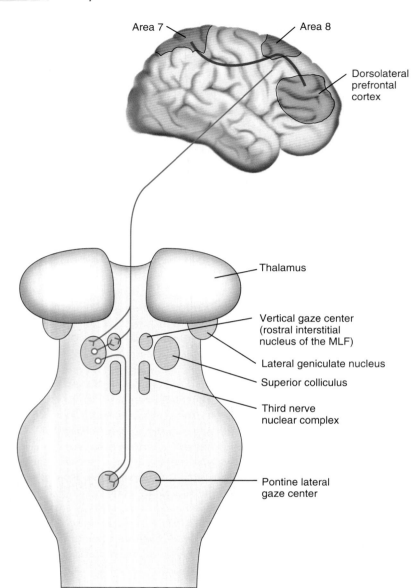

**Figure 8-28** The neuroanatomy underlying gaze mechanisms and the orienting response. MLF, median longitudinal fasciculus.

Two regions of the CNS are responsible for the saccadic eye movements underlying gaze: the frontal eye fields (Brodmann's area 8) and the superior colliculi (Fig. 8-28). Input from other regions of the frontal lobes to the frontal eye fields provides the basis for the deliberate, voluntary direction of gaze to a particular target. Input from the parietal lobes (Brodmann's area 7) to the frontal eye fields provides the basis for reflexive saccades to complex stimuli (reactive gaze). The neural networks of the parietal lobes are linked to visual association cortices in the temporal lobes that enable the sophisticated analysis needed to determine whether

a particular complex stimulus deserves sufficient further investigation to justify a foveating saccade to it. Reflexive saccades to a compelling stimulus, often associated with some component of head movement, constitute the *orienting response*. Deep layers of the superior colliculus, which contain neurons responsive to visual, auditory, and even tactile input (particularly from the face), also generate reflexive saccades to intrinsically important targets—another basis for reactive gaze. However, the superior colliculus responds to far more elementary stimulus attributes than do the parietal and temporal lobes: movement, bright lights, loud noises, and sudden noxious somatosensory stimuli.

The frontal lobes, the parietal lobes, and deep layers of the superior colliculi are engaged in a delicate and constantly shifting balance that defines where we direct our attention and concurrently, where we direct our gaze at any moment. For rats no less than humans, it is important to be able to voluntarily direct attention and gaze to a chosen target, which for rats might be a morsel of food, or for humans might be selected visual aspects of the task at hand. For rats and humans, it is also critical to be able to maintain vigilance and the ability to instantly shift attention and gaze in reactive fashion to important stimuli in the environment. For a rat, this might be a raptor sweeping in for a meal. For humans, it could be an analogous threat, such as a speeding car, or something positive such as the face of an old friend. Patients with diffuse disease of either the cerebral cortex or the hemispheric white matter may exhibit disruption of the delicate balance between voluntary and reactive gaze mechanisms, as illustrated in Case 8-11.

## Case 8-11

### Frontal Systems Dysfunction in Vascular Dementia

*A 70-year-old man with a long history of poorly controlled hypertension is seen in the neurology clinic because of progressive decline in intellectual function. In the course of this evaluation, the examiner assesses the integrity of vision in the four quadrants by having the patient fixate on her nose and indicate the number of fingers she raises in each visual quadrant. Every time she raises one or two fingers, the patient breaks fixation on her nose and saccades to her fingers. This continues despite repeated commands by the examiner to look at her nose, not at her fingers.*

**Comment:** *This patient is exhibiting a visual grasp. He cannot help saccading to the just-moved fingers because he has extensive ischemic demyelination of the deep cerebral white matter (due to many tiny infarcts) that has degraded the connections between the frontal eye fields and the brainstem. Thus, the patient's ability to voluntarily direct his eyes at the examiner's nose, mediated by the frontal eye fields, is overwhelmed by the drive to reflexively saccade toward a movement, mediated by the superior colliculi.*

Superficial layers of the superior colliculi are involved in both directed and reactive saccadic eye movements in a different way. The pattern of activity of the entire population of neurons in these layers of the superior colliculi defines the amount of eye movement that will be needed to saccade from the present position to the new target. This pattern of activity is defined by input from the retinas and visual cortex to the superior colliculi, and by input from the frontal eye fields.

Both the frontal eye fields and the superior colliculi project to regions of the pontine reticular formation ventrally adjacent to the abducens nuclei known as the paramedian pontine reticular formation (PPRF), often referred to as the pontine lateral gaze centers (Fig. 8-28). Frontal eye field-PPRF pathways cross in the dorsal midbrain just caudal to the third cranial nerve nuclear complex. PPRF activity, via complex mechanisms, effectively excites the neurons of the ipsilateral abducens nucleus. Thus, activity in the left frontal eye field leads to increased firing in the right abducens nucleus and a conjugate saccadic movement of the eyes to the right. In the realm of eye movements as in nearly all other movements, each cerebral hemisphere directs movement in or into the contralateral hemispace. The importance of this pathway for localization is illustrated by Case 8-12.

## Case 8-12

### Frontal Lobe Stroke

*A 70-year-old man suddenly develops paralysis of the left side of his body. On neurologic examination, his eyes are tonically deviated to the right, and he cannot be induced to move them to the left past the midline. He has profound weakness on the left, particularly of the left arm, left-sided hyporeflexia, and a left Babinski sign. With an oculocephalic maneuver, conjugate movement of his eyes to the left is easily achieved.*

**Comment:** *This patient's lesion, probably a stroke because of its sudden onset, could be in one of two locations. It could be in the right frontal lobe, simultaneously impairing function of the right frontal eye fields and damaging right hemisphere motor systems, or it could be in the left brainstem, simultaneously damaging the left pontine lateral gaze*

*Continued*

*center (the PPRF) and motor pathways descending in the left basis pontis. A lesion in the right frontal lobe would produce inability to gaze to the left and a left hemiparesis. A lesion in the left pons would produce inability to gaze to the left and a right hemiparesis. Clearly the stroke involves the right frontal lobe. It is a general rule of neurologic localization that the presence of a cranial nerve deficit and a contralateral hemiparesis signals a brainstem lesion.*

Neither a lesion of the frontal eye fields nor a lesion of the PPRF would affect the response to the oculocephalic maneuver (or caloric stimulation), because this response is mediated via direct connections between the medial vestibular nuclei and the abducens nuclei. Case 8-12 contrasts with Case 8-11, in which a patient with chronic lesions of the deep cerebral white matter, disconnecting the frontal eye fields from the brainstem, could not inhibit reactive saccades driven by the superior colliculi. The important difference is that the patient in Case 8-12 has an acute lesion. Under these circumstances, the superior colliculi are temporarily unable to generate reactive saccades to the left. This may reflect a phenomenon similar to the spinal cord shock that occurs after acute injury, a form of diaschisis or physiologic dysfunction related to acute injury to a distant but connected part of the nervous system. If we were to retest the patient in Case 8-12 6 months later, we would find that he had recovered his ability to look to the left and that he had developed a left visual grasp.

## Smooth Pursuit

Two types of eye movements have the general characteristics of smooth pursuit movements. One is voluntary and is actually defined as smooth pursuit. The other is reflexive and is produced by vestibular input to the oculomotor network. Smooth pursuit mechanisms operate when we and a target are moving relative to one another but we are not being accelerated. Vestibular mechanisms operate when we and a target are moving relative to one another and we are being accelerated.

The essential information that drives voluntary smooth pursuit is movement of a visual target across the retina away from the fovea, the point of maximal

visual acuity. This is referred to as retinal slip. Retinal slip is used by the brain to generate conjugate eye movements that are equal in speed but opposite in direction to the slip. Voluntary smooth pursuit movements originate in a region of cortex near the junction of Brodmann's areas 19 and 39 (the angular gyrus) at the divide between the temporal and parietal lobes. Neurons in this region compute the speed and direction of moving visual stimuli. They project to the frontal eye fields and the brainstem. The smooth pursuit pathway descends to the pons without crossing and it projects to the vestibular nuclei, the flocculonodular lobes of the cerebellum, and ultimately, to the ipsilateral abducens nucleus. For this reason, the smooth pursuit center in the left hemisphere controls smooth pursuit to the left. *This is one of the two neurologic functions violating the cardinal principle that each hemisphere generates movements into or within contralateral hemispace (see discussion of CN XII for the other exception).* The localizing importance of the smooth pursuit mechanism is illustrated in Case 8-13.

**Right Hemisphere Stroke**
*A 50-year-old man with a long history of hypertension presents to the hospital with an 8-hour history of left-sided weakness. On examination, he exhibits very mild pronation drift of the supinated left arm, perhaps very slight degradation of fine motor movement in the left hand, and slightly reduced arm swing on the left while he walks. Otherwise his neurologic examination is completely normal. An MRI scan of the head is normal. However, a magnetic resonance angiogram demonstrates probable high-grade stenosis of the right internal carotid artery due to atheromatous disease.*

*The neurologist caring for the patient wishes to ascertain whether this is a cortical infarction, hence a middle cerebral artery event, implicating carotid artery to artery thromboembolism as the cause of the stroke, or whether it is a lacunar infarction related to intracranial microvascular atheromatous disease. If it is the former, he will refer the patient for prompt carotid endarterectomy.*

*He assesses the optokinetic response by moving a 1-m length of cloth, with vertical black stripes at regular intervals, from one side to the other in front of the patient. If the right cortex is intact, when the cloth is moved to the patient's right, the patient's eyes*

## Case 8-13—cont'd

should smoothly pursue each vertical black stripe to the right, saccade back toward the midline (the primary position) to pick up the next vertical stripe, smoothly pursue it to the right, and so on. This regular alternation of slow and fast eye movements constitutes optokinetic nystagmus. The direction of the fast component defines the direction of any nystagmus, including optokinetic nystagmus. Thus, moving the cloth to the right engages the right parieto-occipital smooth pursuit apparatus to generate smooth pursuit movements to the right, and the right frontal eye fields to generate saccadic movements to the left, producing left-beating optokinetic nystagmus. A right hemisphere lesion affecting either of these widely separated locations should produce an abnormal optokinetic response when the cloth is moved toward the side of the lesion. In practice, it is usually difficult to tell whether it is smooth pursuit or saccadic movements that are abnormal. However, an abnormal response of either type (observed in this patient) almost always signals the presence of a cortical lesion. This patient was referred for carotid endarterectomy.

Vestibularly mediated reflexive "smooth pursuit" movements are actually nothing more than the VOR. The VOR, in conjunction with saccadic movements produced by the frontal eye fields, mediates an approximate equivalent of the optokinetic response when the subject is rotating, as opposed to when the visual target is moving, as in Case 8-13. We could observe this phenomenon in a spinning ice skater. Spinning to the right leads to reduced vestibular input to the left abducens nucleus and a smooth conjugate movement of the eyes to the left that is so precisely matched to the velocity of right spin that the skater is able to maintain fixation. This smooth movement of the eyes to the left is followed by a quick, conjugate, saccadic eye movement to the right, enabling the skater's eyes to "catch up" with his head. The cycle is then repeated again and again until the skater stops spinning. Thus, spinning to the right induces right-beating *vestibular nystagmus*. In the course of the spin, the skater sees a series of snapshots of the rink around him, each made during the "smooth pursuit" movement achieved by the VOR between catch-up saccades.

The natural function of the physiology underlying optokinetic nystagmus (Case 8-13), which, as des-

cribed, is elicited in a highly artificial manner, is to enable us to maintain the stability of visual images as we move in a straight line without accelerating, or as the environment moves with respect to us. In these circumstances, the VOR cannot help us. For example, when the skater looks to his left at his audience as he speeds along in a straight line, he fixates on a target, leftward smooth pursuit mechanisms enable him to maintain fixation until the target has passed, and then he generates a rightward saccade to a new target, following which the cycle is repeated—right beating optokinetic nystagmus.

The relationship between pursuit and saccadic eye movement in optokinetic and vestibular nystagmus is summarized in Figure 8-29.

## PRACTICE 8-4

**A.** Return to Practice 8-3C. What would you predict about the nature of this patient's horizontal eye movements? Would you see tonic deviation of the eyes? Would you see limitation of movement? Would you see nystagmus, and if so, what kind of nystagmus and why?

**B.** A 70-year-old man with a long history of hypertension, diabetes, and heavy smoking awakes one morning with right-sided weakness. On examination, he cannot gaze to the left. He has moderate right-sided weakness, worst in his arm, and impairment of fine motor movement in the right hand. He exhibits severe ataxia, dysmetria, and dyssynergia during the right finger-to-nose maneuver. Even though he has only mild weakness in the right leg, he cannot stand because he immediately lurches to the right. He has impaired vibratory and position sense in the right arm and leg. Localize the lesion. What would be the effect of injecting cold water in his left ear? Bonus: what is the likely vascular event?

**C.** A 68-year-old woman with a long history of hypertension awakes one morning with right-sided weakness and double vision. Her examination findings are identical to that of the gentleman described in B except for her ophthalmoplegia. She can look to the left perfectly normally. However, when she looks to the right, the left eye fails to adduct. Localize the lesion. Can you account for the difference in the ophthalmoplegia from the case in B?

**D.** Would a patient with disease limited to the frontal lobes exhibit a visual grasp? Why or why not?

Cranial Nerves and Brainstem Organization

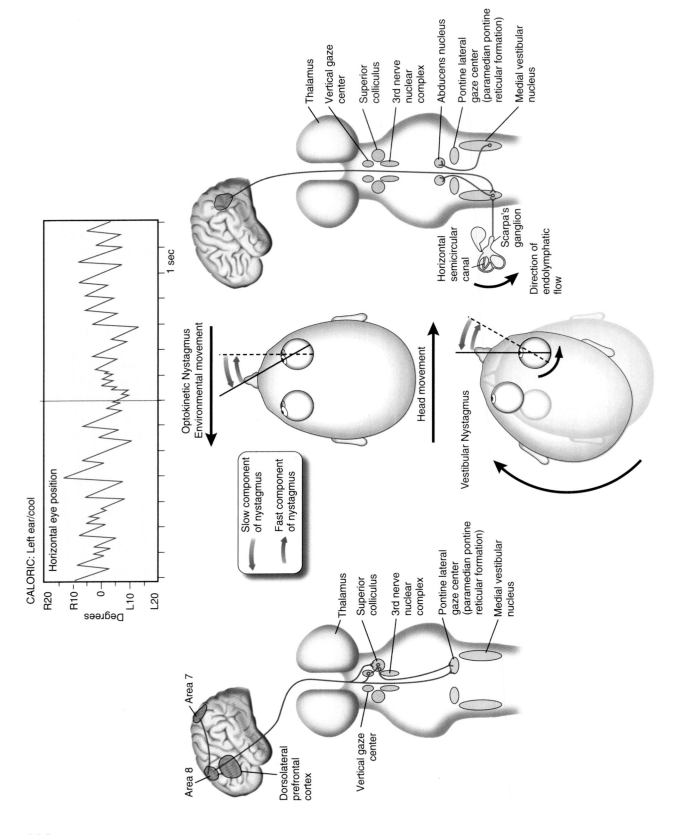

CALORIC: Left ear/cool

Horizontal eye position

Degrees
R20
R10
0
L10
L20

1 sec

Thalamus
Vertical gaze center
Superior colliculus
3rd nerve nuclear complex
Abducens nucleus
Pontine lateral gaze center (paramedian pontine reticular formation)
Medial vestibular nucleus

Horizontal semicircular canal
Scarpa's ganglion
Direction of endolymphatic flow

Optokinetic Nystagmus
Environmental movement

Head movement

Vestibular Nystagmus

Slow component of nystagmus
Fast component of nystagmus

Area 7
Area 8
Dorsolateral prefrontal cortex

Thalamus
Superior colliculus
3rd nerve nuclear complex
Pontine lateral gaze center (paramedian pontine reticular formation)
Medial vestibular nucleus
Vertical gaze center

**Figure 8-29** Summary of the relationship between pursuit and saccadic eye movements underlying optokinetic nystagmus and the vestibulo-ocular reflex. Only movements of the right eye are illustrated in order to simplify the figure.

- The top center drawing of the head illustrates optokinetic nystagmus, in which either the environment moves to the left or the head moves to the right, and there is no head rotation. The eye slowly moves leftward (adduction) so that the visual target remains centered on the fovea, despite the environmental or head movement. At regular intervals, a fast movement (an abducting saccade) moves the eye to the right to foveate the next object in the environment (or the next vertical stripe on an optokinetic tape).

- The bottom center drawing of the head illustrates vestibular nystagmus during head rotation. As the head rotates to the right, the eye moves slowly to the left (adduction) so that the visual target remains centered on the fovea. At regular intervals, a fast movement (an abducting saccade) moves the eye to the right to foveate the next object in the environment.

- Optokinetic nystagmus, vestibular nystagmus, and cold caloric stimulation of the left ear generate the ocular movement waveform (an electro-oculogram) illustrated across the top of the figure.

- The drawing of the brain on the right illustrates the mechanisms of the slow eye movements during both optokinetic and vestibular nystagmus. As we have noted, the actual circuitry involved is quite complicated, so we will describe here only net effects. The left medial vestibular nucleus in effect inhibits the left abducens nucleus. During leftward smooth pursuit movements, an uncrossed pathway from the smooth pursuit center at the left parieto-temporo-occipital junction inhibits the left medial vestibular nucleus. This decreases the inhibitory input to the left abducens nucleus, allowing the eyes to move slowly to the left. During rightward (clockwise) rotation of the head, endolymph in the left horizontal semicircular canal is pushed in a counterclockwise direction. This decreases the excitatory input into the left medial vestibular nucleus, thereby reducing the inhibitory input to the left abducens nucleus and allowing the eyes to move slowly to the left. The velocity of the leftward movement of the eyes is exactly equal in magnitude but opposite in direction to that of the head movement, thus assuring continuous foveation of a visual target. Thus, the final common pathway underlying the slow component of optokinetic and vestibular nystagmus (vestibular nucleus to abducens nucleus) is the same.

- The drawing of the brain on the left illustrates the mechanism of the fast (saccadic) eye movements during both optokinetic and vestibular nystagmus. During either type of nystagmus, the leftward slow eye movement is periodically punctuated by rightward saccades generated via a crossed pathway from the left frontal eye field to the right pontine lateral gaze center (PPRF), which projects in turn to the right abducens nucleus.

- Destruction of the left labyrinthine apparatus, injection of cold water in the left ear, or destruction of the left medial vestibular nucleus, will also diminish the inhibitory input from the medial vestibular nucleus to the left abducens nucleus, allowing the eyes to move slowly to the left. The left abducens nucleus would not be able to distinguish these events from the alteration in input from the medial vestibular nucleus induced by smooth pursuit to the left or rightward head rotation.

- Because the fast component of vestibular nystagmus depends upon a cerebral mechanism, in circumstances in which the cerebrum is substantially dysfunctional (e.g., the comatose patient), this fast component will be lost. In these circumstances, instillation of cold water in the left ear would lead only to tonic deviation of the eyes to the left.

# Cycle 8-5

# Motor Component of Cranial Nerve V

### Objective

Be able to describe the location of the motor nucleus of CN V, the function it subserves, the muscles it innervates, and the pathway the nerve takes to these muscles.

The motor nucleus of CN V is located in the lateral pontine tegmentum at about the junction of the middle and caudal thirds of the pons (Fig. 8-4, V). Its projections follow the mandibular division of CN V (V3) and ultimately innervate the muscles of mastication: the temporalis, the masseter, and the medial and lateral pterygoid muscles. Because contraction of the pterygoid muscles pulls the jaw to the opposite side, a lesion of the motor division of CN V will result in a tendency toward ipsilateral deviation of the mandible and impaired ability to thrust the mandible to the contralateral side. The motor nucleus of CN V receives bilateral supranuclear innervation and hemispheric lesions have no discernible effect on mastication.

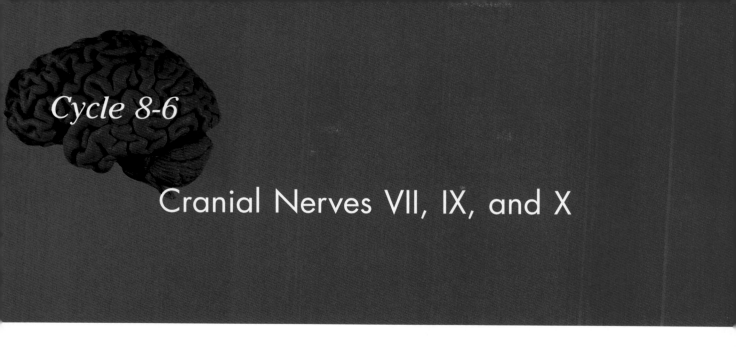

# Cranial Nerves VII, IX, and X

## Objectives

1. Be able to locate the motor nuclei of CN VII, IX, and X; list the muscles they innervate; and describe the pathway these nerves take to these muscles and the consequences of lesions of these nerves.

2. Be able to distinguish between an upper and lower motor neuron CN VII palsy and explain the mechanisms underlying the difference.

3. Be able to describe the pathways underlying the corneal reflex.

4. Be able to describe the somatosensory functions of CN VII, IX, and X, and locate and define the roles of the nuclei involved.

5. Be able to describe the functions of CN VII, IX, and X with respect to taste and the nucleus and neural pathways involved.

6. Be able to describe the autonomic efferent functions of CN VII, IX, and X and locate the nuclei involved.

7. Be able to describe the visceral autonomic afferent functions subserved by CN IX and X and locate the nuclei involved.

8. Be able to define the carotid sinus syndrome and neurocardiogenic syncope and explain their mechanisms.

We will consider the facial (VII), glossopharyngeal (IX), and vagus (X) nerves together because these three nerves, to one degree or another, share duties in somatic motor function, somatic sensation, special sensation (taste), visceral autonomic efferent function, and visceral autonomic afferent function.

## A. SOMATIC MOTOR FUNCTIONS

### Cranial Nerve VII

Somatic motor functions of CN VII are subserved by the motor nucleus, located in the ventrolateral tegmentum of the caudal pons. Fibers of the nerve loop up over the abducens nucleus before passing ventrolaterally to exit along the lateral margin of the pontomedullary junction in the cerebellopontine angle (the CP angle) (Fig. 8-4, VI, VII). The nerve then enters the internal acoustic meatus with the auditory and vestibular branches of CN VIII. It detours into the cancellous bone of the mastoid to exit near the styloid process beneath the mastoid. From there it passes into the parotid gland where it divides into three branches to supply the muscles of facial expression.

The motor nucleus of CN VII is divided into dorsal and ventral components. The ventral component, which supplies the muscles of the forehead, and to some extent the orbicularis oculi, has bilateral supranuclear innervation. The dorsal component of the motor nucleus, which supplies the muscles of the lower face,

401

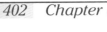 

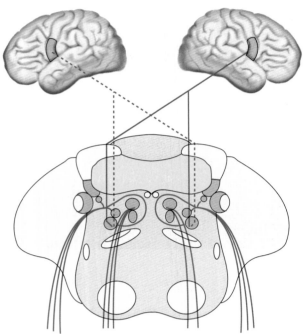

**Figure 8-30** Supranuclear projections to the nucleus of CN VII. Note that only the ventral half of the nucleus, supplying the upper face, gets dual (bilateral) innervation, whereas the dorsal half, supplying the lower face, gets only unilateral, contralateral innervation.

including the orbicularis oculi, receives predominantly unilateral (contralateral) supranuclear innervation. Thus, *a unilateral supranuclear CN VII palsy may produce relatively severe weakness of the muscles of facial expression in the lower face but spares the forehead and typically leaves at least a remnant of orbicularis oculi function. In contrast, because the nerve is undivided between the nucleus of CN VII and the parotid gland, a lesion anywhere along this trajectory will affect the entire hemiface (Fig. 8-30).* This important principle is illustrated in Cases 8-14 and 8-15.

## Case 8-14

### Middle Cerebral Artery Distribution Stroke

*A 69-year-old woman with a history of atrial fibrillation, not receiving anticoagulation therapy, awakes one morning with severe left-sided weakness. On examination, she has a right gaze preference (she tends to look only to the right), and it is difficult to get her to look past the midline to the left. The left lower portion of her face sags slightly, her ability to squeeze her left eye shut is impaired, and she cannot raise the*

## Case 8-14—cont'd

*left side of her mouth when asked to show her teeth. When asked, she raises her eyebrows and wrinkles her forehead perfectly normally. She has profound left-sided weakness, worse in the arm, reduced deep tendon reflexes on the left, and a left Babinski sign.*

**Comment:** *This patient has experienced a right middle cerebral artery distribution stroke as a result of embolization of clot from her left atrium (largely preventable with anticoagulation). The gaze preference clearly indicates that this is a cortical, large vessel distribution infarct and not a lacunar infarct. She has a typical supranuclear CN VII palsy.*

## Case 8-15

### Bell's Palsy

*A healthy 80-year-old right-handed man awakes one morning with severe drooping of the entire right side of his face and aching pain behind his right ear. On examination in the emergency room he is completely unable to move the right side of his forehead. The right side of his face sags and is immobile. The soft tissue beneath his right eye droops so much that he cannot completely close the eye. The remainder of his examination is completely normal. In particular, he has normal language, normal optokinetic nystagmus, not a hint of pronation drift in his right arm, crisp fine motor movement in the right hand, and normal arm swing on the right when he walks.*

**Comment:** *This patient has a "Bell's palsy," an idiopathic paralysis of the facial nerve, probably due to herpes simplex or herpes zoster. Because the lesion affects the facial nerve itself, the entire hemiface is affected. Even though the distribution of weakness is quite manifest in this severe case, and clearly points to a peripheral localization, it is always worth being absolutely certain that there is no evidence of contralateral cerebral hemispheric impairment, which would raise the question of a stroke. The problem this patient is having closing his eye is quite common and potentially serious, as the cornea will rapidly ulcerate as it dries out. Thus, great care is always taken with these patients in the use of artificial tears during the day, eye ointment and eye patching at night, and in some cases, partially suturing the lids together to reduce the palpebral fissure.*

A neural pathway originating in the cornea and ultimately terminating in the orbicularis oculi provides the basis for the *corneal reflex*. Unmyelinated, nociceptive, V1 trigeminal afferent fibers from the cornea synapse on neurons in the spinal nucleus of V. Neurons in the spinal nucleus of V then project to the reticular formation in the immediate vicinity of the facial nucleus. Reticular neurons project to motoneurons in both CN VII nuclei innervating the orbicularis oculi. In this way, stimulation of one cornea elicits a blink reflex involving both eyes. Testing of the corneal reflex, for example, by gently stroking the cornea with a wisp of cotton, is most useful as a test of the integrity of V1. The contralateral corneal reflex is also suppressed following acute hemispheric lesions, such as large strokes, suggesting that the simple reflex arc described above also has a central component. Loud noise and flashes of bright light can also elicit reflex contraction of the orbicularis oculi, suggesting still other projections to the reticular neurons implicated in the blink component of the corneal reflex.

## Cranial Nerves IX and X

CN IX and X exit the lateral medulla (Figs. 8-1, 8-4, VIII, IX/X, XII/sensory decussation), the former as a single nerve, the latter as many rootlets that subsequently coalesce. The nerves leave the cranial vault via the jugular foramen. This places both nerves immediately posterior to the pharynx, to which some neurons in both nerves project. CN IX follows the internal carotid artery (another retropharyngeal structure) down to innervate the carotid sinus (see later discussion) and sends a branch up into the parotid gland (see later discussion). CN X follows the internal and common carotid arteries down into the thorax, where it innervates the heart and lungs and ultimately, the abdominal viscera (see later discussion).

Somatic motor functions of CN IX, the glossopharyngeal nerve, and CN X, the vagus nerve, are subserved by the *nucleus ambiguus*, which is located in the paramedian rostral medulla just dorsal to the inferior olive (Fig. 8-4, VIII, IX). It subserves swallowing. The nucleus ambiguus receives bilateral innervation from the cerebral cortex via corticobulbar tracts. Whereas the bilateral cortical innervation of CN VII neurons supplying forehead muscles is redundant and weakness of one side of the forehead is not seen with unilateral cortical lesions, cortical innervation from both hemispheres is needed to support normal swallowing, and hemispheric strokes are often associated with at least transient dysphagia (difficulty swallowing). Fibers from nucleus ambiguus, via CN IX and X, innervate the musculature of the pharynx and larynx. The division of labor between the two nerves is most unequal, in that CN IX supplies one muscle, the stylopharyngeus (which raises and dilates the pharynx), and CN X supplies the remainder.

Lesions of the nucleus ambiguus produce difficulty swallowing *(dysphagia)*, and alteration of voice *(dysarthria)*. The most common cause of damage is lateral medullary infarction (Practice 8-3C). Dysphagia is commonly a severe problem in patients with this type of stroke, and although this stroke is usually relatively benign and associated with an excellent prognosis for recovery, the rare death is typically related to the development of aspiration pneumonia as a result of inability to keep saliva and food out of the trachea. Occasionally, thoracic surgery is associated with damage to the recurrent laryngeal nerve, which carries fibers from the nucleus ambiguus, via the vagus, to the larynx. These patients develop a very breathy voice as the vocal cord on the side of the injury is paralyzed in abduction.

## B. SOMATIC SENSATION

Cranial nerve IX and to a minor extent CN X subserve sensation in the pharynx and carry the afferent input (via the nucleus of the solitary tract) to the nucleus ambiguus that underlies the swallowing reflex. Cranial nerves VII, IX, and X all innervate the middle ear, the external auditory meatus, and small portions of the pinna. Sensory afferent fibers of VII, IX, and X subserving pain, temperature, and touch sensation, whether from the pharynx or the ear, project to the nuclei of CN V.

## C. SPECIAL SENSATION

Cranial nerves VII, IX, and X all carry afferent fibers from oral tissues subserving taste that ultimately synapse in rostral portions of the *nucleus of the solitary tract*, sometimes referred to as the gustatory nucleus. The nucleus of the solitary tract is composed of a long column of cells and an associated tract located in the dorsolateral tegmentum and extending from the midpontine level well down into the medulla (Fig. 8-1; Fig. 8-4, VI, VII/VIII, IX/X, XII). CN VII carries fibers subserving taste over the anterior two-thirds of the tongue, CN IX the posterior third of the tongue, and CN X the

*Cranial Nerves and Brainstem Organization*

epiglottis. The taste fibers of CN VII project proximally via the chorda tympani, which crosses the superior margin of the eardrum, and only join CN VII in its petrous course. Thus, lesions of CN VII distal to its pathway through the petrous will not affect taste. Components of the nucleus of the solitary tract subserving taste ultimately project, via the contralateral thalamus, to portions of the insula, and via a parallel pathway, to the hypothalamus, the amygdala, and orbitofrontal cortex. The preponderance of limbic projections accounts for our tendency to view tastes, like smells, as either "good" or "bad."

## D. VISCERAL AUTONOMIC EFFERENT FUNCTION

Two major nuclei constitute the sources of visceral autonomic efferent functions subserved by CN VII, IX, and X: *the salivatory nucleus*, located in the dorsal tegmentum of the caudal pons, and the *dorsal efferent nucleus of the vagus*, located in the dorsal medullary tegmentum laterally adjacent to the hypoglossal nucleus (CN XII) (Fig. 8-1; Fig. 8-4, VIII, IX/X, XII/sensory decussation). The nucleus salivatorius actually represents a rostral continuation of the dorsal efferent nucleus of the vagus.

### Salivatory Nucleus

Parasympathetic neurons within the salivatory nucleus project via CN VII to the lacrimal gland of the eye, mucous membranes of the nose and oral cavity, and the sublingual and submandibular salivary glands, and via CN IX to the parotid salivary gland. Because most saliva is produced by the parotid gland, seventh cranial nerve palsies do not produce appreciable oral dryness.

## Dorsal Efferent Nucleus of the Vagus

Axons of neurons of the dorsal efferent nucleus of the vagus travel exclusively in the vagus nerve and provide parasympathetic innervation to essentially all the thoracic and abdominal viscera. The major afferent innervation of the nucleus is from the hypothalamus and the nucleus of the solitary tract. The most conspicuous effects of efferent vagal activity are to slow heart rate and promote gastric and intestinal peristalsis.

## E. VISCERAL AUTONOMIC AFFERENT FUNCTION

CN IX conveys afferent projections from the carotid sinus, a specialized baroreceptor region located in the most proximal portion of the internal carotid artery in the neck. The fibers ultimately synapse in the cardiovascular center located in the reticular formation of the rostral medulla, or they are relayed to this center after synapse in the nucleus of the solitary tract.

Vagal afferent fibers innervate essentially all the thoracic and abdominal viscera and project to caudal portions of the nucleus of the solitary tract, from which there are direct and indirect connections to the dorsal efferent nucleus of the vagus, enabling reflex control of the viscera. Of most relevance to neurologic function are fibers originating from pressure receptors (baroreceptors) in the left ventricle of the heart. There are also vagally innervated baroreceptors in the aortic arch. Baroreceptor afferents project to the medullary cardiovascular center.

The glossopharyngeal and vagal baroreceptor systems play a major role in the etiology of syncope and presyncope (near syncope), as illustrated in Cases 8-16 and 8-17.

---

### Case 8-16

#### Carotid Sinus Syndrome with Syncope
*A 55-year-old truck driver is seen for recurrent syncopal episodes. One episode was heralded by a second or two of dizziness, dimming of vision, and weakness before he lost consciousness. The two other episodes occurred without warning, and the first he realized that something was amiss was when he recovered consciousness. He was standing during one and cracked a rib in the fall. He ran his 18-wheeler*

*off the road in another, demolishing the truck but miraculously escaping serious injury. A 24-hour recording of his electrocardiogram (a Holter monitor) is normal. While being supported against a table tilted to 75 degrees, his carotid sinuses are successively rubbed ("massaged") for several seconds each. The electrocardiogram and blood pressure are continuously recorded. With massage of the right carotid sinus, his heart rate slows to 25 bpm and his*

## Case 8-16—cont'd

systolic blood pressure drops to 50 mm Hg. He becomes extremely dizzy and nearly loses consciousness.

**Comment:** This patient has a hypersensitive carotid sinus, such that mechanical distortion of the sinus elicits excessive glossopharyngeal afferent input, in effect signaling the brain that blood pressure is extremely high. The resultant response is some mix of reduction in heart rate, mediated by the vagus nerve, and reduction in peripheral vascular tone, mediated via sympathetic pathways originating in the intermediate zone of the spinal cord. Recurrent syncope or presyncope (severe dizziness, visual

blurring/dimming, generalized weakness, feeling of imminent syncope), due to a hypersensitive carotid sinus, is known as the carotid sinus syndrome. It is usually caused by largely undefined degenerative processes in the carotid sinus. In 50 percent of people over the age of 65 with syncope, the cause is carotid sinus syndrome. A particularly malignant form may be seen in people with invasion of the carotid sinus by head and neck cancers. To the extent that the syndrome is associated with bradycardia (slowing of the heart), it can be treated by implantation of a cardiac pacemaker. Drops in peripheral vascular tone are much more difficult to treat.

## Case 8-17

### Neurocardiogenic Syncope

A small group of medical students attends a first year seminar in which the clinical features of neurologic diseases are examined and ultimately correlated with neuroscientific aspects of the neural processes involved. The group gathers at the bedside of a 50-year-old man dying of amyotrophic lateral sclerosis (Lou Gehrig's disease), a disorder characterized by degeneration of anterior horn cells and corticospinal neurons in area 4 (see Case 6-2). While the history is being elicited and the patient is examined by one of the seminar leaders, one of the medical students faints. As she collapses, she is caught by her colleagues. She experiences no serious injury and recovers consciousness within a few seconds.

**Comment:** The currently preferred term for the episode experienced by this young woman is neurocardiogenic syncope, more commonly referred to in medical circles as vasovagal syncope. The first clue to the mechanism of this common phenomenon came from trauma victims who had experienced major blood loss. Paradoxically, some of these patients exhibited bradycardia, despite the fact that one would have expected extremely high heart rates to maintain adequate end organ perfusion despite markedly reduced cardiac venous return. Subsequently, left ventricular vagal receptors were discovered. When there is high sympathetic tone, these receptors can be triggered by exceptionally

forceful left ventricular contractions. In the medical student witnessing an emotionally wrenching scene, the stress of what she was experiencing engendered increased sympathetic stimulation of cardiac beta–receptors as a result of increased secretion of epinephrine by the adrenal medulla. Furthermore, standing immobile for a long time led to pooling of blood in her legs and circulating epinephrine stimulated peripheral vasodilatory beta-receptors. The reduced venous return to her heart led to diminished cardiac output, a fall in systemic blood pressure, and further enhancement of sympathetic stimulation of the heart. The resultant simulation of left ventricular vagal receptors due to very brisk left ventricular contractions then elicited bradycardia and a drop in peripheral vascular tone leading to syncope. The enhancement of sympathetic tone as part of the syncopal process and more fully, during the student's recovery from it, were reflected in a rapid heart rate and profuse sweating that were noted as she was lying on the floor recovering. Neurocardiogenic syncope is a common event that occasionally afflicts many normal people, typically young. Even rather minimal interventions may be successful in preventing syncope, for example, repeatedly tightening calf muscles by bouncing on the balls of the feet, thus increasing venous return to the heart. Occasional individuals, who seem to have somewhat exaggerated physiologic responses, may require medical treatment to prevent recurrent syncope.

**Cranial Nerves and Brainstem Organization**

## PRACTICE 8-6

**A.** A 72-year-old man awakes one morning and discovers that he has developed severe swallowing difficulty and chokes whenever he attempts to eat or drink. On examination, when he is asked to say "aaaaah," only the right side of his palate elevates. He has impairment in pain and temperature sensation over the left side of his face and the right hemibody. His left pupil is smaller than the right. He performs the finger-to-nose maneuver quite normally with either hand. His gait is normal. He has normal strength, symmetric deep tendon reflexes, and flexor plantar responses. Localize the lesion. What blood vessel is most likely implicated?

**B.** A 35-year-old man suddenly develops nausea, vomiting, imbalance and difficulty controlling his left upper extremity. His pupils are equal in size. He exhibits right beating nystagmus. He has weakness and sagging of the entire left side of his face. He has diminished pain and temperature sensation over the left side of his face in all three trigeminal dermatomes, but sensation over his right hemibody is normal. His palate lifts symmetrically. He demonstrates ataxia, dysmetria, and dyssynergia during the finger-to-nose maneuver with the left arm. His gait is very unsteady and he tends to fall to the left. Strength is normal, deep tendon reflexes are 1 to 2 and symmetric, and plantar responses are flexor. Localize the lesion.

**C.** A 45-year-old man complains of a 1-year history of insidiously progressive loss of hearing in his left ear. Long habituated to holding the telephone to his left ear, he has recently had to switch to his right because he can no longer understand what people are saying. On examination, he does have markedly reduced auditory acuity on the left, his left corneal reflex is diminished, and he exhibits mild dyssynergia during the finger-to-nose maneuver with his left arm, and a tendency to drift to the left as he walks. The remainder of his examination is completely normal. Which cranial nerves are implicated? Can you localize the lesion? How can you account for the patient's vague imbalance?

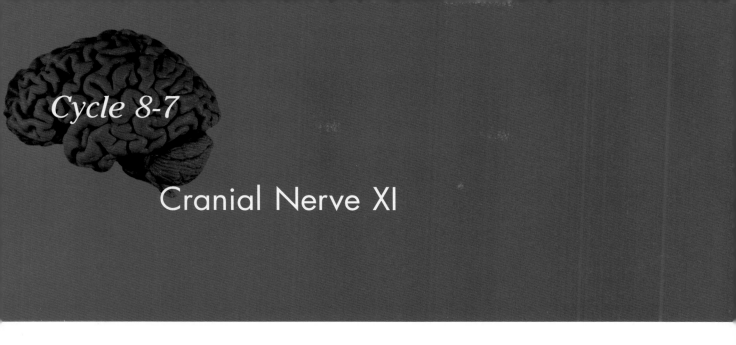

# Cycle 8-7

# Cranial Nerve XI

## Objective

Be able to locate the neurons supplying CN XI, list the muscles innervated by this nerve, describe the pathway the nerve takes to these muscles, and describe the consequences of CN XI lesions.

The axons of CN XI, the accessory nerve, arise from ventral horn neurons in cervical levels C1-C6. They exit the spinal cord laterally, between the dorsal and ventral roots, and course rostrally through the foramen magnum. The nerve then exits the cranial vault via the jugular foramen and innervates the sternocleido-mastoid and trapezius muscles. Its trajectory to the trapezius is very superficial, passing through the sub-cutaneous tissue of the posterior triangle of the neck. Accidental lacerations or tissue biopsies by surgeons may damage the nerve in this region.

The sternocleidomastoid muscle inserts on the clavicle and the mastoid process of the skull. Thus, when it contracts, it rotates the head in the contralat-eral direction. However, the supranuclear innervation of the accessory nerve is organized so that the cardinal rule of hemispheric function, that each cerebral hemi-sphere directs movements in or into the contralateral hemispace, is preserved. In this case, the left hemi-sphere projects to $\alpha$-motoneurons driving the left ster-nocleidomastoid muscle, enabling head turning to the right. The left hemisphere is also responsible for shrug-ging the right shoulder. In practice, sternocleidomastoid and trapezius weakness are usually supranuclear in origin.

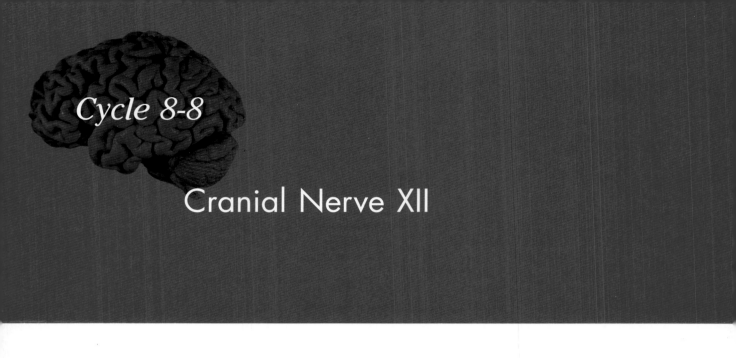

### Objective

Be able to locate the nucleus of CN XII, describe the pathway this nerve takes and the muscles it innervates, and explain the consequences of supranuclear and infranuclear lesions.

The nucleus of cranial nerve XII, the hypoglossal nerve, is located in the dorsomedial medullary tegmentum (Fig. 8-4, X, XII). The nerve courses ventrally through the medulla to exit just lateral to the medullary pyramid. It exits the cranial vault via the hypoglossal foramen, just lateral to the foramen magnum. From there it courses forward to form the major component of the lingual nerve, via which it innervates the muscles of the tongue. The lingual nerve also contains efferent projections of the facial nerve to minor salivary glands and afferent components of CN VII subserving taste. Supranuclear innervation of the hypoglossal nuclei is entirely from the contralateral hemisphere. Because the action of the tongue muscles is largely to thrust the tongue forward and contralaterally, lesions of the hypoglossal/lingual nerve result in protrusion of the tongue to the side of the lesion. The peculiar action of the muscles of the tongue leads to a paradoxic effect of supranuclear CN XII lesions: the tongue deviates to the side opposite the lesion. Tongue movement and ocular smooth pursuit are the only two functions that violate the principle that a cerebral hemisphere directs action in or into the contralateral hemispace.

## PRACTICE 8-8

**A.** A 68-year-old man with a long history of hypertension and heavy smoking awakes one morning with right-sided weakness. On examination, the lower right side of his face moves poorly when he is asked to show his teeth or squeeze his eyes shut, but he is able to wrinkle his brow symmetrically. His ability to turn his head to the right and shrug his right shoulder is impaired. His tongue deviates to the right when protruded. There is no abnormality of visual fields, eye movements, or optokinetic response. He has right hemibody weakness, worse in the arm. Fine motor movement is severely impaired in the right hand. He is too weak to even test for drift on the right or attempt the finger-to-nose maneuver with the right arm. Deep tendon reflexes are slightly hypoactive on the right and there is a right Babinski sign. Sensory examination is normal. Discuss lesion localization and provide a precise account for each of the neurologic signs observed in this patient.

**B.** A 75-year-old woman is found on the floor of her apartment, unable to move, and is brought to the emergency room. On examination, she lies absolutely immobile with her eyes open. She is completely mute. Upon command, she can look up or down but not to either side. Eye movements are conjugate. Pupils are equal and reactive to light. Injection of cold water in either ear fails to elicit any response. Corneal stimulation elicits slight reflexive depression of the eyelids but no contraction of the orbicularis oculi on either side. Painful stimulation of the brow does not elicit any facial movement (i.e., no grimace). She cannot say "aaah" on command, but stimulation of the back of the oropharynx with a cotton-tipped applicator elicits a gag reflex. Her tongue is midline and does not move. She cannot turn her head, shrug her shoulders, or move her limbs. Painful stimulation of the sternum elicits bilateral decerebrate posturing. Deep tendon reflexes are 1 and symmetric, and there are bilateral Babinski signs. She appears to be able to feel the touch of her body, but a detailed sensory examination is not conducted. Localize the lesion. Can you suggest a cause?

**C.** A 27-year-old man complains of numbness in his left leg that progresses over a day to involve his entire left hemibody. He then develops discomfort in the right side of his face, some imbalance, and some diplopia on right gaze. On examination, he has impaired abduction of the right eye. He cannot voluntarily gaze to the right with his left eye but the left adducts normally during an oculocephalic (Doll's eye) maneuver. His right corneal reflex is diminished. He has reduced pain and temperature sensation over his right forehead, cheek, and mandible. He has weakness of the entire right side of his face (including the forehead), and loss of taste over the right side of the anterior portions of his tongue. He has impaired pain and temperature sensation over the left hemibody. He tends to drift to the right when he walks, but he is not grossly ataxic and he performs a finger-to-nose maneuver on the right reasonably well. His motor examination is completely normal. Localize the lesion.

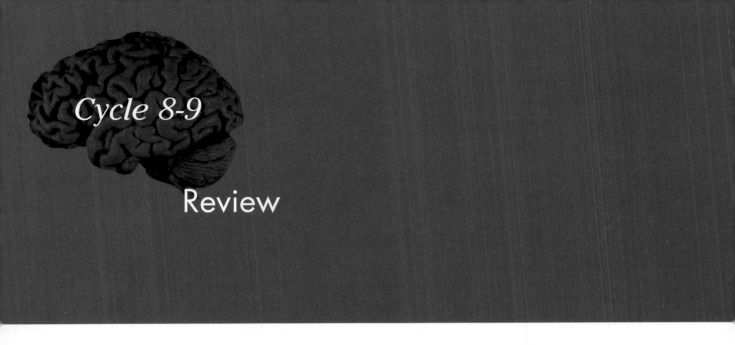

*Cycle 8-9*

# Review

Review Figures 8-1, 8-2, and 8-4 to consolidate your recall of the location of the cranial nerves and their respective nuclei. Table 8-2 summarizes the various functions of the cranial nerves and Table 8-3 summarizes the supranuclear innervation of motor cranial nerves.

## PRACTICE: REVIEW

Draw the levels of CN III, VI-VII, and VIII-IX from memory, depict and identify the major structures as discussed in this chapter. Refer to Figure 8-4 to check your answers.

**TABLE 8-2** Summary of the Cranial Nerves

| Cranial Nerve | Nucleus and Function | | | | |
|---|---|---|---|---|---|
| | **Somatic Motor** | **Somatic Sensory** | **Special Sensory** | **Autonomic Efferent** | **Autonomic Afferent** |
| I Olfactory | | | Olfactory bulb: smell | | |
| II Optic | | | Lateral geniculate nucleus: vision | | |
| III Oculomotor | Oculomotor nuclear complex: SR, IR, MR, IO, and levator palpebrae | | | Edinger-Westphal nucleus: parasympathetic innervation of pupillary sphincter and ciliary muscle | |
| IV Trochlear | CN IV nucleus: SO | | | | |
| V Trigeminal | Motor nucleus of V: muscles of mastication | Mesencephalic, chief sensory, and spinal nuclei of V: somesthesis in the face | | | |
| VI Abducens | Abducens nucleus: LR | | | | |
| VII Facial | Nucleus of CN VII: muscles of facial expression | Chief sensory and spinal nuclei of CN V: somesthesis in external auditory meatus | Nucleus of the solitary tract: taste over anterior 2/3 of the tongue | Nucleus salivatorius: lacrimal gland, sublingual and submandibular salivary glands | |
| VIII Auditory/ Vestibular | | | Cochlear nucleus: hearing; vestibular nuclei: motion | | |
| IX Glossopharyngeal | Nucleus ambiguus: stylopharyngeus muscle | Nucleus of the solitary tract: afferents from pharynx and posterior tongue projecting to n ambiguus—gag reflex; chief sensory and spinal nuclei of CN V: somesthesis in pharynx and external auditory meatus | Nucleus of the solitary tract: taste over the posterior 1/3 of the tongue | Nucleus salivatorius: parotid gland | Nucleus of the solitary tract/ medullary cardiovascular center: baroreceptors in the carotid sinus |
| X Vagus | Nucleus ambiguus: musculature of pharynx and larynx | Chief sensory and spinal nuclei of CN V: somesthesis in external auditory meatus | Nucleus of the solitary tract: taste over the epiglottis | Dorsal efferent nucleus of the vagus: parasympathetic innervation of thoracic and abdominal viscera | Nucleus of the solitary tract/ medullary cardiovascular center: autonomic afferents from thoracic and abdominal viscera |
| XI Accessory | Ventral horn, C1–C6: sternocleidomastoid and trapezius muscles | | | | |
| XII Hypoglossal | Hypoglossal nucleus: tongue | | | | |

*Key*: SR, superior rectus; IR, inferior rectus; MR, medial rectus; IO, inferior oblique; SO, superior oblique; LR, lateral rectus.

Cranial Nerves and Brainstem Organization

**TABLE 8-3** Summary of Supranuclear Innervation of Cranial Nerve Motor Nuclei

| Cranial Nerve/Function | Supranuclear Innervation |
| --- | --- |
| Eye movements (CN III, IV, VI) | |
|    Gaze | Contralateral |
|    Smooth pursuit | Ipsilateral |
| CN V (mastication) | Bilateral, redundant* |
| CN VII | |
|    Forehead | Bilateral, redundant* |
|    Lower face | Contralateral |
| CN IX, X | |
|    Swallowing | Bilateral, dependent† |
| CN XI | |
|    Head turning (sternocleidomastoid) | Ipsilateral (but turns head contralaterally) |
|    Shoulder shrug | Contralateral |
| CN XII | Contralateral (but lesion produces contralateral deviation because of thrusting effect of tongue muscles) |

*Spared by unilateral lesions.
†At least transiently affected by unilateral lesions.

## CYCLE 8-3

**A.** This patient has lesions of right CN V (V2 and V3) and right CN VI. The fact that the remainder of her neurologic examination is normal suggests that the lesion is outside the brainstem (extra-axial). The question is where are V2 and V3 and CN VI in close proximity to each other and yet separated from CN III and CN IV? The answer is in the apex of the petrous bone, where V2 and V3 are passing out of the cranium via the foramen rotundum and ovale, respectively, and CN VI is passing through Dorello's canal. The constellation of symptoms and signs exhibited by this patient constitutes Gradenigo's syndrome. It is most often caused by osteomyelitis of the petrous bone, typically due to infection by *Pseudomonas aeruginosa*. *Pseudomonas* organisms commonly colonize the external ear. Diabetes is associated with reduced ability to combat certain infections, *Pseudomonas* external otitis in particular. In diabetic patients, this is often referred to as "malignant otitis externa" because it is extremely difficult to treat and is often fatal, despite aggressive treatment with antibiotics and surgical debridement. If you answered cavernous sinus, give yourself partial credit. Cavernous sinus involvement probably would also have affected cranial nerves III, IV, and V1 (see Fig. 8-14), and it would have caused thrombosis of the sinus. This would have obstructed venous drainage from the orbit, leading to severe protrusion of the eye (proptosis).

**B.** This patient has a complete, pupil-sparing, right third cranial nerve palsy caused by infarction of the nerve due to diabetic microvasculopathy. Severe ptosis is due to denervation of the levator palpebra. The eye is deviated down and out because of the small but unopposed force of the SO and LR muscles. Infarction spares the pupillary fibers, either because it occurs within the midbrain, where partial third nerve palsies are the rule rather than the exception due to the dispersion of the nerve fibers, or, because when it occurs in the periphery, it primarily affects the core of the nerve, sparing the periphery where the autonomic fibers travel. Intra-axial infarcts causing third nerve palsies are often too small to cause long tract signs. Pupillary involvement with internal carotid—posterior communicating artery junction aneurysms is so reliable that when a patient presents with a complete third nerve palsy with completely normal pupillary function, it is not necessary to perform diagnostic studies to rule out an aneurysm. The loss of sensation in the feet and the missing ankle jerks are due to disseminated damage to peripheral nerves (polyneuropathy) caused by diabetes.

**C.** The loss of pain and temperature sensation in the left hemibody clearly indicates that the lesion is intra-axial; that is, it involves the brainstem or spinal cord, specifically, the lateral spinothalamic tract. Given the presence of an intra-axial lesion, the loss of pain and temperature sensation in the right side of the face implicates the right spinal nucleus and tract of CN V, located in the dorsolateral quadrant of the caudal pons and medulla and extending down to approximately the C2 level of the spinal cord. Such a lesion could also account for the impairment of pain and temperature sensation on the left side of the body, as the right spinal nucleus and tract of V and the lateral spinothalamic tract (which carries crossed fibers) are in close proximity through the caudal half of the brainstem (Fig. 8-4). Epicritic sensation is normal because the medial lemniscus is spared by virtue of its ventromedial location, and the chief sensory nucleus of CN V is rostral to the lesion. The cerebellar signs in the right arm and the gait ataxia implicate cerebellar pathways. The best candidate, given the region of the brainstem implicated so far, is the inferior cerebellar peduncle. Together, these findings suggest a lesion of the right dorsolateral medulla (Figs. 8-31, 8-32). This region also includes descending sympathetic pathways, damage to which would account for Horner's syndrome (ptosis and miosis), and the lateral vestibular nucleus, damage to which would account for both the nausea and vomiting and the strong tendency to fall to the right. This patient has a Wallenberg syndrome as a result of lateral medullary infarction, which is usually caused by

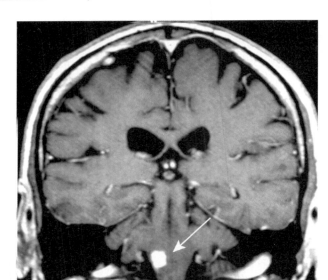

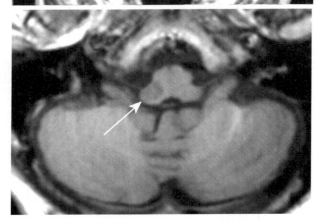

**Figure 8-31** Coronal magnetic resonance image (MRI) after contrast administration (*above*) and axial magnetic resonance image (MRI) of the medulla without contrast (*below*) demonstrating a lateral medullary infarction.

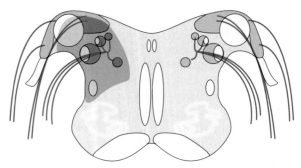

**Figure 8-32** Drawing of cross section of medulla diagramming the lesion in Practice Case 8-3C.

thrombosis of the ipsilateral vertebral artery. This is the second most common cause of Horner's syndrome, after lesions at the pulmonary apex (see Case 8-6).

**D.** This patient has lesions of cranial nerves III, IV, V1-V3, and VI. The absence of any other abnormalities on the examination indicates the lesion is extra-axial. The only place where all these cranial nerves are in close proximity is in the right cavernous sinus (Fig. 8-14). This patient has pituitary apoplexy. He has developed a large pituitary tumor that has grown into the right cavernous sinus. For somewhat uncertain reasons, the tumor has undergone hemorrhagic infarction, which has both compressed the nerves passing through the right cavernous sinus and interfered with their blood supply. The event in the right cavernous sinus caused right frontal headache. The dissemination of blood and necrotic tumor through the meninges produces a chemical meningitis and pancranial headache. The sudden expansion of the tumor upward as a result of the hemorrhage can damage the optic chiasm, impairing vision (more about this in Chapter 9). This situation is life-threatening because of the high likelihood of pituitary insufficiency. Bonus: the pupil is only slightly dilated because both the parasympathetic and the sympathetic innervation to the pupil have been interrupted.

**E.** Left CN VI.

## CYCLE 8-4

**A.** You would not see any impairment of ocular movement because neither the nuclei of CN III, IV, and VI, the gaze centers, or the pathways (mainly the MLF) connecting them are damaged by this very lateral lesion. If you said that you would see tonic deviation to the right, give yourself partial credit. What you would actually see is left beating vestibular nystagmus, which is nystagmus beating away from the lesion. This is because, from the point of view of the brainstem, there is greater vestibular input from the left than the right. This is exactly the situation the brainstem experiences when the head is spinning to the left, and it has no way of knowing that this input pattern is caused not by spinning but by damage to the right vestibular nucleus. The fast component of the nystagmus originates in input from the frontal eye fields. In the comatose patient, this input is lost (because the entire cerebral cortex is not functioning) and one is left with tonic deviation of the

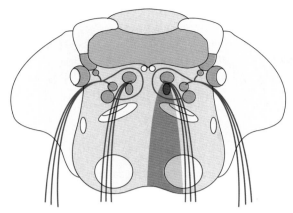

**Figure 8-33** Cross section of caudal pons diagramming the lesion in Practice Case 8-4B.

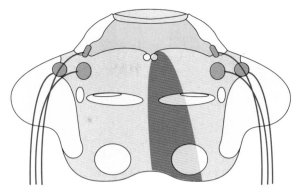

**Figure 8-34** Cross section of mid-pons diagramming the lesion in Practice Case 8-4C.

eyes to the side of the lesion, or the side of injection of cold water during cold caloric testing.

**B.** This patient has an infarction involving the left paramedian basis pontis extending up into the pontine tegmentum to the left PPRF (the left pontine lateral gaze center) (Fig. 8-33). The fact that the gaze paresis and the hemiparesis are on opposite sides tells you that this cannot be a cerebral lesion (see Case 8-12). Remember that the presence of a cranial nerve deficit and a contralateral hemiparesis signals a brainstem lesion.

He has a right-sided ataxic hemiparesis resulting from damage to the left corticospinal tract before it has decussated, and damage to corticopontocerebellar projections destined for the right cerebellar hemisphere. He has loss of epicritic sensation on his right side because of damage to the left medial lemniscus. The results of injection of cold water in the left ear should be normal. If the infarct extended only into the PPRF, then left-sided cold caloric testing would induce right beating vestibular nystagmus. If the infarct extended into the left abducens nucleus, then cold caloric stimulation on the left would have no effect. However, extension of the infarct into the abducens nucleus would have damaged the fibers of CN VII as they loop around the nucleus, producing paralysis of the muscles of facial expression on the left. This is not present, indicating that the infarct extends dorsally only as far as the PPRF. Because this is a single sector infarct (see Chapter 2), it localizes to a single, long, median penetrating artery originating at the basilar artery. It may have become thrombosed either because of a microatheroma or because a large basilar artery plaque expanded and occluded its orifice.

**C.** This patient has essentially the same infarct as the patient in B except that it is slightly more rostral (Fig. 8-34). Thus, instead of damaging the left PPRF, she has damaged the left MLF, causing a left INO. If you are wondering why she doesn't also have a left gaze paresis because of damage to cerebral projections to the left pontine lateral gaze center, you are quite astute. These projections travel relatively near the midline in the dorsal tegmentum (although not in the MLF) and many patients with this type of infarct will indeed have a gaze palsy. The combination of a left gaze palsy and a left INO constitutes the "1½" syndrome.

**D.** He would exhibit a visual grasp. In this case, the ability to voluntarily direct or maintain gaze on a specific target would be overwhelmed by the reflexive orienting mechanisms provided by both the parietal lobes and the superior colliculi.

## CYCLE 8-6

**A.** This patient has a left lateral medullary infarction that is relatively ventral in its distribution (Fig. 8-35). Thus, it involves the nucleus and tract of V, the lateral spinothalamic tract, descending sympathetic fibers, and the nucleus ambiguus, but it spares more dorsal structures. This portion of the brainstem is supplied by one or more twigs from the posterior inferior cerebellar artery (PICA). PICA occlusion is usually associated with vertebral artery thrombosis. The medullary branches of the PICA always supply the dorsolateral quadrant of the medulla, but the exact territory of supply varies somewhat dorsoventrally and along the rostrocaudal axis. In any event, these branches never supply the ventrome-

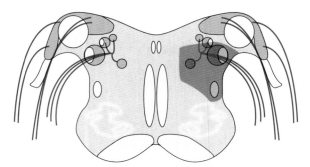

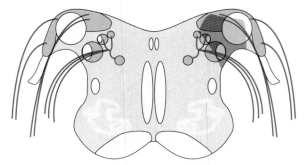

**Figure 8-35** Cross section of rostral medulla diagramming lesion in Practice Case 8-6A.

**Figure 8-36** Cross section of rostral medulla diagramming lesion in Practice Case 8-6B.

dial medulla. Thus, lateral medullary infarctions are never accompanied by weakness, alterations of deep tendon reflexes, or Babinski signs. If one did observe such signs in a patient, it would suggest additional involvement of the anterior spinal artery. This would suggest bilateral vertebral thrombosis, a vascular event associated with a high fatality rate.

**B.** This patient also has a left lateral medullary infarction. However, it is more dorsal and more rostral than the infarct in the patient in A (Fig. 8-36). It is sufficiently rostral to damage the seventh cranial nerve. It involves the nucleus and spinal tract of CN V, the lateral vestibular nucleus (hence the nausea and vomiting and the right beating vestibular nystagmus). The right beating nystagmus reflects the fact that because of the reduced inhibitory input from the left medial vestibular nucleus to the left abducens nucleus, the neurons in the nucleus fire faster, making the eyes deviate to the left. Corticobulbar pathways from the left frontal eyefields projecting to the right pontine lateral gaze center (PPRF) then produce saccades back to the right. The lesion spares the nucleus ambiguus, the descending sympathetic pathway, and the lateral spinothalamic tract. The inferior cerebellar peduncle is involved. This patient's youth makes it unlikely that thrombosis of the vertebral artery, with secondary PICA occlusion, was caused by atheromatous disease. Vascular dissection (separation of the media and adventitia with flow of blood into the resultant space and secondary thrombosis at the site of intimal injury) is a far more likely etiology.

**C.** This patient has a vestibular schwannoma, a benign Schwann cell tumor involving the vestibular portion of left CN VIII (often referred to inappropriately as an acoustic schwannoma) (Fig. 8-37). The tumor compresses CN V and the acoustic portion of CN VIII, leading to reduction of the corneal reflex and hearing

loss. It is quite characteristic for the hearing loss to affect voice frequencies the most, with resultant difficulty in understanding speech. Vestibular function is also affected, but because the brainstem is able to adapt, and there is intact vestibular function on the other side, no vestibular impairment is clinically apparent. CN VII accompanies CN VIII through the CP angle and into the internal auditory meatus. However, it is remarkably resilient, and even with severe stretching of the nerve, these patients seldom present with facial

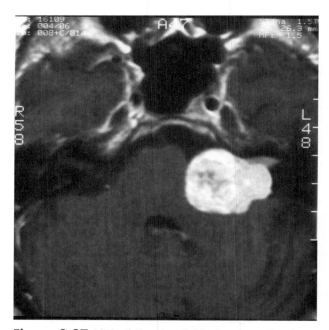

**Figure 8-37** MRI of Practice 8-6C, demonstrating large vestibular schwannoma filling the left cerebellopontine angle cistern, where it compresses the fifth, seventh, and eighth cranial nerves and the cerebellar peduncles.

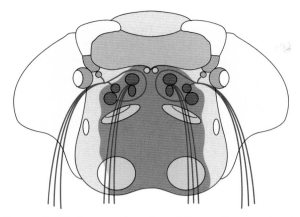

**Figure 8-38** Cross section of caudal pons diagramming the lesion in Practice Case 8-8B.

weakness. The tumor in this case was quite large, filling the CP angle cistern and compressing cerebellar pathways; hence the vague dysequilibrium and mild incoordination of the left arm.

## CYCLE 8-8

**A.** The fact that this patient has a "pure motor stroke" makes it likely that he has experienced a lacunar infarction that is probably located in the posterior limb of the internal capsule or the corona radiata. If it were a left middle cerebral artery distribution infarction, he would probably have some sensory findings, might have abnormalities in the optokinetic response, and almost certainly would have a language disorder (see Chapter 12). The lesion results in upper motor neuron CN VII, XI, and XII palsies. Damage to corticospinal and corticobulbar fibers produces right-sided weakness. The particular involvement of the cerebrum in upper extremity function accounts for the weakness being worse in the arm. Damage to corticospinal fibers is responsible for the impairment in fine motor movement in the right hand. Because of the acuteness of the lesion, he exhibits the cerebral equivalent of spinal cord shock, manifested as temporary depression of deep tendon reflexes on the affected side. Damage to corticobulbar projections to the medullary reticulospinal system produces a Babinski response on the right side.

**B.** This patient has experienced an infarction of much of the basis pontis and the pontine tegmentum due to basilar artery thrombosis (Fig. 8-38). Because she

cannot move even though she is awake and alert and her cerebrum is functioning quite normally, this situation is referred to as a "locked-in" state. Her entire repertoire of voluntary movement is limited to up and down gaze, reflecting preservation of the midbrain, including the vertical gaze center and the third cranial nerve nuclear complex. The gag reflex and decerebrate posturing reflect preservation of tissue in the caudal pons and the medulla. This tragic condition is commonly misconstrued by health care personnel as "coma," leading to insensitive treatment of these patients.

**C.** The presence of cranial nerve deficits on one side and long sensory tract abnormalities on the opposite side tells you this is a brainstem lesion. The abnormalities in sensation and the diminished right corneal reflex clearly implicate the right spinal nucleus and tract of CN V and the right lateral spinothalamic tract. He also has evidence of an infranuclear CN VII palsy (it involves the entire face). The absence of major cerebellar signs tells you that even though the lesion involves the

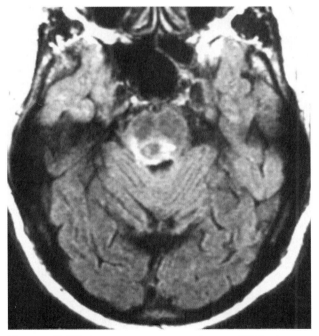

**Figure 8-39** Magnetic resonance image (MRI) demonstrating hemorrhage from a cavernous angioma in the right caudal pontine tegmentum. The hemorrhage is the dark area that is surrounded by an irregular white region (which reflects edema).

dorsolateral quadrant of the brainstem, it has spared the inferior cerebellar peduncle. Thus, it must be rostral to the medulla, most likely in the pons, sufficiently caudal to catch CN VII. The lesion must extend sufficiently medially to involve fibers of CN VI and the PPRF, hence the impaired abduction on the right and the right gaze paresis, respectively. The lesion, shown in Figure 8-39 is precisely in the location predicted by the examination. It is a cavernous angioma, a small vascular malformation that has bled.

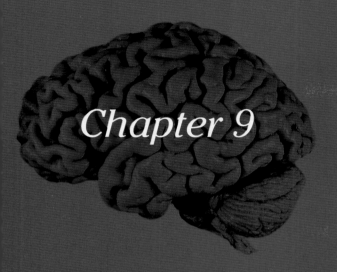

# Chapter 9

# VISION

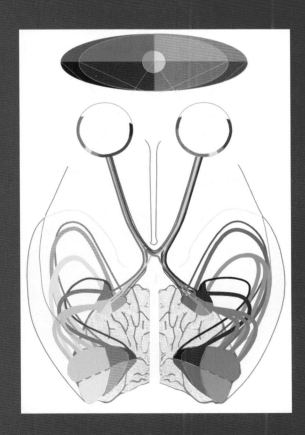

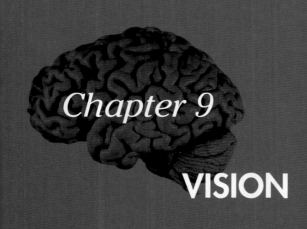

# Chapter 9

# VISION

# Introduction

Visual pathways extend from the eyes backward, past the pituitary gland, around the brainstem, through temporal and parietal lobe white matter to the occipital cortex, and thence forward to temporal and parietal cortex. Because of the extent of these pathways, a clear understanding of visual systems is important to the clinician in localizing and characterizing intracranial disorders.

The optic nerve head, the intraocular portion of the optic nerve, is visible on funduscopic examination. It represents the point at which intraocular pressure is balanced by intracranial pressure. For this reason, the funduscopic examination provides a direct means of detecting certain pathologic processes leading to excessive pressure in either of these two compartments.

The visual system is also of great neuroscientific interest. The neurophysiology of this system exemplifies, better than any other, possibly the single most essential feature of sensory systems in general, that of *feature enhancement*. Thus, light sensitive layers of the retina, lining the back of the eye, might be compared quite reasonably to the film in a camera. However, processes taking place within neural networks of the retina, and further ramified through various stages in the central nervous system (CNS) visual trajectory, serve to enhance selected features of the incoming visual input that are particularly important to our adaptive responses to that input. Stop reading for a moment and gaze at the ceiling of the room you are in. You will notice that your attention is drawn not by the expanses of undifferentiated color and luminance, but rather by the light fixtures and the lines where the walls join the ceiling. This reflects the importance of the shape of objects and their features (both defined by edges) in enabling you to recognize them, and the importance of boundaries between areas of different luminance or color (more edges) in enabling you to navigate in your environment, whether walking about your home, or navigating a narrow pathway along a cliff face. These two examples reflect two other major dimensions of visual systems that are apparent within the retina but become fully ramified only within the temporal and parietal cortices: the division of visual processing into multiple parallel streams, each specialized in a particular type of feature enhancement, and the division of these parallel streams into two major domains, object recognition (the "what" system), and location and movement within the visual environment (the "where" system). As we shall see in Chapter 12, we are capable of focusing our attention upon neural representations within one or the other of these two systems, but in general, our visual experience reflects coordinated neural activity within both of these processing streams and their more highly specialized subcomponents.

Although feature enhancement describes a fundamental emergent property of neural networks in the visual system, the term does not do justice to what the visual brain actually accomplishes. From a two-dimensional, upside-down image cast upon the retina, the brain creates a three-dimensional image that melds what we see with the visual knowledge we already have; that maintains near constancy of visual perception under vastly different lighting conditions and despite sudden movements of the visual field; and that achieves a perception of constancy about the size, shape, and color of objects we see regardless of how near or far, the angle from which we view them, or whether they are moving or still. Thus, the visual system in no way resembles the passive process of a camera—rather, it is a highly creative system.

As important as somesthesis, audition, taste, and olfaction are to our sensory experience and survival, we are primarily visual animals. Over 50 percent of the cerebral cortex is devoted to neural networks involved in processing visual input. For this reason alone, our visual experience (compounded of perception and imagery) plays a dominant role in defining our entire conscious experience.

Vision

*421*

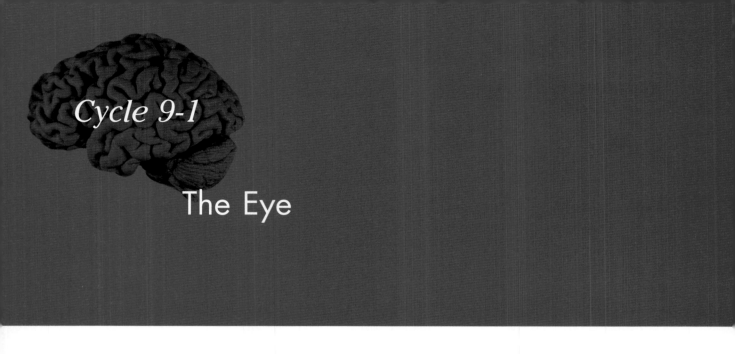

# Cycle 9-1

## The Eye

**Objective**

Be able to identify the major features of the eye.

Figure 9-1 depicts the major features of the eye, and Table 9-1 describes their function. All these features should be considered essential vocabulary.

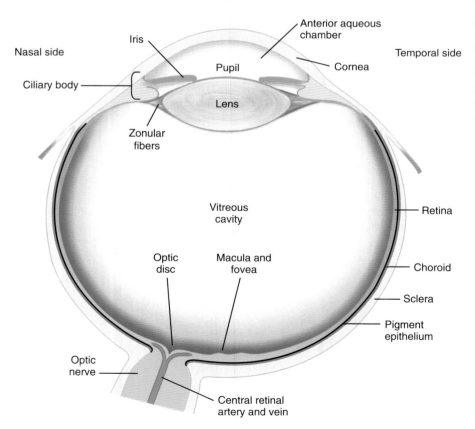

**Figure 9-1** Diagram of a horizontal section through the eye.

**TABLE 9-1** Major Features of the Eye

| Structure | Description/Function |
|---|---|
| Anterior aqueous chamber | Fluid-filled space between the iris and the cornea |
| Central retinal artery and vein | Blood supply and drainage for inner layers of the retina |
| Choroid | Vascularized, nutritive layer between the sclera and retina |
| Ciliary body | Ring of tissue composed of ciliary epithelium, which produces aqueous humor (the fluid in the anterior chamber), and the ciliary muscle, which alters the shape of the lens to enable focusing |
| Cornea | Transparent tissue forming the anterior wall of the anterior chamber; contributes to focusing |
| Fovea | Central, most sensitive portion of the macula, ~700 μm in diameter, subserving the central 2 degrees of vision |
| Fundus | Posterior aspect of the interior of the eye, visualized with an ophthalmoscope |
| Iris | The diaphragm that regulates the amount of light admitted to the eye |
| Lens | Focuses light on the retina |
| Macula | Retinal area providing the highest visual acuity |
| Optic disk | Oval area where the optic nerve enters the eye |
| Optic nerve | Contains the axons of retinal ganglion cells that transmit visual information to the brainstem and thalamus |
| Pigment epithelium | Single layer of pigmented cells behind the sensory retina that absorbs stray light and provides metabolic support to retinal cells |
| Pupil | Opening at the center of the iris that admits light to the vitreous chamber and the retina |
| Retina | Photosensitive receptor layer, associated neurons (the sensory retina) and the pigment epithelium |
| Sclera | Tough, outer covering of the eye that provides the scaffold for the choroid and retina |
| Vitreous cavity | Transparent, jelly-filled space between the lens and the retina |
| Zonular fibers | Fibers that transmit tension from the ciliary muscle to the lens, enabling focusing |

Vision

# Retinal Organization

**Objectives**

1. Be able to describe the layers of the retina in relation to the pathway that light takes to reach the photoreceptors.
2. Be able to describe visual perimetry.
3. Be able to explain the blind spot and account for its location.

Light entering the eye passes successively through the cornea, aqueous humor, pupil, lens, and vitreous humor, and ultimately is focused on the retina. The retina contains the light-sensitive *photoreceptors* (rods and cones). Neural activity elicited by the action of light on these photoreceptors is ultimately transmitted to the brainstem via the optic nerve.

The retina is organized in a peculiar and seemingly illogical manner that nevertheless suffices to support the remarkable visual acuity of which we are capable (Fig. 9-2). The photoreceptors actually form the deepest layer of the retina; they abut the pigment epithelium. The photoreceptors consist of highly specialized intra-cellular material located in long, tubular extensions of cells located immediately above them, forming the outer nuclear layer. The output of these cells is transmitted to a complex network of interneurons composing the plexiform layers of the retina. Axons of cells in the plexiform layers synapse on *retinal ganglion cells*, which constitute the innermost cellular layer of the retina. The axons of retinal ganglion cells compose the nerve fiber layer of the retina and ultimately form the optic nerve. Light must thus pass through the nerve fiber layer, the ganglion cell layer, the plexiform layers, and the cells of the outer nuclear layer to get to the photoreceptors. However, at the fovea, the locus of highest visual acuity, there are relatively few cellular elements between the photoreceptors and the vitreous. Testing of visual acuity assesses only the function of the fovea. Testing of visual fields (Fig. 9-3) is necessary to assess the function of the remainder of the retina.

The point at which the axons of the ganglion cells coalesce to form the optic nerve—the optic nerve head—is also exceptional in that it contains no photoreceptors. This point is the location of the *blind spot* (Figs. 9-3, 9-4).

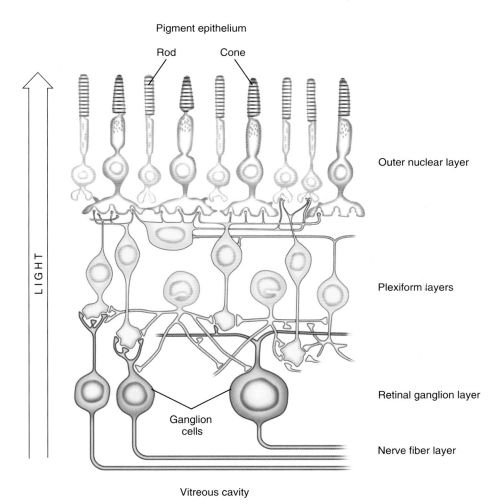

**Figure 9-2** Cellular organization of the retina. (Adapted from Dowling JE. Retina. In Dulbecco R (ed). The Encyclopedia of Human Biology, 2nd ed. Vol. 7. San Diego, Academic Press, 1997, pp 571-587. Copyright 1997 with permission from Elsevier Science.)

Vision

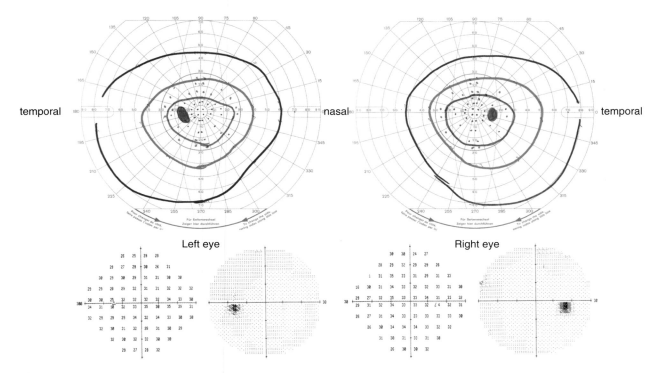

**Figure 9-3** Maps of the visual fields, generally referred to as *visual perimetry*. Each eye is tested individually. The subject places his/her eye at the center of a hemispheric bowl and maintains gaze upon (i.e., *fixates* on) a target point that defines 0° of latitude and longitude. Targets of various size and brightness are then presented systematically at various points on the hemisphere. No matter how perimetry is done, the maps of visual sensitivity that are derived from it always represent what the subject sees. The top two maps (one for each eye) are an example of Goldmann perimetry. The circular lines are derived by connecting points of equal visual sensitivity. The purple lines delineate the most peripheral points at which the subject could see a large, bright stimulus. The red lines define the detection limits for a smaller, dimmer stimulus. The blue lines correspond to a stimulus that is of the same size but lesser luminance than that used to map the red lines. The dots indicate particular additional locations where the ability to detect a target was tested. This study is normal but for a slightly enlarged blind spot in the left eye. Goldmann perimetry is performed "by hand" by a skilled technician. It has the advantage that the technician is constantly able to monitor the subject's compliance, detect instances of deviation of fixation from the 0° point, and retest responses that seem inconsistent. Because of its accuracy, it constitutes the "gold standard." It has the disadvantage of being time-consuming, and labor intensive, and its quality is operator-dependent. The two bottom map pairs are examples of the results of "automated" (computerized) perimetry. To obtain these maps, a computer activates light emitting diodes at various points in the visual fields and the patient presses a button as soon as s/he detects a light. The visual sensitivity in these maps is denoted either as a number (left map of each pair), higher numbers indicating higher sensitivity, or as shading (right map of each pair), lighter shading indicating higher sensitivity. The location of the blind spot is readily evident. *Note that in both the Goldmann and automated perimetric maps, the blind spot is located in the outer or temporal visual hemifield. It is seen here because the optic nerve exits the eye medial to the fovea, which is located at the very back of the eye, and light rays from the temporal hemifield fall on the retina medial to the fovea.*

**Figure 9-4** Cover your right eye and fixate on the cross with your left eye from a distance of about 6 inches. Now gradually move away from the page. At some point, the dark circle will disappear as it is projected onto the blind spot of your left eye. This experiment also demonstrates something very revealing about the consequence of damage to visual pathways—the result is simply the absence of vision rather than black regions. For this reason, patients may be surprisingly oblivious to visual field deficits.

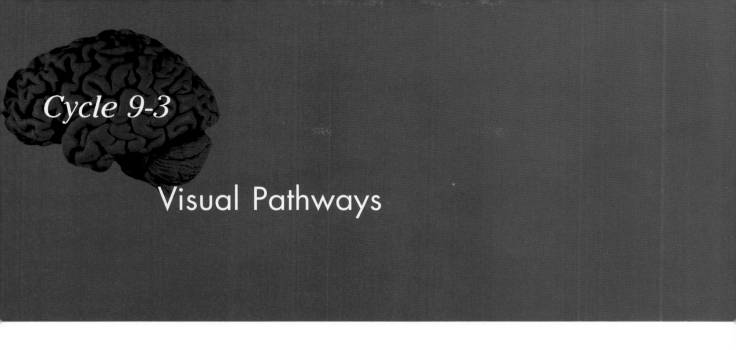

# Visual Pathways

## Objectives

1. Be able to describe the optic pathways from the eyes to the calcarine cortex.
2. Be able to localize lesions of the optic pathways on the basis of specific visual field deficits.
3. Be able to explain the term "retinotopic mapping."
4. Be able to describe the visual association cortices in the brain.

## THE RETINOGENICULATE PATHWAY

The axons of retinal ganglion cells contributing to the retinogeniculate pathway project backward, through an optic nerve, the optic chiasm, and an optic tract, until they finally synapse upon cells in a lateral geniculate nucleus (LGN) of the thalamus. The intraorbital portion of an optic nerve rests in loose fatty tissue within the bony orbit behind the eye and, within this space, has enough extra length to allow the eye free motion (Fig. 9-5). The optic nerve enters the cranial vault through the optic foramen. The two optic nerves come together to form the *optic chiasm* over the sella turcica, just behind the pituitary stalk. The *optic tracts* connect the chiasm to the *lateral geniculate nuclei* of the thalamus. Fibers are redistributed in the optic chiasm so that *each optic tract represents the contralateral visual fields of both eyes*. This distribution is

accomplished as follows: fibers from the temporal halves of the retinas (representing the nasal visual fields) proceed through the chiasm to the optic tracts without crossing, whereas fibers from the nasal halves of the retinas (representing the temporal visual fields) cross in the chiasm to travel in the contralateral optic tract. Each optic tract thus has fibers representing the nasal visual field of the ipsilateral eye and the temporal visual field of the contralateral eye (Figs. 9-5 to 9-9).

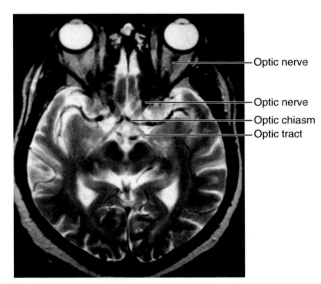

**Figure 9-5** Axial MRI of the head demonstrating the optic nerves as they pass through the fatty tissue of the orbits, through the optic foramina, and into the cranial vault, where they come together to form the optic chiasm.

Vision

Optic nerve         Optic chiasm

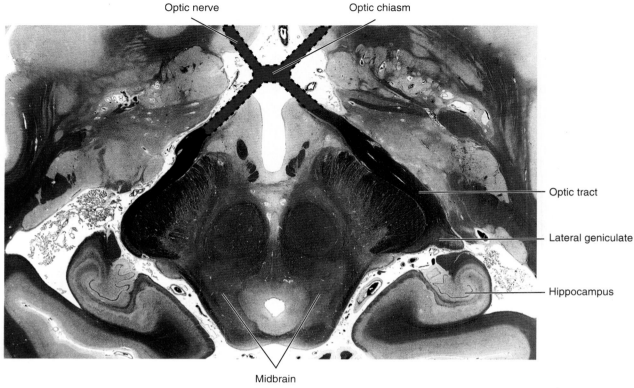

Optic tract

Lateral geniculate

Hippocampus

Midbrain

**Figure 9-6** Axial view of the rostral brainstem demonstrating the optic tracts from the optic chiasm to the lateral geniculate nuclei. This figure employs an inversion of the traditional histologic orientation in order to enable more direct comparison with Figure 9-5. (Modified from Warner JJ, Atlas of Neuroanatomy. Boston, Butterworth Heinemann, 2001, with permission from Elsevier Science.)

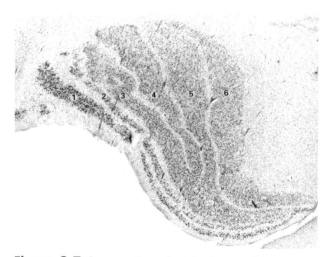

**Figure 9-7** Cross section of a lateral geniculate nucleus, demonstrating the lamina (cresyl violet, ×50). (From Kandel ER, Schwartz JH, Jessel TM (eds). Principles of Neural Science, 4th ed. New York, McGraw-Hill, 2000. Reproduced with permission of The McGraw-Hill Companies, Inc.)

Each optic tract courses around the midbrain and terminates in an LGN (Fig. 9-6). Although the lateral geniculate nuclei are part of the thalamus, they are located so far caudally and laterally that they appear to be separate from the thalamus. Each LGN has six layers or laminae of cells (Fig. 9-7). Fibers from the contralateral eye terminate in layers 1, 4, and 6, and fibers from the ipsilateral eye terminate in layers 2, 3, and 5.

The axons of cells within the LGN ascend through the temporal, parietal, and occipital white matter to synapse on neurons within layer 4 of the cortex along the calcarine fissure on the medial aspect of the occipital lobe. This area is referred to variously as primary visual cortex, *calcarine cortex*, striate cortex, Brodmann's area 17, and *V1*. The visual cortex, like other sensory cortices, is organized into functional columns of neurons. Each column receives input from a single eye and columns responding to input from the same visual field locus but from different eyes are located immediately adjacent to one another. Thus, the func-

A                                              B

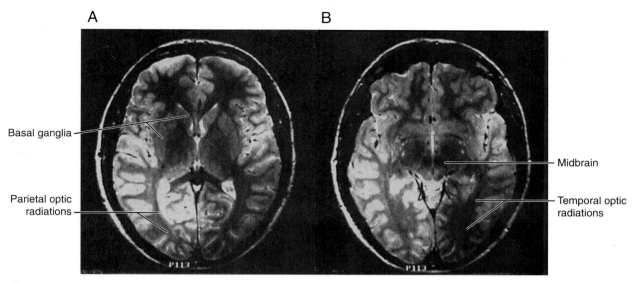

Basal ganglia

Parietal optic radiations

Midbrain

Temporal optic radiations

**Figure 9-8** Axial magnetic resonance image (MRI) of the brain demonstrating the optic radiations. *A* demonstrates the parietal optic radiations. *B* demonstrates the temporal optic radiations.

tional columns in V1 are often referred to as *ocular dominance columns*.

When we look at objects that are relatively near to us, the visual image captured by each retina is not exactly the same. Visual areas of the cerebral cortex use this image disparity to compute distance, thus providing the basis for depth perception (stereoscopic vision). If input from the two eyes to each LGN and calcarine cortex were blended, this capacity for depth perception would be lost. Depth perception is critical to our ability to accurately respond to objects in our immediate vicinity, to our ability to reconstruct three-dimensional perception from two-dimensional retinal images, and to the process of ocular convergence (Chapter 8).

The connections between the LGN and the calcarine cortex are referred to as the optic radiations (Figs. 9-8, 9-9).[1] Fibers corresponding to the inferior

aspects of the retinas (subserving the superior visual fields) loop anteriorly in the deep temporal lobe white matter (Meyer's loop) before coursing posteriorly to synapse on neurons along the inferior bank of the calcarine cortex. Fibers corresponding to the superior aspects of the retinas (subserving the inferior visual fields) course dorsally, through the deep parietal white matter, as they pass posteriorly to synapse on neurons along the superior bank of the calcarine cortex. Thus, the inferior bank of the left calcarine cortex represents the right superior visual field, and the superior bank of the left calcarine cortex represents the right inferior visual field (Fig. 9-9). Fibers representing the central, macular portions of the retinas project to the most posterior aspects of the calcarine cortex, including the occipital pole. Fibers representing peripheral portions of the retinas project to the most anterior portions of the calcarine cortex. Thus, our entire visual field is mapped in a systematic, point-to-point fashion along the calcarine cortex, something referred to as *retinotopic mapping*. The calcarine representation of the macula is disproportionately large, reflecting the extensive cortical resources dedicated to processing visual input to this region of particularly high visual acuity.

The calcarine cortex projects directly or indirectly to over 30 different visual areas in the brain, arranged both in serial (forming hierarchies) and in parallel, each of which enhances certain specific features of visual

[1]We have mentioned only the projections from cells in the LGN to the calcarine cortex. In actuality, for each LGN neuron projecting to the calcarine cortex, one or more neurons in layers 3 and 5 of the calcarine cortex projects back to the LGN. The precise function of these reciprocal connections is not well understood. However, two-way connectivity is the rule rather than the exception in the brain. Among other things, it provides the basis for one of the most useful capacities of neural networks: the ability to use what is already known to help resolve ambiguity or noise in the input. This phenomenon will be discussed at greater length in Chapter 12.

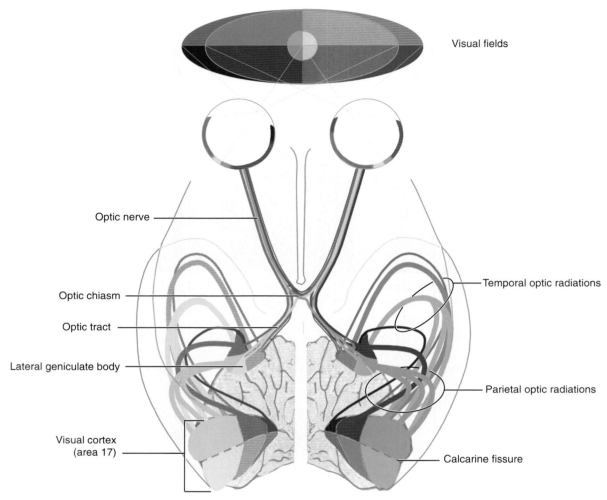

Visual fields

Optic nerve

Temporal optic radiations

Optic chiasm

Optic tract

Lateral geniculate body

Parietal optic radiations

Visual cortex
(area 17)

Calcarine fissure

**Figure 9-9** Summary of retinogeniculate pathways. Note the disproportionately large representation of the (green/yellow) macula in calcarine cortex. The extent of the spread of the optic radiations is exaggerated to enhance clarity.

input. Visual association cortices include the entire occipital lobe (Brodmann's areas 17, 18, and 19), the middle and inferior temporal gyri, and the undersurface of the temporal lobe (Brodmann's areas 20, 21, and 37), and both superior and medial parietal cortex (Brodmann's area 7) (see Fig. 12-1). Most of the specialized visual areas are retinotopically organized. However, in the areas that are most remote from calcarine cortex, particularly those in the temporal lobes, retinal or spatial location no longer constitutes a dimension of visual analysis, as features are analyzed here in the abstract, regardless of location (see following discussion).

## LOCALIZATION WITHIN THE RETINOGENICULATE PATHWAY

Because of the shifting pattern of organization of visual fibers between the optic nerves and the calcarine cortex, lesions at different loci lead to different patterns of visual impairment. These patterns can easily be defined through neurologic examination and, thus, provide a practical basis for neurologic localization. Isolated lesions of the optic tracts and LGN are rare, so in the following cases, we will focus on the impact of lesions of the optic nerves, optic chiasm, optic radiations, and calcarine cortex:

## Case 9-1

### Right Optic Neuritis due to Multiple Sclerosis

*A 25-year-old woman awakes one morning with vague discomfort in her right eye associated with mild blurring of vision. By the next day, she has considerable retro-ocular pain that is exacerbated by eye movement, and she has lost much of the vision in her right eye. Results of examination of her visual fields are shown in Figure 9-10.*

**Comment:** *The lesion in this case involves the right optic nerve. Vision in all four quadrants of the visual field of a single eye is affected. If the lesion were as far posterior as the optic chiasm, visual fields in both eyes would be affected. The rapid but not sudden loss of vision in one eye exhibited by this patient strongly suggests that she has optic neuritis. Most patients with optic neuritis have or will eventually develop multiple sclerosis. The optic nerve is actually part of the CNS (i.e., not a peripheral nerve) and is thus invested by pia and arachnoid (leptomeninges) all the way to its junction with the back of the eye. Whereas inflammation of the nerve itself does not cause pain, inflammation of the associated leptomeninges does because they are heavily supplied by nociceptive nerve fibers. Recovery in this patient can be accelerated by the administration of high-dose corticosteroids and she will probably recover most vision in her right eye.*

## Case 9-2

### Bitemporal Hemianopia due to Chiasmal Lesion

*A 33-year-old woman presents to a neurologist complaining of a 4-month history of headaches. Recently she has noted some vague visual impairment. She feels that her peripheral vision is not as good as it once was. The results of visual field examination are demonstrated in Figure 9-11.*

**Comment:** *This patient demonstrates a bitemporal hemianopia: vision in the temporal half of the visual field in each eye is severely impaired. Therefore, optic nerve fibers originating in the nasal portion of both retinas are involved. These are the fibers that cross at the optic chiasm. Thus, this patient has a lesion in the vicinity of the optic chiasm. In most cases, including this one, this is caused by a pituitary tumor compressing the chiasm from below (Fig. 9-12).*

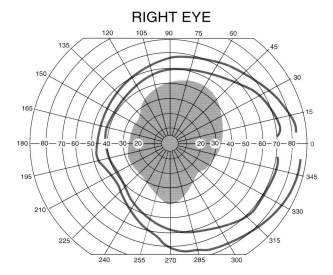

RIGHT EYE

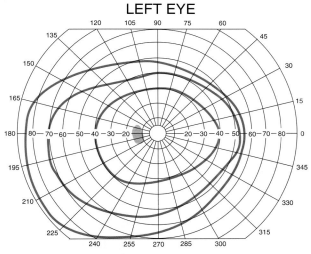

LEFT EYE

**Figure 9-10** Visual fields in Case 9-1. The large pink area in the visual field of the right eye indicates only the region in which the patient could not detect any targets. The patient does not see pink in this region, only an absence of visual features (see Fig. 9-4).

Vision

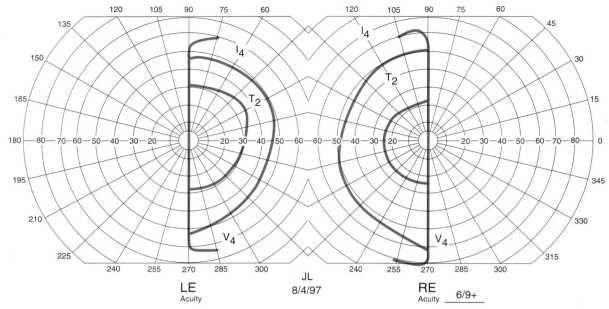

Figure 9-11 Visual fields in Case 9-2.

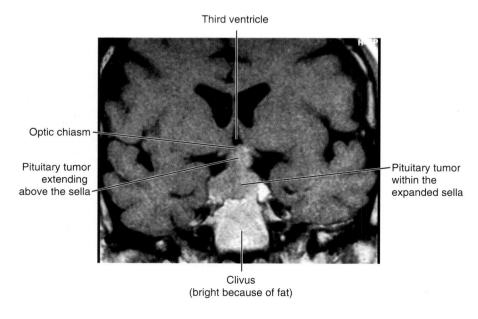

**Figure 9-12** Magnetic resonance image (MRI) of the head demonstrating a large pituitary tumor protruding upward from the sella turcica and compressing the optic chiasm from below (Case 9-2).

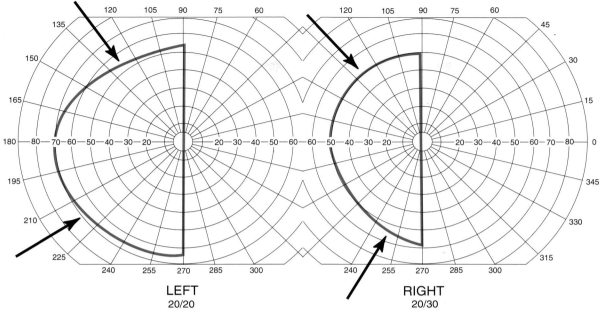

**Figure 9-13** Visual fields in Case 9-3. Isopter lines denoted by arrows.

## Case 9-3

### Right Homonymous Hemianopia due to Left Temporo-occipital Stroke

*A 60-year-old man presents to the emergency room with the chief complaint that he has not been able to see out of his right eye since he awoke that morning. The physician who examines him demonstrates the visual field deficit shown in Figure 9-13. An electrocardiogram shows that the patient is in atrial fibrillation (a cardiac arrhythmia that predisposes to intra-atrial clot formation).*

**Comment:** *This patient has a right homonymous hemianopia. The hemianopia is homonymous because the same field is affected in each eye (in contrast to Case 9-2, in which the visual field defects were heteronymous). It is quite common for patients to misconstrue a hemianopia as loss of vision in the eye with the temporal field defect. The lesion in this case is shown in Figure 9-14. The most likely cause is an infarction caused by embolism of clot formed in the heart as a result of the atrial fibrillation. The infarct has severely damaged the left calcarine cortex and optic radiations.*

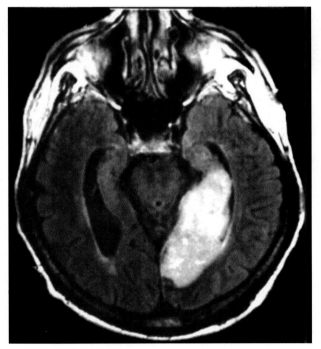

**Figure 9-14** Magnetic resonance image (MRI) of the head in Case 9-3 demonstrating an infarction in the distribution of the left posterior cerebral artery.

Vision

## RETINOCOLLICULAR AND RETINOPRETECTAL PATHWAYS

Retinal ganglion cells also project to the superior colliculus, which subserves processes underlying reactive attention to elemental light stimuli and the associated orienting response (see Chapters 8 and 12), and to the pretectal region, which subserves pupillary responses to light, among other things (see following discussion).

## PRACTICE 9-3

**A.** A 75-year-old man awakes one morning with difficulty seeing to the left. The results of his visual field examination are shown in Figure 9-15. Localize the lesion.

**B.** In the course of a comprehensive eye examination, a 65-year-old man undergoes Goldmann perimetry. The results are depicted in Figure 9-16. Where is the lesion?

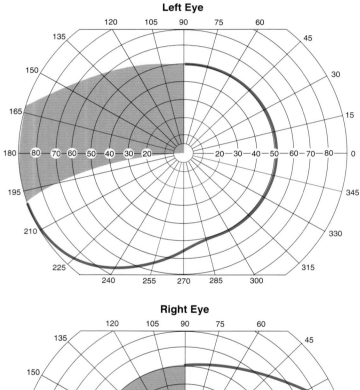

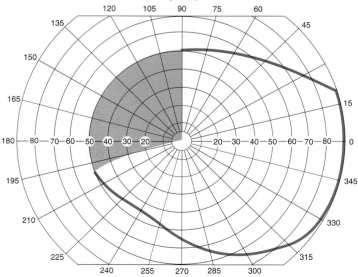

**Figure 9-15** Visual fields in Practice Case 9-3A.

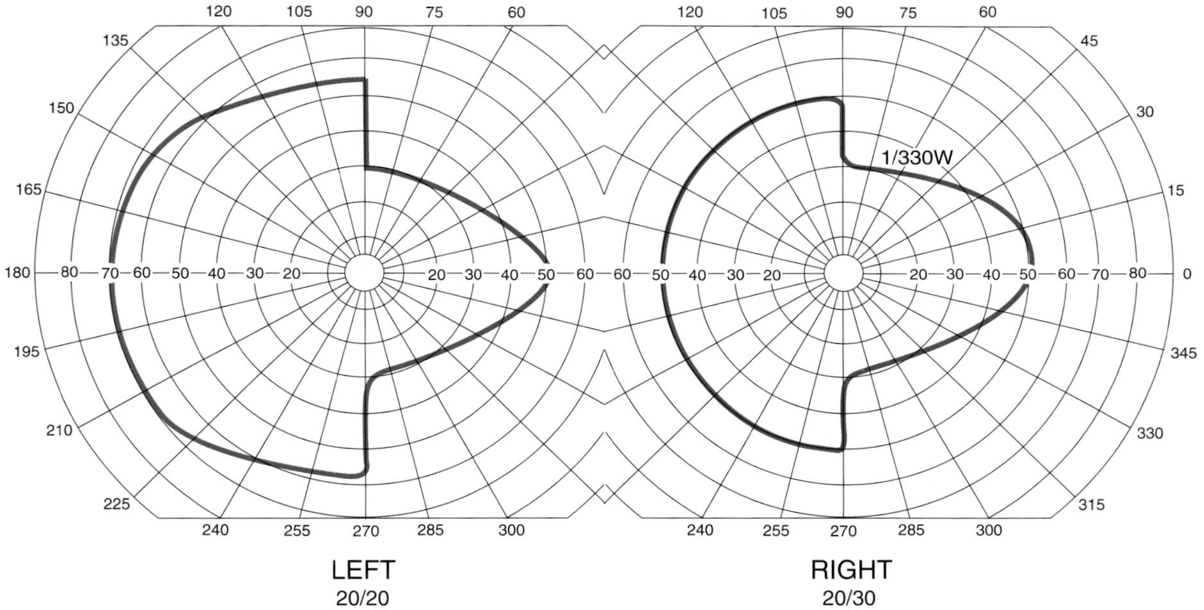

**Figure 9-16** Visual fields in Practice Case 9-3B.

# Neurophysiology and Processes Underlying Feature Enhancement

## Objectives

1. Be able to summarize the processes by which photons entering the eye ultimately elicit action potentials in retinal ganglion cells.

2. Be able to distinguish between rod and cone photoreceptor systems in terms of light sensitivity, color perception, distribution across the retina, and the receptive field sizes of associated retinal ganglion cells.

3. Be able to identify at least three mechanisms by which the eye is able to respond to amounts of ambient light differing by as much as 14 orders of magnitude.

4. Be able to describe briefly the basis for the contrast sensitivity of the visual system.

5. Be able to describe briefly the physiologic basis for color perception and explain color blindness.

6. Be able to describe briefly the basis of motion perception, the location of the lesion that selectively disrupts motion perception, and the consequences of such lesions.

7. Be able to explain the essential properties of the "what" and "where" visual systems, delineate their locations in the cerebral cortex, and describe the consequences of selective lesions.

Light entering the eye is focused on the retina by the cornea and lens. The means by which the shape of the lens is altered to focus light was discussed in Chapter 8. In the normal eye, a perfect right-left reversed, top-down inverted image of the visual field of view is projected in sharp detail upon the retina. Light travels through the transparent cellular layers of the retina to the photoreceptor layer, which consists of tubular extensions of receptor cells aligned parallel to incoming rays of light and abutting the pigment epithelium (Fig. 9-2). Within each of these tubular processes is a stack of disks containing rhodopsin. The presence of stacks of disks maximizes the probability that a photon of light will encounter a rhodopsin molecule before being "lost" in the pigment epithelium. Rhodopsin consists of a membranous protein, opsin, and a small light-absorbing compound, retinal (derived from vitamin A). When retinal changes from a *cis* to a *trans* form in response to light absorption, it induces a conformational change in opsin.

Photoreceptor cells, and indeed most cells within the plexiform layers of the retina, are most peculiar in that they do not produce action potentials. Rather, they tonically release neurotransmitter. When a photon-retinal interaction induces a conformational change in opsin, this engages a cyclic GMP-mediated process that ultimately reduces both the sodium and the calcium conductance of the receptor cell membrane, hyperpolarizes it, and thus reduces the tonic release of neuro-

**TABLE 9-2** Summary of Properties of Rods and Cones

| Feature | Rods | Cones |
|---|---|---|
| Conditions of function | Low light | Moderate to full light |
| Support for color sensitivity | No | Yes |
| Numbers in each eye | 120 million | 6 million |
| Distribution | Throughout retina except fovea | Concentrated in macula; most densely in fovea |
| Receptive fields of target ganglion cells | Large | Small |
| Associated visual acuity | Low | High |

transmitter by the photoreceptor cell.[2] Retinal light detection mechanisms are extraordinarily sensitive. Humans can detect flashes consisting of as few as five photons of light, no more than one of which is likely to strike any given photoreceptor.

The neural networks within the plexiform layers of the retina are complex and the neurophysiologic processes they support are only partially understood. The photoreceptor cells employ glutamate, and most cells in the plexiform layers employ glutamate or GABA as their neurotransmitter. Through circuitry too complex to be elaborated here, the photoreceptor and plexiform layer cells, which rely on graded potentials and tonic release of neurotransmitter, translate photon input into action potentials in ganglion cells. Each ganglion cell responds to light from a restricted portion of the visual field, defined as its receptive field. Through the circuitry of the plexiform layers, most ganglion cells respond maximally when there is a difference between the light striking the center of their receptive fields and light striking the immediately surrounding region. This response is a major contributor to the contrast sensitivity of the visual system, to be discussed in the next section.

There are two classes of photoreceptors: rods and cones (Table 9-2). Rod photoreceptors are capable of functioning under very low light conditions, and they do not support color vision, for reasons to be discussed. Cones function only when there is at least moderate light (they are 1/30 as sensitive as rods) and they support color sensitivity. In each eye, there are 120 million rods and 6 million cones, ultimately supplying input to 1 million ganglion cells. Rods are distributed throughout the retina. Because a relatively large number are associated with any given ganglion cell, the receptive field of rod-linked ganglion cells (the portion of the visual field to which they are responsive) tends to be relatively large. Cones tend to be concentrated in the macula, and they constitute the only receptor type in the fovea. Because relatively few cones are associated with any given ganglion cell (compared to rods), the receptive fields of cone-linked ganglion cells are small, thus providing the basis for the extremely high visual acuity achieved in the portion of the visual field corresponding to the macula.

Although the human eye is capable of detecting just a few photons, it is also capable of functioning in conditions of bright sunlight, in which it receives on the order of $10^{14}$ photons per second. The capacity of the eye to function under different lighting conditions is based upon four fundamental mechanisms: (1) constriction of the pupil can reduce light striking the retina by an order of magnitude; (2) the two types of photoreceptors, rods and cones, differ by an order of magnitude in their sensitivity to incoming light; (3) photoreceptors can adapt to light quite rapidly and alter their sensitivity by up to three orders of magnitude; and (4) neural mechanisms in the retina, LGN, and visual cortices are constructed so as to maximize sensitivity to differences between selected features of ambient light, rather than to absolute magnitude, thus providing the fundamental basis for *feature enhancement*. The specialization of visual systems for detecting changes of features over space and time, rather than for perceiving absolute magnitudes, helps to maintain perceptual constancy over widely varying conditions.

---

[2]A single photon-rhodopsin interaction initiates a biochemical cascade that ultimately leads to the closing of 250,000 sodium ionophores/second. It is this mechanism that accounts for the light amplification capabilities of the retina. The change in sodium current is primarily responsible for the hyperpolarization. The change in calcium current is mainly important for adaptation to bright light.

Vision

We have already discussed the feature of depth perception, which is based upon the analysis of interocular image disparity through interactions between ocular dominance columns. In the following sections, we will discuss other features that are extracted by the visual system.

## A. CONTRAST SENSITIVITY

Neurons throughout the visual system are sensitive to light from a restricted portion of the visual field, their *receptive field*. Receptive fields are very small for retinal ganglion cells (particularly those linked to cones), neurons within the LGN, and most neurons in the calcarine cortex. In contrast, they may be quite large and even bilateral for neurons in higher level visual association cortices.

As small as the receptive fields are for retinal ganglion and LGN neurons, these cells respond better to patterns of light within their receptive fields than to uniform illumination. Specifically, they exhibit a *center-surround* pattern of response: that is, they will respond maximally if illumination is different in the center of their receptive field than in the periphery of their receptive field. For this reason, these cells respond maximally to aspects of the visual scene in which there are sharp spatial gradients in visual attributes, that is, borders of visual features. Such borders may be defined by differences in light intensity or differences in color. As the Nobel laureates Hubel and Wiesel discovered within the calcarine cortex, more integrative cells, which receive input from a number of center-surround responsive cells, are maximally responsive to lines of particular orientations. It is the center-surround responsiveness implicit in the organization of retinal neural networks that provides the fundamental basis for our "attraction" to features within relatively featureless visual domains— for example, our tendency to attend to light fixtures or the junctions of walls and ceiling when we gaze at the ceiling. The "attractiveness" of such features also involves attentional mechanisms, which are discussed in Chapter 12. However, these attentional mechanisms rely on the more elementary processes of contrast sensitivity, a specific form of feature enhancement, built into the lowest levels of the visual system.

## B. COLOR

Cone photoreceptors are maximally responsive to one of three colors: blue-violet, green, and yellow (Fig. 9-17). However, because the spectral sensitivity of photoreceptors is broad, it is preferable to refer to them as short, medium, and long wavelength sensitive receptors, respectively. Our ability to appreciate a continuous spectrum of color actually reflects the existence of retinal circuitry that utilizes relative input from the different classes of photoreceptors to generate responses that are maximal for a particular color. For example, retinal ganglion cells that exclusively receive input from long wavelength photoreceptors provide the basis for perception of red light. Ganglion cells that receive equal input from long and medium wavelength photoreceptors provide the basis for perception of yellow-green light. Ganglion cells that receive equal input from short and medium wavelength photoreceptors provide the basis for perception of blue light. Because color sensitivity reflects the discrimination of differences in input of different types, it constitutes another form of feature enhancement. As long as there is enough light to stimulate cone photoreceptors, this difference discrimination capacity will be present, whether the retina is receiving $10^4$ photons per second or $10^{14}$ photons per second. The existence of photoreceptors sensitive to specific wavelengths of light is genetically determined. Thus, individuals with defects in certain key genes exhibit color blindness (Case 9-4).

### Case 9-4

#### Color Blindness

*Color blindness reflects abnormalities in one or more of the three wavelength classes of cone photoreceptors. The best known are defects related to either the absence of or the presence of an anomalous and dysfunctional form of one of the three classes. Most common are dichromats, that is, people who possess only two functional classes of cone photoreceptors. Between 2 and 6 percent of males of European ancestry have an X-linked recessive defect resulting in the complete absence of, or the presence of a dysfunctional form of, either medium or long wavelength photoreceptors. As a result, they have difficulty differentiating between red and green. Far rarer is an autosomal dominant trait resulting in the absence of a functional form of short wavelength photoreceptors. These individuals have difficulty in making blue-green distinctions. Men and woman are affected with equal frequency. Rarest of all are monochromats, individuals who have only one functioning class of photoreceptor. Because they have no basis for judging the relative amount of light of different frequencies, they are truly colorblind.*

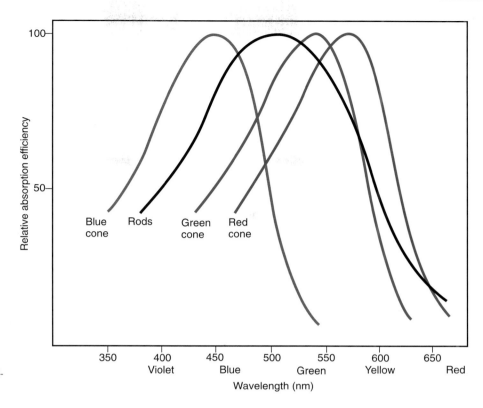

**Figure 9-17** Spectral sensitivities of human cones and rods.

## C. V1 AND V2: LINE ORIENTATION, OCULAR DOMINANCE, AND COLOR PERCEPTION

In calcarine cortex (V1), staining for the mitochondrial enzyme cytochrome oxidase reveals dark, peglike regions most prominent in layers 2 and 3, called "blobs," that are specialized for color vision. However, blobs excepted, the organization of neurons in V1 appears to be defined primarily by two other dimensions: line orientation and ocular dominance. As we noted earlier, through the complex connectivity between retinal ganglion cells and cells in calcarine cortex, the center-surround pattern of response exhibited by retinal ganglion cells is translated into a sensitivity of columns of calcarine neurons to lines of a particular orientation. Furthermore, even though visual input from the two eyes is admixed in the optic radiations, each cortical column of calcarine neurons receives input only from one eye, a principle termed "*ocular dominance.*" In V1, as in other sensory cortices, the neurons are organized in columns, here 30- to 100-μm wide. V1 is divided into alternating strips of cortex corresponding to input from the left or the right eye,

each strip composed of thousands of columns. Within the strips, the columns are organized in repeated groups that form pinwheel shapes approximately 1 mm in diameter (Fig. 9-18). All neurons within a given pinwheel process input from the same location in the visual field. Each radiating arm of each pinwheel consists of a column of neurons specialized for detection of edges or lines of a specific orientation. Thus, the dominant features of V1 seem to be directed primarily toward (1) the detection and amplification of the features—edges—most essential for defining both the form of objects and the most critical aspects of our surrounding environment; and (2) providing the basis for depth perception. Scattered within the pinwheels of columns within each ocular dominance strip are the blobs that are specialized for color vision.

## D. MOVEMENT

Within some cells in the calcarine cortex, center-surround contrast sensitivity is time-delimited. That is, these cells respond maximally when a contrast boundary moves across the receptive field at a certain rate. In

Vision

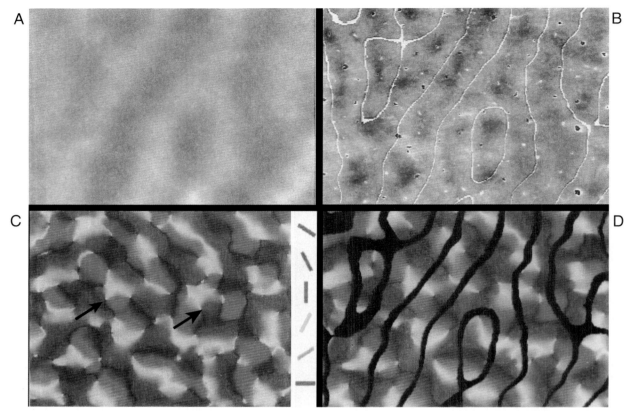

**Figure 9-18** The cortex in V1 is viewed from above. *A,* Alternating strips containing columns (ocular dominance columns) receiving input from a single eye can be vaguely seen as light and dark staining regions. *B,* The borders of ocular dominance strips are delineated by white lines. The tissue has been stained for the mitochondrial enzyme cytochrome oxidase, thus revealing the blobs as dark regions. *C,* The orientation response selectivity of each column of neurons has been determined and mapped as a color (see color legend at right). The transition from one color to another (one direction to another) is gradual except at the points that define the centers of the pinwheels (*arrows*). *D,* The map of pinwheels is superimposed upon a map of ocular dominance strips (borders delineated in black). Any given pinwheel contains a set of columns that together will respond to lines of any orientation. Note that the pinwheels are oriented with respect to each other such that neurons responding to edges of a given orientation at one location in the visual field lie immediately adjacent to neurons responding to that same orientation but at a slightly different location in the visual field. For example, any one green region, representing neurons responding to vertically oriented lines, consists of contiguous vertically responding regions from two adjacent pinwheels. Note also that adjacent pinwheels in different ocular dominance strips share this same economical principle of organization with respect to each other. (From Blasdel GG. Differential imaging of ocular dominance and orientation selectivity in monkey striate cortex. J Neurosci 12:3115–3138, 1992; Blasdel GG. Orientation selectivity, preference and continuity in monkey striate cortex. J Neurosci 12:3139–3161, 1992. Copyright 1992 by the Society for Neuroscience.)

other words, they are specifically sensitive to movement. More integrative cells provide the basis for particular sensitivity to lines (edges) moving in certain directions. The discovery of this property, and indeed the crucial clue to the "vocabulary" of cells in the calcarine cortex, was actually serendipitous. Hubel and Wiesel, after experiencing considerable frustration in the course of fruitless efforts to elicit any responses

from cells in V1, noticed that cells fired briskly as they removed a slide from the projector that served to provide the visual stimulus. The moving edge of the slide proved to be a far more potent stimulus than the various, carefully constructed stimuli that they had been using. Movement perception is one of the most important feature enhancement domains of the visual system because things moving in our environment are usually

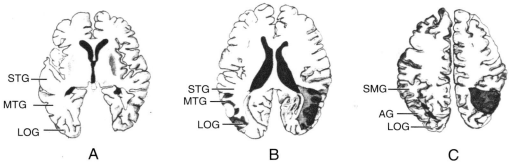

**Figure 9-19** Diagram of computed tomographic (CT) scan slices in Case 9-5. Regions of minor damage are lightly stippled and regions of severe damage are darkly stippled. STG—superior temporal gyrus; MTG—middle temporal gyrus; LOG—lateral occipital gyrus; AG—angular gyrus. (From Zihl J, von Cramon D, Mai N. Selective disturbance of movement vision after bilateral brain damage. Brain 106:313-340, 1983. Used by permission of Oxford University Press.)

important, and because correct perception of environmental movement as we navigate our surroundings is critical. Movement of objects, whether real or only apparent (due to our own movement), also serves to separate these objects from their background.

Sensitivity to movement is a highly prevalent property of neurons in V1. As visual pathways advance forward into visual association areas, there occurs a relative dissociation of various domains of vision (see discussion under Section E, "What" and "Where" Systems). Thus, there is a region of relative specialization for movement detection in the vicinity of the temporoparietal-occipital junction.[3] Case 9-5 describes a patient who experienced bilateral infarction of this region as a result of thrombosis of the superior sagittal sinus and cortical veins (Fig. 9-19).

## E. "WHAT" AND "WHERE" SYSTEMS

The rod and cone photoreceptor systems provide the basis for differential visual processing capabilities along two dimensions: (1) low light and normal or bright light, and (2) black-and-white and color vision, respectively. However, another dimension of feature discrimination cuts across these two and is even more critical to our phenomenal visual processing sophistication: a

---

[3]We perceive motion whether an image moves across the retina, or we follow a moving target with our eyes (smooth pursuit), in which case the image is fixed upon the retina. Thus, it will come as no surprise that this region is also critical to the production of ocular smooth pursuit.

### Case 9-5

**Loss of Motion Perception due to Venous Infarction of Temporoparietal-occipital Junction**
*"She had difficulty, for example, in pouring tea or coffee into a cup because the fluid appeared to be frozen, like a glacier. In addition, she could not stop pouring at the right time since she was unable to perceive the movement in the cup (or a pot) when the fluid rose. Furthermore, the patient complained of difficulties in following a dialogue because she could not see the movements of the face and, especially, the mouth of the speaker. In a room where more than two other people were walking she felt very insecure and unwell, and usually left the room immediately, because 'people were suddenly here or there but I have not seen them moving.' The patient experienced the same problem but to an even more marked extent in crowded streets or places, which she therefore avoided as much as possible. She could not cross the street because of her inability to judge the speed of a car, but she could identify the car itself without difficulty. 'When I'm looking at the car first, it seems far away. But then, when I want to cross the road, suddenly the car is very near.'"* (From Zihl J, von Cramon D, Mai N. Selective disturbance of movement vision after bilateral brain damage. Brain 106:313-340, 1983.)

Vision

dimension that provides the basis for "what" (object perception) and "where" (location/movement perception) processing. Neuroscientists first began to discern this dimension of visual feature discrimination as early as the beginning of the 20th century, but the concept was first fully elucidated by Mortimer Mishkin and Leslie Ungerleider, scientists at the National Institutes of Health, in a famous paper published in 1982.

Even at the retina, there is a latent division into facilities for object vision involving color and form—the "what" system—and for location vision, involving location and movement—the "where" system. Both rod and cone photoreceptors systems project to these two processing pathways. The separateness of the "what" and "where" pathways first becomes readily apparent in the LGN, where ganglion cells particularly adapted for the processing of motion project primarily to layers 1 and 2 (magnocellular ["large cell"] LGN), and ganglion cells particularly adapted for the processing of color, fine texture, and shape project primarily to layers 3 to 6 (the parvocellular ["small cell"] LGN). Edge analysis (Sections A and C) is important for both "what" and "where" vision and the segregation of these two pathways is not easy to discern within V1 or V2 (roughly corresponding to Brodmann's area 18). It is quite clear that at every level of the "what" and "where" systems, there is considerable interaction, and segregation of function is not complete.

Beyond V2, the "what" and "where" systems become widely separate geographically, and their distinctive processing features become manifest (Fig. 9-20). Target neurons in inter-blob (pinwheel) regions of V1 receiving projections originating in the magnocellular neurons of the LGN (layers 1 and 2) project dorsally to visual association areas in the medial and lateral parietal lobes specializing in motion and location processing. Target neurons in both inter-blob (pinwheel) and blob regions of V1 receiving projections originating in both the magnocellular (layers 1 and 2) and the parvocellular (layers 3 to 6) neurons of the LGN project ventrally to visual association areas in the temporal lobes involved in processing color and form.

## The "What" System

The "what" visual system incorporates a process indispensable to perception and recognition of objects located anywhere in the field of vision—the detection of features in the abstract, independent of location. We have noted that cells in calcarine cortex are maximally

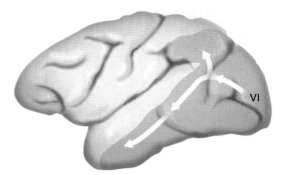

**Figure 9-20** Lateral view of the left hemisphere of a rhesus monkey. The shaded area defines primary and association visual cortices in the occipital, parietal, and temporal lobes. The arrows delineate two visual pathways beginning in occipital cortex (V1), one extending ventrally along inferior temporal cortex, including ventral portions of the temporal lobe (not shown): the "what" pathway; and the other extending dorsally into parietal cortex, including medial hemispheric cortex (not shown): the "where" pathway. (Modified from Mishkin M, Ungerleider LG, Macko KA. Object vision and spatial vision: Two cortical pathways. TINS 6:414-417, 1983.)

responsive to lines of particular orientations. Generally, these neurons (referred to as "simple cells") respond only to lines at a particular locus within the visual field. However, there exist "complex" cells, especially outside V1, that have large receptive fields and will respond to a line of a particular orientation that appears anywhere within their receptive field. This behavior could be explained by a neural network structure in which each complex cell receives input from simple cells with selectivity for bars of a particular orientation whose receptive fields, in aggregate, include the entire receptive field of the complex cell. If the firing of a single simple cell were capable of inducing firing in the complex cell, the complex cell would subserve a logical OR function—if the feature in question were present anywhere (visual locus 1 or visual locus 2 or visual locus 3 or . . .) the complex cell would fire.

Abstract feature detection (detection regardless of visual locus) provides the first step in a hierarchy of neural network processes within the visual system that enables a capacity we all recognize implicitly—that we can recognize an object regardless of where it appears within our visual field. Lesions of the "what" system produce impairment in object recognition, or agnosia, a topic to be discussed further in Chapter 12. Affected patients can see perfectly clearly, but they are unable to name or describe the function of anything they see.

As one proceeds anteriorly through the "what" system to anterior, inferior temporal visual association cortex, several trends are observed, some of which we have touched upon already and we can now summarize:

- Progressive expansion of the receptive fields of visually responsive neurons, until eventually receptive fields become bilateral and cover most or all of the visual field.

- Loss of retinotopic organization.

- Increase in the degree to which particular stimulus features provoke a neural response, regardless of location in the visual field, distance, absolute size, or object orientation.

- Increase in the complexity of stimulus features that induce neural responses, culminating in cells that respond to object configurations and even specific faces.

- An increase in the degree to which our perception of an object represents a mix of what we actually see and what we already know, hence our ability to recognize an object even when we see it from an unusual angle.

- An increase in the degree to which the firing of cells is contingent not just on the nature of the visual input but also on the value of the visual stimulus to the organism—a phenomenon that reflects selective attention (see Chapter 12).

- An increase in the degree to which the visual features of an object that are abstracted in a given cortical area are represented not as isolated activity of a few columns of neurons corresponding to a particular point in retinotopic space, but as a pattern of neural activity involving most of the neurons within that cortical region with little or no retinotopic specificity, in a distributed representation (see Chapter 12).

## The "Where" System

The functions of the "where" system can perhaps be best understood through the behavior of a patient with bilateral lesions of this system—a patient with a syndrome first describe by Balint in 1909 (Case 9-6).

## PRACTICE 9-4

Why does the rod photoreceptor system support only black and white vision?

### Case 9-6

**Hypoperfusion Injury to the Brain Selectively Damaging the "Where" System**

*A 65-year-old woman experiences in-hospital cardiopulmonary arrest in the context of acute myocardial infarction. She is quickly resuscitated but nevertheless experiences a hypoperfusion injury most severe in the region of the terminal distributions of the anterior, middle, and posterior cerebral arteries: the medial and lateral parasagittal parietal cortex of Brodmann's areas 7 and 19 (Fig. 9-21). On reevaluation several months later, neurologic function is remarkably intact except for deficits attributable to damage in this area. When asked to look at specific objects, she has a great deal of difficulty directing her eyes precisely at the target, invariably looking to one side or the other, even as she swears that she "sees it" and is looking straight at it. When asked to reach out and grab an object, she responds promptly and her arm and hand movements are perfectly normal.*

*However, she usually completely misses the object, making repeated groping movements in the general direction of the object but almost always off to one side, or in front of or behind the object. When shown a complex picture, she is able to identify individual items portrayed in the picture but is completely unable to put all the features together and actually describe the entire scene (simultanagnosia). For example, when shown a photograph of an accident scene, replete with mangled cars, backed up traffic on the interstate, police cars, ambulances, and people on stretchers, she identifies individual cars, a stretcher, and a policeman, but she cannot provide a summary description of the picture. She complains that the visual world is fragmented—she is able to see individual things clearly but cannot discern the relationship between them. In attempting to go from her living room to her bedroom by keying on the lamp outside her bedroom door, she crashes into the dining room table. She feels*

*Continued*

Vision

### Case 9-6—cont'd

bewildered when she watches television or movies because she can only see one person at a time and cannot determine who is speaking to whom. Because she is unable to see more than one thing at a time, she is unable to impute causality to the events she sees. During a Western movie, people seem to be suddenly and without warning catapulted across the room because she is unable to see the person who punched them. She is no longer able to write because, as she writes, she sees only the tip of the pencil on the page and not previously constructed letters in the word. (Many of the details of this case are derived from the report of Coslett HB, Saffran E. Simultanagnosia: To see but not two see. Brain 114:1523-1545, 1991.)

**Comment:** The impairments in visually guided eye and hand movements can be explained as a deficit in the translation of the retinotopic coordinates of objects into body-centered coordinates—something that is necessary for us to direct our eyes or our hands to specific spatial locations. The mechanism of simultanagnosia is less clear. The existence of this dramatic disorder suggests that the acquisition of a capability for perceiving features and objects in the abstract, regardless of location, which we observed in more anterior portions of the "what" system, is achieved at considerable cost: only single objects can be perceived. Simultaneous processing is required by the "where" system to give all the other objects in the visual field the "permanence" required to relate them to each other and provide the basis for a cogent analysis of the entire visual scene. Thus, the "what" and "where" systems are fully complementary in their processing specialties and must function in tandem to give us the full experience of normal vision.

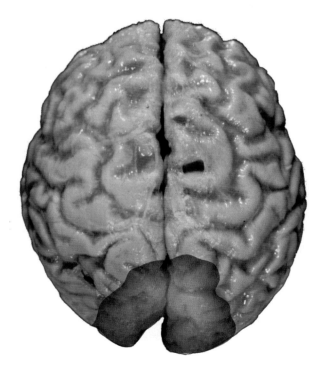

**Figure 9-21** Distribution of the ischemic lesion in Case 9-6.

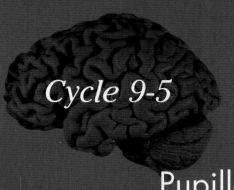

# Cycle 9-5

# Pupillary Responses to Light

Page 581-Edinger Westphal nucleus

## Objectives

1. Be able to describe the neural pathway subserving the pupillary reaction to light.
2. Be able to define a relative afferent pupillary defect and explain its physiologic basis.

Fibers of retinal origin exit the optic tracts to synapse on nuclei within the pretectal region of the midbrain, just rostral to the superior colliculi (Fig. 9-22). Each pretectal nucleus projects to the ipsilateral, ventrally adjacent Edinger-Westphal nucleus of the third nerve nuclear complex (see Chapter 8), and via the posterior commissure to the contralateral Edinger-Westphal nucleus. This circuitry provides the basis for the pupillary response to light. Because each pretectal nucleus projects to both Edinger-Westphal nuclei, shining a bright light into one eye produces constriction of the pupil in that eye—the *direct response*—and constriction of the pupil in the opposite eye—the *consensual response*. Note that the pupillary light reflex has an afferent arc, mediated by the optic nerve, and an efferent arc, mediated by parasympathetic fibers within the third nerves. Occasionally the pupillary light reflexes are impaired by lesions damaging the pretectal region, as illustrated in Figure 8-27. However, the most common and important lesions affecting the pupillary light reflex are those involving the optic nerve itself, as illustrated in Case 9-7.

## Case 9-7

**Abnormalities of Pupillary Function with an Optic Nerve Lesion**

*Return to Case 9-1, a patient with optic neuritis affecting the right eye. Further examination of this patient reveals that when a bright light is shone in the right eye, the right pupil constricts only slightly (Fig. 9-23). When the light is rapidly moved over to the left eye, both the left pupil and the right pupil constrict vigorously. When the light is moved quickly back over to the right eye, the pupil dilates. These reactions indicate that the consensual pupillary response to light*

*in the right eye is greater than the direct response. This response is called a relative afferent pupillary defect (RAPD) (sometimes referred to incorrectly as a "Marcus Gunn pupil"). It is relative because the abnormality of the response can be defined only relative to the other, normal eye. If the patient had bilateral and equal lesions of the optic nerves, we would not see an RAPD. It is afferent because it is caused by a lesion of the afferent arc of the pupillary light reflex. In this case, the presence of an optic nerve lesion was pretty obvious from the history and testing of visual acuity. However,*

*Continued*

Vision

445

## Case 9-7—cont'd

in many cases an optic nerve lesion is clinically silent, and under such circumstances, an RAPD might provide the only evidence of an optic nerve lesion. If the young woman described in Case 9-1 had presented with myelopathy rather than visual loss, the presence of an

RAPD would have strongly suggested that the myelopathy was due to multiple sclerosis, rather than, for example, a compressive lesion like a tumor, because it is characteristic for multiple sclerosis to produce multifocal lesions of the CNS.

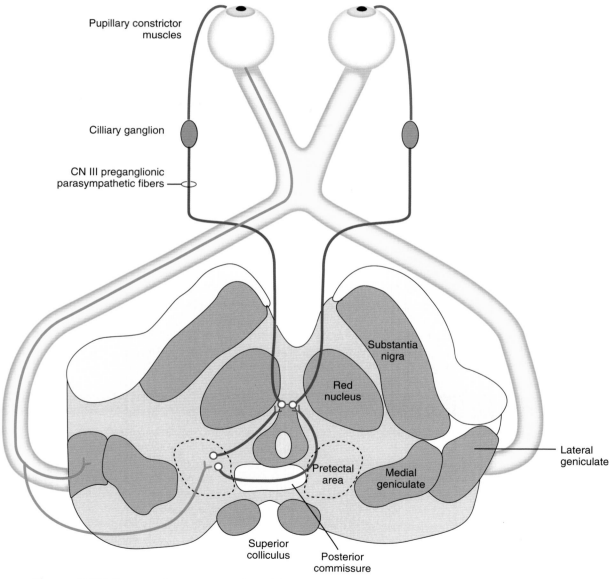

**Figure 9-22** Cartoon of transverse section of the brainstem at the junction of the midbrain and the thalamus, illustrating the pretectal area and the posterior commissure and the pathways involved in the pupillary light reflex.

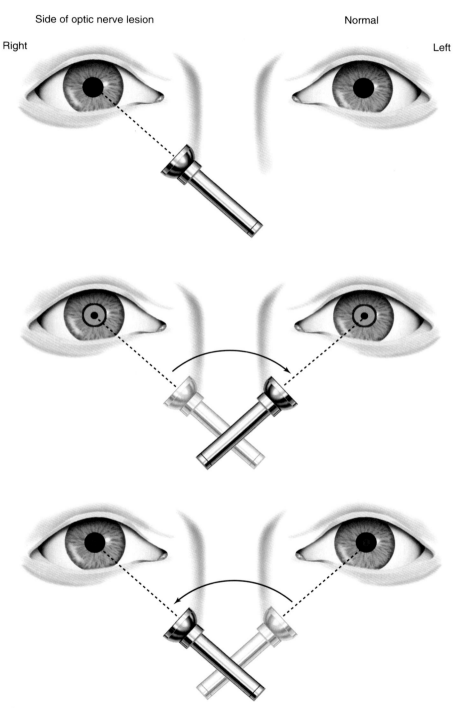

**Figure 9-23** A relative afferent pupillary defect in the right eye (see Case 9-7). For each pair of eyes, the initial position of the flashlight is depicted by the ghost image. The initial size of the pupils is denoted in gray, with the final size in black.

## PRACTICE 9-5

Contrast the pupillary responses one would expect to see in a patient with a right third nerve lesion with what one sees in a patient with a right optic nerve lesion.

# Cycle 9-6

# Intracranial Pressure Transduction and Papilledema

In Chapters 1 and 2, we introduced the concept of increased intracranial pressure and discussed potential mechanisms. The brain is located in a rigid and nearly closed compartment and there is very limited space within that compartment that is not occupied by brain. Large masses, including tumors, hematomas and swelling from extensive infarction, and ventricular enlargement due to obstruction of the outflow of cerebrospinal fluid (CSF) from the ventricular system, can exhaust this limited extra space, thus leading to increased intracranial pressure.

If intracranial pressure exceeds arterial pressure, then blood flow to the brain stops and brain death is immediate. However, long before this occurs, intracranial pressure communicated along the subarachnoid space surrounding the optic nerves may compress the optic nerves sufficiently to interfere with axoplasmic flow along the axons within these nerves. The result is swelling of axons at the optic nerve head— *papilledema* (Fig. 9-24). Because the increase in intracranial pressure is transmitted throughout the cranial vault, both optic nerves are typically affected. Thus, bilateral swelling of the optic disks is likely to indicate increased intracranial pressure (papilledema) rather than inflammation (diskitis), as in Case 9-1. These processes are illustrated by Case 9-8.

Vision

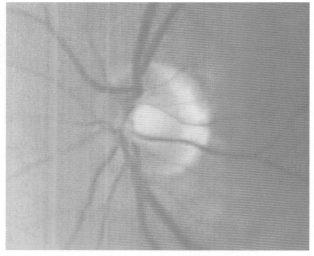

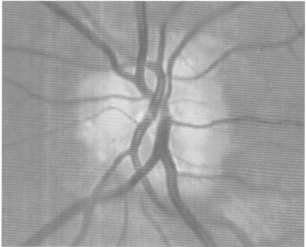

**Figure 9-24** A normal fundus (*top*) and the fundus in a patient with papilledema (*bottom*). Note that in papilledema, the optic disk is elevated and its margins are poorly defined. (Photographs courtesy of P. Kumar Rao, M.D., Associate Professor of Ophthalmology, Washington University/Barnes Retina Institute.)

## Case 9-8

### Papilledema due to Increased Intracranial Pressure from a Brain Tumor

*A 40-year-old attorney develops persistent headaches that are often transiently aggravated by coughing, sneezing, or lifting heavy objects. The headaches become progressively more severe, and he begins to notice that when he does lift something or sneeze, he will suddenly become blind for several seconds. This finding leads him to consult a physician. Examination reveals bilateral papilledema, a subtle right pronation drift, and subtle dedifferentiation of individual finger movements in the right hand. There is subtle reduction of arm swing on the right when he walks. A CT scan of the head reveals a 5-cm diameter tumor involving the left frontal lobe, surrounded by edema. There is left-to-right shift of midline structures and compression of the lateral ventricles so that they are barely detectable slits. Tissue obtained by a stereotactic needle biopsy demonstrates a highly malignant brain tumor, a glioblastoma multiforme.*

**Comment:** *This patient has raised intracranial pressure due to a very large tumor. The chronically increased pressure has led to axonal swelling at the optic nerve heads, or papilledema. Transient further elevations of intracranial pressure, associated with coughing or lifting, are sufficient to cause transient failure of axonal conduction within the optic nerves and temporary blindness. Coughing and lifting also produce sudden traction of the meninges against the inner skull, thus producing sudden worsening of headache.*

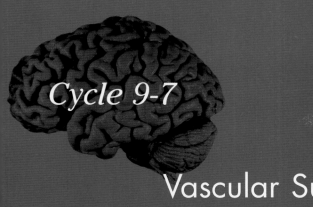

# Cycle 9-7

## Vascular Supply of the Eye

1. Be able to describe the vascular supply to the eye and adjacent orbital contents.
2. Be able to explain the mechanism and significance of amaurosis fugax.
3. Be able to explain the consequences of cavernous sinus thrombosis.

The blood supply to the eye and immediately adjacent tissues is provided by the ophthalmic artery, which is the first branch of the supraclinoid internal carotid artery (see Fig. 2-8). The central retinal artery, which supplies the inner layers of the retina, is a branch of the ophthalmic artery. Because of the origin of the ophthalmic artery from the internal carotid artery, and the extreme sensitivity of the retina to ischemia, symptoms of retinal dysfunction due to ischemia constitute an important clinical signal of thromboembolic events occurring within the internal carotid artery (Case 9-9).

The venous drainage from the eye, the orbit, and adjacent tissues is into the cavernous sinus (see Fig. 2-26). For this reason, infections in or around the eye and nose may seed the cavernous sinus. Infection may lead to cavernous sinus thrombosis, in which case venous drainage from the orbit is severely impeded. These phenomena are illustrated in Case 9-10.

Vision

## Case 9-9

### Transient Monocular Visual Loss

*A 70-year-old man has been experiencing daily episodes of transient loss of vision in his right eye (amaurosis fugax). The patient says it feels as if someone were pulling a window shade down over the eye. A magnetic resonance angiogram (MRA) suggests the presence of severe stenosis of the proximal right internal carotid artery by an atheromatous plaque. A cerebral arteriogram confirms these results and furthermore demonstrates a large crater within the plaque (an ulcer). The patient subsequently undergoes right carotid endarterectomy, in the course of which the atheromatous plaque is removed.*

**Comment:** *Several different processes may cause amaurosis fugax. Most often, amaurosis fugax occurs as large showers of platelet-fibrin emboli and cholesterol crystals originating in an unstable internal carotid artery atheroma traverse the ophthalmic artery as well as major branches of the internal carotid artery supplying the brain. Because the retina is more sensitive to ischemia and has a less adequate collateral blood supply than the brain, the patient experiences only monocular visual symptoms. However, the presence of an unstable atheroma also puts the patient at risk for embolization of a larger clot, which could cause a major stroke. The 2-year stroke risk of approximately 17 percent provides the indication for carotid endarterectomy in selected patients.*

## Case 9-10

### Orbital Venous Congestion due to Cavernous Sinus Thrombosis

*A 65-year-old diabetic man presents with acute swelling around the right eye and injection (redness) of the bulbar conjunctivae. On examination, there is severe protrusion of the eye from the orbit (proptosis). The conjunctivae are pink and severely edematous and there is active transudation of fluid (chemosis). On funduscopic examination, the retinal veins are markedly engorged and have a sausage-like appearance.*

**Comment:** *This patient exhibits the characteristic features of cavernous sinus thrombosis. The obstruction of venous drainage results in engorgement of veins within the orbit and the eye and transudation of fluid with resultant edema. This life-threatening problem is most likely due to a fungal infection.*

## CYCLE 9-3

**A.** This patient has a homonymous left superior quadrantanopia, sometimes referred to as a "pie in the sky" field cut. This deficit localizes either to the inferior bank of the right calcarine fissure, or to the optic radiations projecting from the right LGN through the temporal lobe white matter to this region. He has experienced a stroke in the distribution of the posterior cerebral artery that has spared brain supplied by more superior branches (Fig. 9-25).

**B.** This patient has a peculiar field cut that at first might seem hard to interpret. However, two things tell you that the responsible lesion is "retrochiasmal" (behind the chiasm). First, the field cut is homonymous, indicating that the lesion is on the left side and involves optic nerve fibers from the left side of both retinas, both those that are crossed (from the nasal retina of the left eye) and those that are uncrossed (from the temporal retina of the left eye). Second, the field cut respects the vertical meridian. Because the crossing of optic nerve fibers in the optic chiasm involves only fibers from the nasal retinas, lesions behind the optic chiasm produce field cuts that extend to but not beyond a vertical line transecting the point in the visual fields corresponding to the fovea. Thus, these visual fields are perfectly consistent with a lesion in the left occipital lobe.

## CYCLE 9-4

**A.** Because there is only one wavelength class of rod photoreceptors, there is no basis within the rod system for making judgments about the relative amounts of light of different frequencies, the essential requirement for color perception. Thus, the rod system can make judgments only about relative intensity of light—white, various shades of gray, and black—and luminance contrasts.

## CYCLE 9-5

**A.** With a lesion of CN III, there would be neither a direct nor a consensual response to light in the involved eye.

Vision

*453*

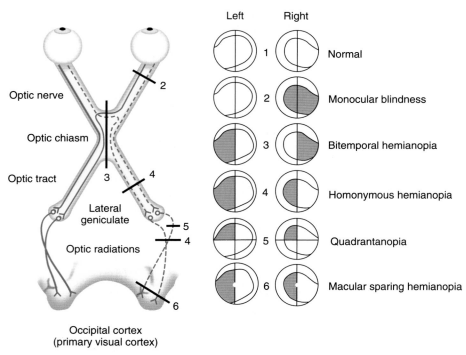

**Figure 9-25** Summary of the visual pathways.

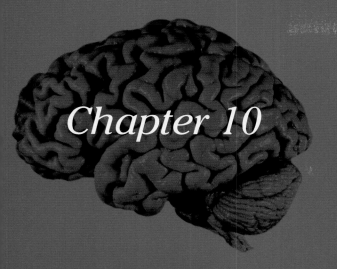

# Chapter 10

# AUDITORY AND
# VESTIBULAR SYSTEMS

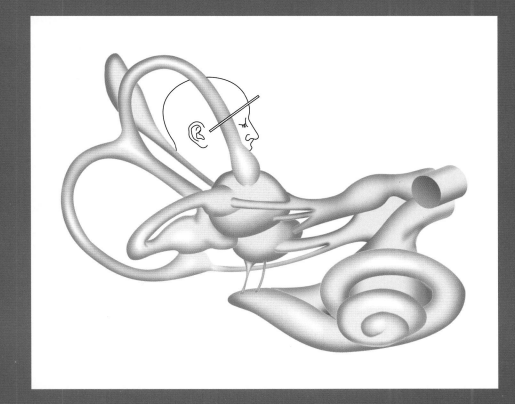

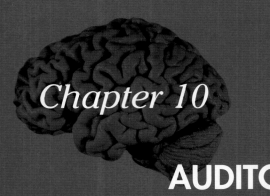

# Chapter 10

# AUDITORY AND VESTIBULAR SYSTEMS

456

# Introduction

Hearing is second only to vision in its importance as a source of human sensory experience. Our general sensitivity to environmental sounds immeasurably enriches our lives, as for example, through music. Sounds serve as crucial cues to important environmental events and readily capture our attention so that we can respond appropriately. Although sign language provides the deaf with a means of communication that is every bit as rich, detailed, and flexible as spoken language, for most of us, hearing provides the primary basis for direct linguistic communication. Furthermore, our ability to hear not just what people say, but how they say it, is crucial to our ability to understand the full meaning of their speech.

Auditory pathways within the nervous system, because of their particular location, and because of the substantial bilaterality of auditory projections, are of considerably less value in localizing disease than are visual or somatosensory pathways. Nevertheless, there are a number of important clinical correlations, which will be demonstrated in cases, as in prior chapters.

Vestibular sensation, to the extent that we are aware of it, is generally unpleasant (note the misery of seasickness). However, as we have seen, vestibular function is absolutely critical to normal motor function, through the maintenance of tone and balance via the vestibular nuclei and the vestibulospinal tracts. Vestibular function is also critical to maintenance of a stable image on the fovea, via the vestibulo-ocular response (VOR), as we move our heads. Because we have already discussed the functional impact of vestibular input in prior chapters, our consideration of vestibular function in this chapter will be limited to the means of generation and propagation of vestibular signals to the brainstem. You should refer to the chapters on the Motor System (Chapter 6) and Cranial Nerves and Brainstem Organization (Chapter 8) to refresh your memory of the impact of vestibular input on motor and ocular function.

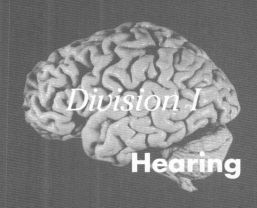

*Division I*

**Hearing**

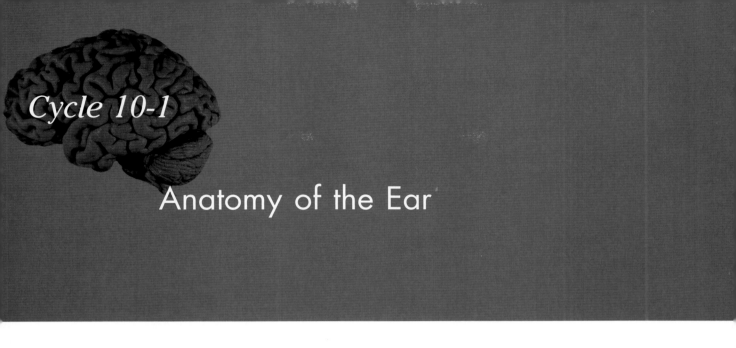

# Cycle 10-1

## Anatomy of the Ear

### Objectives

1. Be able to describe the major anatomic structures of the outer, middle, and inner ear.

2. Be able to explain how the middle ear can become infected.

3. Be able to explain the significance of the finding of blood behind the tympanic membranes and acute hearing loss following head trauma.

4. Be able to describe the mechanism underlying Menière's syndrome.

5. Be able to describe the innervation of the two major components of the inner ear, name two relatively common disorders that affect this innervation, and explain the manifestations of each.

6. Be able to explain and interpret an audiogram.

The ear can logically be divided into three parts: outer, middle, and inner (Fig. 10-1).

### THE OUTER EAR

The outer ear consists of the *pinna*, the visible aspect of the ear, and the *external auditory meatus*, or ear canal. The pinna serves to gather and focus sound waves into the external auditory meatus. Because of the shape of its convolutions and its slightly forward ori-entation, its sound gathering capacity varies with the direction of sound. Our principal means of determining the direction of sound derives from the fact that we have two ears and we are able to detect almost infini-tesimal differences in the timing and loudness of audi-tory events in the two ears—the auditory equivalent of binocular vision. The shape and orientation of the pinna, therefore, provide only a secondary basis for localization of sound, one that is important for local-ization along the vertical axis.

The external auditory meatus provides the air conduit by which sound waves reach the junction between the outer ear and the middle ear: the eardrum or *tympanic membrane*. Obstruction of the external auditory meatus by foreign objects or by buildup of wax (cerumen) reduces the sound energy transmitted to the tympanic membrane.

### THE MIDDLE EAR

The middle ear consists of a small cavity that is bounded on the outer side by the tympanic membrane and on the inner side by the structures of the inner ear. It is linked by the eustachian tube to the nasopharynx. The eustachian tube provides the means by which we can equalize the air pressure on the two sides of the eardrum. Unfortunately, it also provides a means by which infectious organisms can enter the middle ear to cause inflammation (otitis media), a particularly common problem in infants and children. The middle

459

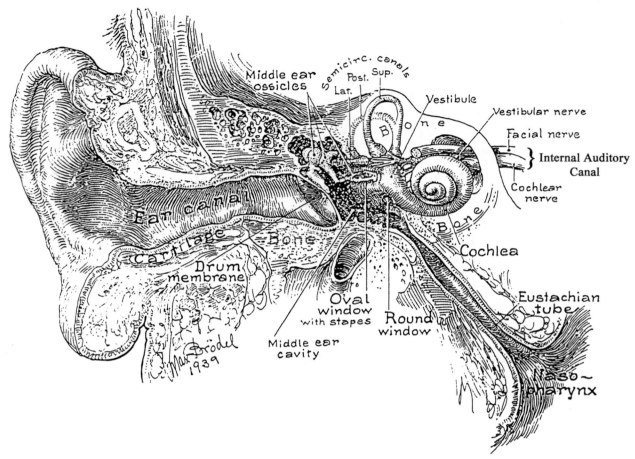

**Figure 10-1** A now-classic diagram of the ear drawn by Max Brödel in 1939, demonstrating the outer, middle, and inner portions of the ear and their relationships to the petrous portions of the temporal bone at the base of the skull and to the nasopharynx.

ear contains three tiny bones, the *malleus* (hammer), *incus* (anvil), and *stapes* (stirrup). The malleus attaches to the eardrum. The three bones are linked in series by typical, albeit very small, cartilage containing joints (Fig. 10-2). The footplate of the stapes covers the oval window, the junction between the middle ear and the inner ear.

## THE INNER EAR

The inner ear is located within a space deep within the petrous portion of the temporal bone, referred to as the bony labyrinth (Fig. 10-3). Although the petrous bone, by virtue of its thickness, generally provides a safe place for the structures of the middle and inner ear, it can be

fractured in major head trauma, as illustrated in Case 10-1.

### Case 10-1

**Syncope with Basilar Skull Fracture**
*A 70-year-old man has been admitted to the hospital for evaluation of episodes of sudden loss of consciousness. While at the nursing station asking directions, he experiences an episode. He falls straight backward, striking the back of his head on the concrete floor. He remains unconscious for 30 minutes. Examination with an otoscope reveals blood behind both tympanic membranes (hemotympanum).*

## Case 10-1—cont'd

**Comment:** *The blood behind the tympanic membranes provides incontrovertible evidence that he has fractured the petrous portion of the skull bilaterally, and that the fracture lines extend through the middle ears on both sides. Such fractures can be confirmed by computed tomographic (CT) scan, which is an exquisitely sensitive technique for defining bony anatomy, but the clinical findings in this case provide more than adequate demonstration of what has happened. Had the fracture lines extended through the inner ears, there would be a high probability that the patient would substantially lose hearing. Basilar skull fractures indicate severe trauma. Because it is not always clear how severely people have been injured in accidents, it is always important to look for hemotympanum during the physical examination.*

## THE MEMBRANOUS LABYRINTH

Within the bony labyrinth lies a complex structure composed of linked sacs and tubes referred to as the *membranous labyrinth* (Fig. 10-4). The membranous labyrinth is filled with *endolymph*. Much of it is suspended entirely within another, slightly larger tubular system, containing *perilymph*, that fills the bony labyrinth. Endolymph has roughly the ionic consistency of intracellular fluid, whereas perilymph has roughly the ionic consistency of extracellular fluid. These differences are critical to the physiologic function of the ear and will be discussed at greater length later in this chapter. Separate cellular structures continuously generate the endolymph and perilymph, much as the choroid plexus produces cerebrospinal fluid. Also like cerebrospinal fluid, both types of fluid must be absorbed continuously. Problems with endolymphatic absorption can result in a very distressing clinical disorder: Menière's syndrome (Case 10-2).

## Case 10-2

**Menière's Syndrome**
*A 55-year-old woman presents with a 2-month history of recurrent episodes of severe dizziness. These episodes are generally heralded by a feeling of pressure over the right temporal region. Within 15 minutes, this suddenly gives way to violent vertigo that*

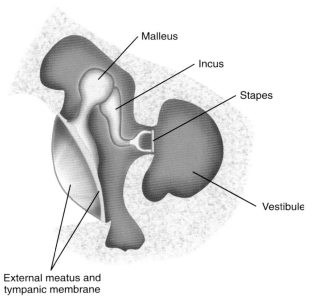

**Figure 10-2** Location of the ossicles within the middle ear.

## Case 10-2—cont'd

*persists for about 30 minutes. During this time, she has such an overwhelming sensation of movement that she feels she must hang on to things around her to keep from being flung about. She experiences violent nausea and vomiting, and a deafening roaring sound (tinnitus) in her right ear. As the vertigo subsides, she is exhausted and drenched in sweat, and she tends to feel fatigued and vaguely dizzy for a couple of days.*

**Comment:** *This patient has a disorder involving the drainage of endolymph, often referred to as endolymphatic hydrops. As a result of intermittent obstruction to fluid egress, the endolymphatic pressure in the right ear transiently becomes very high. This pressure stimulates auditory and vestibular receptors, resulting in tinnitus and vertigo. This disorder is typically treated, not always successfully, with drugs that reduce the production of endolymph.*

The inner ear can be divided into auditory and vestibular portions (Figs. 10-3, 10-4). The auditory portion consists of the *cochlea,* a spiral structure composed of approximately two and one-half turns of the perilymphatic space and its contained endolymphatic space. The vestibular portion consists of the *semicircular canals,* the saccular structure to which they are attached—the *utricle*—and a second, linked saccular structure—the *saccule.*

**Auditory and Vestibular Systems**

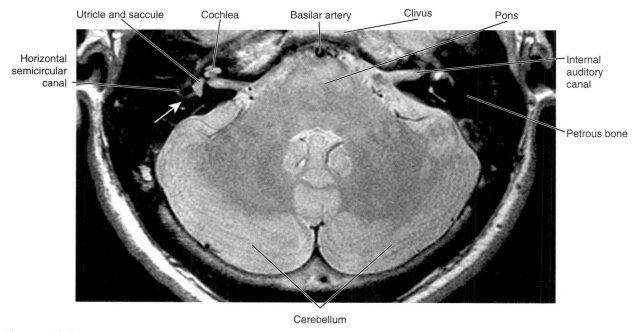

**Figure 10-3** Axial magnetic resonance image (MRI) demonstrating the inner ear (*arrow*) within the petrous portion of the temporal bone at the base of the skull. In this "proton density weighted" sequence, fluid has high signal. Thus, the fluid-filled structures within the inner ear that fill the bony labyrinth appear bright.

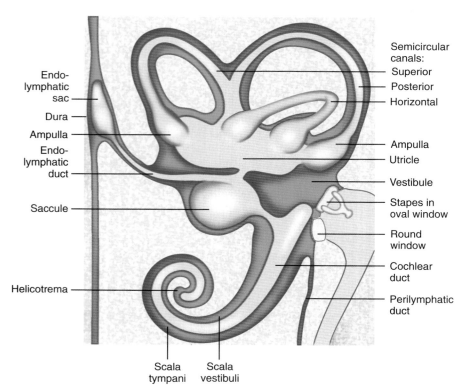

**Figure 10-4** Schematic diagram of cross section through the temporal bone demonstrating the membranous labyrinth within the bony labyrinth.

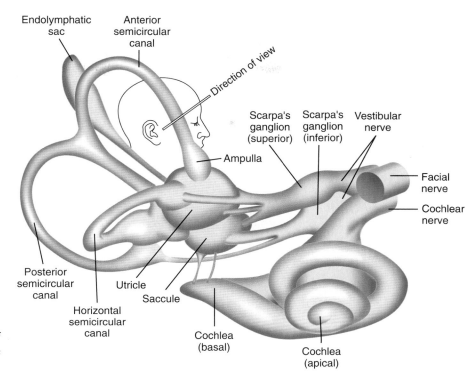

**Figure 10-5** Relationship of the eighth cranial nerve to the inner ear.

## INNERVATION OF THE INNER EAR

The cochlea is innervated by cells in the cochlear or *spiral ganglion*, located within the center of the cochlear spiral. The vestibular portion of the inner ear is innervated by cells in *Scarpa's ganglion* (Fig. 10-5). The cells in these two ganglia generate the fibers of the auditory and vestibular nerves, respectively, which pass through the *internal auditory canal* (Figs. 10-1, 10-3) to eventually terminate in the rostral medulla. Scarpa's ganglion and the auditory and vestibular nerves may be involved by two relatively common pathologic processes, as illustrated in Cases 10-3 and 10-4.

### Case 10-3

**Vestibular Neuronitis**

*A 35-year-old man presents with a 2-day history of severe and constant dizziness. By remaining in bed and holding perfectly still, he manages to keep the dizziness within more or less tolerable limits. However, any movement precipitates a violent wave of vertigo, associated with nausea and vomiting. He has not been able to eat or drink anything since the onset of this problem. Examination is normal but for the presence of vestibular nystagmus beating to the left (i.e., slow phase to the right).*

**Comment:** *This patient has vestibular neuronitis, an inflammation of Scarpa's ganglion, involving the right ear. A viral infection is suspected, and herpes viruses have been incriminated but have not been proved to be the cause of this disorder. Typically,*

*symptoms will gradually subside over the course of about a week, at which point patients can walk again, albeit a little unsteadily. Eventually they completely recover. Residual damage to Scarpa's ganglion has been demonstrated in postmortem studies conducted years later, but the brainstem is readily able to adjust to the inequality in vestibular input from the two ears. The vestibular nystagmus observable during the acute phase reflects the fact that when the brainstem detects asymmetric vestibular input from the two sides, it thinks the head is rotating in the axial plane. It generates an "appropriate" vestibulo-ocular reflex, in this case, slow movements of the eyes to the right with saccades back to the left (see Cycle 8-4B and Fig. 8-29).*

Auditory and Vestibular Systems

## Case 10-4

### Vestibular Schwannoma

*During a routine physical examination, a 65-year-old woman is noted to have a marked reduction in auditory acuity in the left ear (Fig. 10-6). On questioning, she recalls that about 6 months ago, she started holding the telephone over her right ear because she was having trouble understanding people when she held it to the left ear. She also concedes that she has noted some occasional vague imbalance while standing and walking. A magnetic resonance image (MRI) scan reveals a tumor involving left cranial nerve (CN) VIII (Fig. 10-7).*

**Comment:** *This patient has a benign neoplasm resulting from uncontrolled proliferation of the*

*myelin-producing cells, the Schwann cells, of the vestibular portion of CN VIII. These neoplasms are often inappropriately referred to as acoustic neuromas. They impair hearing by compressing the auditory branch of CN VIII. Vestibular dysfunction is usually minimal, despite tumor origin in the vestibular nerve, because of the capacity of the brainstem to gradually adapt to asymmetry in vestibular input. Because of the close proximity of the seventh and eighth cranial nerves in the internal auditory canal, surgical removal of these tumors without damaging CN VII can be quite demanding.*

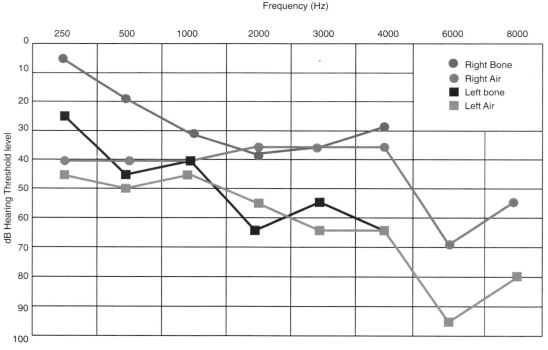

**Figure 10-6** Audiogram of a patient with a left vestibular schwannoma. The lowest amplitude sound the patient is capable of detecting—the hearing threshold—is mapped for each ear at a variety of frequencies (cycles/second or Hertz [Hz]) in relationship to the standardized performance of a normal subject. Both conduction of sound through air and through bone are measured. Hearing loss, like sound levels in general, is measured in decibels (dB). A normal subject would exhibit 0 dB of hearing loss at all frequencies. The relationship of sound levels (*L*) in decibels to sound pressure (the force exerted by the sound) is expressed by the following equation:

$$L = 20 \log_{10} (P/P_{ref})$$

where *P* is the actual pressure and $P_{ref}$ is a standard reference pressure. Thus, an increase in sound pressure by a factor of 10 relative to a reference pressure would correspond to a 20-dB increase in sound level [$20 \log_{10} (10/1) = (20)(1) = 20$]. By the same token, a 20-dB hearing loss corresponds to a 10-fold reduction in sound pressure sensitivity, a 40-dB hearing loss to a 100-fold reduction, and so on. This type of logarithmic relationship appears to reflect a fundamental physiologic principle, as it characterizes all perceptual processes.

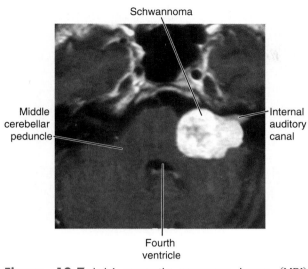

**Figure 10-7** Axial magnetic resonance image (MRI) demonstrating a large vestibular schwannoma filling the left cerebellopontine angle cistern.

## PRACTICE 10-1

**A.** What would be the consequence of losing the pinnas of both ears?

**B.** Audiometry demonstrates 80-dB hearing loss at most frequencies in one ear. What reduction in ability to detect sound pressure does this represent?

**C.** Would you expect patients with meningitis (inflammation of the meninges, usually caused by infection) to experience hearing loss? (Hint: note the relationship of the endolymphatic sac to the dura in Fig. 10-4.)

# Anatomy of the Cochlea

**Objective**

Be able to describe the major anatomic structures of the cochlea.

A slice through the cochlea along the axis of the cochlear nerve and spiral ganglion (Fig. 10-8) reveals that the spiral tube composing the cochlea is divided throughout its length into three chambers, the *scala vestibuli*, the *cochlear duct*, and the *scala tympani*. These parts are depicted in greater detail in Figure 10-9, which displays a cross section through one turn of the cochlea. The scala vestibuli and the scala tympani are filled with perilymph, and the cochlear duct is filled with endolymph. The scala vestibuli represents a direct extension of the vestibule (Fig. 10-4). Thus, movement of the footplate of the stapes, which lies over the oval window of the vestibule, directly moves perilymphatic fluid along the scala vestibuli. The scala vestibuli communicates with the scala tympani at the helicotrema, located at the apex of the cochlea (Fig. 10-4). Thus, perilymphatic fluid shunted forward or backward along the scala vestibuli could, in principle, be shunted along the scala tympani via this communication. Limited movement of fluid along the scala tympani is possible because it terminates in the elastic membrane of the round window. However, as we shall see, movement of perilymphatic fluid in the scala tympani is actually induced primarily by movement of the cochlear duct and its related soft tissue structures (as a result of movement of the fluid in the scala vestibuli), rather than by shunting through the helicotrema.

Whereas the perilymphatic fluid of the scala vestibuli and the scala tympani performs a fluid dynamic function (by virtue of its movement), the endolymphatic fluid of the cochlear duct, although it is buffeted by the events in the scalae, serves a strictly neurophysiologic function. This function will be detailed in the following paragraphs.

A closer look at the cochlear duct reveals the structures responsible for translating sound into neural impulses (Fig. 10-10). The outer wall of the cochlear duct is covered by the stria vascularis, which is responsible for the production of endolymph. Reissner's membrane separates the cochlear duct from the scala vestibuli. The *basilar membrane* separates the cochlear duct from the scala tympani. Appended to the basilar membrane is an intricate apparatus known as the *organ of Corti* (Figs. 10-11, 10-12). The base of the organ of Corti consists of two strips of *hair cells*, the specialized cells directly responsible for translation of movement into neural firing. These cells are stabilized in a matrix of supporting cells. Their apical hairlike processes directly contact a gelatinous but relatively unstretchable overlying membrane, called the *tectorial membrane*. The hair cells receive direct synapses from the dendrites of neurons in the spiral ganglion.

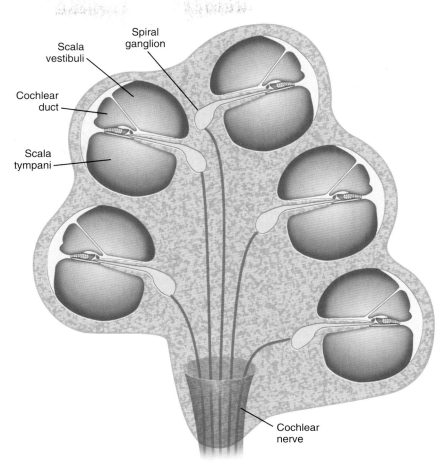

**Figure 10-8** Cross section of the cochlea along the axis of the cochlear nerve and spiral ganglion.

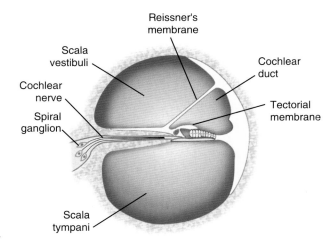

**Figure 10-9** Cross section of one turn of the cochlea.

Auditory and Vestibular Systems

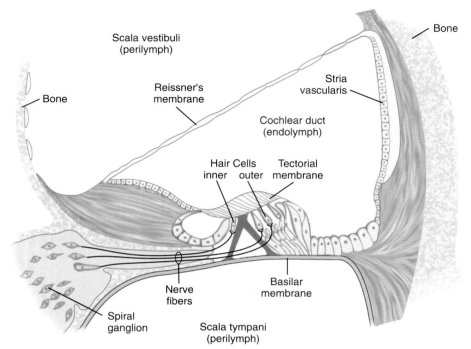

**Figure 10-10** Cross section of the cochlear duct.

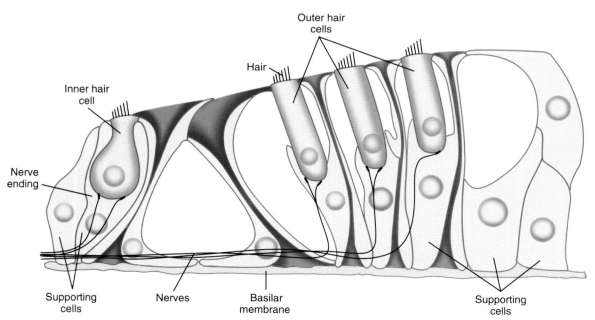

**Figure 10-11** Cross section of the organ of Corti. The orientation of this figure is the same as that of Figure 10-10.

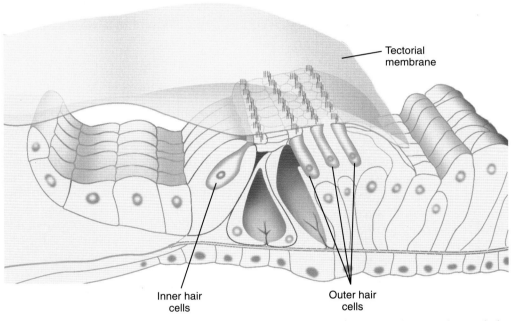

**Figure 10-12** Three-dimensional view of a segment of the organ of Corti, depicting the inner and outer hair cells as they might be seen through a completely transparent tectorial membrane. The orientation of this figure is the same as that of Figures 10-10 and 10-11.

# Cycle 10-3

# Transduction of the Auditory Signal

## Objectives

1. Be able to describe in detail how sound waves are translated into frequency-specific oscillations of discrete parts of the basilar membrane.

2. Be able to explain how oscillation of the basilar membrane is translated into sliding movement of the tectorial membrane across the tips of the cochlear hair cells.

The auditory components of the ear must take the alternating waves of compression and rarefaction of air that constitute sound, translate them into movement, transduce that movement from an air medium to a fluid medium, decompose a complex sound, now manifested as fluid movement, into its component frequencies, and translate movements corresponding to each of these frequencies into frequency-specific neural impulses. Our discussion of the anatomy of the ear in the previous cycles has included all the major structures involved in this complex sequence of processes. We will now consider how this sequence is accomplished.

The tympanic membrane achieves the first step, the translation of sound waves into movement. That movement is conveyed, through the ossicles of the middle ear, to the perilymphatic fluid of the inner ear via the footplate of the stapes in the oval window. One might ask why we need an eardrum and ossicles—why can't we simply translate sound waves directly into fluid

movement at the oval window? The reason we cannot is that waves of energy crossing between two fluids of highly different density (air and water in this case) will tend to be reflected rather than transmitted. This principle is nicely illustrated in the fact that if you are swimming under water, you cannot hear someone shouting at you from above the water—the sound waves produced by their shouting simply bounce off the water's surface. Movements of the tympanic membrane are induced by sound waves. They are very precisely translated by the ossicles into roughly equal movements of the stapes. The tympanic membrane has roughly 35 times the area of the oval window. As a result, the movement of the eardrum is not significantly damped by the linkage to the ossicles, but sufficient force is applied to the fluid at the oval window to produce movement of the fluid beneath that is comparable in magnitude to that of the tympanic membrane.

The effect of fluid movement in the scala vestibuli can be more easily appreciated if we "unwind" the cochlea, as shown in Figure 10-13. As the stapes is pushed in, the perilymph within the scala vestibuli is pushed forward. Because this fluid is incompressible, something must give. The fluid could move into the scala tympani via the helicotrema. However, in practice, the compressed fluid shifts the cochlear duct and its appended structures, most notably, the basilar membrane and the organ of Corti, thereby compressing the scala tympani. The membrane of the round window

470

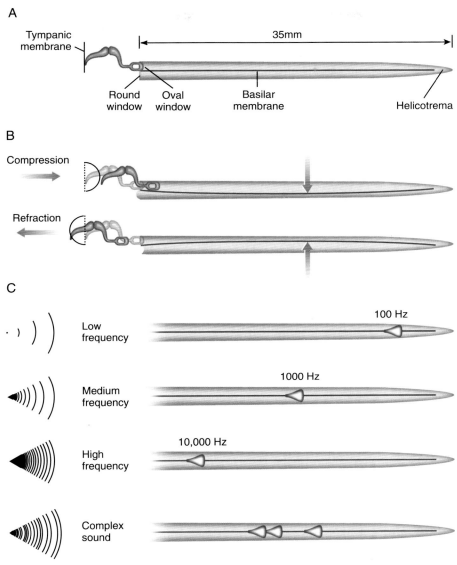

**Figure 10-13** *A,* A highly simplified drawing of an "unwound cochlea." *B,* Effect of insertion and withdrawal of the stapes on a basilar membrane of uniform pliability and thickness. *C,* Effect of vibration of the stapes on a basilar membrane of continuously varying pliability and thickness. Low frequency sounds elicit oscillations maximal in the thin, pliable apical portions of the basilar membrane. High frequency sounds elicit oscillations maximal in the thick, stiff basal portions of the basilar membrane. Complex sounds elicit oscillation at multiple portions of the basilar membrane, which correspond to the multiple component frequencies of these complex sounds. (Adapted from Kandel ER, Schwartz JH, Jessell TM (eds). Principles of Neural Science, 4th ed. New York, McGraw-Hill, 2000, p 595. Reproduced with permission of The McGraw-Hill Companies, Inc.)

**Auditory and Vestibular Systems**

"gives," bulging out to allow this to happen. Exactly the reverse of this process occurs when the stapes is pulled out. In this way, vibratory movements of the tympanic membrane are translated, via vibratory movements of the footplate of the stapes, into vibratory movements of the basilar membrane and its appended structures, the cochlear duct and the organ of Corti.

At this point, it is hard to see what has been gained by translation of vibratory movement at the oval window into vibratory movement of the basilar membrane. This is because the singular function of the cochlea actually owes to the fact that the basilar membrane (which comprises one wall of the cochlear duct) is not a homogeneous structure. At the base of the cochlea, near the oval window, it is thick and stiff. At the apex of the cochlea, near the helicotrema, it is thin and pliable. Between the base and the apex, the thickness and pliability vary continuously. As a result, *at the base of the cochlea, the basilar membrane resonates selectively to high frequencies, whereas at the apex, it resonates selectively to low frequencies*. In this way, a complex oscillatory movement at the oval window is translated into vibration of discrete components of the basilar membrane (and the attached cochlear duct) corresponding to each of the component frequencies of that complex oscillation (Fig. 10-13). In mathematical terms, the basilar membrane performs a Fourier transformation of the waveform introduced at the oval window.

As segments of the basilar membrane move, the adjacent components of the cochlear duct move with them, including the organ of Corti and the tectorial membrane. However, the organ of Corti and the tectorial membrane are anchored at slightly different points, about which they pivot (Fig. 10-10). In this way, up and down movement of the basilar membrane and cochlear duct produces a back and forth sliding movement of the tectorial membrane across the tips of the hair cells, deflecting the hairs. In Cycle 10-4, we will see how deflection of the hairs is translated into neural signals.

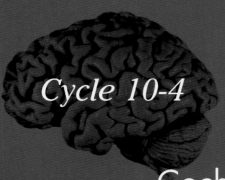

# Cochlear Hair Cells and the Generation of a Neural Signal

## Objectives

1. Be able to describe in detail how movement of hair cells is translated into a change in the firing rate of auditory nerve fibers.

2. Be able to explain the mechanism of aminoglycoside ototoxicity.

Figure 10-14 depicts a hair cell. An array of approximately 100 *stereocilia* up to 100 mm long protrudes from its apex. Each stereocilium is a hollow cylinder with a rigid cytoskeleton composed of actin cross-linked by fibrin. The length of the stereocilia varies systematically across the array from the shortest to the longest, giving the array a beveled appearance. The tip of each stereocilium is attached to the side of its taller neighbor by a fine elastic fiber called a tip link (Fig. 10-15). Tension by the tip link on the shorter stereocilium opens a nonspecific cation channel, thereby converting a mechanical event into an ionic event. When the stereocilia are all pushed by the tectorial membrane in the direction of the tallest stereocilia, the cation channels in each stereocilium spend most of their time in the open state. When the stereocilia are all pushed by the tectorial membrane in the direction of the shortest stereocilia, the cation channels spend most of their time in the closed state.

The intracellular ionic composition of hair cells is similar to that of neurons. In particular, the intracellular potassium concentration is approximately 155 mM.

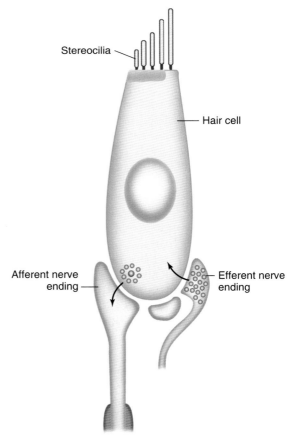

**Figure 10-14** Schematic drawing of a hair cell. Arrows indicate the direction of chemical neurotransmission.

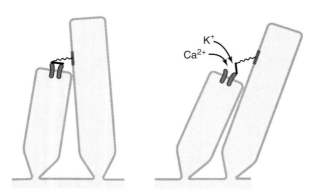

**Figure 10-15** Schematic drawing of the opening of a cation channel by the tip link between two stereocilia as they are pushed toward the taller stereocilium.

The interstitial fluid bathing the bodies of the hair cells, which is contiguous with the perilymph, has a potassium concentration of approximately 4 mM. The movement of potassium ions down their concentration gradient at the cell membrane of the hair cell, as in a neuron, results in a sufficient paucity of positive charge on the inner side of the hair cell membrane to generate a resting membrane potential of approximately −60 mV (see Chapter 5).

The apex of the hair cells, including the stereocilia, is bathed in endolymph. The endolymph is kept separate from the interstitial fluid bathing the bodies of the hair cells by tight junctions between the membrane of the cochlear duct and the hair cell membranes. Endolymph has an ionic composition very similar to that of intracellular fluid. In particular, it has a potassium ion concentration of approximately 140 mM. The endolymph, unlike any other extracellular fluid in the body, has a net charge, a charge of +80 mV, which is referred to as the endocochlear potential. However, unlike the negative charge of intracellular fluid, this positive charge is not achieved by ion flow down a concentration gradient. Rather, it is achieved by an electrogenic pump located in the stria vascularis. This pump produces a slight excess of potassium ions on the inside of the membrane of the cochlear duct, thereby establishing the +80 mV transmembrane potential.

When the cationic channels of the stereocilia are open, even though the potassium ion concentration is roughly the same inside and outside the stereocilia, the potassium ions are drawn into the stereocilia from the cochlear duct by a very large charge gradient (from +80 mV to −60 mV). The sudden resultant influx of positive charge into the hair cell depolarizes its membrane. The tonic, low frequency firing rate of the hair

cell is increased.[1] Because the neurotransmitter of hair cells is glutamate (excitatory), this elicits increased firing in an auditory nerve fiber (Fig. 10-16). When the cation channels of the stereocilia spend more time in the closed state, potassium ion influx into the hair cell decreases, the hair cell becomes relatively hyperpolarized, and its spontaneous firing rate decreases. This results in reduced firing of the auditory nerve fiber.

---

### BOX 10-1 Function of the Outer Hair Cells

In Cycle 10-2, we mentioned that the base of the organ of Corti consists of two strips of hair cells, referred to as inner hair cells and outer hair cells. The task of sound transduction that we have just described is actually carried out by the inner hair cells. Although the role of the outer hair cells is only partially understood, it appears that they solve at least two problems. First, mathematical modeling of cochlear function suggests that a large portion of the acoustic energy is consumed in overcoming the viscous damping effects of cochlear fluids on basilar membrane movement. In fact, it appears that the cochlea should not be able to detect low-intensity sounds. On the other hand, the cochlea is susceptible to saturation at high sound intensity levels. Second, the frequency selectivity of acoustic nerve fibers appears to be too great to be achieved solely through the mechanical properties of the basilar membrane. The outer hair cells appear to be important in adjusting the gain of the hair cells such that low-intensity sounds are selectively amplified and high-intensity sounds are sufficiently attenuated that variations in sound intensity are still detectable. The outer hair cells also appear to be important in increasing the frequency selectivity of inner hair cells. Outer hair cells apparently achieve these effects through their mechanical effects on the tectorial membrane. These cells receive extensive efferent fibers from the superior olivary nucleus in the caudal pons, and they are capable of the modest contraction that modifies tectorial membrane movement, thereby influencing gain and sharpening frequency selectivity. This movement actually generates sound—otoacoustic emissions. Universal screening of ear function in infants is now mandated in Florida and many other states. The most economical way of doing this is to measure otoacoustic emissions.

---

[1]At their resting membrane potential, there is a constant influx of Ca²⁺ through a "leaky" calcium channel, which provides the basis for the tonic, low frequency firing.

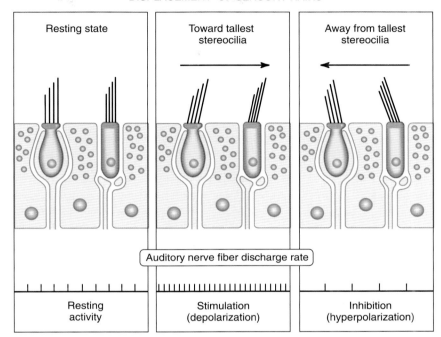

**Figure 10-16** Schematic drawing showing the effect of deflection of stereocilia on the discharge of a cochlear nerve fiber innervating a hair cell.

## Case 10-5

### Aminoglycoside Ototoxicity

*A 75-year-old man is admitted to the hospital with a 2-week history of progressive malaise, fever, and pain in the left lower quadrant of his abdomen. It is ultimately determined that he has diverticulitis (infection and inflammation of multiple, small, pathologic outpouchings or diverticuli of the descending colon). The infection has spread beyond the bounds of the colon, and he has a large, pericolic abscess. He is treated with surgical resection of the involved segment of colon, drainage of the abscess, and the administration of a long course of antibiotics, including the aminoglycoside gentamicin. In the course of this treatment, the patient becomes nearly deaf.*

**Comment:** *Aminoglycosides, for unknown reasons, are concentrated in the endolymph. They are able to pass through the nonspecific cation channel in the stereocilia into the hair cells. There, they damage mitochondria by interfering with protein synthesis by mitochondrial ribosomes, which resemble prokaryotic (e.g., bacterial) ribosomes. As a result, the patient has experienced extensive loss of hair cells in the cochlea. There is evidence that this ototoxicity is increased when patients are in noisy environments. Because the mitochondria are damaged, the hair cells must rely to a greater degree on anaerobic metabolism. This is insufficient to their needs when they are firing rapidly in noisy environments.*

Auditory and Vestibular Systems

**TABLE 10-1** Summary of Sound Transduction in the Ear

| Structure | Function in the Sequence |
|---|---|
| Tympanic membrane | Alternating compression and rarefaction of air (sound) are translated into movement of the membrane. |
| Ossicles | Transduce low force movement of tympanic membrane into high force movement of stapes footplate at oval window, efficiently transferring sound energy to perilymph in the vestibule. |
| Scala vestibuli, scala tympani | Translate longitudinal movement of perilymph along the scala vestibuli into transverse movement of the basilar membrane, cochlear duct, and organ of Corti. |
| Basilar membrane | Graded thickness and pliability provide basis for selective movement of a particular region in response to a particular frequency of perilymph movement. Low frequencies—cochlear apex; high frequencies—cochlear base. |
| Organ of Corti | Translates movement of basilar membrane into movement of tectorial membrane across the stereocilia of the hair cells. |
| Stereocilia | Deflection toward tallest stereocilia opens nonspecific cation channels via tip links. |
| Endolymph | High positive charge of endolymph bathing stereocilia, induced by electrogenic potassium ion pump in stria vascularis, establishes a large charge gradient between endolymph outside stereocilia and intracellular fluid within stereocilia. |
| Stereocilia deflection | Flow of potassium ions down charge gradient from endolymph depolarizes the hair cell, leading to increased firing. |
| Hair cell | Increased firing of hair cell, through release of excitatory neurotransmitter glutamate, induces increased firing in auditory nerve fiber. |
| Tonotopic organization | Relationship between sound frequency and position along the basilar membrane is carried over to hair cells along this membrane, auditory nerve cells, and all CNS projection targets of the eighth cranial nerve. |

The peculiar nature of the nonspecific cation channel of the hair cells renders them susceptible to the effects of other substances that can pass through it (much like anticonvulsants and local anesthetics can pass through voltage-sensitive sodium channels—see Chapter 5). Case 10-5 illustrates this susceptibility.

Because each hair cell is associated with a particular portion of the basilar membrane, fluctuations in its discharge rate reflect the presence or absence of a sound component of a particular frequency.[2] The organization of hair cells along the length of the basilar membrane, with each cell responding to a narrow range of frequencies that depends upon its particular position along the basilar membrane, is referred to as tonotopic organization. Because each auditory neuron synapses on a single hair cell, this tonotopic organization is replicated in the spiral ganglion. It is further replicated at each waystation along the central auditory pathways, all the way to and including the primary auditory cortex.

The entire sequence of sound transduction through the ear is summarized in Table 10-1.

## PRACTICE 10-4

**A.** Disorders of the ear can produce hearing loss in two ways. Dysfunction of the tympanic membrane or the ossicles produces *conductive* hearing loss. Dysfunction of the inner ear or its innervation produces *sensorineural* hearing loss. Simple bedside tests can distinguish these two disorders. Simply rubbing one's fingers together near the ear, at first very lightly, and gradually more firmly, enables one to identify the side of the hearing loss. A second test, the *Weber test*, can

---

[2]Because stereocilia move back and forth with each sound wave, fluctuations in the release of glutamate by hair cells could, at least in principle, encode the sound frequency. However, there are physiologic limitations on the ability of the hair cells to do this, at least at high frequencies, and it is presently unclear to what extent sound wave entrainment by hair cells adds to the frequency decoding achieved through the properties of the basilar membrane. The entrainment of frequency by stereociliary oscillation may be particularly important in the analysis of the temporal evolution of complex sounds, and it is almost certainly important in the detection of the small differences in the time of arrival of sound wave fronts in the two ears that enable us to locate sound (see Cycle 10-6A and B).

distinguish between conductive and sensorineural loss. In the Weber test, a vibrating 512 Hz tuning fork is placed firmly against the forehead. The vibration is transmitted through the bone to both inner ears equally. However, if there is conductive hearing loss in one ear, sound transmitted through bone will be perceived as relatively louder in this ear. The reason for this is not agreed upon, but one hypothesis is that sounds transmitted through bone are relatively louder because competing environmental sounds are reduced as a result of limitation of movements of the tympanic membrane and ossicles. In the case of sensorineural hearing loss, sensitivity to sound conducted by air or bone is reduced and the sound is heard as louder in the opposite, normal ear. Using these principles, answer the following questions:

1. In Case 10-4, on which side would the patient hear the sound during the Weber test (i.e., to which side would the Weber test lateralize)?

2. A child with acute otitis media (inflammation with fluid accumulation in the middle ear) has reduced hearing in the left ear. On which side would this patient hear the sound during the Weber test?

3. A 70-year-old man complains of hearing impairment in his right ear. You confirm this with a bedside test of auditory acuity. The Weber test lateralizes to the right (the patient reports that the sounds seems to come from the right). Does this patient have conductive or sensorineural hearing loss?

**B.** How do you think language will develop in children with hearing impairment (sensorineural or conductive)?

**C.** Menière's syndrome eventually results in loss of hair cells that is maximal in the apex of the cochlea. Describe the pattern of hearing loss that would result.

**D.** Aging is associated with loss of hair cells and decline in the endocochlear potential (the positive charge of the endolymph). Explain what effect these changes would have and why.

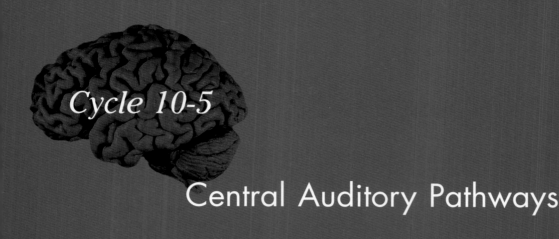

# Central Auditory Pathways

The auditory nerve exits the spiral ganglion, passes through the internal auditory canal, and terminates in the *dorsal* and *ventral cochlear nuclei* in the dorsolateral medulla (Figs. 10-3, 10-17). These nuclei project via a number of structures in the ventral pontine tegmentum to the inferior colliculi, which then project to the *medial geniculate nuclei* of the thalamus (Fig. 10-18). Each medial geniculate nucleus projects, via the auditory radiations in the temporal lobe white matter, to *primary auditory cortex (Heschl's gyrus, AI).* Heschl's gyrus lies on the dorsal surface of the temporal lobe, buried deep within the Sylvian fissure (Fig. 10-19). Auditory projections from the cochlear nuclei to Heschl's gyrus are predominantly but far from exclusively contralateral. Thus, *hearing is not perceptibly altered by unilateral lesions anywhere along the ascending trajectory from the cochlear nuclei to and including Heschl's gyrus.* Neurons in Heschl's gyrus project to adjacent auditory association cortices.

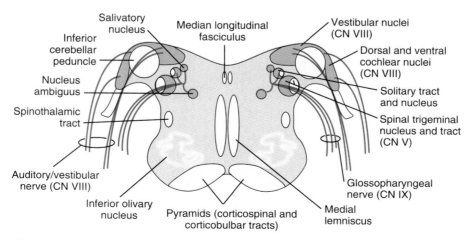

**Figure 10-17** Diagram of axial section of rostral medulla showing the location of the dorsal and ventral cochlear nuclei.

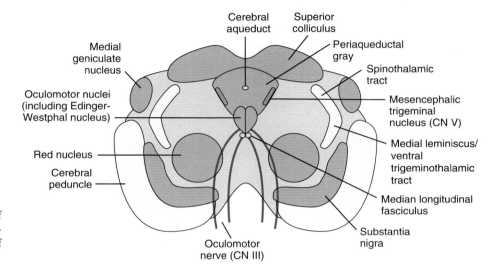

**Figure 10-18** Diagram of axial section of rostral midbrain showing the location of the medial geniculate nuclei.

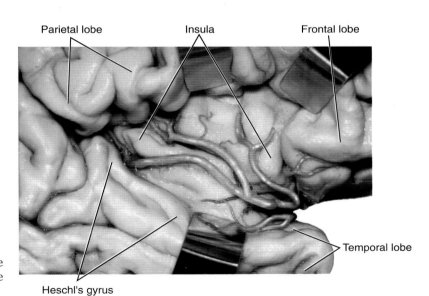

**Figure 10-19** Heschl's gyrus on the dorsal surface of the temporal lobe, and the insula.

Auditory and Vestibular Systems

# Signal Processing in the Ascending Auditory Pathways and the Auditory Cortex

## *Objectives*

1. Be able to describe briefly the basis for sound localization.
2. Be able to describe briefly the basis for sound sequence decoding and explain the relationship of this capacity to language.
3. Be able to describe briefly an example of neural plasticity in auditory cortex.

Signal processing in the auditory system is far less well understood than it is in the visual system. However, recent intensive research has yielded some key insights. We will focus on three areas: (1) the brainstem system that enables sound localization; (2) the neural networks in auditory cortex that enable sound sequence decoding; and (3) neural plasticity in auditory cortex.

## A. SOUND LOCALIZATION

Neural structures in the ventral pontine tegmentum known collectively as the superior olivary nuclei are exquisitely sensitive to differences between the two ears in the timing of sound arrival and in sound intensity, both of which are used to locate sounds. The supe-

rior olivary nuclei are capable of distinguishing sound arrival differences of as little as 10 microseconds. This corresponds to an ability to detect differences in sound direction of as little as 3 degrees. Differences in the sound intensity detected by the two ears are related primarily to the fact that with sound sources located to one side, sound to one ear is going to be partially attenuated by the sound absorptive properties of the head. Neurons involved in the detection of interaural differences in the timing of arrival of sound wave fronts respond primarily to lower frequency sounds. Neurons involved in detecting interaural differences in sound intensity respond primarily to higher frequency sounds. This is logical because only high-frequency sounds are significantly absorbed by the head.

## B. SOUND SEQUENCE

Studies of neuronal responses in the primary auditory cortex (Heschl's gyrus, AI) in experimental animals have demonstrated a tonotopic organization—the highest frequencies represented at one end of AI, the lowest frequencies at the other end. Perpendicular to the frequency axis of AI is a response latency axis. Thus, within each band of neurons responding optimally to a given sound frequency, there is a systematic variation in the time to respond, ranging, for example, in the squirrel monkey, from 8.6 to 20 ms. This range provides the basis for representing information not just about individual tones, but also about the sequential relationships between tones. In this way, a burst of complex sound might elicit a pattern of neural activity involving the entirety of AI that represents both the frequency of all the components of that sound burst and the temporal relationship of these components to each other. Within a given frequency band, some (short latency) neurons will be responding to one sound while other (long latency) neurons are still responding to the previous sound. Interactions between short and long latency neurons in AI presumably provide the basis for AI responses that depend on the interrelationship between sounds occurring at slightly different times.

Consider an experiment in which responses of neurons in AI to repeated, fixed frequency, pure tones are recorded, responses of these same neurons to repeated clicks are recorded, and then responses to alternating tones and clicks are recorded. If AI represented only frequency, one would expect the responses in the alternating click and tone experiment to be simply a mix of those observed in the pure tone and pure click trials. However, the actual responses are quite different, reflecting the fact that a response to a pure tone is markedly different when it follows a click than when it follows another pure tone. These experiments provide a dramatic demonstration of the sequence information represented in the pattern of neural activity in AI.

One of the greatest challenges to deciphering the neural representation of complex behaviors like language and skilled movement has been to understand how the brain encodes perceptions and movements that change continuously over time (as in heard and spoken language). The most essential attribute of language cortex appears to be the ability to decode and encode particularly rapid sound transitions, as occur with consonant use.[3] Studies of AI in primates tell us that one way the brain has approached this problem is to convert a temporal distribution of sound sequence into a cortical geographic distribution of sound sequence.

---

[3]Anderson, Southern, and Powers found, in an autopsy study of human brains, that the axons of neurons in the posterior superior temporal gyrus on the left (Wernicke's area—a major site of language processing) were larger and more heavily myelinated than those on the right. Greater axonal size and heavier myelination enhance the speed of processing.

## BOX 10-2 Language Devoid of Tones—Still Understandable

Robert Shannon and his colleagues have performed experiments in which sound-editing equipment was used to remove most of the sound frequency information from normal spoken language, leaving only the changes in rhythm and the fluctuations in amplitude. Normal subjects are able to interpret this grotesquely altered speech with astonishing success. This work suggests that temporal information is at least as important as sound frequency information in understanding spoken language. It also helps to understand the success of cochlear implants in enabling the deaf to hear. The placement of a cochlear implant involves the insertion of a small number of microstimulation electrodes into the center of the basal spiral of the cochlea, where they directly stimulate auditory nerve fibers innervating the basal turn. These electrodes are connected to a small amplifier that receives input from a microphone. Because the electrodes of the cochlear implant stimulate only the basal auditory nerve fibers, patients hear an extremely limited sound frequency range. Nevertheless, many are able to comprehend spoken language with remarkable facility, reflecting the importance of temporal information in language decoding and comprehension, as suggested by the experiments of Shannon and his colleagues.

## C. PLASTICITY

Until relatively recently, it was thought that the brain had very limited capacity to reorganize in response to experience or injury, at least in adults. In Chapters 6 and 7, on the Motor System and Somesthesis, we cited some dramatic evidence that this view is incorrect. Nevertheless, there is still a tendency to view the association cortices as the main venue of neural plasticity, and to perceive primary cortices as being relatively fixed and impervious to change. In Chapters 6 and 7, we reviewed some evidence that this view is fundamentally incorrect, at least in motor cortex and somatosensory cortex. An experiment reported by Kilgard and Merzenich in 1998 showed that it is not correct for the auditory system either. This experiment involved the auditory cortex of adult rats. In all the rats (experimental and control), a tiny electrode was placed in the nucleus basalis of Meynert (located just below the globus pallidus in the basal forebrain). The function of the nucleus basalis will be discussed at greater length in Chapter 12, Higher Neural Function. Here we need point out only that, by generating a surge of acetylcholine in the cerebral cortex, the neurons in nucleus basalis inform active cortical neurons, in effect, that "what you are doing is important, so learn it." All rats (experimental and control) were repeatedly exposed every 8 to 40 seconds to a pure tone stimulus (e.g., 9 kHz) as they wandered about their cages. This tone did not signal that anything was about to happen, or that the rats had to do something. In experimental rats, each occurrence of the pure tone was paired with brief electrical stimulation of nucleus basalis. In control rats, the nucleus basalis was never stimulated.

At the conclusion of a long period of exposure to the pure tones, the frequency representation within primary auditory cortex was mapped in control and experimental rats using single neuron recording techniques. In the control animals, as expected, there was a more or less evenly distributed representation of frequencies between 1 kHz and 40 kHz (the hearing range of normal rats). In the experimental group, Kilgard and Merzenich discovered something remarkable. Most of the neurons in AI now responded preferentially to tones near 9 kHz, and neurons responding to all other frequencies were located in small regions at either end of AI. AI, a primary sensory cortex, heretofore thought to be substantially immutable, had, in a very brief time, been effectively converted from a broad-spectrum sound processor to a 9 kHz tone processor. These dramatic results suggest the scope of the neural plasticity that might be engaged to help humans to recover from brain injury.

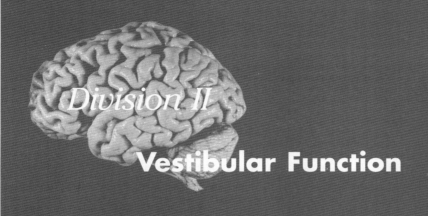

# Division II

# Vestibular Function

# The Vestibular Component of the Inner Ear

## *Objectives*

1. Be able to describe the major anatomic structures of the vestibular component of the inner ear.
2. Be able to describe in detail how linear acceleration (including that due to the effect of the gravitational field) is sensed by the inner ear.
3. Be able to describe and explain the clinical consequences of loss of vestibular function.
4. Be able to describe in detail how angular acceleration is sensed by the inner ear.
5. Be able to describe the mechanism of benign positional vertigo and explain the principles underlying its treatment.

The vestibular portion of the inner ear consists entirely of membranous labyrinth. It is composed of two saccular structures, the *saccule* and the *utricle*, and three *semicircular canals*, all filled with endolymph (Figs. 10-3, 10-4, 10-5). The three semicircular canals are attached to the utricle. The saccule and the utricle are connected by a thin passage, and the saccule and the membranous labyrinth of the cochlea are connected by another thin passage. Thus, the endolymph produced by the stria vascularis of the cochlea circulates throughout both the cochlear and vestibular portions of the membranous labyrinth.

Vestibular function involves the sensation of acceleration. Acceleration may be linear or angular. The saccule and the utricle each contain an *otolithic organ* that is sensitive to linear acceleration. The fluid within each of the semicircular canals, coupled with an apparatus to detect movement of that fluid, the *crista ampullaris*, provides the basis for sensation of angular acceleration (Table 10-2).

## A. LINEAR ACCELERATION

Each otolithic organ consists of a flat sheet of hair cells (the *macula*), the stereocilia of which insert in an overlying gelatinous membrane, the *otolithic membrane* (Fig. 10-20). Calcium carbonate crystals ("stones" or otoliths) are embedded in the otolithic membrane, giving it significant mass. Because of this mass, the membrane has some inertia. Thus, when the head is accelerated in a certain direction, the membrane tends to lag behind, thereby deflecting the hair cells, increasing or decreasing their firing rate, and giving us a sense of the acceleration. The mass of the otolith-studded membrane, in the context of the gravitational field, also makes it heavier than the endolymph. Thus, the membrane will always be pulled downward within the gravitational field, thereby providing the basis for our sensation of what is down and what is up. Alterations in the firing rates of hair cells in the otolithic

**TABLE 10-2** Summary of Auditory and Vestibular Systems

| Feature | Auditory | Vestibular | |
|---|---|---|---|
| | | Utricle and Saccule | Semicircular Canals |
| Sensory modality | Sound | Linear acceleration | Angular acceleration |
| Inner ear apparatus | Cochlea | Otolithic organs of utricle and saccule | Cupulae of semicircular canals |
| Stimulus detector | Hair cells of organ of Corti | Hair cells of maculae | Hair cells of crista ampullaris |
| Mechanism of hair cell deflection | Oscillatory sliding of tectorial membrane | Effect of inertia/gravitational field on otolithic membrane | Effect of intertial lag of endolymphatic fluid on cupula |
| Inner ear innervation | Spiral ganglion | Scarpa's ganglion | Scarpa's ganglion |
| Signal transduction to CNS | Auditory nerve | Vestibular nerve | Vestibular nerve |
| Brainstem target of primary afferents | Cochlear nuclei (medulla) | Vestibular nuclei (medulla and caudal pons) | Vestibular nuclei (medulla and caudal pons) |
| Major CNS projections and functions | Medial geniculate nucleus, primary auditory cortex (sound analysis); superior olivary nuclei (sound localization) | Vestibulospinal tract (postural reflexes, antigravity tone); cerebral cortex (various) (perception of down and up) | Abducens nuclei, flocculonodular lobe of cerebellum (vestibulo-ocular reflex), cerebral cortex |

organs are relayed to neurons in Scarpa's ganglion just as alterations in the firing rates of hair cells in the cochlea are relayed to neurons in the spiral ganglion. The otolithic membrane in the saccule is oriented in the sagittal plane and the otolithic membrane in the utricle is oriented in the axial plane. Thus, between the two organs, we are capable of sensing linear acceleration (due either to increasing speed or the gravitational field) in any direction. The importance of our capacity to sense the direction of the gravitational field is dramatically illustrated in patients who have lost this capacity, for example as a result of the toxic effects of

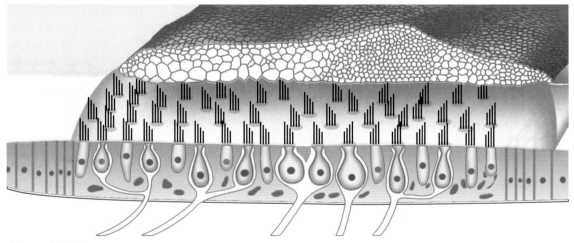

**Figure 10-20** An otolithic organ and its otolithic membrane. Note the opposite orientation of the two groups of hair cells depicted here. In fact, within a given macula, there are hair cells oriented in all possible directions within the plane of the macula. This enables the otolithic organ to detect movement of the otolithic membrane in any direction tangential to the macula.

Auditory and Vestibular Systems

aminoglycoside antibiotics on the hair cells of the vestibular component of the inner ear (Case 10-6).

---

### Case 10-6

#### Aminoglycoside Vestibular Toxicity

*65-year-old man receives a prolonged course of antibiotics, including gentamicin, for the treatment of a heart valve infection with Staphylococcus aureus ("staph" endocarditis). When he finally recovers to the point that he is able to get out of bed, he finds that his balance is abysmal and that he can barely walk. His gait is wide-based and extremely unsteady, and he is in constant imminent danger of falling.*

**Comment:** *This patient has experienced extensive damage to the hair cells of the vestibular component of the inner ear because of the toxic effects of the aminoglycoside, gentamicin. It is not clear why some patients experience preponderantly cochlear damage while others experience preponderantly vestibular damage (see Case 10-5). Because of the vestibular hair cell damage, tipping of his body and head, with attendant tipping of his otolithic organs in the gravitational field, no longer elicits a significant change in the firing rate of vestibular neurons in Scarpa's ganglion. Consequently, there is no alteration in the activity of systems within the brainstem and spinal cord (e.g., the vestibulospinal tract—see later discussion) that would serve to counteract the tipping. He has to rely solely on proprioceptive input, from position receptors in his ankles, and visual input. When vestibular impairment is severe, these other systems are not adequate to the job of maintaining balance. Fortunately, such patients typically show substantial recovery. Vestibular function is also commonly degraded in otherwise normal elderly people. This impairment is commonly an important contributing factor to their problems with balance (see Case 8-9).*

---

## B. ANGULAR ACCELERATION

The three semicircular canals are nearly perpendicular to each other (Figs. 10-4, 10-5). The plane of the horizontal canal is located in the axial plane of the brain (Fig. 10-3). The planes of the anterior and posterior canals are oriented at a 45 degree angle to the coronal and sagittal planes of the brain. Thus, between them,

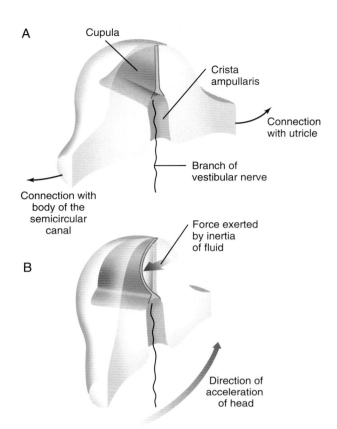

**Figure 10-21** The crista ampullaris of a semicircular canal.

the three semicircular canals of each ear are capable of sensing angular acceleration in any direction.

One end of each semicircular canal communicates freely with the utricle. The other end, defined by the ampulla (Fig. 10-4), is occluded by the crista ampullaris and an attached deformable membrane, the *cupula* (Fig. 10-21). The cupula is linked to hair cells within the crista ampullaris. Thus, the crista ampullaris of the semicircular canals is analogous to the macula of the otolithic organs in the saccule and utricle, and the cupula is analogous to the otolithic membrane of the otolithic organs.

As the head begins to turn within the plane of a particular semicircular canal, the endolymph within that canal tends to lag behind slightly because of inertia associated with its mass. This lag results in deformation of the cupula, which then leads to an alteration in the firing rate of the linked hairs cells in the crista, thus providing us the basis for our sensation of the initiation of rotational movement. If the rate of rotation becomes constant, the movement of the head will eventually be transferred to the endolymph in the semicircular canal, and cupular deflection will gradually cease. The function of the semicircular canals is revealed in a particularly clear way in a common disorder of the inner ear known as *benign positional vertigo* (Case 10-7).

## Case 10-7

### Benign Positional Vertigo

*A 45-year-old woman is seen for a 1-month history of episodic dizziness. Every episode is very brief, lasting perhaps 15 seconds. Episodes are exquisitely associated with movement, particularly rising to a standing position or rolling over in bed. She may experience a dozen episodes in a day, and then go for days without any episodes. Her neurologic examination is normal. When her physician sits her on the side of the examining table, has her turn her head to the right, and suddenly pushes her backward into a supine position (Nylen-Barany maneuver), she experiences an episode of severe vertigo that begins within 2 seconds and persists for approximately 10 seconds. At the height of the vertigo, some rotatory nystagmus is observed.*

**Comment:** *Benign positional vertigo is caused by the accumulation of cellular debris and dislodged otoliths within the vestibular portion of the membranous labyrinth (canalolithiasis). Normally this material floats loosely within the utricle, where it causes no problem. However, it has a tendency to accumulate within the posterior semicircular canal. If a sufficient quantity has accumulated, it may settle into a plug that fills a segment of the canal. When the plug moves under the influence of gravity (it is heavier than the endolymph by virtue of the otoliths within it), the endolymph cannot flow freely around it. Consequently, the pressure of the endolymph between the plug and the cupula is transiently increased or*

## Case 10-7—cont'd

*decreased, leading to deflection of the cupula. This results in a sensation of spinning. Eventually (within about 10 seconds) the plug settles to the lowest portion of the posterior semicircular canal and enough endolymph is able to leak past it that the fluid pressure on each side equalizes and deformation of the cupula ceases. The frequency with which the episodes occur probably reflects in part the tendency of repeated head movement to break up the plug into a cloud of loose debris that will pose no obstacle to the flow of endolymph past it as it settles in the gravitational field. In addition, head movements probably serve to dump some of the debris out of the posterior semicircular canal into the utricle, until there is no longer sufficient debris to produce a plug.*

## PRACTICE 10-7

**A.** Given your understanding of the mechanism of benign positional vertigo, and what tends to happen to the intracanalicular debris naturally in the course of various daily movements, can you think of a way of treating the disorder that involves moving the debris using the force of gravity?

**B.** In one of the more popular entertainments at amusement parks such as Disneyworld, visitors are strapped into chairs attached to a platform that can be tipped in any direction but cannot be moved laterally. As they sit in complete darkness, they view a movie projected on one end of the room. The movie might emulate the view from the front of a rocket ship careening up, down, and around the canyons and mountains of a barren alien planet. Explain, using what you know about the structure and function of the otolithic organs, how the viewer in this show is given a sense of violently accelerating, decelerating, and turning to narrowly escape collisions with rapidly looming obstacles.

Auditory and Vestibular Systems

# Cycle 10-8

# Central Vestibular Function

## Objectives

1. Be able to describe vestibular pathways from Scarpa's ganglion to the termination point of vestibular nerves in the brainstem.

2. Be able to explain the effect of acute loss of vestibular input from one ear on balance.

3. Be able to explain the vestibulo-ocular reflex (VOR) and the consequences of reduction of vestibular input from one ear, either because of a lesion or the injection of cold water in the external auditory meatus.

Bipolar neurons within Scarpa's ganglion synapse on the hair cells of the otolithic organs and the crista ampullaris. Their axons project via the vestibular branch of the eighth cranial nerve through the internal auditory canal to enter the dorsolateral medulla to synapse on the various vestibular nuclei located there and in a similar location in the caudal pons (Fig. 10-22). The vestibular nuclei project to several cortical areas, most notably Brodmann's area 7, which is important to our ability to align our own body-centered coordinate system with environmental coordinates (see Chapter 12, Higher Neural Function).

The tonic input to the vestibular nuclei from the hair cells of the vestibular labyrinths subserves two major functions: (1) the maintenance of postural sta-

bility within the gravitational field through postural reflexes and the maintenance of antigravity muscle tone (Cycle 6-6A), and (2) the vestibulo-ocular reflex (VOR) (Cycle 8-4B).

## PRACTICE 10-8

**A.** Review Case 10-6. Tested visual acuity in this gentleman is 20/30 (he sees at 20 feet what a normal person would be able to see at 30 feet). His visual acuity is then retested as he slowly rotates his head from side to side at a frequency of 1 Hz. His visual acuity is now 20/200. Why?

**B.** 70-year-old woman with a history of hypertension, diabetes, and heavy smoking awakes one morning feeling dizzy and nauseated. She notes problems using her right upper extremity and cannot walk because she keeps falling to the right. On examination, she has ptosis and miosis of the right eye (Horner's syndrome). Sensation of pain and temperature is diminished over the right face and the left hemibody. Extraocular movements are full, but she has left beating nystagmus. The right side of her palate does not elevate when she opens her mouth and says "aaaah." She exhibits dyssynergia, dysmetria, and ataxia during a right finger-to-nose maneuver. When she stands, she tends to fall to the right. Localize the lesion. Explain why she tends to fall to the right and has left beating nystagmus. Explain the other findings on the neurologic examination.

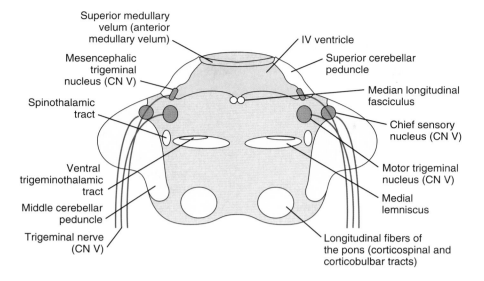

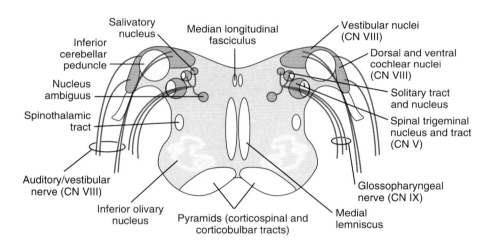

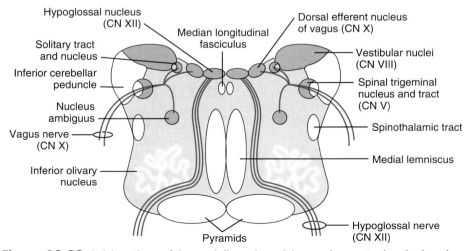

**Figure 10-22** Axial sections of the medulla and caudal pons demonstrating the location of the vestibular nuclei.

## CYCLE 10-1

**A.** The ability to localize sound along the vertical axis would be lost. Sound localization in the horizontal plane would be preserved because this depends on the ability to detect differences between the ears in the timing and loudness of arriving sound. This is discussed further in Cycle 10-6.

**B.** Sensitivity to sound pressure is reduced to 1/10,000 of normal.

**C.** Hearing loss, at times severe, is a common sequel to bacterial and fungal meningitis because of the existence of only a thin barrier between the perimeningeal spaces and the endolymphatic sac. This provides an avenue for extension of the infection and inflammation into the endolymphatic sac.

## CYCLE 10-4

**A.**

1. Right. Because of damage to the eighth cranial nerve producing sensorineural hearing loss on the left, the auditory nerve input to the brainstem produced both by sound conducted by air (generated by finger rubbing) and by bone (Weber test) will be reduced. Thus, the patient will hear both better on the right.

2. Left. The fluid and inflammation within the middle ear will dampen the movements of the left tympanic membrane. This will reduce sensitivity to the sounds of fingers rubbed beside the left ear, but it will also reduce environmental sounds that compete with sound transmitted through bone during the Weber test. Thus, during the Weber test, sound transmitted by bone will be heard better on the side of the otitis.

3. The fact that he hears sound transmitted by bone during the Weber test better on the pathologic side indicates that the patient's hearing loss must be conductive (sound transmitted by bone is not

masked by environmental sound). This distinction is important because there is a high likelihood that this patient's conductive hearing loss can be corrected, rather than simply being compensated with a hearing aid. Case 10-4 (Fig. 10-6) exhibits evidence of a conductive hearing loss in the right ear—the ear not involved by the tumor.

**B.** Spoken language development may be severely impaired. Because the neural network encoding of spoken language facilitates the development of ability to read and write, development of these skills will also tend to be severely impaired. Affected children are often thought to be mentally retarded and consigned to special education classes. For these reasons, routine testing of hearing in young children is of utmost importance.

**C.** A selective deficit in ability to hear low frequency sounds.

**D.** Decline in the endocochlear potential will reduce the charge gradient across the nonspecific cation channels in the stereocilia, thereby reducing the influx of potassium associated with opening of these channels by tip links. This will reduce glutamate release by hair cells. Both reduced glutamate release by hair cells and hair cell loss will result in loss of afferent input to auditory nerve fibers, thereby decreasing auditory nerve responses to acoustic stimuli. This hearing loss associated with aging is called presbyacusis.

## CYCLE 10-7

**A.** This is a hard question intended to get you to think about the structure of the posterior semicircular canal and its orientation with respect to the head. In fact, a description of the most effective maneuver, the Semont maneuver, was only widely disseminated in 1994. If you thought something along the line of having the patient do slow somersaults in order to pull the canalicular debris around the posterior semicircular canal until it fell out the top end into the utricle, give yourself full credit. You have captured the essential principle of the

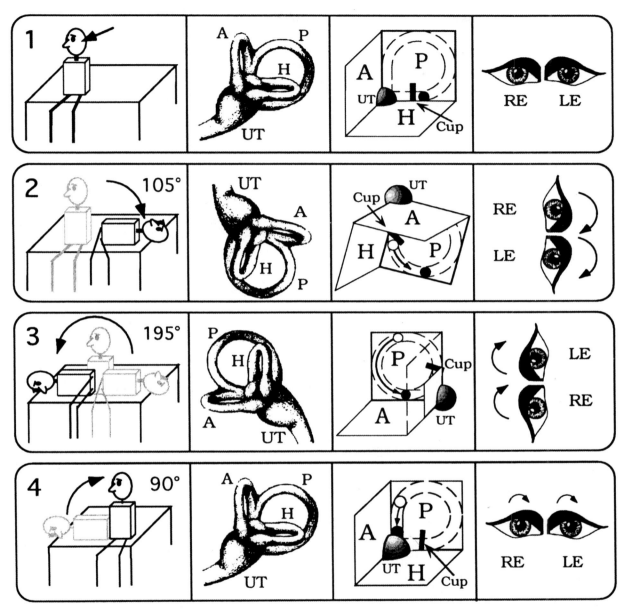

**Figure 10-23** Schematic drawing of the Semont maneuver in a patient with typical benign positional vertigo from left ear canalolithiasis. Boxes from left to right: position of body and head, position of the labyrinth in space, position and movement of the plug in the posterior canal and resulting cupula deflection, and direction of the rotatory nystagmus. The plug of debris is depicted as an open circle within the canal and a black circle represents the final resting position of the plug. A, P, and H = anterior, posterior, and horizontal semicircular canals, respectively; Cup = cupula, UT = utricle, RE = right eye, and LE = left eye. (From Brandt T, Steddin S, Eng D, Daroff RB. Therapy for benign paroxysmal positioning vertigo, revisited. Neurology 44:796-800, 1994. Reproduced with permission of Lippincott Williams & Willkins.)

Semont maneuver (and other analogous therapeutic maneuvers). The Semont maneuver achieves the somersault effect in a way that is a little easier on the patient (Fig. 10-23). It is at least 80 percent effective in curing benign positional vertigo.

**B.** The essence of the illusion is that the otolithic organs are simply detectors of linear acceleration. Therefore, given appropriately coordinated visual input, the brain can be fooled into thinking that a change in the direction of gravitational force (achieved by tilting the viewer) is a change in speed of movement. Thus, if the visual scene depicts a rapid turn to the right, the viewer is tilted in a precisely coordinated fashion to the left. The otolithic membrane of the utricle is pulled to the left by the force of gravity. However, because of the visual input, the brain concludes that the otolithic membrane is being pulled to the left by centrifugal force. So long as the tipping movement is sufficiently gradual, stimulation of the semicircular canals is too subtle to give away the artifice. The combination of congruent visual and vestibular input is so compelling that the viewer tends to hang on for dear life for fear of being thrown out of the seat.

## CYCLE 10-8

**A.** By producing compensatory eye movements, the VOR keeps the eyes fixed in such a way that objects of fixation are projected steadily on the fovea. Because this patient has lost nearly all input from the vestibular labyrinths, his VOR is severely degraded. He can no longer maintain the steady projection of images on the fovea during head movement. The test described in this problem is a convenient means of quantitatively assessing vestibular function at the bedside (see Case 8-9).

**B.** This patient has a right lateral medullary infarction ("Wallenberg" syndrome), which in most cases is caused by thrombosis of the ipsilateral vertebral artery with concomitant occlusion of the branch artery supplying the dorsolateral medullary region, usually the posterior inferior cerebellar artery (PICA). The infarct has damaged the vestibular nuclei on the right. Because of the right vestibular lesion, her brainstem has the illusion that she is tilted to the left and generates appropriate compensatory reflex movements. Direct damage to the right vestibulospinal system may also compromise the maintenance of antigravity tone on the right. Damage to the right inferior cerebellar peduncle may also contribute to the problem with balance and the tendency to fall to the right.

Because of damage to the right medial vestibular nucleus or its input from Scarpa's ganglion, vestibular input to the abducens nuclei from the right side is reduced. The abducens nuclei perceive all asymmetries in vestibular input as evidence that the head is rotating, in this case to the left. Therefore, they generate slow, smooth, compensatory eye movements to the right (the slow phase of the nystagmus)—the VOR. The frontal eye fields then intermittently generate saccades back to the left—the fast phase of the nystagmus. In Chapter 8, in an oversimplification used to aid understanding, we said that the input from the right medial vestibular nucleus to the right abducens nucleus could be viewed as inhibitory. In the presence of a right vestibular lesion, the inhibitory input to the right abducens nucleus is reduced, leading to slow movement of the eyes to the right (the VOR). The effects of a lesion of the vestibular nuclei can be reproduced by injection of cold water into the right ear (cold caloric testing), which will reduce tonic input from the vestibular portion of the labyrinth to the vestibular nuclei.

As for the other findings in this case: the Horner's syndrome results from damage to the sympathetic autonomic fibers descending in the dorsolateral quadrant of the brainstem; the failure of palatal elevation on the right from damage to nucleus ambiguus; the loss of pain and temperature sensation in the right face from damage to the nucleus and tract of the spinal nucleus of CN V; the loss of pain temperature sensation over the left hemibody from damage to the right lateral spinothalamic tract; and the impairment of the finger-to-nose maneuver on the right from damage to the right inferior cerebellar peduncle.

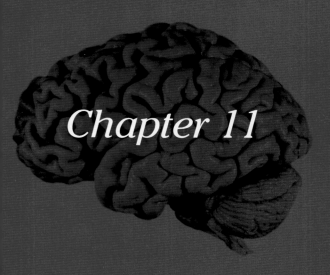

# Chapter 11

# AUTONOMIC, NEUROENDOCRINE, AND REGULATORY FUNCTIONS

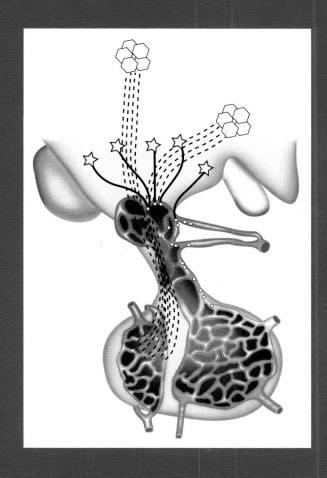

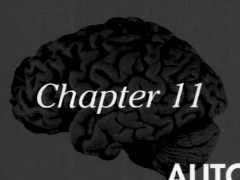

# *Chapter 11*

# AUTONOMIC, NEUROENDOCRINE, AND REGULATORY FUNCTIONS

Our focus in Chapters 1 through 10 and 12 of this book is on perceptual and motor functions that, with few exceptions, are accessible to consciousness. Motor responses are readily observable even when not conscious (e.g., deep tendon reflexes). The systems underlying these functions subserve the design and execution of behavior, much of it voluntary. In this chapter, we focus on functions that are automatic and largely inaccessible to consciousness, many of which subserve homeostasis. Although the systems underlying these functions interact extensively, they can conveniently be divided into five categories: the autonomic nervous system, neuroendocrine systems (adrenocortical function, thyroid function, growth hormone, endocrine support of sexual and reproduc-tive function, and lactation), hypothalamic regula-tory systems (preservation of plasma osmolality and intravascular volume, circadian rhythms, control of body temperature and mass), drive systems (appetite, thirst, sexual drive), and cardiorespiratory regulatory systems. Although the term "homeostasis" implies the maintenance of one state, the five major systems we will discuss actually serve to maintain stable and, for the most part, optimal bodily function under an enor-mous variety of states imposed upon the body. In these systems, as in the purely neural systems discussed else-where in this book, there are bottom-up and top-down interactions. To the extent that one region of the brain can be said to direct these various disparate systems, it is the hypothalamus.

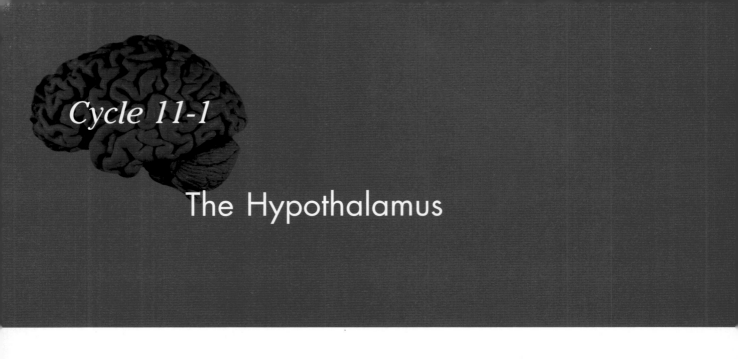

# Cycle 11-1

# The Hypothalamus

## Objectives

1. Be able to describe the location of the hypothalamus.

2. Be able to define the two major mechanisms by which the hypothalamus sends and receives signals.

3. Be able to define the two major routes by which the hypothalamus exerts its influence on the body.

4. Be able to list the major efferent components of the autonomic nervous system that receive hypothalamic projections.

5. Be able to list the major cerebral structures projecting to the hypothalamus and briefly describe some circumstances under which this input to the hypothalamus is important.

6. Be able to describe the essential difference between the neurohypophysis and the adenohypophysis in mechanism of function.

7. Be able to list the major hypothalamic regulatory functions.

8. Be able to give some examples of the substantially hypothalamically mediated motivational phenomena referred to as drives.

The hypothalamus consists of a population of nuclei lying on either side of the rostral, ventral portions of the third ventricle (Fig. 11-1). The upper margin of the hypothalamus can be defined roughly by a line drawn from the posterior margin of the anterior commissure to the posterior margin of the mammillary bodies. The hypothalamus extends anteriorly as far as the *lamina terminalis*, a membrane that forms the inferior anterior wall of the third ventricle. It extends ventrally to the inferior surface of the basal forebrain. Three major landmarks define the inferior border: the optic chiasm, the *median eminence*, and the *mammillary bodies* (the latter two being part of the hypothalamus itself). The median eminence is a small protuberance located on the ventral midline of the hypothalamus, immediately posterior to the optic chiasm. It gives rise to the *infundibulum*, or *pituitary stalk*, which joins the hypothalamus to the pituitary gland lying within the sella turcica. The hypothalamus extends laterally to the sagittal planes defined by the medial temporal lobes.

The hypothalamus is unique in that efferent and afferent information is conveyed by both neural and hormonal mechanisms. Neural efferent and afferent connections link the hypothalamus to cerebral, brainstem, and spinal cord structures. Hormonal efferent and afferent information is chiefly conveyed by the *circumventricular organs (CVOs)*, clusters of neurons located at various loci along the midline ventricular system, and the pituitary gland (some in the hypothalamus itself) (Fig. 11-2). In CVOs, the blood-brain barrier is attenuated, permitting proteins to be released by hypothalamic neurons into the blood, or proteins cir-

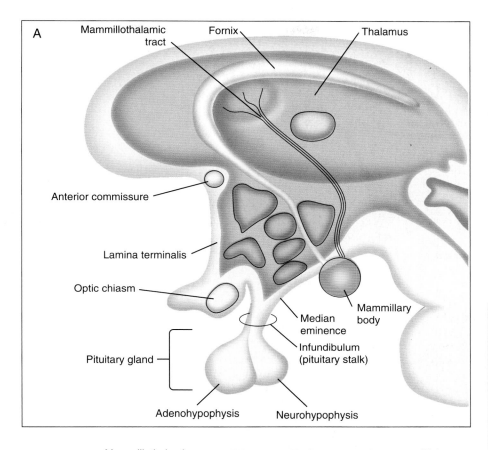

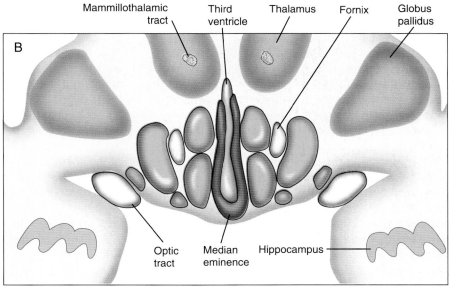

**Figure 11-1** *A*, Midsagittal view of the diencephalon demonstrating the relationship of the hypothalamus (darkly shaded nuclei) to adjacent structures. *B*, Coronal view of the hypothalamus.

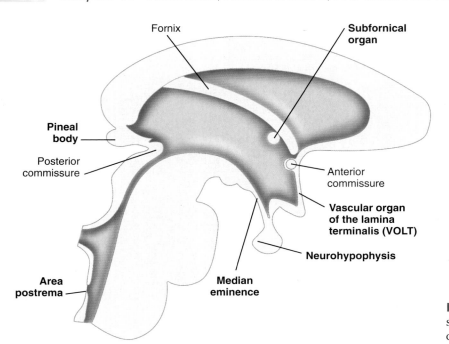

**Figure 11-2** Diagram of a midsagittal section of the brain showing the circumventricular organs (in bold type).

culating in the blood to directly influence neural function. For example, the CVO in the median eminence region of the hypothalamus serves to convey proteins released by hypothalamic neurons to the anterior lobe of the pituitary via the *hypothalamic-pituitary portal system*. The neurons of the subfornical organ (a CVO located adjacent to the fornix at the point where it divides into pre- and postcommissural fibers) have receptors for circulating angiotensin II. Via projections of these neurons to the hypothalamus, they mediate the generation of thirst, which serves to generate drinking to correct hypovolemia. Steroid hormones from the gonads and the adrenal cortex are not dependent on CVOs for entry into the CNS because they are lipid-soluble, and therefore diffuse readily across the blood-brain barrier into target neurons in the hypothalamus.

Hypothalamic function can be divided into four partly overlapping domains: autonomic, neuroendocrine, regulatory, and drive and emotions. *Hypothalamic connections to the autonomic and neuroendocrine systems provide the two major tools by which the hypothalamus exerts its influence on the body.* As will become evident, these two output systems interact with each other. The four functional domains will be discussed in greater detail in later cycles. In the remainder of this cycle, we provide an overview.

## A. AUTONOMIC NERVOUS SYSTEM

### Brainstem and Spinal Cord

Portions of the hypothalamus, particularly the paraventricular nucleus, located immediately adjacent to the wall of the third ventricle, project, via monosynaptic and multisynaptic routes, to both major efferent components of the autonomic nervous system: sympathetic (intermediate zone of the thoracolumbar spinal cord) and parasympathetic (cranial nerves [CN] III, VII, IX, and X and the intermediate zone of the sacral spinal cord) (Fig, 11-3). These portions of the hypothalamus also project to the neuronal targets of autonomic afferent projections in the nucleus of the solitary tract and the intermediate zone of the spinal cord. The nucleus of the solitary tract (which receives input from CN IX and X) conveys information regarding visceral, cardiovascular, and respiratory activity. In this way, activity in the paraventricular nucleus exerts a strong influence on both sympathetic and parasympathetic activity, efferent and afferent, throughout the body.

Despite the geographic extent of central nervous system (CNS) autonomic systems, focal disorders of autonomic function are rarely evident with discrete CNS lesions. The one major exception is Horner's syndrome

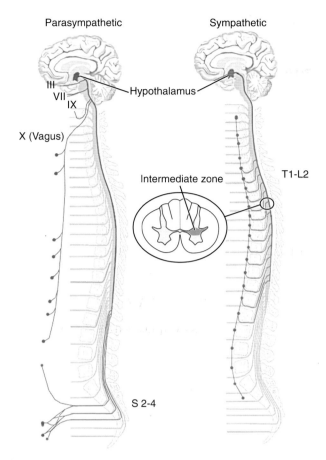

Parasympathetic

Sympathetic

III
VII
IX

Hypothalamus

X (Vagus)

Intermediate zone

T1-L2

S 2-4

**Figure 11-3** Central nervous system portions of the sympathetic and parasympathetic components of the autonomic nervous system. Roman numerals indicate cranial nerves.

(ptosis and miosis). This syndrome occurs commonly with lateral medullary (Wallenberg) infarctions, which interrupt the sympathetic fibers descending from the hypothalamus in the dorsolateral quadrant of the medulla.

## Cerebrum

The hypothalamus has efferent and afferent connections with several brain regions, predominantly within the limbic system. These regions, which include the amygdala, the lateral septal nuclei, and the insular cortices, influence hypothalamic input to the autonomic nervous system. The hypothalamus is able to thereby

establish the autonomic prerequisites for demanding activity, such as preparation for fight or flight, and sexual activity. Lesions of the limbic system, particularly the insula, may be associated with prominent autonomic dysfunction.

## B. NEUROENDOCRINE SYSTEM

The hypothalamus is linked via the infundibulum to the pituitary gland. Axons of hypothalamic neurons traverse the infundibulum to the posterior portion of the pituitary gland (the *neurohypophysis*), where they terminate upon blood vessels. At these termination sites, the hormones *oxytocin* and *vasopressin* are released directly into the systemic circulation. The axons of other hypothalamic neurons terminate upon branches of a portal venous system that originates at the median eminence in the proximal infundibulum. A number of hormones are released into this portal blood and travel downstream to receptors located in venous sinusoids within the anterior portion of the pituitary gland (the *adenohypophysis*). These hypothalamic hormones regulate the release by the adenohypophysis of *adrenocorticotropic hormone (ACTH), thyroid-stimulating hormone (TSH), growth hormone (GH), gonadotrophins (luteinizing hormone [LH] and follicle-stimulating hormone [FSH])*, and *prolactin* into the systemic circulation.

CVOs, most notably in the median eminence, the vascular organ of the lamina terminalis, and the intermediate and posterior lobes of the pituitary gland, provide the route for protein hormonal feedback on hypothalamic neuroendocrine function. Steroid hormonal feedback is mediated by diffusion of these hormones across the blood-brain barrier.

## C. REGULATORY FUNCTIONS

Major hypothalamic regulatory functions include the maintenance of body mass, body temperature, blood volume, plasma osmolality, and circadian rhythms. Input from CVOs is important to regulation of body mass, body temperature, blood volume, and plasma osmolality, and efferent neuroendocrine activity provides the basis for control of these functions. Retinal input to the suprachiasmatic nuclei of the hypothalamus contributes to the regulation of circadian rhythms.

**Autonomic, Neuroendocrine, and Regulatory Functions**

## D. DRIVES AND EMOTIONS

The limbic system, in conjunction with the hypothalamus and its links to the autonomic nervous system, provides the basis for emotions (see Chapter 12). Emotions correspond to the values we attach to perceptions, memories, and plans. They provide the basis for motivation. Many emotions are complex and subtle and reflect as yet poorly understood patterns of activity in the limbic system and hypothalamus. Others are sufficiently elemental that they are commonly referred to as drives and include hunger, thirst, and sexual drive. Drives are substantially the province of the hypothalamus itself. Connections between the hypothalamus, limbic structures, and the cerebral cortex, particularly the frontal lobes, and input from CVOs, translate hunger, thirst, and sexual drive into complex behavior.

## PRACTICE 11-1

What is the single focal neurologic deficit that can be observed with damage to hypothalamic projections to the autonomic nervous system in the brainstem? In what stroke syndrome is this most commonly observed? What is the other location at which this focal autonomic function is commonly disrupted?

- Horner's Syndrome
- Lateral medullary infarcts
    (AKA wallenbuy)
- Interrupt sympathetic fibers

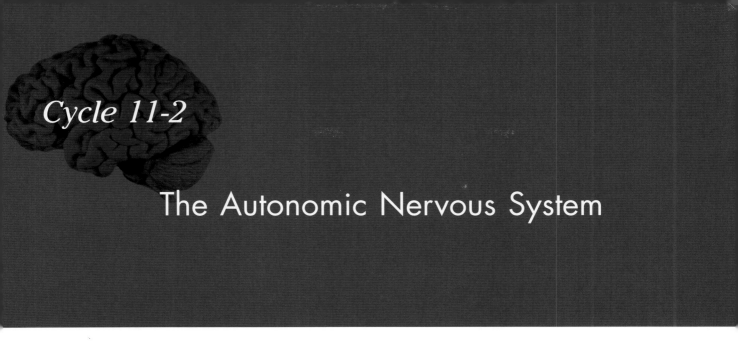

# Cycle 11-2

# The Autonomic Nervous System

## Objectives

1. Be able to describe the location of preganglionic sympathetic and parasympathetic neurons within the central nervous system.

2. Be able to list the neurotransmitters of pre- and postganglionic sympathetic and parasympathetic neurons.

3. Be able to give a general description of the various anatomic relationships of sympathetic and parasympathetic ganglia to the nervous system and to target organs.

4. Be able to list the two major CNS targets of autonomic afferent projections.

5. Be able to briefly summarize the general functions of the sympathetic and parasympathetic nervous systems.

6. Be able to describe the consequences of loss of preganglionic sympathetic nervous system neurons and the most common clinical setting in which this occurs.

7. Be able to describe the manifestations of inadequate and excessive parasympathetic activity and list potential causes.

The autonomic nervous system is divided into sympathetic and parasympathetic component (Table 11-1). In both components, a preganglionic neuron within the brainstem or spinal cord projects to a peripheral ganglion, where it synapses on a postganglionic neuron. The postganglionic neuron then projects directly to target tissues. Most axons of preganglionic neurons are lightly myelinated, whereas those of postganglionic neurons are unmyelinated and therefore conduct impulses quite slowly (e.g., 1 to 2 m/sec). In both components, the preganglionic neuron is cholinergic, and the postsynaptic receptor on the postganglionic neuron is nicotinic. Postganglionic neurons in the sympathetic nervous system (SNS) are predominantly noradrenergic with the single major exception of those innervating sweat glands, which are cholinergic. The postganglionic neurons of the parasympathetic nervous system (ParaSNS) are uniformly cholinergic and their postsynaptic receptors are muscarinic. The entire autonomic nervous system, both central and peripheral, is somatotopically and viscerotopically organized.

Preganglionic neurons of both the SNS and the ParaSNS receive projections, via monosynaptic and multisynaptic routes, from the hypothalamus. They also receive projections from other sources, to be detailed later. Links between the hypothalamus and the autonomic nervous system provide the hypothalamus one of its major tools in executing its roles in homeostasis, regulatory function, and drive. These same links assure that hypothalamic actions mediated through the autonomic nervous system are coordinated with hypothalamic neuroendocrine activity and hypothalamic interaction with cerebral structures.

**TABLE 11-1** Summary of Sympathetic and Parasympathetic Nervous Systems

| Characteristic | Sympathetic | Parasympathetic |
|---|---|---|
| Location of preganglionic neuron | T1-L2 | Edinger-Westphal, salivatory, dorsal motor nucleus of CN X, nucleus ambiguus, S2-S4 intermediate zone |
| Location of ganglia | Paravertebral: trunk, limbs: vascular tone, sweat glands, piloerector muscles<br>Superior cervical ganglion: head and neck<br>Middle and inferior cervical ganglia: heart, lungs<br>Prevertebral ganglia (celiac, superior and inferior mesenteric, pelvic-hypogastric): abdominal and pelvic viscera, genitalia<br>Adrenal medulla: endocrine | End-organ<br>Pelvis |
| Neurotransmitter: preganglionic neuron | Acetylcholine (nicotinic receptor) | Acetylcholine (nicotinic receptor) |
| Neurotransmitter: postganglionic neuron | NE (except sweat glands: acetylcholine) | Acetylcholine (muscarinic receptor) |
| Function | Fight/flight<br>Peripheral/splanchnic vasoconstriction<br>Tachycardia, increased cardiac contractility<br>Sweating<br>Mobilization of glycogen stores | Increase gastrointestinal peristalsis, blood flow<br>Bradycardia<br>Bladder emptying |

Our focus will be primarily on efferent components of the autonomic nervous system. However, it is important to note that efferent components are substantially paralleled by afferent components. Two-way connectivity is a general feature of the nervous system, one that is an essential prerequisite for important properties of neural network function (see Chapter 12). Afferent projections also provide the basis for feedback systems and reflex arcs. Finally, afferent autonomic activity may be a major contributor to emotional function (see Chapter 12). For the most part, autonomic afferent input is provided by dorsal root ganglion neurons that also subserve somesthesis. This role is particularly true for neurons supplying the vital organs, hence the commonly used term, visceral afferent fibers. Neurons subserving autonomic afferent function for the body project to several lamina of the spinal cord, particularly in the intermediate zone, providing a basis for autonomic reflex arcs. Neurons providing afferent input pertinent to autonomic cranial nerve functions (all parasympathetic) are located in cranial nerve sensory ganglia and most project to the *nucleus of the solitary tract*.

The functions of the two components of the autonomic nervous system are far too complex to be easily subsumed under any simple dichotomy. However, the SNS can be roughly characterized as providing the basis for vigorous action, such as fight or flight. Thus, it mediates tachycardia, increased cardiac contractility, vasoconstriction of visceral vasculature, vasodilation within muscular vascular beds, sweating (to dissipate heat), and mobilization of glycogen stores. The ParaSNS, on the other hand, mediates bradycardia, increased peristaltic activity in the gut (and indirectly, increase in blood flow to the gut), and salivation in the process of digestion. Both systems contribute to autonomic components of sexual function. The ParaSNS supplies only the viscera, external genitalia, glands in the head, and the eye.

## SYMPATHETIC NERVOUS SYSTEM

Presynaptic neurons of the SNS are located in the intermediate zone of the spinal cord from the T1 to L2 levels

(Fig. 11-3).[1] Some of these neurons project to paravertebral ganglia located adjacent to the vertebral column at each of these levels. Postganglionic neurons in these ganglia then join peripheral nerves to terminate on blood vessels (skin and muscle), sweat glands, and piloerectile muscles of the trunk and limbs.

Axons of other preganglionic neurons from the T1 through T5 levels pass through their respective paravertebral ganglia without synapse and travel rostrally to terminate in the inferior, middle, and superior cervical ganglia (Fig. 11-4). The most rostral of these, the superior cervical ganglion, located high in the anterior cervical compartment and supplied from the T1 and T2 levels, innervates the tissues of the head and neck (recall that a lesion of this pathway causes Horner's syndrome). Postganglionic neurons located in the middle and inferior cervical ganglia innervate the heart, lungs, and bronchi. The inferior cervical and first thoracic ganglia are often united, in which case they are referred to as the stellate ganglion.

Axons of some preganglionic neurons located at lower levels of the thoracolumbar intermediate zone also pass through their respective paravertebral ganglia, without synapse, to terminate in one of five more distal ganglia: three prevertebral ganglia named for their respective locations near major branches of the aorta (celiac, superior mesenteric, inferior mesenteric), the pelvic-hypogastric prevertebral ganglion, and the adrenal medulla. Neurons in the celiac, superior mesenteric, and inferior mesenteric ganglia innervate, via splanchnic nerves, various portions of the gut and other abdominal viscera. Neurons of the inferior mesenteric ganglion innervate distal portions of the large bowel as well as pelvic organs. Neurons of the pelvic-hypogastric ganglion innervate the urinary and genital tissues. Neurons of the adrenal medulla release norepinephrine and epinephrine directly into the blood stream.

Autonomic dysfunction is a concomitant feature of most serious diseases. In addition, some syndromes can be attributed entirely to autonomic dysfunction. Case 11-1 is an example of pure SNS dysfunction.

---

[1]Although preganglionic sympathetic neurons are scattered throughout the intermediate zone of the spinal cord, they are particularly concentrated in a lateral excrescence of the spinal gray matter located at the junction of the dorsal and ventral horns, known as the intermediolateral column. Although the term intermediolateral column is widely used to refer to the location of the sympathetic preganglionic neurons, we will use the more anatomically accurate designation, intermediate zone.

## Case 11-1

**Degeneration of Sympathetic Preganglionic Neurons in the Intermediate Zone with Orthostatic Hypotension**

*A 70-year-old man with a 10-year history of Parkinson's disease complains of a 1-year history of progressively worsening problems with dizziness. He characterizes it as a feeling of lightheadedness or impending loss of consciousness, and he has actually lost consciousness and fallen on a couple of occasions. Symptoms occur exclusively when he is standing. They are particularly bad when he first awakes in the morning and in the early afternoon, and they are worse in the heat. On examination, blood pressure while supine is 120/70 mm Hg. Three minutes after standing, blood pressure is 60/0 mm Hg, and he complains of severe dizziness.*

**Comment:** *Although the features of Parkinson's disease primarily reflect dopamine deficiency in the putamen as a result of loss of dopaminergic neurons in the substantia nigra, this disease also may be associated with degeneration of neurons in a number of other loci within the CNS. This patient has experienced extensive loss of preganglionic sympathetic neurons in the intermediate zone. Thus, when he is erect, he cannot produce sufficient constriction of peripheral vessels to maintain his blood pressure as the force of gravity pulls blood into the capacitance vessels of the lower extremities. He becomes dizzy when there is insufficient perfusion of the brain to maintain normal function. Symptoms are worse when he first gets up in the morning because his blood volume is relatively depleted as a result of nocturnal diuresis (urine production). Symptoms are worse in early afternoon because he consumes his major meal of the day at noon and thereafter shunts a considerable amount of blood to the splanchnic circulation. Symptoms are worse in the heat because he then shunts blood to his skin in order to control body temperature, and he loses fluid because of sweating.*

## PARASYMPATHETIC NERVOUS SYSTEM

Preganglionic neurons of the ParaSNS are located in two separate regions: within specific autonomic nuclei

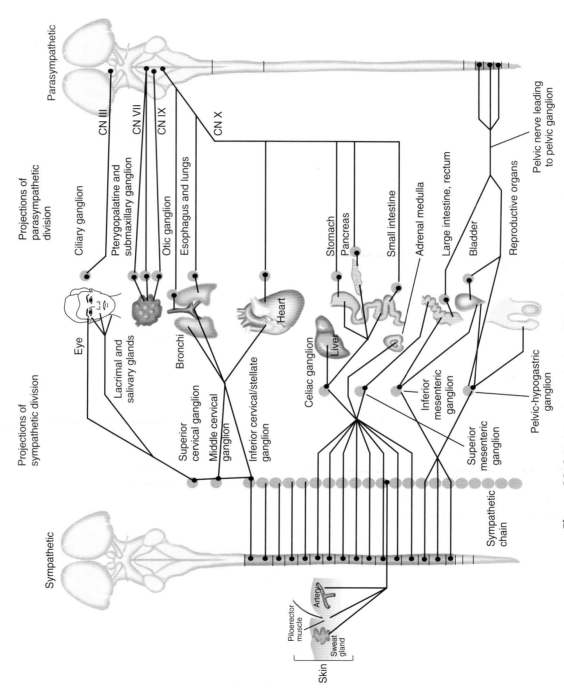

**Figure 11-4** Peripheral organization of the autonomic nervous system.

504

within the brainstem, and in the intermediate zone at the S2 to S4 levels (Fig. 11-3). The autonomic nuclei within the brainstem include the Edinger-Westphal nucleus in the midbrain, which projects via CN III to the ciliary ganglion of the eye, mediating accommodation and pupillary constriction; the salivatory nucleus in the pons and medulla, which projects via CN VII to the lacrimal glands and submaxillary and sublingual salivary glands, and via CN IX to the parotid gland; and the dorsal motor nucleus of CN X and ventrolateral nucleus ambiguus, which project via the vagus nerve to the thoracic and abdominal viscera. Preganglionic neurons from S2 to S4 project via pelvic splanchnic nerves to postganglionic neurons innervating the kidneys, bladder, transverse and distal colon, the reproductive organs, and genitalia.

Unlike the SNS, preganglionic neurons of the ParaSNS generally do not terminate in discrete para- or prevertebral ganglia. Rather, most terminate on neural plexuses located in the target organs themselves. However, preganglionic parasympathetic neurons destined for the external genitalia synapse on postganglionic parasympathetic neurons located in the pelvic-hypogastric ganglion, which also contains the sympathetic postganglionic neurons innervating the genitalia. *Common ganglion*

Within the gastrointestinal tract, there exists a complex array of neural plexuses located in the muscularis (the myenteric plexus), and within the submucosa (the submucosal plexus). The number of neurons in this system may exceed the number in the spinal cord. Because of the extent of this system, and evidence that it exhibits considerable autonomy of function, it is often referred to as the third component of the autonomic nervous system—the enteric nervous system. However, because there are extensive vagal terminations on this system, it probably makes more sense to regard it as a very complex postsynaptic ganglion of the vagus nerve.

Many drugs have prominent anticholinergic (antimuscarinic) or cholinomimetic properties and, as a result, produce side effects that reflect associated dysfunction of the ParaSNS. Cases 11-2 and 11-3 illustrate these effects.

## Case 11-2

### Anticholinergic Effects

*A 25-year-old man with a 3-year history of paranoid schizophrenia is hospitalized for a flareup of psychotic symptoms. He is treated with haloperidol, a dopamine D-2 receptor blocker, and benztropine, an anticholinergic agent that somewhat ameliorates the Parkinsonian side effects of haloperidol. He complains of constipation, dry mouth, difficulty initiating a urinary stream, and inability to read.*

**Comment:** *His complaints reflect side effects of benztropine: reduced peristaltic activity in the intestine, reduced salivation, reduced contractility of the detrusor muscle of the urinary bladder, and inability to accommodate, respectively.*

## Case 11-3

### Cholinomimetic Effects

*An 80-year-old man complains of a 3-month history of waxing and waning diplopia (double vision) and dysphagia (difficulty swallowing), and a 1-month history of generalized weakness. On examination, he has moderate bilateral ptosis, dysconjugate gaze, and at least some impairment in moving his eyes in any direction. He also has moderate weakness of limb girdle muscles that gets worse with repeated effort. When given edrophonium (Tensilon), a short-acting acetylcholinesterase inhibitor, for a few minutes his ptosis disappears, his eye movements improve, and his strength seems to improve. He is then put on pyridostigmine, a long-acting acetylcholinesterase inhibitor, four times a day. At a follow-up visit, he is pleased with the improvement in his original symptoms, but he complains of abdominal cramping and diarrhea.*

**Comment:** *This patient has myasthenia gravis, an autoimmune disorder that results in destruction of the postsynaptic acetylcholine receptor at the*

*Continued*

## Case 11-3—cont'd

*neuromuscular junction. By inhibiting the breakdown of acetylcholine in the neuromuscular junction with pyridostigmine, we increase the probability that sufficient miniature end plate potentials will be generated at each neuromuscular junction to depolarize the muscle fiber to the point of eliciting an action potential. Unfortunately, we also increase the amount of acetylcholine at muscarinic receptors in the gut, leading to the gastrointestinal side effects. Precisely these same symptoms occur when we give acetylcholinesterase inhibitors that cross the blood-brain barrier, such as donepezil, to patients with Alzheimer's disease, in order to improve their memory function.*

## PRACTICE 11-2

A 60-year-old man with an extensive history of heavy smoking develops a small cell carcinoma of the lung. This tumor (which is of neuroepithelial origin), expresses N-type voltage-gated calcium channel proteins. This engenders an antibody response to these proteins, which then becomes directed at similar proteins on all neural endings on CNS neurons projecting to the periphery. As a result, these N-type calcium channels are destroyed, preventing uptake of the calcium needed for neurotransmitter release. Predict this patient's symptoms.

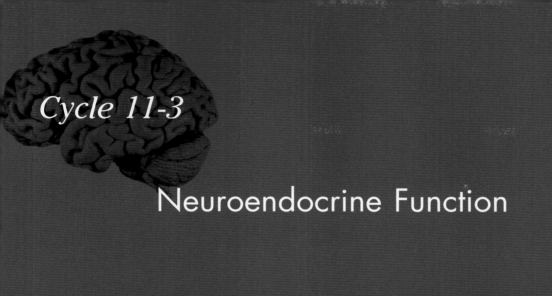

# Cycle 11-3

# Neuroendocrine Function

**Objectives**

1. Be able to define the primary purpose of the hypothalamic-pituitary-adrenocortical system; list its major components; and describe briefly the basis for its regulatory control.

2. Be able to describe briefly and explain the major manifestations of pituitary apoplexy.

3. Be able to define the two major roles of the thyroid gland; very briefly describe the basis for its regulatory control; and explain how thyroid function might be influenced by time of day, cold exposure, and sepsis.

4. Be able to list the major effects of growth hormone; very briefly describe the basis for regulatory control of this hormone; and briefly characterize the syndrome in adults that results from growth hormone excess.

5. Be able to describe briefly the hypothalamic regulation of gonadotrophin secretion, and the effect of LH, FSH, estrogen, and testosterone on target organs in men and woman; list the alterations in

sexual function through the life span that are related to GnRH activity; and briefly describe the mechanism by which low body mass and physical stress impact reproductive function in women.

6. Be able to describe briefly the regulatory control of prolactin, the clinical consequences of pituitary prolactinomas in women of reproductive age, and the means and mechanism of medical treatment of these tumors.

7. Be able to summarize the mechanisms by which AVP (arginine vasopressin) regulates plasma osmolality. Be able to describe the clinical consequences of impairment of hypothalamic production of AVP.

8. Be able to summarize the mechanisms underlying regulation of blood volume and explain what is meant by inappropriate and partially inappropriate secretion of AVP.

9. Be able to list the roles of oxytocin in reproductive function.

Autonomic, Neuroendocrine, and Regulatory Functions

Neuroendocrine functions of the hypothalamus are mediated through the pituitary gland, which can be divided into anterior and posterior portions. The regulation of the anterior pituitary, or adenohypophysis, is via a portal system (Fig. 11-5). This begins as arteriolar branches of the superior hypophyseal artery (a branch of the internal carotid artery) in the median eminence region of the hypothalamus (a CVO). The capillaries

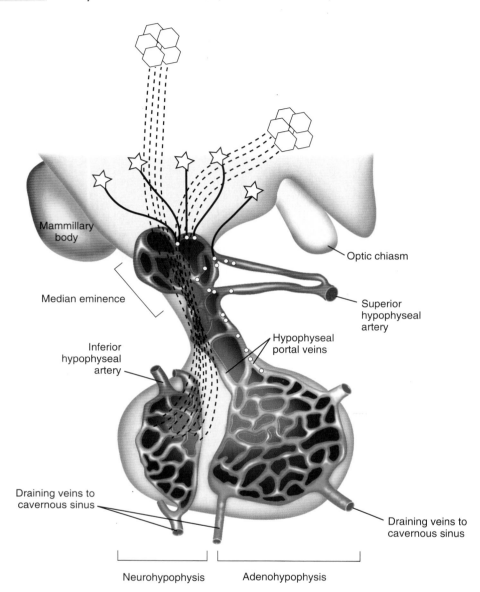

Mammillary body

Median eminence

Inferior hypophyseal artery

Draining veins to cavernous sinus

Optic chiasm

Superior hypophyseal artery

Hypophyseal portal veins

Draining veins to cavernous sinus

Neurohypophysis          Adenohypophysis

**Figure 11-5** The hypothalamus, adenohypophysis, neurohypophysis, and the hypothalamic-pituitary portal system.

and veins derived from these arterioles ultimately drain into remote venous sinusoids located in the adenohypophysis. Releasing and inhibiting hormones produced from nerve terminals in the median eminence region traverse the portal system, bind to specific receptors in the venous sinusoids, and thereby regulate the secretion of secondary stimulating hormones by cells in the adenohypophysis. Stimulating hormones are released into veins draining into the cavernous sinus. The hypothalamic releasing and inhibitory hormones and their corresponding pituitary stimulating hormones are summarized in Table 11-2 and are discussed individually in

the following sections. The secretion of hypothalamic releasing and pituitary stimulating hormones is controlled by neural input to the hypothalamus and hormonal feedback to the brain, the hypothalamus, and the adenohypophysis.

The posterior portion of the pituitary, or neurohypophysis, receives the axon terminals of neurons located in the supraoptic and paraventricular nuclei of the hypothalamus. These terminals release the hormones oxytocin and vasopressin (AVP) directly into the systemic circulation, without an intervening portal system.

**TABLE 11-2** Hypothalamic Releasing Factors, Pituitary Hormones, Their Target Organs, and Their Functions

| Hypothalamic Releasing Factor | Pituitary Stimulating Hormone | Target Organ | Hormone Produced by Target Organ | Regulation of Hormone Production | Effects of Pituitary Hormones |
|---|---|---|---|---|---|
| Corticotropin releasing hormone (CRH) | Adrenocorticotropic hormone (ACTH) | Adrenal cortex | Glucocorticoids | Neural input to hypothalamus<br>Negative feedback by glucocorticoids on CRH and ACTH release | Mediation of responses to stress |
| Thyrotropin releasing hormone (TRH) | Thyroid-stimulating hormone (TSH) | Thyroid gland | Thyroxin ($T_4$), Triiodothyronine ($T_3$) | Neural input to hypothalamus from brain, suprachiasmatic n., and thermoregulatory neurons of hypothalamus<br>Negative feedback by $T_4$ and $T_3$ on TRH and TSH secretion<br>Influence of tumor necrosis factor-$\alpha$ and IL-1 on TRH release | Regulation of protein synthesis and metabolic activity<br>Growth of neural processes, synapse formation, myelination, axonal transport in early life |
| Growth hormone releasing hormone (GHRH) (stimulatory)<br>Somatostatin (SS) (inhibitory) | Growth hormone (GH) | Various | Insulin-like growth factor 1 (IGF-1) | Neural input to hypothalamus<br>Negative feedback on GHRH and GH production by GH and IGF-1 | Enhances protein synthesis, increases lipolysis, promotes glucose uptake, stimulates organ growth, metabolism, skeletal growth and maturation, and immune function |
| Gonadotropin releasing hormone (GnRH) | Luteinizing hormone (LH), follicle-stimulating hormone (FSH) | Ovary, testis | Estrogen, progesterone testosterone | Negative feedback on GnRH, LH, and FSH secretion by testosterone (males)<br>Negative and positive feedback on GnRH, LH, and FSH release by estrogen (females) | Support of secondary sex organs, sex-specific body features<br>Support of spermatogenesis<br>Participation in hormonal processes orchestrated by ovary underlying the menstrual cycle<br>Regulation of behavioral components of sexual dimorphism<br>Puberty; body mass and stress effects on menstruation<br>Suspension of ovulation during lactation |
| Dopamine (inhibitory) | Prolactin | Breast | | Hormonal milieu of pregnancy<br>Neural input to hypothalamus induced by nursing | Preparation, maintenance, and secretory activity of the mammary gland |

# ADENOHYPOPHYSIS

## Adrenocortical Function

The primary function of the adrenocortical system appears to be the mediation of responses to stress. Cells in the paraventricular nucleus of the hypothalamus release corticotropin releasing hormone (CRH) into the hypothalamic-pituitary portal system. The paraventricular nucleus receives input from many sources: (1) brainstem noradrenergic neurons in the vicinity of the nucleus of the solitary tract (which receive input from CN IX and X concerning autonomic afferent activity) and in the locus ceruleus; (2) serotonergic neurons from the raphe system; (3) the periaqueductal gray (a projection target of nociceptive sensory systems); (4) the midbrain reticular formation (the basis for level of arousal); (5) orbitofrontal cortex, the amygdala and lateral septal nuclei (indirectly mediating input pertinent to emotional state); (6) CVOs transmitting afferent hormonal feedback (adrenocorticotropic hormone [ACTH], angiotensin II); (7) the adrenal cortex (glucocorticoids); (8) other hypothalamic nuclei. The details of this input are less important than the logic of the system: the hypothalamic site of release of CRH receives input pertinent to the state of the autonomic nervous system, the level of arousal, painful sensory input, and hormonal feedback, as well as from trans-system neurotransmitter systems (norepinephrine and serotonin) involved in multisystem coordination within the brain. Among the most important hypothalamic inputs to the paraventricular nucleus is that from the suprachiasmatic nuclei, which are responsible for circadian rhythms within the brain.

Both suprachiasmatic input and the pattern of food intake provide the basis for the circadian pattern of CRH release. CRH release precedes ACTH release. ACTH is maximal in the morning, minimal in the evening and night. Other inputs to the paraventricular nucleus modify CRH release according to the demands upon the organism.

On exposure to CRH, corticotrophes in the anterior pituitary synthesize and release ACTH. Circulating ACTH binds to receptors on cells in the adrenal cortex, thereby leading to the synthesis and release of glucocorticoids. Circulating glucocorticoids provide negative feedback, primarily affecting CRH release, but also ACTH release, by slow (gene transcription) and fast (direct) mechanisms. Numerous other regions of the brain express glucocorticoid receptors, but the effects

---

> ### BOX 11-1 Glucocorticoids and Stem Cells
>
> Glucocorticoids are necessary for the replication of pluripotent stem cells in the vicinity of the temporal horn that are capable of differentiating into neurons or glia. The hippocampus has particularly dense glucocorticoid receptors. The hippocampus is the crucial neural structure for the learning of new fact memories (see Chapter 12), and the high glucocorticoid receptor density could conceivably reflect that facts to which one is exposed in stressful situations are particularly likely to be important, and worth remembering.

of glucocorticoids on these systems are complex and as yet poorly understood.

The administration of glucocorticoids (e.g., prednisone), as in the treatment of autoimmune disease, suppresses CRH production, and if continued for long periods of time (greater than 4 months), will lead to atrophy of ACTH-secreting cells in the anterior pituitary. Sudden cessation of glucocorticoid medication under these circumstances can lead within hours to a state of profound and life-threatening adrenocortical insufficiency known as Addisonian crisis (Case 11-4).

Of all hypothalamic-pituitary neuroendocrine functions, the CRH-ACTH axis is most resistant to damage. However, hemorrhagic infarction of tumors of the pituitary gland (adenomas), can lead to acute collapse of this system, as in Case 11-4.

---

> ### *Case 11-4*
>
> **Panhypopituitarism with Addisonian Crisis due to Hemorrhagic Necrosis of a Pituitary Adenoma (Pituitary Apoplexy)**
>
> *A 78-year-old man presents to the hospital with a 1-day history of severe, persistent headache, malaise, nausea, vomiting, and diplopia. On examination, his complexion is pasty and he appears acutely ill. Blood pressure is 90/60 mm Hg. The skin over his extremities is cool and mottled. He has a stiff neck and he is mildly lethargic. He has a complete right third cranial nerve palsy. The left pupil is 4 mm and normally reactive. The right pupil is 6 mm and unreactive. Analysis of electrolytes the next day reveals a serum sodium of 133 mEq/L (normal range is 138 to 142 mEq/L). Cerebrospinal fluid obtained by lumbar puncture has a protein content of*

## Case 11-4—cont'd

210 mg/dL (normal level being <45 mg/dL), a glucose level of 45 mg/dL (normal, >60 mg/dL), white blood cell count of 75/dL (normal, <6), predominantly neutrophils, and red blood cell count of 50/dL (normal, 0).

**Comment:** This patient has a large pituitary tumor (macroadenoma) (Fig. 11-6). These tumors may grow in any direction, presumably following the path of least resistance. This one shows evidence of expansion upward, placing the optic chiasm at risk, and into the right cavernous sinus, producing the cranial nerve III palsy.

Pituitary adenomas, which are fundamentally benign neoplasms, typically present insidiously with predominantly neuroendocrine manifestations (see Case 11-5). The neuroendocrine function that is most susceptible to disruption by pituitary lesions is reproductive. However, this dysfunction is most likely to be evident in a woman during reproductive years as interruption of menses; even loss of libido may be inapparent in an old man. Tumors of all types depend upon the growth of new blood vessels (neovascularization) to nourish them. These new blood vessels are not always of the best quality, setting the stage for ischemic infarction of portions of tumor, at times with hemorrhage into the infarcted tissue. Under these circumstances, the tumor can undergo rapid expansion, which is what has happened in this case. Compressive effects of the tumor are responsible for the cranial nerve III palsy. The release of hemorrhagic and necrotic material into the subarachnoid space has produced a low-level chemical meningitis, hence the cerebrospinal fluid abnormalities, headache, and stiff neck. The acute hemorrhagic infarction of the tumor has seriously interfered with essentially all functions of the adenohypophysis, most critically the production of ACTH and TSH. This patient exhibits signs and symptoms of adrenal collapse (Addisonian crisis): malaise, lethargy, his pasty appearance and the coldness and mottling of his skin, his hypotension, and the low serum sodium level. Unless he is promptly administered corticosteroids and thyroid supplement, he will die. On the other hand, with immediate medical treatment, and surgical removal of the pituitary tumor, his prognosis for living and regaining normal neurologic function is quite good. He will require chronic administration of corticosteroids, thyroid supplement, and testosterone to compensate for the permanent loss of pituitary function.

Many pituitary adenomas do not produce hormones, as in this case of pituitary apoplexy. Of all the hormones produced by pituitary adenomas, prolactin is the most common (see discussion of Lactation). Rare tumors produce ACTH, leading to the highly characteristic Cushing's syndrome (Case 11-5).

## Case 11-5

### Cushing's Syndrome due to ACTH-Producing Pituitary Adenoma

A 60-year-old woman presents with a 2-year history of insidiously progressive weight gain, generalized weakness, and fatigue. During this time she has also experienced insomnia, increased anxiety, and emotional lability. Treatment of hypertension was initiated 18 months ago. She has experienced two vertebral compression fractures in the past year. On examination she weighs 250 lb. Her obesity is mainly truncal. Her face is round and puffy. She has prominent fat deposition in the supraclavicular fossae and in the midline over her upper back ("buffalo hump"). Neurologic examination is noteworthy only for mild weakness in all proximal muscles.

**Comment:** This patient's disorder, named for Harvey Cushing, the man who almost single-handedly defined the entire field of neurosurgery, is caused by an ACTH-secreting microadenoma of the anterior pituitary. As a result of chronically elevated glucocorticoid levels, she has developed the characteristic pattern of obesity, osteoporosis, hypertension, psychiatric symptoms, and corticosteroid-induced muscle disease (myopathy). To this day, pituitary tumors continue to be surgically resected by some variation of the approach, known as transphenoidal hypophysectomy, originally developed by Cushing in the 1930s. Via an entry point either through an incision high in the gum-line above the front teeth, or through one nostril (using an endoscope), the surgeon passes through the retronasal region to enter first the floor and then the ceiling of the sphenoid sinus (which, in part, forms the floor of the sella turcica). By resecting the tumor through the floor of the sella turcica, the brain is left undisturbed and the operative intervention is so minimal that patients can often leave the hospital in a day.

## Thyroid Function

The primary role of the thyroid gland appears to be the regulation of protein synthesis and metabolic activity throughout the body. Cells in the periventricular nucleus of the hypothalamus release thyrotropin releasing hormone (TRH) into the hypothalamic-pituitary portal system in the region of the median eminence. TRH binds to specific receptors on TSH-secreting cells

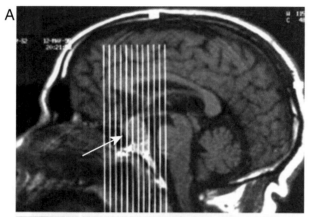

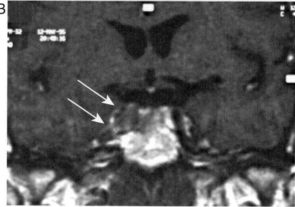

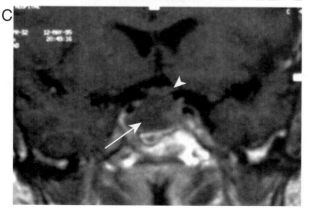

in the anterior pituitary, leading to synthesis and release of TSH. TSH in turn stimulates the synthesis and release of thyroxin ($T_4$) and triiodothyronine ($T_3$) by the thyroid gland. Both TRH and TSH secretion are inhibited by circulating levels of $T_4$ and $T_3$. TRH cells in the periventricular nucleus also receive input from the suprachiasmatic nucleus of the hypothalamus, providing the basis for the circadian pattern of TRH release; from cells in the hypothalamus that are sensitive to core temperature, providing the basis for the responsivity of TRH release to cold exposure; and from ascending brainstem noradrenergic projections (as for paraventricular neurons producing CRH). The thyroid gland is densely innervated by both the SNS and the ParaSNS, providing a route other than the direct hypothalamic connection by which thyroid hormone production is influenced by the autonomic nervous system. TRH release is sensitive to certain circulating cytokines, most notably tumor necrosis factor-α (TNF-α) and interleukin 1 (IL-1), a fact that helps to explain alterations in thyroid activity observed during sepsis.

Clinical disorders of thyroid function almost invariably involve the thyroid gland itself (primary hypo- or hyperthyroidism). Disorders of thyroid function related to hypothalamic or pituitary dysfunction (secondary hypothyroidism) are rare. TRH and TSH production are nearly as resistant to hypothalamic and pituitary lesions as are CRH and ACTH production. However, catastrophic lesions of the pituitary gland, as in pituitary apoplexy (Case 11-4), may have an impact on thyroid function, and secondary hypothyroidism contributes to the clinical picture observed in pituitary apoplexy. Normal thyroid function in early life is critical to normal brain development. Severe hypothyroidism leads to impaired growth of axons and dendrites, reduced synapse formation, decreased myelination,

**Figure 11-6** Magnetic resonance image (MRI) of a pituitary macroadenoma. *A,* The top (sagittal) image shows a large tumor (*arrow*) filling the sella turcica and extending upward into the suprasellar space. The vertical lines indicate the planes of the coronal cuts taken through the region of the tumor. *B,* In the middle MRI, extension of the tumor into the posterior right cavernous sinus can be seen (*arrows*), accounting for the third cranial nerve palsy. *C,* On the lower coronal cut, the tumor (*arrow*) abuts the optic chiasm (*arrowhead*); thus, although visual fields are normal, the patient is at risk for developing a bitemporal hemianopia. Extensive areas of necrosis and hemorrhage were apparent at the time of surgery, but the hemorrhage is not evident on this scan because of the particular stage in the evolution of MR signal generated by blood.

and delayed axonal transport, with clinical consequences of mental retardation and impairment in motor function.

## Growth Hormone

Growth hormone (GH) is the principal anabolic hormone. It enhances protein synthesis, increases lypolysis, produces insulin-like effects in promoting uptake of glucose and amino acids during eating, but also has insulin-antagonistic effects in opposing the lipogenic effects of insulin. GH stimulates organ growth, metabolism, skeletal growth and maturation, and immune function.

The synthesis and release of GH by the anterior pituitary is promoted by cells in the arcuate nucleus of the hypothalamus, which release growth hormone releasing hormone (GHRH) into the portal system in the region of the median eminence. Although GHRH is the principal regulator of GH production, a second hormone produced by the hypothalamus, somatostatin (SS), acts to inhibit GH release by modulating GHRH action in the anterior pituitary. GH exerts a host of effects on peripheral tissues, one of which is to elicit the production of insulin-like growth factor 1 (IGF-1). Both GH and IGF-1 act on the hypothalamus and the adenohypophysis to inhibit release of GHRH and GH. Most of the effects of GH on peripheral tissue can be elicited by IGF-1, but the two hormones act synergistically.

GH secretion is pulsatile, occurring at roughly 2-hour intervals, and 70 percent of secretion occurs at night. GH production is influenced by physical and emotional stress, protein deprivation (during which production is reduced), hypoglycemia (during which production is increased), glucocorticoids, and thyroxin. GHRH secretion is stimulated by noradrenergic, dopaminergic, serotonergic, and enkephalinergic systems.

GH is of critical importance in the neonatal period and it plays a major role in the growth spurt of adolescence. Clinically significant disorders of GH production are rare. In children, GH deficiency leads to impaired growth and short stature and excess GH production induces gigantism. In adults, GH deficiency is often inapparent, and GH excess causes acromegaly, as described in Case 11-6.

## Reproductive Function

Men and women have fundamentally the same hypothalamic-pituitary mechanism underlying reproductive

---

### Case 11-6

**Acromegaly**

*A 50-year-old man presents with a history of many years of insidiously progressive change in his physiognomy, marked mainly by coarsening of features and increasing prominence of his brow. He has developed spaces between his teeth where he had none before. He now wears size 13 shoes when much of his life he wore size 10. His hands have also increased in size. His voice has deepened, his skin has become somewhat oily, he now sweats a great deal, he has gained 30 lb, and he fatigues easily. He has developed arthritic pain affecting many joints. Despite being happily married, he has had little interest in sexual activity for years. He has had operations on both wrists to relieve carpal tunnel syndrome (episodic pain in the forearm and tingling paresthesias in the lateral aspect of the volar hand and fingers, occurring mainly during sleep and while driving, as a result of entrapment of the median nerve at the wrist).*

**Comment:** *This patient exhibits many of the characteristic features of acromegaly. Entrapment neuropathies such as carpal tunnel syndrome occur frequently in this condition because enlarging joints result in narrowing of adjacent passages through which nerves pass. Forty percent of patients with GH-secreting pituitary adenomas have a point mutation in the G protein that mediates the GHRH effect on GH-producing cells in the adenohypophysis. This mutation leads not only to GH hypersecretion, but also to proliferation of GH-producing cells.*

---

function. Gonadotropin releasing hormone (GnRH) cells scattered through much of the hypothalamus release GnRH into the portal system in the region of the median eminence, and thereby elicit the release of the gonadotropins, luteinizing hormone (LH), and follicle-stimulating hormone (FSH), by cells in the anterior pituitary. Unique among the hypothalamic-pituitary neuroendocrine systems, the gonadotropin system is susceptible to both negative and positive feedback by sex hormones produced by gonadal tissues (see later discussion). Under most circumstances (and uniformly in males), the feedback is negative. Reductions in sex hormone levels at the hypothalamus lead to an increase in the rate of GnRH and associated gonadotropin pulses, whereas reductions in sex hormone levels at the pituitary act to increase the amplitude of LH and FSH pulses by increasing the sensitivity of gonadotrophs to GnRH.

Sexual differences in reproductive function derive almost entirely from the structure and function of the gonads. In males, LH stimulates testosterone production in the Leydig cells of the testes. FSH and testosterone, in coordination, stimulate spermatogenesis in the testicular seminiferous tubules. Testosterone also supports the sex organs in the male, including penis, prostate, and seminal vesicles, and it acts on other tissues in the body to variously increase muscle mass, facial and body hair, and produce the changes in the larynx that underlying deepening of voice. In the female, FSH and LH act to stimulate the production of ovarian steroid hormones estrogen and progesterone, FSH acts at the beginning of each ovarian cycle to stimulate follicle development, and a surge in FSH and LH at midcycle acts to stimulate ovulation in the middle of the cycle. Ovarian hormones also act on sexual organs in the female, including the uterus, cervix, fallopian tubes, and external genitalia, and they act on various other tissues to increase breast development and produce a patterned increase in subcutaneous deposition of fat.

Although the hypothalamic contribution to sexual dimorphism is poorly understood, some evidence suggests that such a contribution exists. A region in the preoptic area of the hypothalamus is approximately twice as large in males. Furthermore, the cytoarchitecture of the rostral hypothalamus may be different in homosexual males than in heterosexual males.

The function of the hypothalamic-pituitary-gonadal circuit in men is relatively simple, characterized by stereotyped pulsatile production of GnRH, LH, FSH, and more constant production of testosterone, which suppresses secretion of GnRH, LH, and FSH. The function of this circuit in women is more complex, involving both negative and positive feedback components. To provide a sense of this complexity, the sequence of events in women is summarized in Table 11-3; the ovary, not the hypothalamus, is the timekeeper of this cyclic process.

Neural input to GnRH secreting neurons of the hypothalamus is scant relative to that of other hypothalamic neurons. However, there is evidence of input from noradrenergic, serotonergic, dopaminergic, β-endorphinergic, and a number of other systems. Remarkably, GnRH neurons appear to lack receptors for gonadal steroid hormones, and the feedback effects of these hormones appear to be mediated entirely by

their effects on neural systems that project to GnRH neurons.

Many alterations in reproductive function through the course of life appear to be mediated by changes in GnRH neuronal activity. During childhood, there is virtually no production of LH or FSH, and puberty appears to be precipitated by an increase in activity of GnRH neurons. The necessary and sufficient conditions for this to occur are unclear. Body size and fat mass appear to be major contributory factors. This is a teleologically satisfying explanation, as a minimum in body size is necessary for a female to successfully sustain pregnancy and delivery, and a minimum in body size is necessary for males to compete for mates. By the same token, reduced body mass, as in starvation (whether due to environmental circumstances or anorexia nervosa) suppresses GnRH secretion, leading to secondary amenorrhea in women. The adverse impact of reduced body mass on GnRH neuronal activity is potentiated by vigorous exercise. Women with low body mass who exercise vigorously (e.g., long distance runners, ballerinas), who often develop amenorrhea, may experience rapid re-instatement of menstrual cycles during periods of inactivity, as occurs during injury. GnRH secretion is also suppressed by stress. This effect may be mediated by β-endorphinergic and CRH projections to GnRH neurons.

Two major events in reproductive function, pregnancy and menopause, are mediated not by primary alterations in GnRH neuronal function, but by uterine and gonadal events. During pregnancy, the placenta produces human chorionic gonadotropin (hCG), which binds to LH receptors on the corpus luteum, thereby sustaining luteal activity during early stages of embryonic growth. Later, the placenta produces massive quantities of estrogen and progesterone, as well as GnRH, thereby assuring the uterine conditions necessary to sustain the pregnancy. Menopause is caused by depletion of ovarian follicles. However, the suppression of ovarian cyclic activity during lactation is related to reduced activity of GnRH neurons; the mechanism underlying this phenomenon is unclear, and is probably multifactorial, but appears to reflect in part the effects of secretion of prolactin by the pituitary (see next section).

## Lactation

In all mammals, the primary role of the pituitary hormone prolactin appears to be in the preparation,

**TABLE 11-3** Reproductive Cycle in Women

| Phase | Ovarian Process | Change in Sex Hormones | Change in LH, FSH |
|---|---|---|---|
| Onset of menses | Developing follicles begin to secrete estrogen in response to FSH | | LH and FSH pulses every 60–90 min |
| Onset of follicular phase | | | |
| | | ↑ estrogen and inhibin production by follicles | ↓ LH, FSH |
| | Most developed follicle develops LH, FSH receptors, enabling continued development despite ↓ LH, FSH | | |
| | Less developed follicles undergo atresia | | |
| | Dominant follicle | ↑ production of estrogen and possibly ↓ production of inhibin | Positive feedback on hypothalamus and pituitary: ↑ frequency and magnitude of FSH and LH pulses |
| Ovulation, beginning of luteal phase | Surge in LH, FSH → final maturation of follicle, ovulation | | |
| | Initiation of luteal phase | | |
| | Support of CL maintained by high LH | | LH pulses every 6–12 h |
| | | ↑ estrogen and progesterone production by CL | Negative feedback on hypothalamus: ↓ LH pulse frequency |
| | If no fertilization, implantation: CL involution | ↓ progesterone, estrogen | ↑ FSH, LH preparing for new follicle development |

*Key:* CL, corpus luteum; FSH, follicle-stimulating hormone; LH, luteinizing hormone.

maintenance, and secretory activity of the mammary gland. Maternal serum prolactin levels rise throughout pregnancy, and in the postpartum period each act of nursing induces a further marked transient elevation within minutes. The hormone induces ductal and alveolar outgrowth in the breast, increases mRNA levels for the milk protein casein, and increases the rate of translation of casein mRNA into protein. Suckling, via induced prolactin release, can delay implantation of a fertilized ovum. By complex and not yet well understood mechanisms, it may be associated with prolonged anovulation. At least in part this appears to be due to the suppressive effect of prolactin on GnRH neurons of the hypothalamus and on the gonadotrophs of the adenohypophysis, which reduces the frequency and amplitude of LH and FSH release.

Although a number of substances, including TRH, vasoactive intestinal peptide (produced by the brain), and estradiol promote prolactin release by the anterior pituitary, a primary releasing hormone has not yet been identified. Rather, the principal regulatory hormone dopamine acts to inhibit prolactin secretion. Dopamine is produced by cells in the arcuate nuclei of the hypothalamus and is released into the portal system via axon terminals in the median eminence region.

To the extent that pituitary tumors are hormonally active, they most often produce prolactin. These tumors are associated with a characteristic clinical picture (Case 11-7).

Autonomic, Neuroendocrine, and Regulatory Functions

## Case 11-7

### Secondary Amenorrhea and Galactorrhea due to Pituitary Tumor

*A 35-year-old sexually inactive woman reports to her gynecologist that she has not had a menstrual period in 6 months and that over the past 2 months she has been experiencing watery discharge from her breasts (galactorrhea). Her neurologic examination is normal. An MRI scan of the brain reveals a 1-cm tumor of the pituitary, and serum prolactin levels are markedly elevated. Following treatment with bromocriptine, galactorrhea ceases and her menstrual periods resume.*

**Comment:** *This patient has a pituitary prolactinoma. Serum levels of prolactin may become somewhat elevated with any pituitary tumor to the extent that the tumor interferes with the inhibition of lactomorphs in the adenohypophysis by hypothalamic dopamine. However, in this case the tumor secretes prolactin. The gonadotropin system is the most susceptible of the hypothalamic-pituitary systems to disruption by local pathology, and this may account for the amenorrhea in this case. However, as we have noted, prolactin also has direct suppressive effects on GnRH, LH, and FSH producing cells. Bromocriptine is a dopamine $D_2$ receptor agonist. It suppresses prolactin production by the pituitary tumor, and furthermore, generally induces a dramatic reduction in the size of these tumors, thereby sparing many patients the need for surgery.*

## NEUROHYPOPHYSIS

The neurohypophysis (posterior pituitary) is primarily involved in the regulation of plasma osmolality and blood volume through the actions of arginine vasopressin (AVP).[2] AVP is produced by neurons in the supraoptic and paraventricular nuclei of the hypothalamus. Axons of these neurons traverse the pituitary stalk and terminate in the posterior pituitary in what is effectively a CVO, where AVP is released into the systemic circulation.

The other major neurohypophyseal hormone, oxytocin, potentiates uterine contractions during parturition and contracts the myoepithelial cells of the mammary alveoli, causing them to expel milk from the secretory tissue to the nipple ("milk let-down"). Uterine muscle cells and mammary myoepithelial cells develop significant responsivity to oxytocin only in the context of the specific hormonal environment of late pregnancy.

## Plasma Osmolality

AVP acts on renal receptors to increase the water permeability of the distal convoluted tubules of the kidney through insertion of water channels into the apical membranes of tubular epithelial cells. Because of the high osmolality in this region of the kidney, water is reabsorbed from the urine into the blood, thereby acting to reduce plasma osmolality. In a sense, this response is a temporizing measure, because the real solution to plasma hyperosmolality is to increase free water consumption. Thirst, too, is stimulated by increased plasma osmolality.

AVP secretion is induced by the activity of neurons in a CVO located in the anterior hypothalamus, the vascular organ of the lamina terminalis (VOLT), which project to the supraoptic and paraventricular nuclei of the hypothalamus. High plasma osmolality results in flow of water from the intracellular to the extracellular space throughout the body. In the VOLT, this leads to increased neuronal firing, and thereby, excitation of AVP-producing cells in the hypothalamus. This mechanism provides for a strong, linear AVP secretory response to hyperosmolality (Fig. 11-7).

Hyperosmolality can be corrected by (1) retention of free water (via the action of AVP); (2) the potentiation of natriuresis (excretion of sodium in the urine); (3) the reduction of salt intake; or (4) stimulation of free water intake (thirst). Atrial natriuretic peptide, which is secreted by cells in the left atrium of the heart and in the brain, acts on the kidney to increase natriuresis. However, this is most evident in response to hypervolemia (see later discussion). Other renal mechanisms also tend to correct hyperosmolality, for example, via reduction in aldosterone (see next discussion). Secretion of atrial natriuretic peptide in the brain acts, by uncertain mechanisms, to inhibit salt appetite. The neural circuitry controlling thirst is largely unknown. Hypothalamic control of osmolality is summarized in Table 11-4.

Reduced or absent secretion of AVP can occur with destructive lesions of the anterior hypothalamus that interfere with the input from the VOLT to the supraoptic and paraventricular nuclei. The result is a dramatic

---

[2]Often referred to simply as vasopressin; also called antidiuretic hormone (ADH).

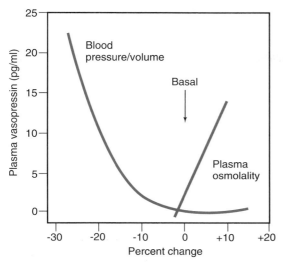

**Figure 11-7** Plasma concentrations of AVP (vasopressin) as a function of plasma osmolality (green) and intravascular volume (blue). (Modified from Robertson GL. Posterior pituitary. In Felig P, Baxter J, Frohman LA (eds). Endocrinology and Metabolism. New York, McGraw-Hill, 1986, pp 338–385. Reproduced with permission of The McGraw-Hill Companies, Inc.)

condition called diabetes insipidus, in which very large volumes (up to a liter/hour) of very dilute urine are produced. Diabetes insipidus can occur in association with a rare systemic inflammatory disease, sarcoidosis, that sometimes affects the central nervous system, particularly at the base of the brain, or as a result of cancer that has metastasized to the hypothalamus. However, more commonly, it is a transient result of surgery in the region of the hypothalamus. Diabetes insipidus can be treated with a synthetic, long-lasting form of AVP, desmopressin acetate (DDAVP).

**TABLE 11-4 Summary of Hypothalamic Control of Osmolality**

| Hyperosmolality | Hypo-osmolality |
|---|---|
| ↑ VOLT →↑ AVP | ↓ VOLT →↓ AVP |
| ↑ AVP →↑ renal retention of free water | ↓ AVP → diuresis |
| ↑ Atrial natriuretic peptide in brain →↓ salt appetite | ↓ Atrial natriuretic peptide in brain →↑ salt appetite |
| ↑ Thirst (unknown mechanism) | ↓ Thirst |

*Key:* AVP, arginine vasopressin; VOLT, vascular organ of the lamina terminalis.

## Blood Volume

Hypovolemia, whether due to dehydration combined with sodium loss, or to loss of blood, also elicits several compensatory mechanisms, nearly all of which involve the hypothalamus (summarized in Table 11-5):

1. Loss of blood volume is first detected by stretch receptors in the superior and inferior vena cava. Decreases in blood volume sufficient to drop arterial pressure also reduce stretch of baroreceptors in the aortic arch and carotid sinus. Autonomic afferent fibers traveling in CN IX and X convey this information to the nucleus of the solitary tract, from which it is relayed by several pathways to the hypothalamus. This directly elicits secretion of AVP, which reduces diuresis, thereby helping to conserve volume. It also elicits thirst.

**TABLE 11-5 Homeostatic Responses to Hypovolemia**

| Inciting Event | Mechanism | Consequence |
|---|---|---|
| ↓ venal caval receptor stretch | CN IX, X → NST → hypothalamus | ↑ AVP, thirst |
| ↑ AVP | kidneys | ↓ diuresis |
| ↑ renin | ↑ angiotensin II | vasocontriction |
| ↑ angiotensin II | subfornical organ | ↑ AVP, ↑ thirst |
| ↑ angiotensin II | adrenal cortex | ↑ aldosterone → renal salt retention |
| ↑ NST activity, stress | ↑ CRH →↑ ACTH | potentiation of aldosterone release |
| ↓ ANP secretion by heart | | ↓ natriuresis |
| ↓ ANP secretion in brain | | ↑ salt appetite |

*Key:* ACTH, adrenocorticotropic hormone; ANP, atrial natriuretic peptide; AVP, arginine vasopressin; CRH, corticotropin releasing hormone; NST, nucleus of the solitary tract.

Autonomic, Neuroendocrine, and Regulatory Functions

2. In response to hypovolemia, the kidneys secrete the enzyme renin, an action that is in part mediated by stimulation of β-adrenergic receptors in the kidney. Renin initiates an enzymatic cascade that results in the formation of angiotensin II, a potent vasoconstrictor. Angiotensin II acts on a CVO, the subfornical organ (SFO), which projects to the hypothalamus and stimulates AVP release and elicits thirst.

3. Angiotensin II stimulates the adrenal cortex to release aldosterone, which induces salt retention by the kidneys. The secretion of aldosterone is potentiated by the action of ACTH. ACTH release is elicited by increased production of CRH, which is induced both by the stress that frequently accompanies hypovolemia and by input to the hypothalamus from the nucleus of the solitary tract in response to decreased stretch of baroreceptors.

4. Hypovolemia reduces secretion of atrial natriuretic peptide by cells in the left atrium of the heart, thereby reducing natriuresis. There is recent evidence of secretion of atrial natriuretic peptide by the brain as well. When injected into the CSF, it inhibits salt appetite.

Hyponatremia occurs fairly commonly in acutely ill patients. It is often attributed to the "syndrome of inappropriate secretion of antidiuretic hormone (SIADH)." True SIADH may occur in the context of aneurysmal subarachnoid hemorrhage, by uncertain mechanisms. However, much more commonly, ADH (AVP) secretion only appears to be inappropriate. Understanding that AVP production is at least partially appropriate under such circumstances can be crucial to proper clinical management, as illustrated in Case 11-8.

## Case 11-8

**Partially Inappropriate Secretion of ADH (AVP)**

*A 70-year-old man with a long history of hypertension is in the hospital recovering from a minor ischemic stroke. A routine check of serum electrolytes demonstrates a sodium level of 128 mEq/L (normal, 136 to 142 mEq/L), a blood urea nitrogen (BUN) of 40 mg/dL (normal, 8 to 15 mg/dL), and a creatinine (Cr) level of 1.5 mg/dL (normal, 0.8 to 1.2 mg/dL).*

## Case 11-8—cont'd

*Urine sodium is high. The resident says this is evidence of inappropriate secretion of ADH, possibly related in some way to the patient's stroke, and that intake of water should be severely restricted. Is this correct?*

**Comment:** *No. The elevated BUN/Cr ratio indicates that the patient is dehydrated; that is, he has a reduced intravascular volume. This volume depletion is sufficiently severe that it outweighs the inhibitory effect of hyponatremia on AVP secretion. In short, the patient is preserving volume over osmolality, and his secretion of AVP is appropriate to his volume status (though inappropriate to his hyponatremia). The hyponatremia is a strong inducement to sodium conservation mechanisms and the hypovolemia leads to reduced secretion of atrial natriuretic peptide. Under these circumstances, urine sodium should be close to zero. The fact that it is elevated indicates that this patient has impaired renal resorption of sodium—renal "salt wasting"—a common phenomenon in the elderly. It is often aggravated by the prescription of diuretics (which potentiate renal sodium loss), either as a measure to control hypertension, or to deal with edema in the legs. Ischemic stroke per se is rarely, if ever, a cause of inappropriate AVP secretion.*

## PRACTICE 11-3

**A.** A patient with orthostatic hypotension experiences particularly severe orthostatic dizziness when he gets up in the morning. He is also getting up three or four times a night to urinate. What measures might be taken to alleviate both these problems, giving him a full night's sleep and reducing his morning dizziness?

**B.** A 50-year-old woman has Hashimoto's thyroiditis, an autoimmune inflammatory disease that results in progressive destruction of the thyroid gland. Would you expect her TSH level to be reduced or elevated?

**C.** What level of LH would you expect in a post-menopausal woman?

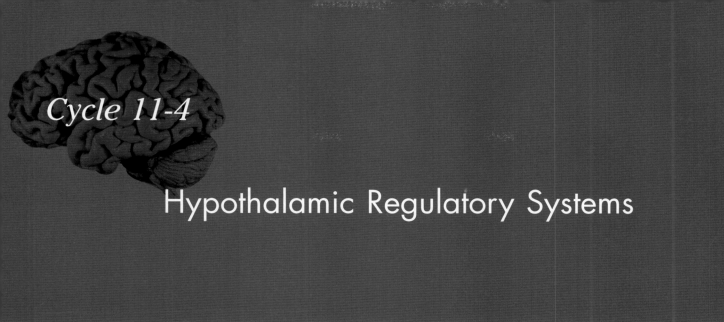

# Hypothalamic Regulatory Systems

## Objectives

1. Be able to describe briefly the regulatory control of circadian rhythms.
2. Be able to describe briefly the hypothalamic basis of thermoregulation and a mechanism for fever.
3. Be able to describe briefly the mechanisms underlying satiety and weight control.

In the preceding two cycles, we have seen how the hypothalamus participates, through its autonomic and neuroendocrine functions, in a host of systemic physiologic processes. The role of the hypothalamus and neurohypophysis in maintaining blood osmolality and volume can be viewed as regulatory functions. In this section, we review three other regulatory functions—those involving circadian rhythms, temperature, and weight—that cannot easily be subsumed within discrete autonomic or neuroendocrine functions but in which the hypothalamus plays a major role.

## REGULATION OF CIRCADIAN RHYTHMS

Experiments in which humans have volunteered to live in quarters deep underground, completely isolated from any input from the outer world and deprived of clocks, have shown that they exhibit a natural rhythm with a cycle duration of between 24 and 25 hours—an endogenous circadian rhythm. Organisms as primitive as *Drosophila* and the bread mold *Neurospora* also exhibit circadian rhythmicity, indicating that this is one of the most fundamental physiologic attributes of living species. In mammals, several areas in the brain appear to exhibit endogenous circadian activity, but by far the most important is the suprachiasmatic nuclei (SCN) of the hypothalamus.

Each neuron of the SCN exhibits an intrinsic pattern of activity, minimal at night, maximal during the daytime, that cycles once a day (once per 24–25-hour period). This endogenous cycle is modified by a variety of stimuli (zeitgebers), which serve to reset both the phase and the period of the SCN pacemaker. By far the most important zeitgeber is exposure to light. Neuronal responses to light exposure are conveyed to the SCN from retinal cone cells (and their target retinal ganglion cells) via a retinal-hypothalamic pathway that diverges from the optic nerves proximal to the optic chiasm and terminates on cells in the SCN. The cyclicity of the SCN is, to a lesser extent, influenced by diurnal locomotor activity, and by patterns of sleep (conveyed by serotonergic input from the raphe system to the SCN).

The SCN are linked in a reflex arc with melatonin-producing neurons in the pineal gland. This circuit appears to be critical to the sexual behavior of many animals. For example, hamsters reproduce only in the spring, during which time days are getting longer, thus providing the opportunity for the pups to be raised during the more hospitable spring and summer months. Under the influence of melatonin-driven mechanisms, the testes of male hamsters actually become atrophic at other times of the year, and it is only during the advancing days of spring that they grow and the males become fertile and sexually active. This melatonin influence on reproductive behavior is not evident in humans. However, there is evidence that the feedback effect of the pineal melatonin system on the SCN can be utilized by giving people melatonin to treat jet lag.

The SCN project mainly to other hypothalamic nuclei, thereby providing the basis for circadian rhythmicity in the production of TRH, CRH, and GHRH, and for diurnal fluctuations in body temperature (see next section). The SCN also project widely to other regions of the brain, providing one basis for diurnal variations in psychomotor performance, sensory perception, eating, and sleep-wake cycles.

## THERMOREGULATION

Thermoregulation is maintained by a variety of mechanisms, including general metabolism (mediated by hypothalamic and pituitary systems), thermogenesis, regulation of muscle activity, vasomotor tone in the skin, and sweating. Thermogenesis involves variable uncoupling of mitochondrial electron transport from adenosine triphosphate (ATP) production in adiposites. When body core temperature is low, vasoconstriction of skin vessels and minimization of sweating (both mediated by the sympathetic nervous system) help to minimize heat loss, and increased muscle activity, if not shivering, generates heat. Thermoregulatory control is chiefly the province of thermosensitive neurons in two regions of the hypothalamus, one in the preoptic region of the anterior hypothalamus and the other in the posterior hypothalamus. The anterior region promotes heat dissipation, whereas the posterior region promotes heat generation and conservation. Both regions are influenced by projections from the SCN. Thus, there is a circadian body temperature pattern in which temperature is maximal in the late evening and minimal at dawn.

Systemic immunologic processes, most often those elicited by infection, lead to the production by mononuclear cells of a variety of cytokines, most notably interleukin-1 (IL-1). IL-1 crosses the blood-brain barrier at the VOLT (a CVO), where it elicits the production of prostaglandins, which stimulate the anterior hypothalamic thermoregulatory center, leading to elevation of its set point (to above 37°C) and the generation of fever. The intermediary prostaglandin mechanism provides the basis for the antipyretic effects of aspirin and acetaminophen, which inhibit the synthesis of prostaglandins. "Central fever" is often invoked as an explanation for fever of unknown origin. However, this phenomenon is extremely rare, and the most common disorder of hypothalamic thermoregulatory control is encountered in patients who are essentially brain dead and exhibit inability to maintain normal body temperature.

The anterior hypothalamic thermoregulatory center has a very high density of estrogen receptors. This may provide the mechanism for "hot flashes" experienced by many women during the profound estrogen decline of menopause.

## REGULATION OF WEIGHT

Throughout evolutionary history, organisms have had to struggle nearly constantly to find adequate food. Thus, systems regulating food intake can usefully be viewed as existing in a long-term state of hunger and nutritional need that is intermittently punctuated by periods of satiety and nutritional adequacy.

Satiety is defined as the short-term satisfaction of need for food intake in the course of a meal. Satiety is induced by several factors, all of which act on vagal afferent fibers terminating in the nucleus of the solitary tract: gastric distention, cholecystokinin produced upon the introduction of food into the small bowel, elevated glucose and plasma osmolality within the hepatic portal system, and possibly elevated insulin levels. Taste receptor afferents also terminate in the nucleus of the solitary tract, providing the basis for modification of satiety-related behavior under certain circumstances (e.g., there is always room for dessert). Cessation of eating in response to these factors will occur even in decerebrate animals (animals in which the brainstem is completely severed from the cerebrum) because all the neural mechanisms underlying the satiety response are located in the medulla in the vicinity of the nucleus of the solitary tract.

Long-term nutritional adequacy is signaled by a hormone, leptin, which is secreted by adiposites and actively transported into cells within the hypothalamus.

Leptin acts by as yet poorly defined mechanisms to suppress appetite and to increase thermogenesis.

Hypothalamic control of food intake is mediated by a number of neurotransmitters, particularly neuropeptide-Y (NPY). NPY-producing neurons in the arcuate nuclei of the hypothalamus project to the hypothalamic paraventricular nucleus. Increased release of NPY into the paraventricular nucleus elicits eating. Rarely, tumors of the hypothalamus may result in disinhibition of these neurons, resulting in hyperphagia and obesity. NPY neuronal activity has a circadian pattern (higher during normal feeding times); it is increased by food depriva-tion; and it is reduced by insulin (which is actively transported across the blood-brain barrier) and by leptin.

The leptin-NPY mechanism appears to be essential to the set point at which body weight is maintained. Obese people have elevated serum leptin levels, and the precise nature of the dysfunction in this system that underlies obesity remains unclear. Obesity could be the result of reduced leptin transport into the CNS (as appears to occur with aging), defective leptin associated signal transduction, dysfunction in the NPY system, or alteration of thermogenesis and the systems that regulate it.

**Autonomic, Neuroendocrine, and Regulatory Functions**

# Cycle 11-5

# Hypothalamic Drive Systems

## Objective

Be able to give three examples of hypothalamic drive systems and summarize the functional relationship between the hypothalamus and other components of the nervous system as reflected in the physiologic and behavioral manifestations of one of these drives.

Hunger, thirst, and sexual attraction are commonly referred to as drives. Clearly, hypothalamic events are important in defining the impulse to eat, drink, or engage in sexual activity; eating and drinking are associated with complex autonomic and endocrine processes (reviewed previously); and sexual activity is associated with complex yet stereotyped events mediated by the autonomic nervous system and through a characteristic repertoire of somatic behavior. However, hunger, thirst, and sexual activity occur in the context of processes that engage the entire brain, and the hypothalamically mediated impulse to such behaviors is usually but a small contributory part. For example, a starving person will eat almost anything. However, under common circumstances, eating behavior depends upon the particular foods that are available,

the amount of trouble it will take to acquire the food, the appearance, texture and aroma of the food, consideration of the implications of this particular food for one's health, the social context in which eating occurs, and the anticipated cost of the meal, among other things. Eating is also associated with a feeling of pleasure. Thus, eating engages, in addition to the hypothalamic impetus, perceptual components (implicating sensory cortices), knowledge components (implicating association cortices throughout the brain), goal-oriented activity (implicating the frontal lobes), and a sense of positive value (pleasure) (implicating the limbic system). Drinking behavior and sexual behavior involve cerebral systems in analogous manner. As simple as the hypothalamic impulse to such behaviors might seem, the behaviors themselves may become so complex that the impulses are inapparent. The precise neural mechanisms underlying these processes are poorly understood.

There is evidence that drug addiction can usefully be viewed as reflecting a hypothalamic drive mechanism. Like the drives we have discussed, it involves a strong, sometimes overwhelming impetus to a particular behavior, and like other drives, fulfillment is associated with pleasure and lack of fulfillment with discomfort if not craving (reflecting limbic-hypothalamic links).

# Brainstem Regulatory Systems

## Objectives

1. Be able to locate the principal CNS centers for regulation of cardiovascular function.

2. Be able to summarize the effects of increased parasympathetic tone on cardiovascular function and the means by which this is mediated.

3. Be able to summarize the effects of increase sympathetic tone on cardiovascular function and the means by which this is mediated.

4. Be able to summarize the major afferent projections to the CNS that provide the basis for regulation of cardiovascular function.

5. Be able to provide two examples of CNS lesions that produce major alterations in cardiovascular function and describe the underlying mechanisms.

6. Be able to describe the phenomenon of autonomic dysreflexia and briefly describe its mechanism.

7. Be able to describe briefly the CNS structures involved in voluntary and automatic respiration.

8. Be able to describe briefly the peripheral neural mechanisms underlying respiration.

9. Be able to describe briefly the three major afferent systems that modulate breathing.

## CARDIOVASCULAR SYSTEM

Central nervous system influence on cardiovascular function is accomplished through a number of centers in the rostral and caudal medulla, including the nucleus of the solitary tract. Both afferent and efferent components of this apparatus receive hypothalamic projections. Therefore, although medullary cardiovascular systems have considerable autonomy, they are susceptible to hypothalamic influence and, indirectly, the influence of cerebral activity, most particularly that of the limbic system. It is via this connectivity that the autonomic requisites for dealing with threatening conditions, demanding either fight or flight, are established.

Central nervous system influence on cardiovascular function is exerted almost entirely through the autonomic nervous system (Table 11-6). Parasympathetic influence on cardiovascular function occurs through projections from the dorsal motor nucleus of the vagus and portions of the nucleus ambiguus, via the vagus nerve, to the heart. Increased vagal tone results in bradycardia and reduced contractility. Increased vagal tone is also usually associated with reductions in sympathetic tone, resulting for example, in reduction of peripheral vascular resistance.

Sympathetic projections from medullary cardiovascular centers terminate on cells in the intermediate zone at the T1-L2 spinal cord levels. Intermediate zone cells at the T1 through T5 levels project to postsynaptic neurons in the middle and inferior cervical ganglia.

**TABLE 11-6** Summary of Cardiovascular Regulatory Function

| System | Localization | Effect |
|---|---|---|
| Parasympathetic | Dorsal motor nucleus of X, nucleus ambiguus via vagus → cardiac muscarinic receptors | Bradycardia<br>↓ myocardial contractility |
| Sympathetic | T1 and T2 level intermediate zone cells via inferior and middle cervical ganglia → cardiac $\beta_1$-receptors | Tachycardia<br>↑ myocardial contractility |
|  | T3-L2 level intermediate zone cells via para- and prevertebral ganglia |  |
|  | → $\alpha$-receptors on precapillary arterioles in viscera, skin | Vasoconstriction |
|  | → $\beta_1$-receptors on precapillary arterioles in muscle | Vasodilation |
|  | Thoracic level intermediate zone cells → adrenal medulla → epinephrine, norepinephrine → $\beta > \alpha$ stimulation | Skin and visceral vasoconstriction, muscle vasodilation |
|  | Thoracic and lumbar intermediate zone cells → renal $\beta$-receptors | Renin release → angiotensin II → vasoconstriction |
| Afferent | Aortic arch stretch receptors, pressure receptors in left atrium → vagus → N. solitary tract |  |
|  | Carotid sinus stretch receptors → CN IX → N. solitary tract |  |

Postsynaptic neurons in these ganglia project to the heart, which has predominantly $\beta_1$-adrenergic postsynaptic receptors. Increased sympathetic input to the heart is associated with both inotropic (increased contractility) and chronotropic effects (increased heart rate). Cells in the intermediate zone at lower levels project to paravertebral and prevertebral ganglia. Postsynaptic neurons in these ganglia project to resistance blood vessels (precapillary arterioles) in the viscera (including the kidneys), skeletal muscle, and skin. Vessels in skeletal muscle contains predominantly $\beta$-receptors, which when stimulated have vasodilatory effects, whereas vessels in other tissues contain predominantly $\alpha$-receptors, which when stimulated have a vasoconstrictive effect. Sympathetic vasomotor tone is also exerted indirectly via the adrenal medulla (also innervated by intermediate zone projections). Because the adrenal medulla releases more epinephrine than norepinephrine, and $\beta$-adrenergic receptors are more sensitive to epinephrine, the effect of increases in adrenal medullary activity is increased blood flow to muscles and reduced blood flow to other body tissues (precisely what is needed for fight or flight). Sympathetic outflow also acts on $\beta$-receptors in the kidneys, where is elicits the release of renin, which catalyzes the generation of angiotensin II, a potent vasoconstrictive peptide.

Reduced intravascular volume elicits the release of AVP. In Cycle 11-3, the antidiuretic effect of AVP (medi-ated via V2 vasopressin receptors in the kidneys) was discussed. AVP also has vasoconstrictive effects, mediated by vasopressin V1 receptors on arterioles.

Central nervous system regulation of heart rate and contractility and peripheral vascular tone is influenced by afferent input from aortic arch stretch receptors, relayed via the vagus nerve, carotid sinus stretch receptors, relayed via the glossopharyngeal nerve, and pressure-sensitive receptors in the left ventricle, relayed by the vagus nerve. Input from all three of these sources ultimately projects to the nucleus of the solitary tract,[3] from which it is relayed to other medullary regions involved in cardiovascular function. Increased stretch at the receptors leads to an acute increase in parasympathetic tone and reduction in sympathetic tone. Common clinical disorders involving this feedback circuit are described in Cases 8-16 (carotid sinus syndrome) and 8-17 (neurocardiogenic syncope). Unmyelinated afferent fibers from chemosensitive receptors in muscles provide an additional basis for increased cardiac output and blood pressure in response to physical exertion.

---

[3]The nucleus of the solitary tract is viscerotopically organized: taste afferent fibers project to the most rostral portions, gastrointestinal afferent fibers to intermediate regions, cardiovascular afferent fibers to caudomedial regions, and respiratory afferent fibers to caudolateral regions.

# DISORDERS OF CARDIOREGULATORY FUNCTION

Breakdown in the autonomic control of blood pressure sufficient to cause syncope as a result of a critical drop in systemic (and cerebral) perfusion pressure is almost always due to processes initiated outside the central nervous system. Carotid sinus syndrome and neuro-cardiogenic syncope are exemplary, as are cardiogenic syncope (due to cardiac arrhythmias), micturition syncope, syncope during effortful bowel movements, and syncope due to orthostatic hypotension. Syncope due to central nervous system pathology is extremely rare, and when it occurs, it suggests pathology involving cardioregulatory centers in the medulla, as in Case 11-9.

## Case 11-9

### Cough Syncope due to Medullary Compression

*A 30-year-old man complains of severe dizzy spells and occasional loss of consciousness precipitated by sneezing or bouts of coughing. An MRI scan (Fig. 11-8) reveals an Arnold-Chiari malformation. This congenital anomaly of the central nervous system is characterized by caudal displacement of the cerebellar tonsils into the foramen magnum or even into the upper cervical spinal canal.*

**Comment:** *Cough syncope is a relatively common disorder most often seen in overweight, elderly men with a history of chronic obstructive pulmonary disease. Prolonged bouts of coughing increase intrathoracic pressure and reduce pulmonary venous return until cardiac output drops to a level insufficient to maintain adequate cerebral perfusion. Clearly, this explanation cannot be the cause of cough syncope in the present case. In this patient, the combined mass of the cerebellar tonsils and the rostral medulla tightly fills the foramen magnum. When he coughs, the increased intrathoracic pressure is transmitted to the intracranial compartment via the venous system. This leads to downward thrust of the brainstem with each cough, increasing the compression of the medulla. Transient medullary ischemia causes dysfunction of medullary cardioregulatory centers, which is manifested as a sudden drop in systemic blood pressure and syncope. This problem can be treated surgically by removing some of the bone around the foramen magnum.*

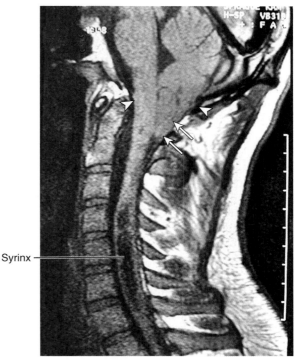

Syrinx

**Figure 11-8** Magnetic resonance image (MRI) of the brain illustrating an Arnold-Chiari malformation. Portions of the cerebellum (*arrows*) extend well below the foramen magnum (*arrowheads*) into the cervical canal. (Contrast with Figure 6-34.) This MRI also reveals a syrinx, a cavity that has formed within the spinal cord, in this case asymptomatic. Arnold-Chiari malformations and syrinxes are often associated with each other, reflecting the tendency for neurodevelopmental abnormalities to occur along the midline neuraxis.

Whereas the central nervous system is only rarely implicated in the causation of hypotension, CNS pathology is fairly commonly responsible for acute hypertension. By far the most common example is acute, large vessel distribution, ischemic stroke. In these circumstances, although the precise mechanisms are unknown, the response may be homeostatic. The acute thrombotic occlusion results in a region of brain, the ischemic penumbra, in which blood flow is just barely adequate to maintain metabolic requirements. Under these circumstances, cerebral resistance vessels are maximally dilated, and blood flow is a linear function of systemic blood pressure. Thus, elevated systemic pressures serve the useful purpose of maximizing perfusion of the ischemic penumbra, and thereby saving brain until the occluding thrombus is recanalized by thrombolytic processes. Aggressive treatment to

**Autonomic, Neuroendocrine, and Regulatory Functions**

normalize blood pressure in this situation may result in catastrophic enlargement of the stroke.

Some rare clinical syndromes involving CNS mediated sympathetic hyperactivity with hypertension also serve to emphasize the capacity of hypothalamic and medullary autonomic centers to acutely influence cardiovascular function: the *Cushing response*, *neurogenic pulmonary edema*, and *neurogenic sudden death*. The Cushing response consists of the triad of hypertension, bradycardia, and slow, irregular breathing. It can be elicited experimentally by mechanical distortion of certain regions of the caudal medulla. It is most often observed in children with large posterior fossa tumors associated with tonsillar herniation and associated mechanical distortion of the medulla, but it can be seen in adults with massive intracranial hemorrhage causing acute central herniation, or subarachnoid hemorrhage leading to increased pressure in the fourth ventricle (from acute communicating hydrocephalus).

Pulmonary edema is almost invariably associated with some combination of fluid overload and left-sided heart failure, which leads to increased pressure in the veins draining the lungs into the left atrium (hence transudation of intravascular fluid into pulmonary interstitial tissue and alveoli). Rarely, pulmonary edema may occur with normal heart function and intravascular volume in the context of intracranial catastrophes such as severe head trauma, subarachnoid or intracerebral hemorrhage, bacterial meningitis, or generalized status epilepticus. This phenomenon, known as neurogenic pulmonary edema, results from hyperactivity of the sympathetic nervous system, which causes extreme peripheral vasoconstriction leading to massive shunting of blood to the central circulation (heart and lungs). It is uniformly associated with severe acute hypertension, against which the left ventricle must pump to reduce pulmonary venous pressure. It is also possible that heightened sympathetic activity increases pulmonary capillary permeability. The precise mechanisms underlying neurogenic pulmonary edema are unknown. However, it can be produced in animals by stimulation of selected regions in the caudal hypothalamus or destruction of the nucleus of the solitary tract, and it has been described in humans with lesions of the medullary tegmentum.

We use the term "neurogenic sudden death" to describe death due to cardiac arrhythmias resulting from hyperactivity of the sympathetic nervous system caused by brain lesions. It is well established that catecholamine infusions in normal animals will induce cardiac arrhythmias in conjunction with a peculiar and characteristic histologic abnormality of the heart known variously as contraction band cardiomyopathy or myofibrillar degeneration, in which myocardial cells die in a state of intense contraction. Similar observations have been made in humans with pheochromocytomas—a rare catecholamine-producing tumor. Prominent electrocardiographic abnormalities and cardiac arrhythmias are common in patients with aneurysmal subarachnoid hemorrhage and may be seen in patients with ischemic stroke or other cerebral lesions. Patients with epilepsy may experience sudden, unexplained death. These phenomena constitute a clear demonstration that cerebral events, mediated through the hypothalamus and medulla, and ultimately through sympathetic and parasympathetic innervation of the heart, can have a profound influence on cardiac function. Contraction band cardiomyopathy has been documented in victims of assault who died despite the fact that they had not sustained serious injury. In a very real sense, it appears that these people were frightened to death. The concept that an emotional reaction, reflecting a particular pattern of activity in the limbic system, can induce intense and potentially fatal sympathetic hyperactivity finds further support in animal studies showing that stimulation of certain regions of the insula will induce lethal cardiac arrhythmias and contraction band cardiomyopathy, and observations in stroke patients that insular lesions, particularly those on the right side, are associated with a heightened risk of sudden death.

## HIERARCHICAL CONTROL OF AUTONOMIC ACTIVITY

One of the recurring themes in this text has been the hierarchical organization of neural systems, first elucidated by Hughlings Jackson. In this conceptualization, higher neural centers not only add sophistication to particular functions, but they also inhibit lower centers involved in these functions. Disconnection of higher from lower centers may lead to "release" phenomena, such as release of the nociceptive flexion reflex (the Babinski sign) by lesions of the spinal cord damaging the medullary reticulospinal tract, or brain lesions disrupting input to the medullary reticular formation (see Chapter 6). An analogous release phenomenon involving the autonomic innervation of the bladder was described in Cycle 6-7. More generalized release of spinal components of the autonomic nervous system can occur, as illustrated in Case 11-10.

## Case 11-10

**Autonomic Dysreflexia due to Spinal Cord Injury**

*A 30-year-old man is left with a chronic, C6 level quadriplegia after fracturing his neck in a motorcycle accident. He develops malaise and fever, and from past experience, he suspects he has a urinary tract infection. Later that day he is observed by family members to be severely agitated. He complains of headache and nausea. His blood pressure is 200/100 mm Hg, his heart rate is 40 bpm, and he is hyperventilating. His face is flushed, his pupils are dilated, he is sweating profusely, and he has "goose-bumps." His legs are rigidly extended and his abdomen is rock-hard. He has a penile erection. He suddenly experiences bowel incontinence.*

**Comment:** *This patient is exhibiting the full panoply of manifestations of autonomic dysreflexia, which is seen quite commonly in patients with chronic spinal cord lesions. Some kind of noxious stimulus, often a distended bladder (caused, as in this case, by infection-induced bladder outlet obstruction), triggers a massive sympathetic response that is uninhibited below the level of the lesion. Secondary hypertension leads to marked enhancement of vagal tone, hence the bradycardia, nausea, and increased bowel activity.*

## RESPIRATORY SYSTEM

Breathing is accomplished by the coordinated contraction and relaxation of the diaphragm, innervated by the phrenic nerve, and intercostal muscles, innervated by intercostal nerves. The phrenic nerve derives from $\alpha$–motoneurons at the C3-C5 levels, and the intercostal nerves derive from $\alpha$–motoneurons at the T1-T12 levels. Expiration is aided by $\alpha$–motoneurons at the low thoracic and high lumbar levels innervating abdominal musculature. These various $\alpha$–motoneurons receive afferent input from two sources: the corticospinal tract, which provides the basis for voluntary modulation of breathing (most critical during speech), and neurons in the rostral and caudal medulla, which provide the basis for automatic breathing. The fundamental rhythm of automatic breathing is established by medullary pacemaker neurons. Extensive lesions of the medulla can be associated with highly irregular ventilatory patterns and respiratory insufficiency. Drugs, most notably

opiates, barbiturates, and general anesthetics, can sufficiently depress the activity of these neurons to cause apnea. Predominantly parasympathetic autonomic output to bronchial smooth muscles, relayed via the vagus nerve, controls airway resistance (hence the value of inspired anticholinergic drugs such as ipatropium [Atrovent] in alleviating bronchospasm).[4]

Three major afferent systems modify breathing: (1) oxygen-sensitive receptors in the carotid body (located at the carotid artery bifurcation); (2) $CO_2$-sensitive receptors of uncertain location, most probably the medulla[5]; and (3) pulmonary mechanoreceptors sensitive to various perturbations of breathing and pulmonary chemoreceptors sensitive to irritants.

Neurons in the carotid body project via the glossopharyngeal nerve to the nucleus of the solitary tract. Respiration is relatively insensitive to $P_{O_2}$. Breathing 100 percent oxygen reduces respiratory drive by only about 15 percent, and reduction in $P_{O_2}$ to below 60 mm Hg is necessary to increase respiratory drive.

In contrast, respiration is very sensitive to $P_{CO_2}$. Given a resting respiratory rate of 5 L/minute, a 1 mm Hg increase in $P_{CO_2}$ from a baseline of 40 mm Hg will result in a 40 percent increase in respiratory rate. However, under pathologic conditions, the medullary $P_{CO_2}$ set point will gradually increase, as exemplified in Case 11-11.

## Case 11-11

**Amyotrophic Lateral Sclerosis**

*A 50-year-old man with a 1.5-year history of amyotrophic lateral sclerosis (ALS, a degenerative disease of anterior horn cells), has become so weak that he is wheelchair-bound. Nevertheless, he is still able to eat, independently take care of personal hygiene, and work at his computer. Over the course of several weeks, he becomes progressively more lethargic. A test of arterial blood gases reveals a $P_{CO_2}$ of 90 mm Hg.*

**Comment:** *This man's respiratory muscles have become so weak that he does not maintain adequate ventilation at night while he sleeps and respiratory*

*Continued*

---

[4]Airway smooth muscle cells also have $\beta$-adrenergic receptors but are relatively sparsely innervated by sympathetic neurons.
[5]Strictly speaking, these are pH sensitive receptors. Carbonic anhydrase catalyzes the conversion of $CO_2$ and water to $H^+$ and $HCO_3^-$.

## *Case 11-11—cont'd*

drive is somewhat diminished. With consequent hypoventilation and retention of $CO_2$, he has gradually increased his medullary $CO_2$ set point. Eventually, his arterial $CO_2$ concentration becomes sufficiently high to produce narcosis, which further depresses respiratory drive, setting in motion a vicious cycle. The decision as to whether or not to employ respiratory support in patients with ALS is always an agonizing one. However, respiratory support may be worthwhile to patients who can still manage to enjoy a high quality of life despite profound weakness. The theoretical physicist Stephen Hawking has made most of his extraordinary contribution to our understanding of the universe during a period in his life when he has been essentially incapable of movement and has been respirator-dependent. For the patient described, exclusively nocturnal respiratory support will probably be adequate, at least for a time, in resetting and maintaining his $CO_2$ set point at a normal level, thereby enabling him to continue his daytime activity unfettered by a mechanical respirator.

The most important pulmonary mechanoreceptors are the slowly adapting stretch receptors, which, through their central projections via the vagus nerve to the nucleus of the solitary tract, provide the basis for the Breuer-Hering reflex. This reflex assures that breath to breath changes in lung volume are appropriate for exchange of gas. For example, if the lungs are inhibited from emptying after a normal inflation, the subsequent expiratory period is greatly lengthened. If the lungs are prevented from filling during an inspiratory period, the next inspiratory period is lengthened and the magnitude of inspiratory muscle activity is greatly increased. The Breuer-Hering reflex provides the basis for adaptation of breathing to environmental circumstances such as changes in body position (lying or standing) or alterations in respiratory resistance (e.g., breathing while carrying a heavy backpack, breathing through a snorkel or during bronchospasm). Other pulmonary mechanoreceptor systems alter respirations in response to sudden interference with inspiration or expiration. Chemosensitive systems alter respirations in response to pulmonary irritants and may precipitate coughing. These systems also provide the basis for hiccups. Hiccups, when pathologic, are typically precipitated by diaphragmatic irritation, but may be seen with medullary lesions, for example, in lateral medullary (Wallenberg) infarction.

## PRACTICE 11-6

**A.** Predict respiratory function in a patient with complete destruction of the spinal cord at the T2 level. What if the cord lesion were at the C3 level?

**B.** Suppose that in Case 11-11, the patient was also found to be hypoxic at night. Comment on the advisability of providing him supplemental oxygen (Hint: think about what mechanisms are providing his respiratory drive).

## CYCLE 11-1

Horner's syndrome (ptosis and miosis). The descending autonomic fibers travel in the dorsolateral quadrant of the brainstem and are most often damaged by (dorso-) lateral medullary infarctions, which produce the Wallenberg syndrome. The pathway providing sympathetic innervation to ocular and periocular tissue involves a preganglionic neuron that sends its axon via the T1 root, upward through the inferior and middle cervical ganglia to terminate in the superior cervical ganglion (Fig. 8-23). Thus, it is susceptible to damage by cancer affecting the pulmonary apex (Case 8-6).

## CYCLE 11-2

**A.** You may have recognized this as a case of Eaton-Lambert syndrome (see Case 4-1). Reduced acetylcholine release at the neuromuscular junction by anterior horn cells causes generalized weakness. Reduced acetylcholine release by preganglionic autonomic neurons produces a host of symptoms reflecting both sympathetic and parasympathetic dysfunction: orthostatic hypotension, reduced sweating, impotence, dry mouth, and constipation.

## CYCLE 11-3

**A.** Elevating the head of the bed 30 degrees at night will reduce the pressure in the left atrium, thereby reducing the production of atrial natriuretic peptide, nocturnal natriuresis, and diuresis. Administration of desmopressin acetate (DDAVP) at bedtime will reduce renal loss of free water and nocturnal diuresis. Both measures will therefore reduce nocturia, and result in the patient starting the day with a larger intravascular volume, hence reduced orthostatic dizziness.

**B.** The TSH level will be elevated because of reduced negative feedback on TRH and TSH production by thyroxin and triiodothionine.

**C.** The LH level will be increased because of reduced negative feedback of estrogen on both the hypothalamus (reduced GnRH pulse frequency) and the pituitary gland (reduced LH pulse magnitude).

## CYCLE 11-6

**A.** A T2 level lesion would interrupt central innervation of α–motoneurons supplying intercostal and abdominal muscles; patients with lesions at this level often experience some respiratory distress but are capable of adequate ventilatory function. A C3 level lesion would interrupt input to α–motoneurons supplying the phrenic nerve and produce apnea.

**B.** Given the pathologic insensitivity of this patient's $CO_2$-mediated respiratory drive, he may be relying on oxygen-mediated drive. Thus, the provision of supplementary oxygen could further suppress his respiration.

Autonomic, Neuroendocrine, and Regulatory Functions

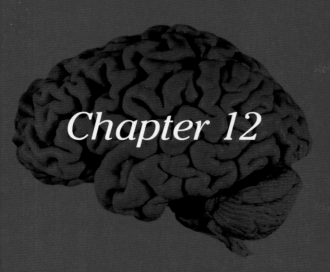

# Chapter 12

# HIGHER NEURAL FUNCTIONS

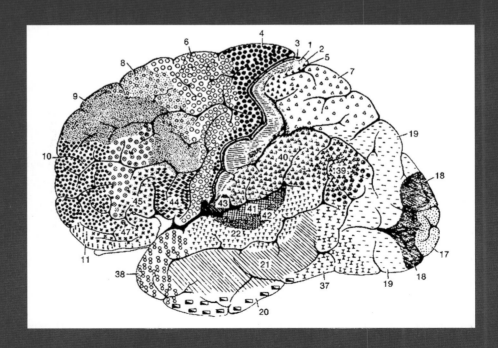

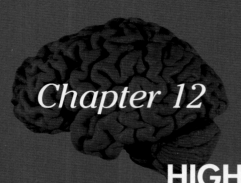

# Chapter 12

# HIGHER NEURAL FUNCTIONS

532

# Introduction

In this chapter we will explore the neural basis for higher functions such as language, skilled motor function, visuospatial and emotional function, memory, attention, and goal-directed activity. Each of these functions involves specific neural network systems and specific regions of the brain. Also, a great deal of interaction takes place between the systems underlying these functions. For example, in order to speak, not only do we need a language apparatus, but we also need to formulate a plan for what we are going to say and we need to engage the neural representations of concepts as we talk, which involves some of the mechanisms underlying attention. The concepts may include emotional components and we may convey that emotion in our tone of voice. What we say and the responses we get will engage memory mechanisms that enable us to recall the conversation at a later date. We will consider the ways in which specific disruptions of this complex array of interlinked systems may lead to major neurobehavioral and psychiatric disorders. Our ultimate goal is to present a model of brain function that will help you to evaluate, understand, and treat the clinical disorders you will encounter.

The first seven cycles of this chapter follow the model used through much of the text: a discussion of anatomy and physiology supplemented by clinical cases that both help to elucidate basic scientific principles and serve to link basic and clinical science. The many practice cases at the end of each cycle, in conjunction with cycle objectives, provide a precise guide to the most important concepts and to problems you are likely to encounter in future clinical practice.

The discussion of the neural mechanisms underlying several major psychiatric disorders in Cycle 12-9 takes this same approach. However, more generally, the last two cycles of this chapter take a broader, more conceptual approach, one that harks back to our cautions in the Preface about the need to acquire graded knowledge in this course. These two cycles will attempt to give you a glimpse of the answer to perhaps the most fundamental question in neuroscience: how is it possible for neurons, whose currency is electrical impulses and squirts of neurotransmitter, to generate the astonishingly complex behaviors discussed throughout the text but particularly in this chapter? This material will be difficult for many students. Indeed, it is difficult even for those of us committed to research in basic or clinical neuroscience to transcend the gap between conventional neuroanatomy and physiology and the realm of statistical physics, which provides the mathematical underpinnings necessary to answer this question with precision. Clearly, we do not expect you to gain the sort of understanding that can be explicitly tested. We do hope that you emerge with a sense of how it all works; a sense of the implications of the mathematical properties of neural networks for the functions they subserve; a sense of awe about the emergence of an intricate and powerful order from a source, chaos—the principles of self-organizing systems—whose existence you may not have even suspected; and perhaps enough curiosity to look further into this fascinating emerging science.

# Cerebral Cortical Anatomy

In Chapter 1 we identified the major targets of afferent input to the cerebrum, the *primary sensory cortices*. These cortices include visual cortex along the upper and lower banks of the calcarine fissure on the medial aspect of the occipital lobe (area 17), somatosensory cortex along the postcentral gyrus (areas 3, 1, and 2), and auditory cortex (areas 41 and 42) in Heschl's gyrus on the superior surface of the temporal lobe deep within the sylvian fissure (Fig. 12-1). We also identified the major source of cerebral efferent projections, the primary motor cortex (area 4) in precentral gyrus. At this point we will quickly survey the remaining cerebral cortical surface, which is composed of *association cortices*, the fundamental substrate for higher neural functions. Visual association cortex includes the entire medial surface of the occipital lobe beyond the banks of the calcarine fissure, the lateral surface of the occipital lobe (Brodmann's areas 18 and 19), the middle and inferior temporal gyri, and the entire inferior surface of the temporal lobe (areas 20, 21, and 37). Auditory association cortex includes areas surrounding Heschl's gyrus and adjacent portions of superior temporal gyrus (area 22). Somatosensory association cortex includes

Brodmann's area 5 in the superior parietal lobe. Premotor cortex (area 6), immediately anterior to the precentral gyrus in the frontal lobes, can reasonably be viewed as "motor association cortex."

All the association cortices discussed thus far process neural signals in a single modality. Some areas of the brain are best viewed as *polymodal cortices*. Area 7 in the superior parietal lobe, which receives both visual and somatosensory projections, is a good example. Parahippocampal gyrus, which overlies the hippocampus and serves as the hippocampal receiving area for projections from nearly the entire cerebral cortex, is another. Other areas are better viewed as *supramodal cortices* because the neural processes they subserve are not directly linked to sensory or motor functions. These cortices include the entirety of prefrontal cortex (all frontal cortex anterior to area 6), limbic association cortex (insula, cingulate gyrus, and the temporal poles), and perisylvian cortex bilaterally (parts of areas 22, 39, and 40, and areas 44 and 45). The perisylvian cortex is a region unique to humans. In the dominant hemisphere it subserves language function.

## PRACTICE 12-1

In Figure 12-2, locate primary visual, auditory, and somatosensory cortices; motor cortex; visual, auditory, somatosensory, and motor association cortices; limbic association cortex; and other supramodal cortices until you have a ready grasp of cortical geography.

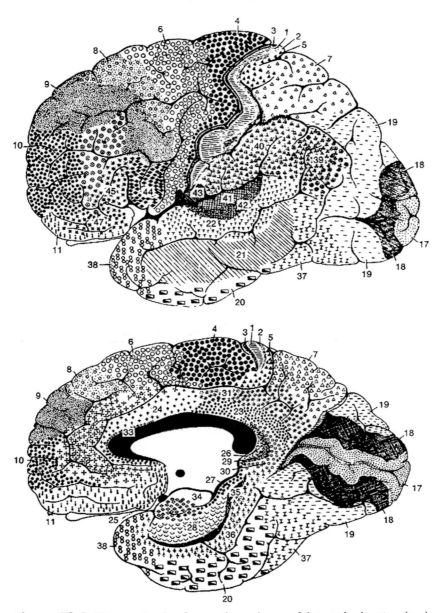

**Figure 12-1** This drawing is a frequently used map of the cerebral cortex developed early in this century by Brodmann on the basis of the characteristic cytoarchitecture of different regions of the brain. The durability of his scheme is a tribute to the astounding quality of his work. The fundamental underlying hypothesis behind this work is that particular functions must reflect the peculiarities of local neural organization. This hypothesis continues to drive extensive research. You are not expected to learn Brodmann's areas, only to use the numbered areas cited in the text to help you relate function to anatomy.

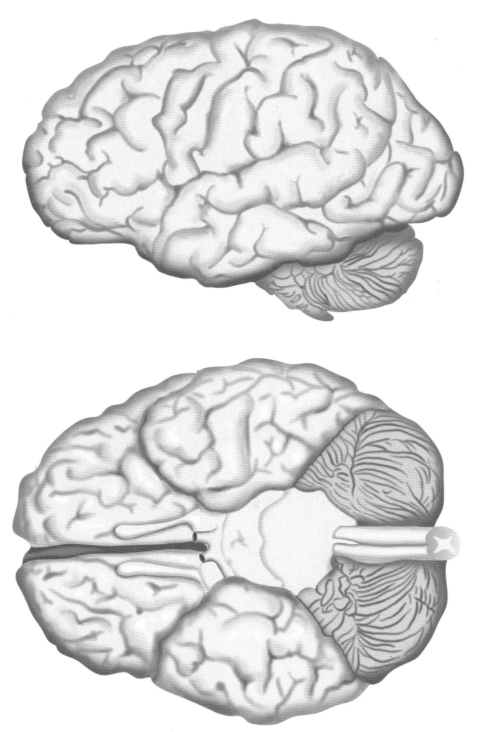

**Figure 12-2** Practice 12-1

# Functions of Sensory Association Cortices

## Objectives

1. Be able to describe how sensory association cortices are organized as:
   a) Hierarchical multistage processors of afferent sensory input;
   b) Parallel processors that analyze different attributes of a given sensory modality;
   c) Way stations to polymodal and supramodal cortices.
2. Be able to describe the concept of a distributed representation and be able to relate it specifically to visual ("what" and "where" systems), auditory, and somatosensory modalities.

*One somewhat simplistic way of viewing a sensory association cortex is as a multistage hierarchical processor that carries out successively more sophisticated analysis of neural activity in primary sensory cortex.* Case 12-1 illustrates the consequences of dysfunction in higher visual association cortices, notwithstanding substantial preservation of elementary visual function.

## Case 12-1

**Visual Agnosia due to a Stroke Involving Visual Association Cortices**

*An elderly gentleman suddenly loses all his vision due to a stroke involving the occipital and posterior*

## Case 12-1—cont'd

*temporal lobes bilaterally, caused by bilateral posterior cerebral artery occlusion (Fig. 12-3). He ultimately regains some rudimentary vision and is able, for example, to accurately point to objects held up in front of him and to avoid bumping into things as he walks. Visual acuity is nearly normal. He can discriminate objects that differ in size or luminance but has great difficulty when they differ only in shape. He has difficulty naming brightly colored objects and he is completely unable to name any line drawings of objects, copy drawings of objects, or match drawings to each other. He cannot point to objects named by the examiner. When allowed to feel an object, he readily identifies it and describes its function.*

**Comment:** *This patient has apperceptive visual agnosia. His normal visual acuity attests to the integrity of at least the macular representation at the occipital pole, and his ability to avoid walking into things suggests that he has preservation of some aspects of vision in his peripheral fields. However, higher order visual processing is clearly severely impaired as he is rarely able to identify things that he sees. He has a fundamental impairment in visual shape discrimination. His visual perception is sufficiently disordered that he cannot even copy drawings of objects. However, his touch perception is normal.*

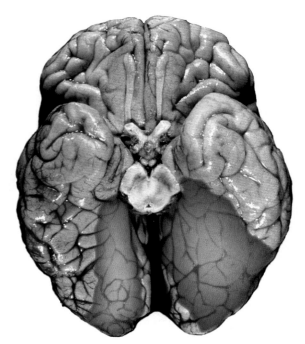

**Figure 12-3** Inferior view of the cerebrum demonstrating the lesions in Case 12-1.

*A sensory association cortex supporting a particular modality (e.g., vision) is more accurately viewed as a group of hierarchies that are to some degree interlinked but operate substantially in parallel, each individual hierarchy developing some aspect of sensory input. Our perception of sensory input consists of the sum total of the different types of analysis that are distributed across the hierarchies.* Thus, our actual perception corresponds to a grand representation composed of a number of subrepresentations, each generated by one hierarchy or a segment of a hierarchy. We refer to this grand representation as a *distributed representation*. Destruction of the neural substrate for a subrepresentation will deplete our perception by eliminating the corresponding perceptual component, but it will not eliminate the overall perception. Case 12-2 illustrates the result of damage to a lower level component of one of the functional hierarchies in the visual system.

## Case 12-2

### Selective Loss of Color Vision due to a Stroke Involving Visual Association Cortices

*A 60-year-old gentleman awakes to find that he has lost all color vision. Otherwise his visual function seems to be relatively normal. A magnetic resonance image (MRI) of the brain reveals bilateral strokes limited to the medial portions of the posterior temporal lobes (Fig. 12-4).*

**Comment:** *This patient provides evidence of divisions in the visual system that, as we discussed in Chapter 9, actually begin at the retina in the cone photoreceptors. Interactions between retinal ganglion cells receiving input from cones sensitive to different wavelengths of light provide the basis for color perception. Neural input supporting this color perception is projected to the "blobs" of the primary visual cortex (V1). Within V1, the blobs are located within the interstices of cortex primarily made up of columns of neurons characterized by the eye of predominant input and the angle of lines to which they are maximally sensitive. Beyond V2 (roughly Brodmann's area 18), the visual system divides into the geographically separate "what" and "where" systems, the "what" system located in the inferior and lateral temporal cortices, the "where" system in the parietal cortices (Fig. 12-5). Within the "what" system, there is further geographic separation into color and forms subsystems. Cortex supporting color analysis (V4), which was selectively damaged in this patient, is located in the most medial portions of the temporal lobes (Fig. 12-4).*

Actual visual perception consists of the distributed representation of visual input across the "what" and "where" pathways. In Case 12-2, we saw the result of damage to a lower component of the "what" system

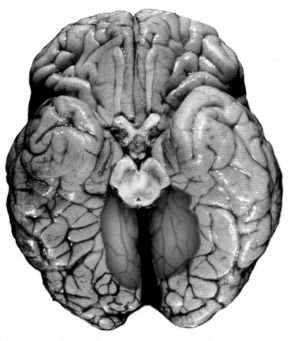

**Figure 12-4** Inferior view of the brain demonstrating the lesions in Case 12-2.

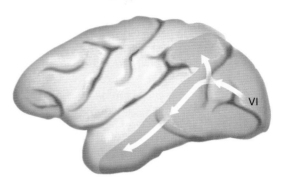

**Figure 12-5** Lateral view of the left hemisphere of a rhesus monkey. The shaded area defines primary and association visual cortices in the occipital, parietal, and temporal lobes. The arrows delineate two visual pathways beginning in primary visual cortex (V1), one extending ventrally along inferior temporal cortex (the "what" pathway), and the other dorsally into parietal cortex (the "where" pathway). (Modified from Mishkin M, Ungerleider LG, Macko KA. Object vision and spatial vision: two cortical pathways. TINS 6:414–417, 1983.)

## Case 12-3

**Loss of Form Vision but Preservation of Movement Vision due to a Stroke Involving Visual Association Cortices**

*A 65-year-old retired teacher suddenly experiences severe impairment of vision due to bilateral occipitotemporal strokes (Fig. 12-6). She is able to accurately point to objects but cannot name them or describe their purpose or function. However, when an object is swung like a hammer (even if it is actually a screwdriver or a pen), she readily identifies it as a hammer. When a comb is gripped and turned about its long axis, she identifies it as a screwdriver.*

**Comment:** *Damage to the color/form "what" visual system prevents this patient from deriving any useful information merely by looking at objects. However, relative preservation of the location/movement "where" visual pathway allows her to take advantage of her knowledge of the motion attributes of objects. (From Schwartz RL, Barrett AM, Crucian GP, Heilman KM. Dissociation of gesture and object recognition. Neurology 50:1186–1188, 1998.)*

subserving only the color component of vision, in effect a subhierarchy within the "what" hierarchy. In Case 12-3 we see the results of much more extensive damage to higher levels of the "what" system with preservation of the "where" system.

*Sensory association cortices serve as way stations to supramodal cortices.* This connection is exemplified in Case 12-4, in which there is a traumatic disconnection of higher level "what" system visual cortices and the limbic system.

Higher Neural Functions

## Case 12-4

### Visual-Limbic Dissociation due to Bilateral Temporal Lobe Hematomas

*A 30-year-old architect experiences severe head trauma as his motorcycle collides with an automobile that failed to yield right of way. A computed tomographic (CT) scan reveals bilateral hematomas (accumulations of blood) within the posterior portions of the temporal lobes (Fig. 12-7). After a long recuperative period, the patient attempts to return to his prior life. He finds that he can no longer work as an architect because, although his technical skills appear to be relatively intact, he no longer has any aesthetic appreciation of architectural drawings. He cancels his Playboy subscription because photos of nudes no longer elicit any feelings. (From Bauer RM. Visual hypoemotionality as a symptom of visual-limbic disconnection in man. Arch Neurol 39:702–708, 1982.)*

**Comment:** *This patient has lesions of the ventral "what" visual pathway bilaterally that substantially disconnect color/form representations from the limbic system, most notably the amygdala, which provides the basis for the affective responses to visual input (see Cycle 12-4). This represents the disconnection of a unimodal sensory association cortex from the limbic system, which can be considered as functionally equivalent to a supramodal cortex. Viewed from another perspective, the normal perception of a drawing of a beautiful building consists of a distributed representation across visual and limbic neural systems; this patient has lost part of that distributed representation because of a disconnection.*

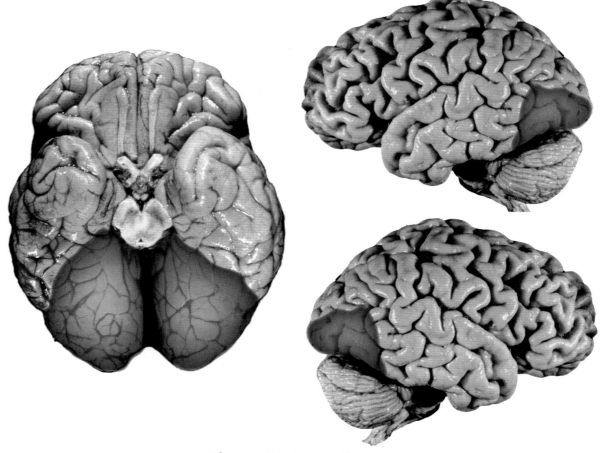

**Figure 12-6** Lesion in Case 12-3.

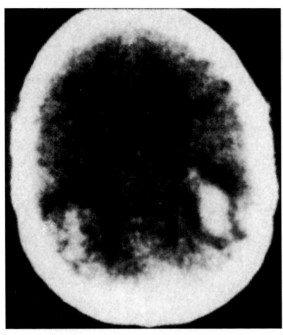

**Figure 12-7** Axial computed tomographic (CT) slice of the brain in Case 12-4 demonstrating bilateral inferior temporal hematomas. The poor quality of this image reflects the limited imaging technology available in 1980. Nevertheless, the ability to "see inside the brain" represented a revolutionary advance.

## PRACTICE 12-2

**A.** You test sensory function in a patient by stimulating him over various parts of the body with either a Q-Tip or a toothpick. You ask him to tell you whether the stim-ulus is sharp or dull and where you are stimulating him. Discuss the cerebral processing of this sensory input in terms of distributed representations. Can you draw an analogy to visual systems?

**B.** A 70-year-old woman is brought in by family members alarmed that she seems to have suddenly lost her hearing. She demonstrates no comprehension whatsoever of things said to her and the nurses are getting frustrated because she will not obey any commands despite the fact that she is able to speak perfectly normally. She readily comprehends even very complex written commands. When someone drops a glass she jumps as she is startled and immediately looks to the direction of the accident and comments. When her physician's pager goes off, she points to it and suggests that he better go answer the page. Discuss this case in terms of distributed representations.

**C.** A 65-year-old woman experiences bilateral superior occipital and parietal strokes due to hypotension experienced in a cardiac arrest (Fig. 12-8). Predict (a) her visual field cuts; (b) her ability to recognize, describe, and name objects she sees; and (c) her ability to point to things.

**D.** A 68-year-old man experiences a stroke due to embolism to the left posterior cerebral artery. The stroke destroys the left calcarine cortex and the splenium of the corpus callosum (Fig. 12-9). Because there was no embolism to the left middle cerebral artery, the patient's language cortex in the left perisylvian region is completely normal. What predictions do you make about the patient's reading ability? Why?

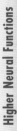

**Higher Neural Functions**

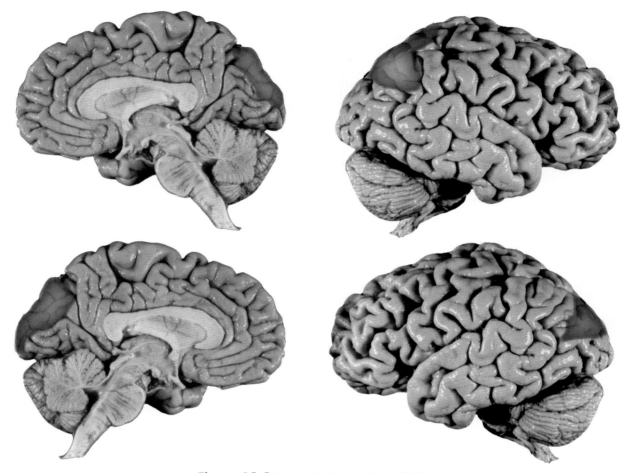

**Figure 12-8** Lesion in Practice Case 12-2C.

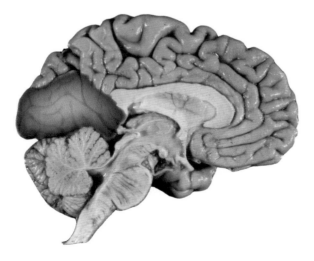

**Figure 12-9** Lesion in Practice Case 12-2D.

# Functions of Polymodal and Supramodal Cortices

## Objectives

1. Be able to define the distributed representations of phonology and meaning and describe the effects of lesions of parts of these representations.

2. Be able to define the major components of the distributed representation of praxis and describe the consequence of lesions of components of this representation.

3. Be able to define constructional apraxia and locate lesions likely to cause it.

4. Be able to describe briefly the basis for our ability to orient our bodies in space.

## LANGUAGE

In the previous section we discussed the idea that the processing of various sensory modalities was parallel and distributed with multiple association cortices working simultaneously on different aspects of a particular sensory input. This principle also applies to higher neural functions that take place in cortices receiving sensory input in a variety of modalities (polymodal cortex) and in supramodal cortices, which perform functions that cannot readily be defined in terms of a sensory modality. Language, the best understood of higher neural functions, provides a perfect example of parallel and distributed processing in higher neural function.

The neural core of language function is the specialized cortex that enables us to understand spoken (heard) and written (seen) language, enables the blind to understand braille (felt language), and enables us to speak and write. It consists primarily of supramodal cortex in the perisylvian region of the *left* "dominant" hemisphere: posterior area 22 (Wernicke's area), area 40 (supramarginal gyrus), and areas 44 and 45 (Broca's area) (Fig. 12-10). To a variable but much lesser extent, there is some language representation in nondominant perisylvian cortex.

Nearly all left-handed people have more bilateral representation of language, but only a minority of left handers have "situs inversus" brains. The dominant perisylvian cortex, which has no homolog in the most advanced primates for which we have adequate data (macaque monkeys), provides us with the ability to convert knowledge of meaning (which other animals have) into symbolic representations.

The fundamental symbolic unit represented by left perisylvian cortex is the *phoneme*. Phonemes are the smallest discrete units of language. Most can be symbolically represented as letter sounds, such as /b/, /t/, /k/. We enclose the letters in slashes to indicate that we mean the sound of the phoneme, for example, the "b" sound of "bat" and not the letter sound "bee." Some phonemes cannot be represented by single letters, as /th/ of "this." Dominant perisylvian cortex, via its links with association cortices, enables a distributed

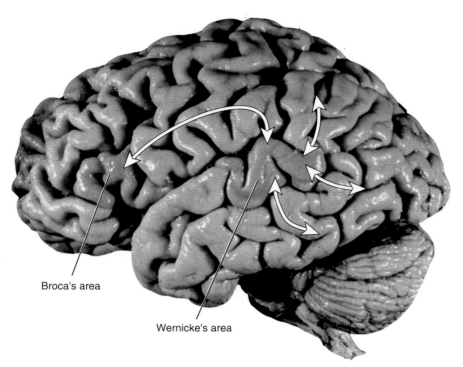

Broca's area

Wernicke's area

**Figure 12-10** Lateral aspect of the left hemisphere diagramming the perisylvian cortex that supports the distributed representation of phonemes and its links to association cortices. All connections are indicated as two-way, as they actually are in the brain. This has important consequences for how the brain functions, as we shall see in Cycle 12-8.

representation of phonemes in their various forms: motor (the movement programs necessary for us to actually produce the sound of phonemes or write letters corresponding to phonemes), auditory (the acoustic representations of phonemes), visual (the visual representations of letters), and in the blind, somatosensory (the tactile representation of the braille form of letters). The motor representations are supported by links to inferior premotor and motor cortex from Broca's area (Fig. 12-10). The auditory representation is supported by links to auditory association cortex in the vicinity of Heschl's gyrus on the superior surface of the temporal lobe, deep within the Sylvian fissure. The visual representation is supported by links to inferior visual association cortices (a subcomponent of the ventral "what" system). The somatosensory representation is supported by links to somatosensory association cortex (presumably area 5 or the secondary somatosensory area in the parietal lobe). The sensory association links (auditory, visual, somatosensory) are presumably with Wernicke's area or cortex immediately posterior to it (areas 37 and 39). The representation of an individual phoneme consists of a particular pattern of neural activity in the dominant perisylvian cortex and the linked association cortices.

We have discussed the means by which an abstract representation of a phoneme, defined by some pattern of neural activity in dominant perisylvian cortex, is translated into various "real" representations of phonemes, such as speech, writing, heard language, read language, or felt language, via links to association cortices. Perisylvian cortex also supports sequence knowledge that provides the means for combining phonemes into various orderly "clumps" corresponding to common phoneme combinations (such as, /str/), syllables, and words. However, for clumps of phonemes to have any value, they must be linked to cortex that represents meaning.

*Meaning corresponds to the particular pattern of neural activity distributed across association cortices throughout the brain that actually represents a particular concept.* Thus, the meaning of "dog" is represented as a pattern of neural activity in ventral visual association cortices bilaterally corresponding to our "mind's eye" image of dogs in general as well as various particular dogs we have known; a pattern of neural activity in auditory association cortices corresponding to our "mind's ear" image of dogs (e.g., barking, whining, pleading); a pattern of neural activity in limbic association cortices corresponding to our feelings about dogs we have known, mainly as our own pets; perhaps still other patterns of neural activity in somatosensory and olfactory association cortices; and patterns of neural activity in various supramodal cortices representing our knowledge about the behavior of dogs, their relationship to other animals, and so on. Case 12-3 involved a stroke patient who had lost the visual form aspect of the meaning of objects she saw; her "mind's eye" image would also lack this form aspect of meaning. Case 12-4 involved a patient who had lost the limbic aspect of the meaning of seen objects because of a disconnection between visual association cortex and the limbic system. However, because this patient had an intact limbic system, he was able to access emotional meaning by any route other than the visual one. In fact, his interest in music increased substantially after his unfortunate accident. In Cases 12-5, 12-6, and 12-7, we will see how various acquired lesions disrupt different aspects of the language processor.

## Case 12-5

### Broca's Aphasia

*A 75-year-old man experiences a large left hemisphere stroke that extensively damages the frontal lobe including Broca's area and inferior premotor and motor cortex (Fig. 12-11). He is unable to produce much language and what he does produce is extremely labored and slurred (dysarthric). Pictured in Figure 12-12 is a recording of electrical activity in muscles of his face and tongue as he attempts to say "peep" compared with that of a normal person.*

*We see in the recording of the normal person two very discrete contractions of the perioral musculature as the lips are brought together to form the /p/ sounds. Furthermore, the perioral contractions are almost the same every time. In contrast, the motor activity corresponding to /p/ is very prolonged in the patient and it varies from time to time.*

**Comment:** *This patient has a type of language impairment referred to as Broca's aphasia. The cortex supporting the oral motor representation of phonemes has been extensively damaged. Would he be able to write? In principle he might be able to, because the oral motor representations of phonemes and the hand motor representations of letters (graphemes) are different and physically separate. However, because these two representations are closely adjacent in the brain, we rarely see only one affected. Would he be able to comprehend language? Of course he would, because posterior portions of dominant perisylvian cortex and their links to sensory association cortices supporting meaning are intact.*

## Case 12-6

### Conduction Aphasia

*A 70-year-old woman experiences a small stroke involving area 40 and the posterior portion of area 22 (Fig. 12-13). She has reasonably good comprehension of written and spoken language and is able to produce a fair amount of speech that is well articulated (not dysarthric). However, both her spontaneous language (Table 12-1) and language she repeats are full of phonemic substitutions (phonemic paraphasias).*

**Comment:** *This patient has a conduction aphasia, so-called because it has traditionally been conceptualized as impaired ability to conduct neural impulses from cortex supporting "word representations" in an abstract form to cortex supporting the translation of word representations into actual speech. However, it is more likely that it represents damage to the hierarchical processor within perisylvian language cortex that is responsible for converting words as distributed concept representations into sequences of phonemes. As a result, errors in phonemic selection are common. Because the patient retains the capability for generating patterns of neural activity corresponding to "word images," she recognizes the errors she makes and repeatedly tries to correct them.*

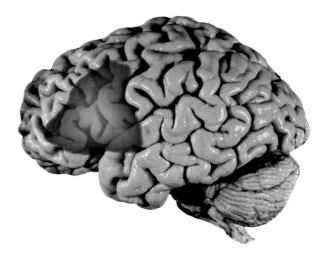

**Figure 12-11** Lesion in Case 12-5.

## Case 12-7

### Transcortical Sensory Aphasia

*A 55-year-old man experiences a stroke involving left temporoparietal cortex (Fig. 12-14). His ability to repeat is excellent and his speech is not dysarthric. However, his comprehension is poor and his spoken language is lacking in content. Often he exhibits word finding difficulty (inability to actually come up with the word even though it seems as if it is on "the tip of his tongue") and circumlocution (attempts to explain a single word by other means). When asked to describe what he had for breakfast (pancakes, sausage, orange juice, and coffee), he responds:*

*"I had ah ah . . . to drink . . . in a cup . . . and . . . and . . . [gesturing with hands] syrup . . . no, no . . . it was . . . I had . . . eggs . . . no, no . . . brown . . . You know . . . things . . . things for breakfast . . . ah, I ate . . ."*

**Comment:** *This patient has what is traditionally referred to as a transcortical sensory aphasia. The idea is that he has damaged transcortical links between perisylvian cortex supporting phonologic representations and association cortices supporting meaning. One gets the sense that he really knows what he had for breakfast; that is, cortex supporting meaning is intact. However, he has extraordinary difficulty using the pattern of neural activity representing meaning to generate a pattern of neural activity in left perisylvian cortex corresponding to the phonologic representation of that meaning. Thus, he often fails to come up with the word he is looking for, and he sometimes makes semantic paraphasic errors—substitution of a related word, for example, eggs for either pancakes or French toast. He makes inappropriate use of terms of nonspecific reference, here "things" and "things for breakfast." He is able to repeat normally because his perisylvian cortex supporting phonologic processing is intact. He has poor comprehension because his ability to link word sounds to meaning is as impaired as is his ability to link meaning to speech output.*

The scientific literature on language now includes thousands of papers. In this brief introduction, we have had the opportunity to discuss only the most fundamental aspects.

**TABLE 12-1 Sample Speech Production by a Patient with Conduction Aphasia***

I've been retired since 1972 with /cardimiapesun/ (cardiomyopathy).
Ten per cent [of] the people [with] the /catraps/ (cataracts) has the [problem with the] retina.
I was in the /bizzet/ (business) of records . . . /fotegraph/ (phonograph) records . . . for the /shusta/ (distribution?) . . . In other words, I was a /eksiev/ (executive).
Look, I think it's /porten/ (important).
I can't [say] /tivelsha/, /diveltsher/ (television), uh TV.

*Missing words are in brackets, neologisms (nonwords) in slashes, and translations of neologisms in parentheses.
*Source:* From Pate DS, Saffran EM, Martin N. Specifying the nature of the production impairment in a conduction aphasic. Lang Cogn Processes 2: 43–84, 1987. Reprinted by permission of Psychology Press.

## PRAXIS

*Praxis* consists of our knowledge of objects as tools. This concept at first seems pretty straightforward. However, tool knowledge has a number of different aspects, which correspond to the various distributed representations of tools: (1) Looking at a hammer, we can name it because the pattern of neural activity in ventral visual association cortex (the "what" system) elicits a pattern of neural activity in left perisylvian cortex corresponding to /hamr/. (2) We can also conjure up a "mind's eye" image of a hammer being used. Case 12-3 had lost the first of these aspects of tool knowledge (because of bilateral damage to the "what" visual pathway) but retained the second. (3) We also have a "mind's hand and arm" sense of holding a hammer and swinging it to strike a nail, most likely represented in premotor cortex. This particular aspect of tool knowledge is nearly always represented in the hemisphere opposite the dominant hand and constitutes a major factor determining handedness. (4) Finally, we have a rather abstract concept of a hammer as a mass on the end of a lever. Thus, lacking a hammer, we can improvise using any heavy object, such as a rock or a heavy pair of pliers. Normally we use all parts of this distributed representation of tool knowledge. Cases 12-8 and 12-9 illustrate ways in which praxis can be affected when various portions of this distributed representation are damaged.

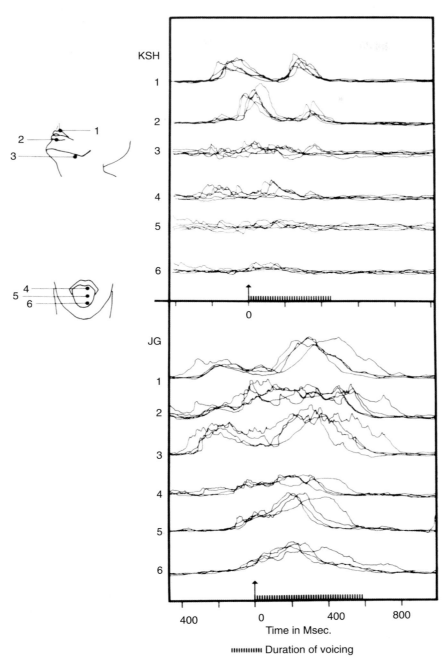

**Figure 12-12** Recording of electrical activity about the mouth and tongue (electrode locations indicated at upper left) as a normal subject (*top*) and the aphasic patient (*bottom*) say "peep." The hash marks denoting duration of voicing indicate the time over which the subjects produced the "ee" sound. (From Shankweiler D, Harris, KS, Taylor ML. Electromyographic studies of articulation in aphasia. Arch Phys Med Rehab 49:1–8, 1968. © W.B. Saunders Company.)

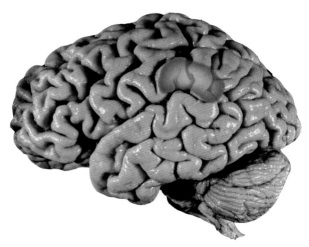

**Figure 12-13** Lesion in Case 12-6.

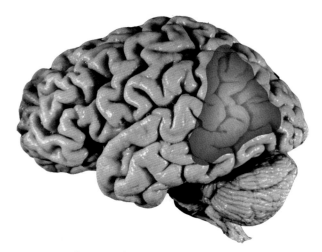

**Figure 12-14** Lesion in Case 12-7.

## Case 12-8

### Ideomotor Apraxia due to a Stroke

*A 65-year-old man experiences a left hemisphere frontoparietal stroke (Fig. 12-15). His language function, although impaired, is sufficient for us to engage him in complex tasks. He has a right hemiparesis so we ask him to demonstrate movements using his left hand. When asked to pantomime the use of a screwdriver, he sticks out his index finger and rotates the hand about the axis defined by the extended finger, something referred to as a body-part-as-tool error. When told to pretend he is actually holding the screwdriver as he demonstrates its use, he looks confused, makes some variously incorrect rotatory movements of the hand, and ultimately returns to the finger-extended rotatory gesture he used in the first place. When asked to demonstrate the use of a pair of scissors, he extends his index and middle fingers and repeatedly moves them apart and together in a scissoring motion, another body-part-as-tool error. When told to actually pretend he is holding the scissors, he again looks confused and ends up*

*repeatedly opposing his thumb to the tip of his index finger. When the examiner demonstrates the correct and several incorrect pantomimes of scissors, the patient readily identifies the correct gesture.*

**Comment:** *This patient has experienced damage to the cortex supporting the "mind's hand and arm" representation of tools. Thus, his ability to demonstrate tool use is severely impaired. He has an ideomotor apraxia. He frequently substitutes tool knowledge that he retains, namely, his "mind's eye" image of what the tool looks like as it is being used—hence his tendency to use his index finger as the shaft of the screwdriver or his index and middle fingers as the blades of the scissors. This preserved "mind's eye" representation in visual association cortex also enables him to distinguish the correct gesture when it is performed by the examiner. It is worth noting that this man's "normal" left arm function is not as useful as one might have thought, because he is impaired in tool use as a result of the left hemisphere lesion.*

## Case 12-9

**Conceptual Apraxia due to Alzheimer's Disease**
*A 75-year-old man has Alzheimer's disease. This neurodegenerative disease is associated with diffuse damage that is maximal in the temporal and parietal unimodal, polymodal, and supramodal association cortices (Fig. 12-16). When asked to demonstrate the use of tools, he looks confused and produces repetitive movements of his right hand that only vaguely resemble the desired gesture. He sometimes makes body-part-as-tool errors. When given a variety of tools and a board with a screw partly advanced into a hole and asked to finish the job, he looks at all the tools (including a screwdriver) for a while and ultimately ends up trying to advance the screw with his fingers alone. As he is observed eating, he prepares a glass of iced tea by pouring in some sugar, holding a knife blade submerged in the tea with his right hand and rotating the glass with his left hand.*

**Comment:** *This patient has an ideomotor apraxia quite similar to that seen in Case 12-8. We can infer that even in the absence of any impairment in more elementary aspects of motor function (he does not have a hemiparesis), he has lost his "mind's hand and arm" representation of tool knowledge. However, there is evidence of degradation of other aspects of tool knowledge—other portions of the distributed tool representations. His knowledge of associations between tools and the objects upon which they operate is defective, possibly because of damage to association cortex in the "what" visual system, hence his inability to select the correct tool to advance the screw or to stir the iced tea. Furthermore, although he retains vestiges of general concepts of tool use, such as the twisting involved in advancing a screw and rotation involved in stirring, the iced tea performance indicates that these concepts are quite degraded. Thus, he has what has been referred to as a conceptual apraxia. This mixed apraxia is an almost universal feature of Alzheimer's disease, often one of the first problems to develop, and it is one of the most debilitating features as it seriously interferes with the patient's ability to perform the myriad overlearned motor activities needed to carry out activities of daily living.*

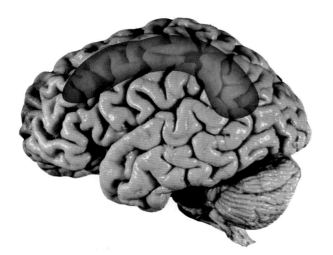

**Figure 12-15** Lesion in Case 12-8.

## VISUOSPATIAL FUNCTION

Visuospatial functions include a large variety of complex cognitive processes, most not well understood. We will focus on only two, *constructional praxis* and *bodily orientation in space*, because they provide insight into two particularly important aspects of brain function. These functions are best explained through descriptions of patients with lesions affecting them.

**Higher Neural Functions**

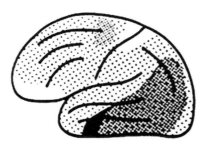
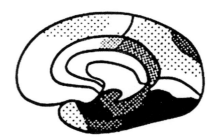

**Figure 12-16** The distribution of pathology in Alzheimer's disease. Darker shading indicates more severe pathology. (From Brun A, Gustafson L. Limbic lobe involvement in presenile dementia. Arch Psychiat Nervenkr 226:79–93, 1978. Reproduced with permission of Springer Verlag.)

## Case 12-10

### Constructional Apraxia

*A 65-year-old man experiences a large right hemisphere stroke. When asked to copy a simple drawing of a house, his production is so abnormal it is not even recognizable as a house (Fig. 12-17).*

**Comment:** *This patient has constructional apraxia: he has lost his ability to draw and construct, in this case largely because of an inability to capture the overall aspect or "Gestalt" of the house in his drawing. This disorder is common in patients with right hemisphere damage. To produce even a simple drawing like this, one must capture the defining spatial qualities of the image. The all-at-once, parallel processing implicit in this analysis stands in contrast to the fundamentally more linear and sequential nature of processes represented predominantly in the left hemisphere, such as language and praxis. All known cognitive functions, even the most strongly lateralized, demonstrate at least some bilaterality of representation, and the degree of functional asymmetry varies substantially from person to person. Nevertheless, there is consistent evidence of a difference in the general flavor of the expertise brought to cognitive processing by the left and right hemispheres, the left being more involved in predominantly sequential processes, the right in processes requiring simultaneous, all-at-once analysis. Note also that many features are missing from the left side of the patient's drawing, reflecting hemispatial neglect, a disorder of attention that we will discuss in Cycle 12-7.*

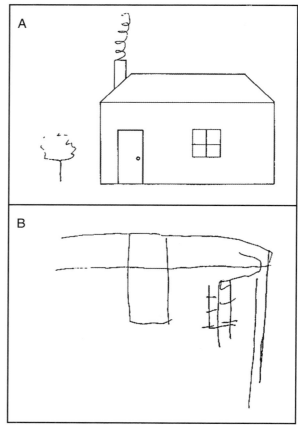

**Figure 12-17** Drawing of a house (*A*) and reproduction by patient in Case 12-10 (*B*).

## Case 12-11

### Disorder of Correlation of Personal and Environmental Coordinate Systems

*A 55-year-old woman is referred to a behavioral neurologist because of a series of unaccountable automobile accidents and an embarrassing incident at a public social function. She is an extraordinarily bright person, heavily engaged in charitable organizations and political activities, an officer in many organizations, often called upon to make public speeches. Over the past 6 months, she has had a total of six automobile accidents, several while trying to park her car. One night, after giving a speech, she found herself unable to sit down in her chair without guidance from those sitting beside her. She undergoes extensive neurologic and neuropsychological testing. In one test, she is asked simply to walk up to a bed and get in it. She looks vaguely intimidated by the task but attempts to comply. She climbs on to the bed on her hands and knees and after interminable moving around, ends up sitting cross-legged facing to one side of the bed. She says to the examiner "I suppose you want my head on the pillow," as if this were an unreasonable requirement. She tries to comply several more times but is ultimately unsuccessful. In a second test, she sits facing the examiner and is asked to move her right hand back and forth between her nose and the examiner's upheld index finger (the "finger-to-nose" test). She manages to do this reasonably accurately, albeit somewhat slowly and with continual correction of the trajectory of her movement. The examiner then tells her to repeat the maneuver, this time with her eyes closed, relying only on her memory of the position of his finger. She makes wide searching movements with her hand and ultimately succeeds only in grabbing the examiner's knee. A CT scan reveals evidence of a focal degenerative process (known as a lobar atrophy) remarkably delimited to area 7 (Fig. 12-18). (From Stark M, Coslett HB, Saffran EM. Impairment of an egocentric map of locations: Implications for perception and action. Cognitive Neuropsych 13:481–523, 1996.)*

**Comment:** *The essential nature of the bizarre disorder exhibited by this patient is not entirely clear, but it appears that she has lost a critical part of the neural representation of her internal spatial map. In order for us to position our bodies in space, we must correctly align our body/head coordinate system with the coordinate system defined by the world around us. This patient has severe impairment in this capacity, hence her difficulty in getting into parking spaces, getting her body into a chair at the meeting, and getting into bed. When doing the finger-to-nose maneuver with eyes open she is able to rely on constant visual guidance to get her finger to the target. However, with eyes closed, she must rely on the relationship of her own coordinate system to her memory of the environmental coordinate system and the place of the examiner's finger in it and she fails miserably. Area 7 appears to be particularly crucial to the alignment of internal and external spatial coordinate systems. Area 7 is a polymodal cortex receiving input from visual and somatosensory association cortices. This is precisely the type of input that would be most useful to aligning our bodies in space.*

## EMOTIONAL PERCEPTION AND EXPRESSION

Emotions are complex processes that incorporate a number of major functional components and represent another example of a distributed representation. In a later section (limbic system) we will discuss the genesis of emotional feeling. Here we will consider only emotional expression (*affect*) and emotional perception. The neural processes involved and the anatomic location are not nearly so well understood as in language. Thus, our discussion will be limited to things we are reasonably sure of.

Emotional perception derives not just from the meaning of the words people say to us but also from the meaning conveyed in tone of voice and facial expression. If someone says "I really like you" in a sarcastic tone of voice, we know to disregard the linguistic content and not expect any favors from this person. If they say it in a tone consistent with the linguistic content but their facial expression is at odds with both, we will be suspicious about the sincerity of the statement. These judgments reflect processing of speech *prosody* (modulation of tone of voice and vocal emphasis) and facial expression. This decoding of affective content occurs substantially in the right hemisphere. Different neural networks in the right hemisphere appear to be crucial to our ability to endow our speech with emotional prosody and to generate appropriate facial expressions, that is the encoding of affective content. Case 12-12 illustrates the effects of severe deficits in affective decoding and encoding.

**Higher Neural Functions**

## Case 12-12

### Loss of Expression and Comprehension of Emotion due to Right Hemisphere Stroke

*A 55-year-old woman experiences a large right hemisphere stroke. When seen in clinic 3 months later, she demonstrates remarkable recovery of motor function and has only subtle impairment in dexterity of her left hand. She does not seem especially happy about this recovery. In fact, her affect in general seems to be quite flat. Her responses to your greetings as you say hello and to your enthusiasm about her recovery are perfunctory, she shows little change in facial expression throughout the clinic visit, and she speaks in a near monotone. Her husband is deeply troubled. He takes you aside after the clinic visit and tells you his wife is no longer the same woman. She seems cold and indifferent. Since her hospitalization, he lost his job but a month later managed to get a new one with better opportunities and a higher salary. His wife's response on each occasion was perfunctory. He feels guilty about criticizing her given the tragic event that has occurred and he wonders what he has done to offend her. He cannot understand their difficulty in communicating because before the stroke they always had an extraordinarily close*

*relationship. (We are indebted to Kenneth M. Heilman for this case.)*

**Comment:** *This patient exhibits phenomena very common after right hemisphere strokes. She has severe impairment in her ability to decipher speech prosody and read facial expression and comparable loss of ability to endow her own speech and facial expression with appropriate emotional tone. These "receptive" and "productive" components of affective expression can be dissociated. That is, perception may be much more severely impaired than production, or vice versa. The disorders in affective function exhibited by patients with right hemisphere strokes often make them seem cold and indifferent to the examiner. Close family members are likely to impute psychological explanations, as in this case, leading to guilt and endless rumination over possible causes. The lay public is generally not aware that personality is encoded in the brain, no less than language or motor function. As personality is a complex, extensively distributed brain function, it may be altered in various ways by lesions in a variety of locations. It is very important for clinicians to explain the ramifications of these lesions to family members.*

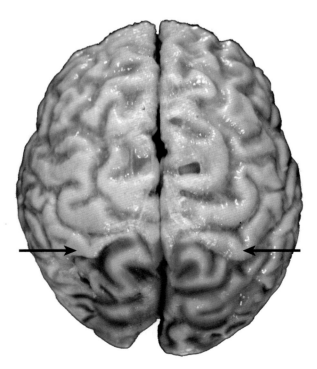

**Figure 12-18** Lesion in Case 12-11 (the postcentral gyri are indicated by arrows).

# PRACTICE 12-3

**A.** An 80-year-old right-handed man suddenly develops language impairment due to a stroke. He talks constantly but his language consists almost entirely of incomprehensible *neologisms* (words with one or more phonemic substitutions). He cannot name objects and his comprehension is poor. Locate his lesion. Would you expect him to be hemiparetic?

**B.** A 35-year-old right-handed woman experiences an intracerebral hemorrhage as a result of an arteriovenous malformation of the corpus callosum. Much of the corpus callosum is destroyed. Ultimately she enjoys a dramatic recovery and to the casual observer she appears perfectly normal. Do you think her ability to use tools with her left hand will be normal (allowing for her lesser left hand dexterity)? Why or why not?

What about her ability to identify numbers traced on her left hand (*graphesthesia*)?

**C.** A 72-year-old man develops insidiously progressive anomia. His elemental neurologic examination is normal. The referring physician is concerned about the possibility of a left temporoparietal brain tumor. You additionally elicit a history of getting lost, first in relatively unfamiliar parts of town, most recently in his own neighborhood. This problem is most likely due to damage to what part of the brain? Does this increase or decrease your concern regarding a brain tumor?

**D.** Consider again Case 12-12. You say to her "The man won the lottery," but you say it in a very sad tone of voice. When you ask her how you sound, what do you expect her answer to be? Discuss these observations in terms of distributed representations.

# Cycle 12-4

# The Limbic System

## Objectives

1. Be able to describe the role of the limbic system in defining the subjective properties of perceptions and the evidence of this role in our sense of value and emotional experience.

2. Be able to describe briefly the relationship of the limbic system to the fight/flight response.

3. Be able to list the major structures of the limbic system.

4. Be able to list the primitive drives that are related largely to hypothalamic function.

5. Be able to describe briefly the consequences of lesions of the amygdala and the lateral septal nuclei.

6. Be able to describe briefly the James theory of definition of limbic values in terms of patterns of autonomic activity, together with the neuroanatomy implicated in this theory.

## LIMBIC FUNCTION: THE ASSIGNMENT OF VALUE

Our senses provide the means by which we define the *objective* properties of stimuli about us. The limbic system provides the means for defining *subjective* properties. Implicit in the term "subjective" is the *assignment of value*. The limbic system does precisely this but it does so on myriad dimensions that neuroscience has yet to define in any principled way. The sound of a few bars from a familiar tune evokes the memory of an intimate moment experienced perhaps decades ago, together with the rush of pleasure that accompanied that experience. Witnessing an athletic triumph evokes one's own recall of the feeling of athletic accomplishment together with admiration, vicarious enjoyment, a sense of human courage, and myriad other feelings. Hearing the word "Auschwitz" evokes not just recalled images from photographs one has seen but also a sense of unspeakable evil and horror. The feelings underlying love, altruism, generosity, ethics, and morals, as well as hate, resentment, jealousy, and greed, are all generated by the limbic system. We commonly refer to many of these feelings as emotions. Our perception or recall of a stimulus actually corresponds to a distributed representation composed of two major parts. One part, our inner "feeling" about the perception, corresponds to a particular pattern of neural activity within the limbic system. In many ways, it is the most important part because it conveys a sense of value. The other part, which provides the basis for those aspects of the perception that we can actually describe to others, is defined by a particular pattern of activity in sensory and polymodal association cortices.

Although limbic-generated value immeasurably enhances our sensory experiences with an enormous pallet of emotional color, its principal adaptive function undoubtedly lies in the criteria it provides for a number of productive brain processes. These processes include deciding what is important to remember, what stimuli to attend to, and what actions to take. We will discuss each one of these in later cycles of this chapter. However, at this point it is worth noting a potentially crucial adaptive response that depends in a critical way upon the limbic system: the fight/flight response. As Walter Cannon originally theorized, the limbic system endows certain perceptions with the sense of extreme urgency that leads to fight or flight. Obviously, any organism that took a casual approach to life-threatening situations would not survive long.

## LIMBIC ANATOMY

At this point we will review the major structures composing the limbic system and what is known about their function. The principal effector organ of the limbic system is the hypothalamus. It is to the limbic system what the precentral gyrus is to motor systems. The hypothalamus is linked via multisynaptic pathways to the sympathetic and parasympathetic components of the autonomic nervous system (Fig. 12-19; see Chapter 11). Sympathetic projections from the hypothalamus ultimately synapse on preganglionic cells within the intermediate zone of the spinal cord extending from spinal level T1 to L2. Cells in the intermediate zone of the cord project to postganglionic neurons in the vertebral and more distal chain ganglia. Cells within these ganglia then project to viscera, blood vessels, exocrine glands, and skin.

Parasympathetic projections from the hypothalamus ultimately project to the dorsal efferent nucleus of the vagus nerve and to parasympathetic neurons in the sacral spinal cord. Cells at these loci in turn project to viscera via parasympathetic ganglia. All the targets of autonomic projections reciprocate with afferent autonomic projections that supply the central nervous system with data on the autonomic tone of the body. These afferent pathways ultimately project to the limbic system, many by way of the nucleus of the solitary tract.

The hypothalamus is also implicated in a host of complex neuroendocrine functions including adrenocortical, thyroid, and gonadotropin function. These hormonal systems, while serving crucial biologic functions, also act directly on receptors in the central nervous system, some of which are involved in autonomic and limbic functions.

*Hypothalamic circuitry provides the basis for value judgments related to some very basic functions*

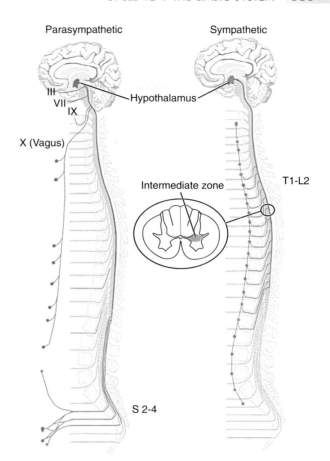

**Figure 12-19** Hypothalamic-autonomic system pathways.

*such as hunger, thirst, and primitive components of sexual drive.* However, the rich palette of value judgments we have already alluded to is based on links between the hypothalamus and more complex intermediate limbic effector organs, the amygdala and the lateral septal nuclei (Fig. 12-20). These nuclei are in turn linked to what might be viewed as limbic association cortices: the cingulate gyrus, the temporal poles, and portions of the insula. Limbic nuclei and limbic association cortices are also linked to other brainstem nuclei involved in autonomic function, to brainstem structures implicated in responses to pain (an emotion-provoking stimulus), such as the periaqueductal gray, and to brainstem structures that define arousal or the degree of wakefulness, which are critical to preparing us for definitive action in response to a threatening stimulus (see Cycle 12-7). Finally, the limbic system is connected to association cortices throughout the brain. These connections provide the means by which perceptions and memories are accorded a value component.

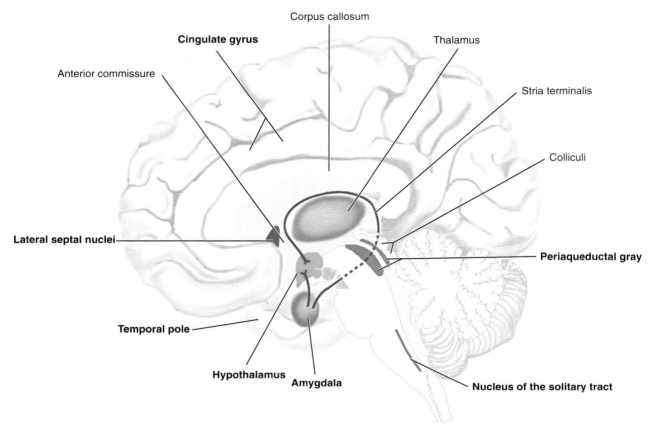

**Figure 12-20** The limbic system (structures are in bold type). The insula is not illustrated because of its more lateral location. With the exceptions of amygdalar connections to the hypothalamus via the stria terminalis and the ventral amygdalofugal pathway, connections between structures are not indicated.

## EFFECTS OF LIMBIC LESIONS

The precise ways in which these various components of the limbic system function are not well understood. The general flavor of the function of the amygdala and the lateral septal nuclei has been best captured in animal experiments. For decades free-roaming macaque monkeys on the island of Cayo Santiago in the Caribbean have provided investigators an opportunity to study these animals in a relatively unrestricted setting. It is clear from these studies that macaque society is strongly and rigidly ordered. Early on, individual monkeys learn their status within the group and develop the repertoire of behaviors appropriate to that status. The penalties for status-inappropriate behavior are very high: immediate vicious attack by the offended superior with general acquiescence, if not support, by

other members of the colony of both higher and lower rank. In this setting, an experiment was performed in which monkeys who had undergone bilateral amygdalectomy were reintroduced to their tribes. As these amygdalectomized animals are unusually placid and easily handled, there was no particular reason to believe there would be difficulty when they again mingled with other colony members. Against all expectation, however, they rapidly came under repeated attack. Careful observation provided some clues to this seeming paradox. In interacting with other colony members, the amygdalectomized monkeys no longer seemed to be restricted by social mores. They unhesitatingly took food from their superiors, and males courted females claimed by monkeys of superior rank. They seemed absolutely fearless in the conduct of these behaviors even though they were repeatedly attacked. Obviously we cannot be absolutely sure what transpired in these monkeys' brains during these encounters. However, it is not likely that they lost all knowledge of correct behavior because this knowledge is probably widely distributed. Instead, they seem to have lost the complex feelings, normally derived from amygdalar activity, that would normally constrain their behavior. Consequently, their behavior was largely governed by more elementary feelings defined by the hypothalamus itself, such as hunger and sexual drive. The hypothalamic "drive" was in effect released by the loss of amygdalar input. This general pattern of release of lower centers following damage to or disconnection from higher centers, first explicated by British neurologist Hughlings Jackson early in this century, has been demonstrated repeatedly throughout the nervous system. The Babinski response discussed in motor systems is another excellent example.

Other animal experiments have provided some clues to the function of the lateral septal nuclei. Animals such as cats and rats that are maintained in laboratory environments are generally not handled frequently and shown the affection given to domestic pets. If they are extensively handled, they will behave very much like pets. However, more typically their behavior reflects to some degree the mix of fear, vigilance, and defense that characterizes feral creatures. When given the opportunity to flee from human contact, they will do so. When cornered, they will demonstrate rage-like behavior and defend themselves very effectively. After ablation (destruction) of the lateral septal nuclei, these animals will demonstrate such rage and propensity for attack under far less provocative circumstances, often leading investigators to characterize them as vicious. A more reasonable interpretation is that the normal feelings in these animals evoked by the experimental situation are magnified such that they are provoked to fight behavior by far less threatening stimuli. Presumably this reflects, in part, the release of behavior driven by the amygdala and the hypothalamus. Recall that amygdalectomized animals are unnaturally placid.

Neither of these examples of animal behavior following ablation of limbic effector organs provides detailed insight into the functions of the amygdala and the lateral septal nuclei, which are complex and very difficult to study. Nevertheless, they provide a sense of the role of the feelings generated by these structures, the crucial nature of such feelings in behavior, and the level of complexity these organs bring to the relatively simpler behaviors founded in hypothalamic circuitry.

## THEORIES OF LIMBIC MECHANISMS

One of the major challenges of limbic system research has been to determine how emotional feelings are actually generated. In 1890, William James proposed that emotion-provoking stimuli induce changes in autonomic outflow from the central nervous system that are in turn monitored via visceral afferents that define, through the pattern of activity evoked in the brain, the actual emotional feeling. Even today, this theory remains compelling. Various attempts to test it, for example, by measuring emotional responses in patients with transections of the cervical spinal cord, have always been imperfect but nonetheless have suggested that the long autonomic circuit from brain to body and back to brain probably does at least influence emotional feeling. Other experiments suggest that emotional feelings are strongly colored by the cognitive state of the individual. This conclusion comes as no surprise as we now recognize that all our perceptions reflect widely distributed representations. An appealing adaptation of James' theory was that proposed by Mandler, namely, that although emotional feeling continues to be modulated by the long autonomic circuit throughout life, much of our emotional feeling as adults consists of the evocation of primitive memories formed in infancy and early childhood via feedback through the autonomic circuit. Presumably these memories are represented in limbic association cortices such as the insula, the temporal poles, and the cingulate gyrus.

Because of the particular importance of the value component of perception that is generated by the limbic system, disorders of the limbic system have a profound impact on perceptual experience and behavior. This impact is amply demonstrated in psychiatric disorders. However, because psychiatric disorders are best viewed as multisystem disorders, we will not consider them until Section 12-9.

## PRACTICE 12-4

**A.** A 45-year-old man presents to clinic with a complaint, chiefly by family members, of sudden and unpredictable mood swings. He is a successful businessman, happily married with three children, all of whom are doing well. There is neither a history nor evidence by examination of depression or any other psychiatric disorder. He is a warm and engaging person who immediately wins the friendship and respect of the physician examining him. However, near the end of the examination, he suddenly becomes surly and hostile, to the point that he is almost unmanageable, and is ushered by his embarrassed wife out to the waiting room. She returns to assure the physician that he is already calming down. She notes that this is precisely the type of episode that has been occurring more and more often lately. An electroencephalogram (EEG) reveals evidence of epileptiform activity. An MRI scan reveals an approximately 1-cm diameter lesion. Given the information that an acute epileptic discharge usually has the effect of a temporary destructive lesion, locate this patient's lesion.

**B.** A number of years ago, neuroscientists discovered that stimulation of certain portions of the hypothalamus in experimental animals would induce "rage." Cats would arch their backs, hair on end, snarling and hissing, and strike viciously if approached. Would you expect similar results of such stimulation in a pet? Why or why not?

**C.** Can one be frightened to death, or is this just an old saying? Why or why not?

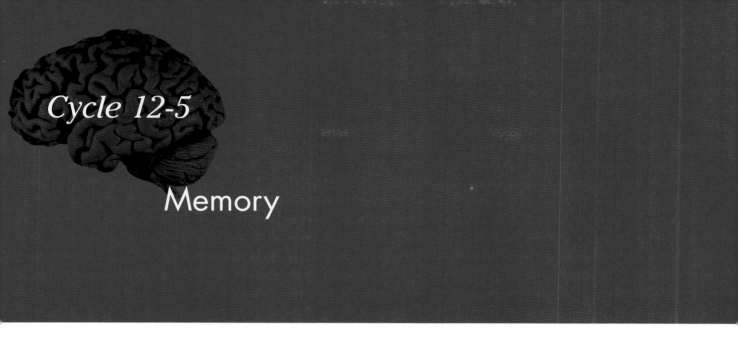

# Cycle 12-5

# Memory

## Objectives

1. Be able to define the neuronal loci of information storage in the brain.

2. Be able to define the following terms and relate them to cerebral structures or neural phenomena: Hebbian learning, remote memory, declarative memory, semantic memory, episodic memory, recent memory, immediate memory, working memory, procedural or skill memory, and classical conditioning.

3. Be able to name the major structures in the hippocampal system, describe the roles of this system in memory acquisition and consolidation, and note the consequences of lesions of this system.

4. Be able to explain why thiamine deficiency and disseminated white matter disease may affect the hippocampal system.

## THE NEURAL BASIS OF MEMORY

Ramón y Cajal and Tanzi independently proposed over 100 years ago that information is stored in the brain in terms of the strengths of interneuronal connections. However, it was Donald Hebb who, in the 1940s, really developed this idea. In particular, Hebb proposed that learning occurs through alteration in the strength of neuronal interconnections and that the strength of the connection between any two neurons grows to the extent that those neurons are simultaneously active. This "Hebbian" learning algorithm has been widely adopted in one form or another in computer models of the brain (see Cycle 12-8). A large body of circumstantial evidence suggests that it accurately, if somewhat simplistically, represents what actually happens in the brain. There is, for example, a large amount of literature on a process known as long-term potentiation (LTP) whereby interneuronal connection strengths in various parts of the brain are enhanced by electrical or natural stimulation.

## TYPES OF MEMORY

There are several forms of memory in the brain, all based on interneural connection strengths (Table 12-2). *Remote memory* consists of the sum total of information stored in the brain. Remote memory can be conveniently divided into declarative and nondeclarative memory. *Declarative memory* consists of discrete pieces of information. Declarative memory composed of information unrelated to any particular place or time, such as the material you are reading right now, is referred to as *semantic memory*. Declarative memory that is time- or place-tagged, such as your memory of who is with you as you read this and where you are reading it, is referred to as *episodic memory*. Declarative memory is stored in association cortices

*559*

**TABLE 12-2 Types of Memory**

| Type | Nature | Substrate | Locus |
| --- | --- | --- | --- |
| Remote | Stored information | Interneuronal connection strengths | Association cortices |
|   Declarative | Pieces of infomation | | |
|     Semantic | Generic information | | |
|     Episodic | Time- and place-specific information | | |
|   Nondeclarative | | | |
|     Procedural | Skill memory | | Motor and premotor cortices, cerebellum |
|     Classical conditioning | Associations | | Various |
| Recent | Declarative memory storage | Interneuronal connection strengths | Hippocampal system |
| Immediate/working | Declarative memory buffer | Specific maintained patterns of neural activity | Association cortices |

throughout the brain. Because any one memory is variably distributed across a number of cortices, it will not be eliminated completely by damage to a part of the brain.

Nondeclarative memory includes a variety of different types of information. One major category is *procedural or skill memory*. As you improve your tennis game, you acquire procedural memory. Procedural memory is probably stored largely in motor systems in the brain, including motor and premotor cortex (Brodmann's areas 4 and 6) and the cerebellum.

Another major category is memory acquired through classical conditioning. The prototypic example is the association Pavlov's dogs learned between a bell ringing and imminent food. Associations acquired through conditioning are stored in various places within the central nervous system according to their particular nature.

The term "*recent*" memory is often used to refer to the process of acquisition of new declarative memory. The term "*immediate*" memory is often used to refer to information that is being temporarily held in mind. A good example would be a phone number or street directions. In general, immediate memory consists of *working memory*, which is generally defined by the transient activation of groups of neurons in parts of the brain specific to the memory. Thus, immediate or working memory of a phone number corresponds to a particular pattern of activity (not connection strengths) in auditory association cortex (or ventral visual association cortex if we looked at the written number). The human brain has a special device for enhancing

auditory-verbal recent memory—the process of silent rehearsal. Thus, we can keep refreshing our working memory of a phone number by repeating it silently over and over. No comparable device exists for working memory involving other domains of higher neural function. Because immediate or working memory corresponds to temporary patterns of activity, rather than connection strengths, it is not a true memory. We will discuss these entities at greater length later in the chapter when we talk about attention and selective engagement. Finally, the phrase "short-term memory" is used in varying ways by different neuroscientific disciplines; for this reason, we will avoid using this term.

## MEMORY ACQUISITION

It appears that conditioning and the acquisition of procedural memory occur by relatively simple processes not far removed from the Hebbian principle. Both these types of learning develop through many repetitions, each of which incrementally adjusts connection strengths. However, declarative memory clearly incorporates an additional component because it can be established through a single exposure to a piece of information. The establishment of declarative memories seems to absolutely require the participation of a special system, the core of which is the hippocampus. The hippocampal system is intimately connected to immediately adjoining structures, such as the subiculum and the parahippocampal gyrus, as well as the

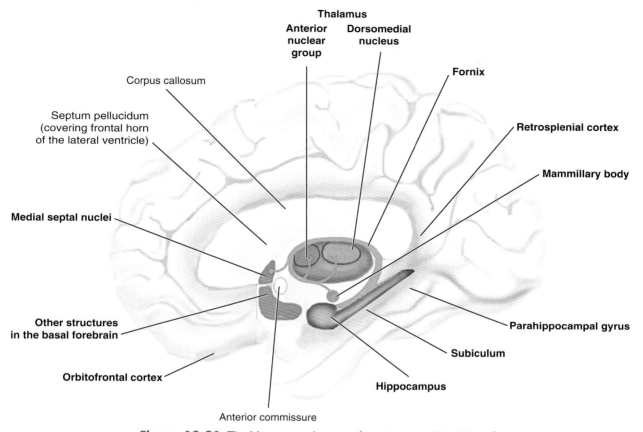

**Figure 12-21** The hippocampal system (structures are in bold type).

cortex overlying the amygdala, two major nuclear groups in the thalamus (the dorsomedial nucleus and the anterior nuclear group), the mammillary bodies, cortex immediately posterior to the splenium of the corpus callosum (retrosplenial cortex), the medial septal nuclei, and the basal forebrain—the neural tissue on the undersurface of the frontal lobes immediately anterior to the pituitary stalk (Fig. 12-21). Because declarative memories are predominantly represented as strengths of neuronal interconnections in the cerebral cortex, the hippocampal system depends on long efferent and afferent white matter pathways to and from association, polymodal, and supramodal cortices to achieve the changes in connection strengths necessary to encode new memories. For this reason, any disease affecting cerebral white matter will be associated with impairment in declarative memory function.

The hippocampus and its associated structures have long been considered part of the limbic system. However, recent research has clearly dissociated the functions of these two systems (despite their phys-ical proximity), except to the extent that the limbic system helps to distinguish what is important to remember.

The hippocampal system appears to be crucial both to the *acquisition* of new declarative memories and to their *consolidation*. Consolidation consists of the process whereby the most central aspects of a complex of memories become more and more entrenched over time even as many of the details are lost. The bulk of memory consolidation appears to occur over the first 2 to 3 years after we acquire a memory.

Recent advances in the science of neural network function (see Cycle 12-8) have provided considerable insight into the purpose and mechanisms of hip-pocampal function. Declarative memory, as we have noted, can be acquired all at once, in a single exposure. Unfortunately, if new information is added all at once to a neural network that already stores many pieces of old information, much of the old information will be lost. Only if the network is able to repeatedly rehearse old information between exposures to new

**Higher Neural Functions**

information will it eventually be able to encode both old and new without significant losses. The hippocampus enables this through its capacity for almost instantly (within 1 second) forming new connections between cortical neurons, albeit very long ones looping from the cortex to the parahippocampal gyrus, the hippocampus itself, the subiculum, the parahippocampal gyrus again, and back to the cerebral cortex. These incredibly long connections serve as the temporary basis of new memory. They also serve as teachers to the cortical neuronal networks involved, repeatedly exposing them to the new information between rehearsals of old memories. There is now accumulating evidence that this interleaved teaching and rehearsal process, which constitutes memory consolidation, occurs during dream sleep. Long cortical-hippocampal-cortical connections probably serve as the permanent basis for memories that are not readily consolidated, such as memories of autobiographic events (which are episodic memories).

Because declarative and nondeclarative memories rely on completely different systems, it is common to see disorders of one system at the same time that the other is perfectly preserved. The patients described in the next two cases demonstrate problems with recent memory encoding (Case 12-13) and remote memory consolidation (Case 12-14) caused by lesions of the hippocampal system.

## Case 12-13

### Amnesia due to Bilateral Temporal Lobe Resection

HM (the most famous and extensively studied patient in the history of behavioral neuroscience) was a young man when Henry Scoville performed bilateral temporal lobectomies on him at the Montreal Neurological Institute in an effort to treat his intractable epilepsy. Temporal lobectomy remains a mainstay in the treatment of intractable epilepsy, but largely due to the experience with HM, bilateral lobectomies are never done. HM was never able to acquire a single new piece of information. He had anterograde amnesia. For example, many years after his surgery, he still remembered the way to the place he lived before the operation but he had no idea of the location or address of his new home. On the other hand, he was able to acquire considerable skill on the rotor-pursuit task, a test of procedural memory acquisition. The device used in this task looks like a

## Case 12-13—cont'd

phonograph with a small metal spot on the turntable. The experimental subject is given a "wand" and his task is to keep the tip of the wand in contact with the spot as much as possible as the turntable spins at different speeds. HM acquired his skill at the rotor pursuit task even though every time he had another session with the device, he swore he had never seen it before and he had to be given complete instructions again.

**Comment:** HM underwent surgical removal of both hippocampi. Thus, he had no means for encoding new declarative memories. However, skill on the rotor pursuit task involved the development of procedural memory, which does not depend on the hippocampal system. Patients with degenerative diseases such as Huntington's disease, which at least initially involve motor systems to a greater degree than the hippocampus, demonstrate impairment in the acquisition of procedural memory with relative preservation of ability to acquire declarative memory.

## Case 12-14

### Amnesia due to Hippocampal Damage from Prolonged Seizures

A 35-year-old engineer developed encephalitis complicated by continuous seizure activity (status epilepticus). To control his seizures, he had to be kept in deep pentobarbital coma for 3 weeks. Eventually his seizures subsided to the point that they could be controlled with high doses of conventional anticonvulsants, thus allowing him eventually to leave the hospital. Unfortunately, the prolonged seizures caused extensive damage to the hippocampi. When he left the hospital, he had severe impairment in his ability to learn new pieces of information. He also remarked in amazement to his wife on the strange appearance of many of the automobiles he saw. He had little or no recollection of the appearance of models manufactured over the prior 2 to 3 years. He recognized his young children (aged 2 and 4) but could not remember the experience of their births or any of the things he had done with them. He also had impaired recall of personal events throughout his life.

## Case 12-14—cont'd

**Comment:** *This patient, like HM, lost his ability to acquire new declarative memories (anterograde amnesia) because of severe bilateral hippocampal damage which was clearly demonstrable when he died about a year later due to aspiration of gastric contents during a grand mal seizure. He also demonstrates the fact that the hippocampus was necessary to maintain memories acquired over the prior 2 to 3 years which were only partially consolidated at the time of his encephalitis. Finally, he demonstrates the fact that the hippocampus instantiates the connections representing storage of long-term episodic memories of personal life events, which may not lend themselves to consolidation in cerebral association cortices. This is because, very often, a memory of a particular event at a particular place and time can be integrated to a very limited degree with one's general knowledge. Thus, lesions of the hippocampal system produce both an anterograde and a selective retrograde amnesia.*

## PRACTICE 12-5

**A.** A 50-year-old chronic alcoholic has had repeated bouts of Wernicke's encephalopathy (lethargy or stupor and ophthalmoplegia) caused by thiamine deficiency. This disorder causes hemorrhagic necrosis of the tissue along the Sylvian aqueduct and immediately adjacent to the third ventricle. Would you expect him to have memory impairment? What type? (Hint: What gray matter structures critical to memory formation are immediately adjacent to the third ventricle?)

**B.** A patient undergoes left temporal lobectomy for treatment of a refractory seizure disorder. How would you expect him to perform on a test requiring memorization of word lists? On a test of ability to remember complex drawings? Why?

**C.** Patients with multiple sclerosis may develop extensive demyelinative lesions in the deep cerebral white matter. Would you expect this to affect memory? What types? Why?

**D.** A 60-year-old man recovers from herpes simplex encephalitis following treatment with acyclovir. Nevertheless, he has sustained extensive damage to the inferior surface of his temporal lobes bilaterally. When he is asked to name pictures of things, would you expect him to have more trouble remembering the names of tools or of animals (refer back to Cycle 12-2 if you need to).

**E.** Patients with an unusual degenerative central nervous system disorder known as corticobasal degeneration or Rebeiz syndrome have Parkinsonian symptoms due to basal ganglia disease and apraxia due to damage to premotor and parietal cortex. Would you expect them to have memory impairment? What type? Why?

**F.** An overconfident world-class tennis player is a little too casual during the week before Wimbledon, misses a fair amount of practice, and suffers an ego-deflating debacle at the tournament. What does this tell you about procedural memory?

**G.** Explain the provocative effect of certain smells on memory in terms of the anatomic proximity of the olfactory apparatus to the parahippocampal gyrus.

# Frontal Systems

## Objectives

1. Be able to define the fundamental role of frontal lobe systems and the circumstances under which their role is most crucial.

2. Be able to describe the two major plan formulation subsystems within prefrontal cortex, their major connections, the way in which they define behavior, and the consequences of lesions of these systems upon behavior.

3. Understand the concept of dynamic balance between dorsolateral and orbitofrontal systems, provide a clinical example of imbalance, and explain it.

4. Be able to describe the Jacksonian concept of release of function and account for utilization behavior in terms of this concept.

5. Be able to describe the functions of dorsomedial frontal cortex and the consequences of lesions in this region.

Frontal systems consist of prefrontal cortex and its links via white matter pathways to association cortices throughout the brain and to a number of subcortical structures (most of the limbic system, hippocampal input and output structures, the basal ganglia, and the thalamus). Injuries to the prefrontal cortex, many of these connected structures, or the intervening white matter pathways may produce features of frontal systems dysfunction.

The purpose of frontal systems is to develop, choose, and carry out plans, a process we will refer to as *intention*. These may be elaborate, long-range plans sustained over months or years, such as a decision to prepare for a certain career, or they may be very simple, short-range plans, such as what direction to look in the next 500 ms. These plans may be reflected in overt behavior or they may be inapparent, as in the processes comprising thinking. To choose a plan, one must carefully analyze the requirements of the situation and tailor the plan to those requirements, a process that defines judgment. To carry out a plan requires initiative, which combines linkage of the plan to a source of motivation and the engagement of motor systems to start the execution of the plan.

In the course of daily life, we generate thousands of plans and actually execute a large percentage of them. Most of these plans involve heavily overlearned routines that come to us automatically. For example, we can get up in the morning, shower, groom, get dressed, prepare and eat breakfast, and travel to work with very little thought beyond perhaps the choice of clothes for the day. All the plans that enable us to do this are represented in memories instantiated in sensory and polymodal association cortices, supramodal cortices, and premotor cortex. The only thing that frontal systems need to do is to participate in the release of the appropriate plan at the appropriate time. As simple as this sounds, we do see disorders in this aspect of frontal function in patients with certain brain lesions, as Case 12-15 demonstrates.

---

### Case 12-15

#### Utilization Behavior in a Patient with a Frontal Lobe Lesion

*A famous French neurologist, Francoise Lhermitte, described the behavior of several patients with very large lesions of one of the frontal poles. One older gentleman was presented at grand rounds at Salpêtrière in Paris. In Europe these presentations are formal affairs involving a large number of people, all paying great deference to the professor. Lhermitte had placed a number of objects on the table in front of the patient, including a drinking glass, a pitcher of water, a pen and some writing paper, several pairs of eyeglasses, and a urine receptacle (a "duck"). Without invitation or suggestion and in front of the grand entourage including the esteemed Professor, the patient helped himself to a glass of water, wrote a brief letter, successfully put on two pairs of eyeglasses (simultaneously) and attempted to put a third on top of the other two, and then dropped his trousers and urinated into the duck.*

*Lhermitte subsequently brought another patient to his apartment. Lhermitte had taken down some of his artwork and left it lying about. As the patient entered he remarked "Oh wonderful, an art gallery." When he noticed the paintings sitting around, he requested a hammer and some nails, which he proceeded to drive into the walls here and there in order to hang the pictures. As he entered Lhermitte's bedroom and noticed the turned-down bed with neatly folded pajamas, he promptly got undressed, put on the pajamas, and got into bed.*

**Comment:** *The behavior exhibited by these patients is known as utilization behavior. It represents well-developed plans requiring essentially no thought in their execution, executed properly but at an inappropriate time or place. Prefrontal damage led to improper release of these behaviors, just as spinal cord damage leads to the release of the nociceptive reflex, thereby producing Babinski signs. Both utilization behavior and Babinski signs are examples of the Jacksonian principle that higher neural systems both add a capacity for more complex function and act to inhibit lower systems.*

---

The most important function of frontal systems is the development of new plans to deal with *novel situations*. These plans need to be tailor-made to the precise requirements of the situation. Patients with frontal lesions, impaired in their ability to develop such plans, will often use a previously learned approach even though it is not exactly appropriate. When confronted with the less than perfect results of their actions, these patients will often remark "Oh, it's close enough," even when the results are quite poor. They have lost a capacity for the close, directed examination of their actions, self-criticism, and attempts at correction that are so critical to the success of the trial-and-error approach we normally take to novel problems.

## PREFRONTAL SYSTEMS THAT PARTICIPATE IN PLAN FORMULATION

In developing solutions to novel problems, we make use of two major types of criteria. One type is founded in the specific requirements of the task itself, that is, in *external* criteria. We use our senses to evaluate the situation and from this sensory analysis, develop a motor plan designed to deal with the problem. This sensory-linked planning process takes place in dorsolateral prefrontal cortex. *Dorsolateral prefrontal cortex* (Fig. 12-22) is well equipped for this role because it is heavily interconnected with sensory association cortices. Dorsolateral prefrontal lesions are associated with deficits in novel task performance that can readily be detected using specific neuropsychological tests.

The other major type of criteria we use in developing plans to deal with novel situations is *internal*. These criteria are the subjective judgments we bring to bear in defining our responses to stimuli. They include such relatively primitive criteria as fear, hunger, thirst, and sexual urge as well as more complex criteria such as love, envy, or jealousy. They also include complex and seemingly emotionless criteria such as ethics and morals. The drive that invests all these criteria is generated by the pattern of neural activity in the limbic system. This limbic-linked planning process occurs in *orbitofrontal cortex* (Fig. 12-22), which is well equipped for this aspect of behavior through its extensive connections to the limbic system. The overall pattern of behavior that is shaped by the orbitofrontal-limbic system defines a major component of *personality*. Lesions of orbitofrontal cortex result in deficits in

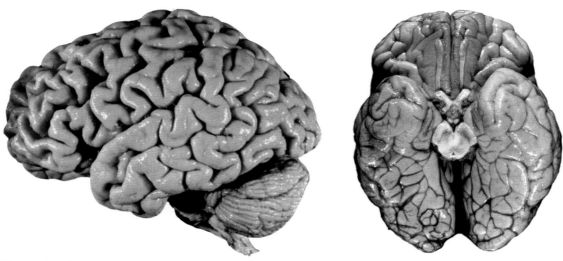

**Figure 12-22** *Left,* Dorsolateral prefrontal cortex (Brodmann's areas 9, 10, 46, 47). *Right,* Orbitofrontal pre-frontal cortex (Brodmann's areas 11 and 12).

behavior involving those novel situations that require subjective judgments and an assay of inner value (recall that the peculiar contribution of the limbic system is to provide a sense of value). By far the most common such situation is interaction with other human beings. Thus, patients with orbitofrontal lesions often exhibit inappropriate social behavior. They often also fail at complex tasks, the execution of which depends on ambition or sense of responsibility. In Case 12-16, we describe a patient with a lesion of left dorsolateral pre-frontal cortex and in Case 12-17, a patient with extensive lesions of orbitofrontal cortices.

## Case 12-16

### Frontal Systems Dysfunction due to Dorsolateral Frontal Lobe Damage

*A 45-year-old businessman is brought in by his wife because of problems he is experiencing at work. Although he remains enthusiastic about the future of his business, he has become somewhat lackadaisical in his daily work. He also seems to be having problems executing his work responsibilities and has become progressively more reliant on his administrative assistant. A review of systems uncovers the fact that he has been experiencing mild but persistent headaches for the last 6 months. His elementary neurologic examination is completely normal. An MRI scan reveals a 6-cm malignant tumor of the left frontal lobe.*

**Comment:** *This patient exhibits a classic dorsolateral frontal lobe syndrome, in this case caused by an infiltrating glial tumor. Even though his long-range work plans continue to be appropriately driven by internal value, he has a problem attaching that drive to his*

*daily work chores, something referred to as abulia—hence his lackadaisical behavior at work. His ability to develop novel strategies to deal with his various work responsibilities is impaired, hence his increasing reliance on his administrative assistant.*

*He is administered a modification of the Thurstone word fluency test: He is asked to produce in 1 minute as many words as he can think of beginning with the letter F; proper nouns and derivations (fast, faster, fastest, fasting) are not permitted. He immediately produces four words and then sits silently for the remainder of the minute.*

**Comment:** *The Thurstone word fluency test requires that the neural representation of one's dictionary be intact, and it requires the development and maintenance of a strategy to systematically search that dictionary in the peculiar fashion required by this test. This patient's performance is very poor (normal for a person in his*

## Case 12-16—cont'd

position would be >15) and quite characteristic of patients with dorsolateral frontal lobe impairment, particularly on the dominant or language side of the brain. It reflects failure to develop a search strategy and maintain that search.

He is administered the Trailmaking Test part B (Fig. 12-23). On this test he is required to draw a line from "1" to "A" to "2" to "B" and so on. He makes many mistakes in which he continues a numeric or alphabetic sequence, such as 1-2-3-4.

**Comment:** On the Trailmaking Test he is unable to regularly shift set from number to letter to number, and so forth. He is unable to resist the more natural tendency to follow a number or letter sequence.

Finally, he is administered the Wisconsin Card Sort Test (Fig. 12-24). On this test the examiner turns up 64 cards, one at a time. Some of the cards perfectly match one of the four cards shown in Figure 12-24. However, most provide only a partial match, being similar in color, form, or number of objects. For example, in Figure 12-24, the next card shows two red crosses. The subject could sort according to color, placing this card beneath the red triangle; he could sort according to number, placing this card beneath the two green stars; or he could sort according to form, placing this card beneath the three yellow crosses.

At the beginning of the test, the patient is supposed to sort according to the form of the objects. However, he is given no instructions and must discover the correct sorting criterion as the examiner pronounces "correct" or "incorrect" as the patient places each successive card in what he believes to be the appropriate stack. Once the patient has caught on and made 10 successive correct choices, the sorting criterion is changed without warning to color. After another 10 correct choices, it is changed again to number and so on. The patient being tested here takes about 10 trials before he catches on that the sorting criterion is form. When it eventually changes to color, he never succeeds in changing his strategy and makes erroneous choices for the remainder of the test.

**Comment:** On the Wisconsin Card Sort he fails to adequately scrutinize his mistakes and learn from them and thus is slow to figure out the first sorting criterion. Once he does figure it out, he is unable to give it up and develop a new set, that is, he tends to perseverate.

## Case 12-17

### Frontal Systems Dysfunction due to Orbitofrontal Damage

This famous case was reported by Eslinger and Damasio. The patient was a 35-year-old businessman, smart, rising rapidly in his business, highly respected by his peers, and regarded by his siblings as the family leader. He was happily married and had two children. He began to exhibit some behavioral problems that eventually led to the discovery of an enormous olfactory groove meningioma. This tumor and the surgery to resect it resulted in extensive damage to much of his frontal lobes, sparing only some of dorsolateral frontal cortex. Orbitofrontal cortex was obliterated (Fig. 12-25).

Following a prolonged recuperative period the patient underwent extensive neuropsychological testing, including tests of frontal function. He performed at well above average level on all these tests. Eventually he went back to work. Within a short time he was fired because of constant tardiness and lack of responsibility. He and his wife also soon divorced and he had a number of brief casual affairs. Eventually he married an older woman who evinced a somewhat maternal relationship with him. He put his life savings into a rather dubious "get rich quick" venture and lost the entire investment.

One night he went out to dinner with Drs. Eslinger and Damasio. They allowed him to choose the

*Continued*

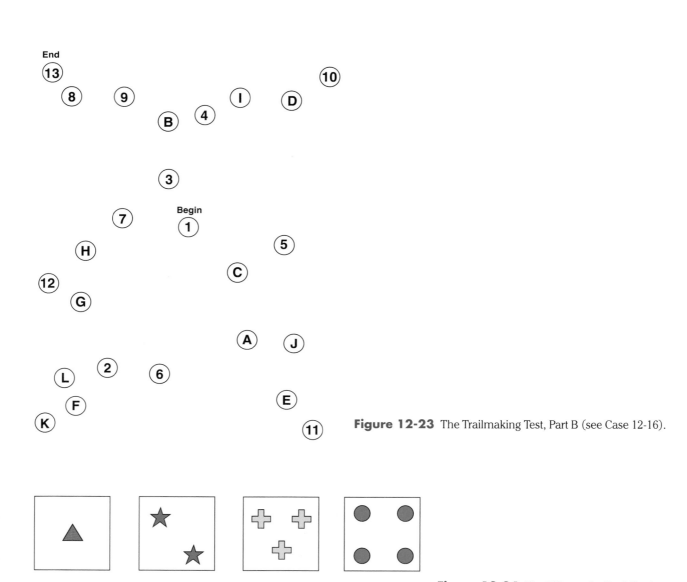

**Figure 12-23** The Trailmaking Test, Part B (see Case 12-16).

**Figure 12-24** The Wisconsin Card Sorting Task (see Case 12-16). (From Milner B. Some effects of frontal lobectomy in man. In Warren JM, Akert K (eds). The Frontal Granular Cortex and Behavior. New York, McGraw-Hill, 1964. Reproduced with permission of The McGraw-Hill Book Companies, Inc.)

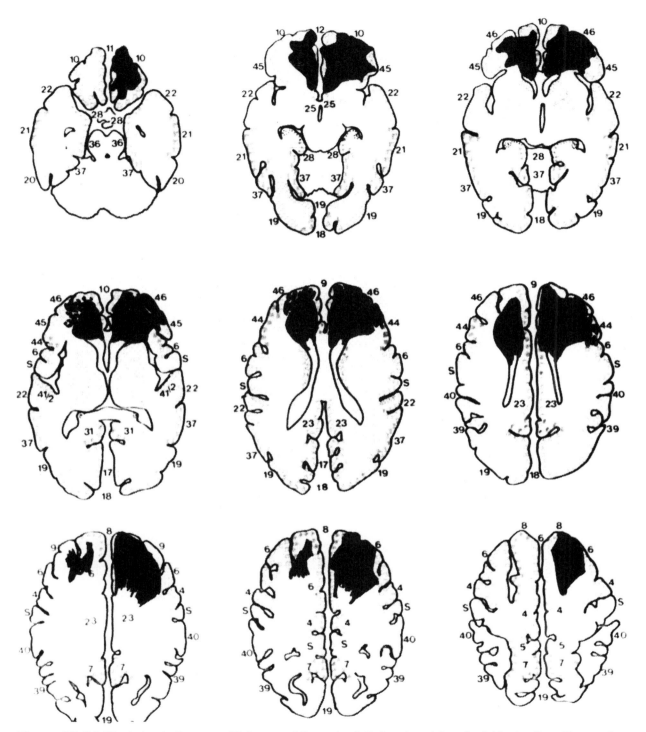

**Figure 12-25** The lesion in the case of Eslinger and Damasio plotted on templates of axial brain slices. The numbers designate Brodmann's areas (see Case 12-17). (From Eslinger PJ, Damasio AR. Severe disturbance of higher cognition after bilateral frontal lobe ablation: Patient EVR. Neurology 35:1731–1741, 1985. Reproduced with permission of Lippincott Williams & Willkins.)

## Case 12-17—cont'd

restaurant. On the way he described the establishment in detail, relishing the various items on the menu and features of the decor. When they finally arrived, he proceeded to tell them about another restaurant, again elaborating on its features as they drove to this establishment. This process continued until Drs. Eslinger and Damasio, quite hungry and tired of their experiment, decided to dictate a restaurant choice.

**Comment:** This patient exhibits a syndrome quite characteristic of patients with extensive orbitofrontal damage. The key feature is that even though he still has an intact limbic system and experiences a normal

palette of values in response to his various perceptions, he is unable to link these values to his plans for behavior. Thus, ambition and a sense of responsibility no longer govern his work behavior. He has lost the motivating force of the deep and complex value system that originally drove the loving relationship he had with his first wife and children. As often happens in such patients, his interpersonal relationships became relatively shallow. He was lured by the appeal of a get-rich-quick scheme because he could no longer bring to bear a plan that would inhibit or replace the "knee-jerk" response he made. On the other hand, when he was obliged to make the subjective decision necessary for a restaurant choice, he could not.

In thinking about frontal systems, it is natural to view the value-driven orbitofrontal subsystem as the ultimate arbiter of behavior. However, optimal behavior actually depends on a dynamic balance between orbitofrontal and dorsolateral systems articulated through a cascade of white matter connections between these two areas of the brain. Utilization behavior (Case 12-15) reflects, in part, behavior driven by dorsolateral frontal systems and inadequately inhibited (in effect, released) by orbitofrontal systems. The patient of Eslinger and Damasio (Case 12-17) attempted to make a restaurant choice strictly via criteria generated

through dorsolateral systems when in fact, orbitofrontal judgement is critical to this task.

## THE DORSOMEDIAL SYSTEM AND PLAN EXECUTION

Whereas dorsolateral and orbitofrontal systems are involved in the definition of behavior, a third major region of the frontal lobes, *dorsomedial cortex*, is involved in *initiating* and *sustaining* behavior, as demonstrated in Case 12-18.

## Case 12-18

### Frontal Systems Impairment due to Dorsomedial Damage

A 75-year-old gentleman is brought in by his family because of a 6-month history of progressive difficulty with walking and balance and a 4-month history of urinary incontinence. Further inquiry reveals that, whereas he was once gregarious, quite a raconteur, and invariably busy with any one of dozens of projects, he now spends his days quietly sitting alone, staring off into space (akinesia). He generally answers appropriately when asked a question, but only with a single word or short sentence without elaboration. If given several things to do, he will at best complete one of them (motor impersistence). For example, if asked to write a brief note, fold the paper, put it in an envelope,

and seal the envelope, he may simply write one word on the piece of paper. He cannot rise to a standing position without assistance. As he attempts to walk, his feet appear to be glued to the floor. Eventually he gets going with tiny steps and finally, under way, his stride lengthens and approaches normal. However, when required to turn, his walking again breaks down into a flurry of tiny steps and he nearly loses his balance (gait apraxia). His MR scan is shown in Figure 12-26.

**Comment:** The clinical features in this case indicate compromise of dorsomedial frontal systems. Thus, the patient has impairment in initiating and sustaining behavior (yielding akinesia and motor impersistence,

## Case 12-18—cont'd

respectively). He also exhibits compromise of motor systems subserving the legs and midline function in general, hence the gait disorder, termed a gait apraxia. Finally, he has urinary incontinence, reflecting compromise of structures in the parasagittal region important for urinary control, or their descending projections. These clinical features localize but they do not tell us the etiology. The MR scan (Fig. 12-26),

however, demonstrates that the likely etiology is obstruction of the flow of cerebrospinal fluid. Because this fluid is produced by the choroid plexus within the ventricles, the obstruction causes an increase in fluid pressure which, although intermittent in this type of hydrocephalus, causes progressive enlargement of the ventricular system. This in turn compresses the cerebral structures adjacent to the ventricles.

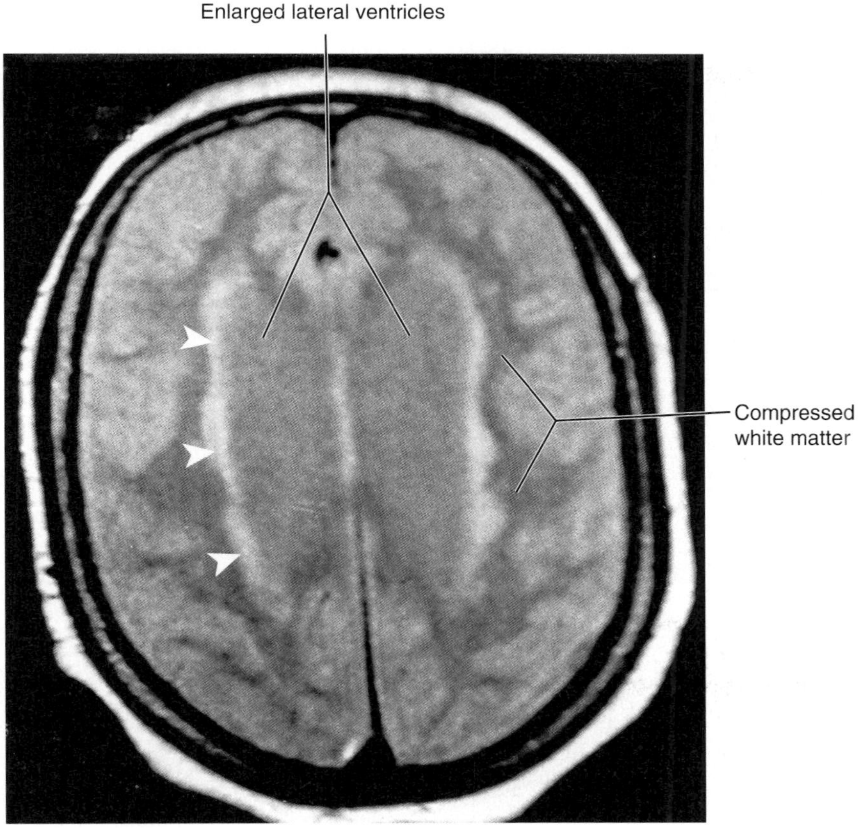

**Figure 12-26** Communicating hydrocephalus. The ventricular system is dilated and adjacent deep cerebral white matter is compressed. Intermittently increased pressure within the ventricular system results in direct flow of cerebrospinal fluid across the lining of the ventricles (the ependyma) into the adjacent periventricular tissue (*arrowheads*) (see Case 12-18).

Enlarged lateral ventricles

Compressed white matter

## PRACTICE 12-6

**A.** A 40-year-old patient has undergone surgical removal and radiation therapy of a frontal lobe tumor. When asked to copy a drawing of a house (Fig. 12-27), his production is barely recognizable as a house and it is characterized by perseverative retracing of lines. When this behavior is interrupted and he is asked whether his drawing resembles the target, he responds "close enough." He is asked to perform a task in which he holds his right hand lightly closed in a fist opposite the examiner's. When the examiner raises one finger, the patient is to immediately raise two. When the examiner raises two fingers, the patient is to immediately raise one (*contrasting programs*). The patient is absolutely unable to resist mimicking the examiner's movement (*echopraxia*). Where is this patient's lesion?

**B.** You are asked to evaluate a 30-year-old man with a known brain tumor. One glance at your name badge and he proceeds to address you by your first name. He is in fine humor and jokes about everything, including your choice in clothes. He leers at a passing nurse and speculates about what it would be like to have sex with her. He indicates that he has been hospitalized against his will as a result of chicanery by his wife who is putatively after his money. Where is this patient's lesion?

**C.** A 75-year-old man with a lifelong history of hypertension is brought in by his family because of a 3-year history of insidiously progressive loss of spontaneous activity (akinesia) and speech. He now spends his days sitting, staring off into space. Once garrulous, he is now difficult to engage in conversation. On being asked to detail his experiences in Europe during World War II, he responds "marched." In general, he answers all questions, however open-ended, with a single word or a short sentence. When given two-step commands, he will perform only one, usually the second. On a Thurstone word fluency test he produces one word in a minute. Locate this man's lesion(s). What elemental neurologic deficits would you expect, if any?

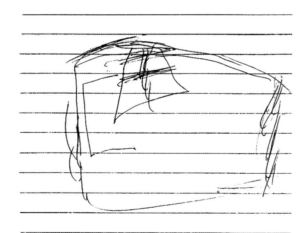

**Figure 12-27** See Practice 12-6A.

# Arousal, Attention, and Selective Engagement

## Objectives

1. Be able to describe the general function of the mid-brain reticular formation and the consequences of lesions of this structure.

2. Be able to describe the major stages of sleep.

3. Be able to describe the role of the major structures involved in sleep including the basal forebrain, the locus ceruleus, the caudal pontine reticular formation, and the suprachiasmatic nuclei. Be able to explain major sleep disorders in terms of dysfunction or failure of coordination of these structures, or decomposition or bad timing of components of REM and deep slow wave sleep.

4. Be able to explain the difference between reactive and intentional attention and the function of the major neural structures involved in the orienting response.

5. Be able to describe the major features of the neglect syndrome and explain it in terms of attentional and intentional systems.

6. Be able to explain the concept of selective engagement and relate it to attention and working memory.

7. Be able to list the major biogenic amine systems and their chief respective nuclei, and broadly describe their projection targets.

8. Be able to briefly contrast and explain the effects of reserpine and antidepressants on biogenic amine function, and the clinical consequences of using these drugs.

9. Be able to briefly contrast and explain the effects of dopaminergic agents, cocaine, amphetamines, and neuroleptics, and the clinical consequences of using these drugs.

In this section we review some of the most basic processes underlying cerebral function. Although it might seem more logical to have introduced this material earlier, it has been left until now because, to understand the role of these processes, it is necessary to have a reasonably comprehensive sense of cerebral function.

## AROUSAL

The arousal system defines our state of wakefulness and alertness. The core of this system lies in the *mid-brain reticular formation (MRF)*. In 1949, in one of the most famous neuroscientific experiments of the twentieth century, Moruzi and Magoun reported that electri-

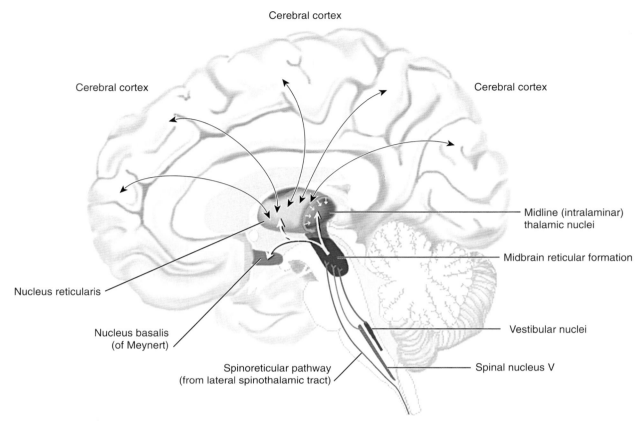

**Figure 12-28** Thalamic, basal forebrain, and cortical connections of the midbrain reticular formation (MRF).

cal stimulation of the MRF in animals induced both behavioral characteristics of wakefulness and the electroencephalographic (EEG) features of wakefulness.[1] On the other hand, damage to the MRF produces

varying degrees of lethargy up to actual coma, a state in which a patient appears to be deeply asleep and will not respond to any stimuli, however noxious. The MRF receives heavy input from the vestibular nuclei and from ascending pain pathways—hence the profound arousing effect of these stimuli.

How the MRF interacts with the cerebrum to produce the various manifestations of arousal is only partly understood. Three major components have been defined (Fig. 12-28): (1) The MRF projects to the midline nuclei of the thalamus, which in turn send diffuse projections to the entire cerebral cortex. (2) The MRF projects directly to the neurons throughout the thalamus that send information to the cerebral cortex via focal projections, thereby directly regulating thalamocortical transmission. (3) The MRF projects to the thalamic reticular nucleus (NR), a thin sheet of neurons that envelops the thalamus and projects onto thalamic neurons. NR is a particularly important device for regulating thalamocortical relay. The MRF, via its extensive connections with NR, opens the thalamic gate, allowing free flow of transmission through the thala-

---

[1]To obtain an EEG, electrodes are placed at standard locations over the scalp so that they sample the electrical activity over the full extent of the cerebral convexity. Voltage differences are measured either between neighboring pairs of electrodes, or between each scalp electrode and a reference electrode placed, for example, at the ear. The actual voltages measured reflect the voltage differences that develop between the dendritic trees and the cell bodies of cortical pyramidal cells as afferent input (e.g., from the thalamus) depolarizes the dendritic trees of large numbers of these neurons. The cortical voltages are attenuated by the insulating properties of the skull such that potentials measured at the scalp range from 3 to $50\,\mu V$. The EEG is most useful in detecting the paroxysmal discharges that characterize seizures. However, it also provides useful information about the state of cortical function. Characteristic patterns define the different stages of sleep (see text). Certain abnormal patterns may be seen with focal lesions of the brain such as brain tumors or strokes, or with diffuse cerebral dysfunction due to the effects of drugs, toxins, or metabolic abnormalities.

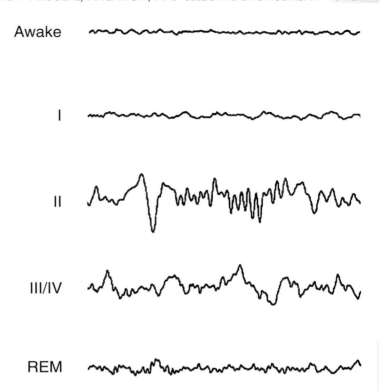

Awake

I

II

III/IV

REM

**Figure 12-29** Electroencephalogram (EEG) in the waking state and during the various stages of sleep. Note the large, negative potential (downward) spike followed by a 1.2-second run of sinusoidal oscillation (sleep spindle) in stage II sleep.

mus. The thalamus functions as a major relay station in the brain, relaying activity in sensory systems from the brainstem and the optic nerves to the cerebral cortex, and relaying transthalamic corticocortical transmission. *Thus, the MRF has direct effects on the cerebral cortex, via the midline thalamic nuclei, and it indirectly affects activity in the cerebral cortex by enabling the free flow of information through the thalamus.*

## SLEEP

In the previous section, we noted that damage to the MRF may produce lethargy, stupor, or coma. MRF function is also altered naturally in the course of sleep.

At first glance sleep seems like a simple affair of shutting down the brain. However, even the most superficial examination suggests that brain activity during sleep is every bit as complex as during wakefulness, perhaps more so.

Sleep studies employing a combination of behavioral observation, subject inquiry, EEG monitoring, and measurement of muscle tone define five different sleep stages. In the eyes open-awake state, the EEG is dominated by unsynchronized, low-voltage, high-frequency activity (Fig. 12-29). With stage I sleep, slower, more

synchronized rhythms appear. Subjects awakened from this stage of sleep will often have the perception that they were not really sleeping. The advent of stage II sleep is marked by the appearance of large negative-potential spikes across the midline, known as vertex waves. These waves are often followed by 1- to 2-second runs of high-frequency regular sinusoidal oscillations known as sleep spindles. Stage III sleep is marked by the appearance of very slow, relatively synchronized rhythms. When these very slow rhythms take up more than 50 percent of the ongoing record, this defines stage IV sleep. During these four stages of sleep, the person lies quietly and muscle tone is moderately reduced. The threshold for arousal becomes progressively higher with advancing stages of sleep. During a fifth stage of sleep, known as rapid eye movement (REM) sleep, or paradoxic sleep, the EEG reverts to the pattern of an awake person, frequent irregular saccadic eye movements appear, muscle tone declines to very low levels, and there may be intense autonomic activity. Dreaming may occur during any stage of sleep, but it is most prominent during REM sleep, and dreams are most likely to be recalled if subjects are awakened during REM sleep. A normal night is characterized by repeated cycling through the five sleep stages. Non-REM sleep tends to predominate during the first hours of sleep, when REM episodes are very brief, whereas

**Higher Neural Functions**

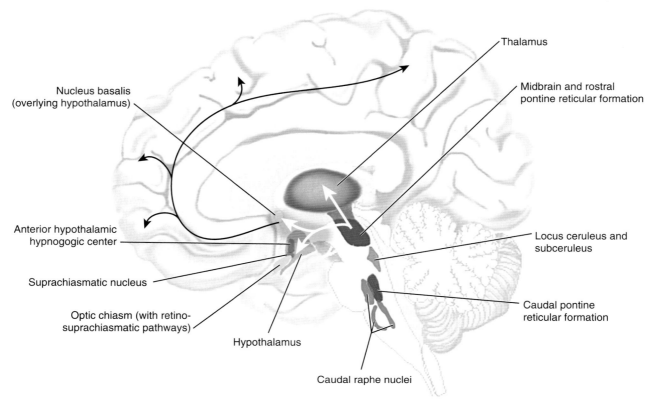

**Figure 12-30** The neural apparatus underlying sleep.

**TABLE 12-3 Major Structures Implicated in Arousal and Sleep**

| Structure | Function |
|---|---|
| Midbrain reticular formation (pedunculopontine nucleus (cholinergic), laterodorsal tegmental nucleus (cholinergic)), tuberomammillary nucleus (histaminergic) | Arousal/wakefulness |
| Caudal pontine reticular formation | Hypnogenic center |
| Rostral pontine tegmentum | REM sleep architecture |
| Basal forebrain anterior to hypothalamus (ventrolateral preoptic nucleus) | Hypnogenic center |
| Nucleus basalis of Meynert | High frequency, unsynchronized pattern of EEG in awake, eyes-open state |
| Peri-locus ceruleus | Suppression of muscle tone during REM sleep |
| Suprachiasmatic nuclei | 24 hour awake-sleep cycle |

EEG, electroencephalogram; REM, rapid eye movement.

during the latter part of the night, REM sleep is more frequent and prolonged.

We do not yet have a comprehensive understanding of the anatomy and physiology of sleep. However, many of the sleep phenomena we have just reviewed have been linked to particular regions of the brain, or even in some cases to certain physiologic events (Fig. 12-30, Table 12-3). As we have noted, the MRF (as well

**TABLE 12-4** Summary of Major Disorders of Sleep Architecture

| Disorder | Functional/Structural Abnormality |
|---|---|
| Narcolepsy tetrad | |
|    Narcolepsy | Entry into REM sleep directly from waking state |
|    Sleep paralysis | Paralysis due to suppression of muscle tone by locus ceruleus during waking state |
|    Cataplexy | Paralysis due to suppression of muscle tone by locus ceruleus precipitated by emotional arousal during wakefulness |
|    Hypnogogic/hypnopompic hallucinations | Dreams occurring in Stage I sleep |
| REM sleep behavior disorder | Acting out of dreams because of failure of locus ceruleus to suppress muscle tone |
| Sleep terrors | Acting out of dreams because they occur in Stage IV sleep, during which there is normally minimal suppression of muscle tone |
| Fatal familial insomnia | Persistent wakefulness, presumably due to destruction of prehypothalamic hypnogenic center by prion disease |
| Persistent wakefulness in locked in state following pontine stroke | Damage to/disconnection of caudal pontine reticular hypnogenic center |

REM, rapid eye movement.

as rostral portions of the pontine RF and extensions of the MRF up to the posterior hypothalamus) provides the basis for arousal or wakefulness. It appears that sleep involves not simply an attenuation of activity in the MRF but the active involvement of hypnogenic centers in the caudal pontine reticular formation and in the basal forebrain just anterior to the hypothalamus (the ventrolateral preoptic [VLPO] nuclei). Cells in the VLPO nuclei inhibit cholinergic and histaminergic cells in the reticular formation of the rostral pons, midbrain, and posterior hypothalamus responsible for arousal. The neural apparatus responsible for REM sleep phenomena lies in reticular nuclei in the rostral pontine tegmentum. Neurons in the vicinity of the locus ceruleus are responsible for the profound suppression of muscle tone during REM sleep. Whether the rapid eye movements of REM sleep are generated exclusively at the brainstem level or reflect saccades to dream images generated within the cerebral cortex is unclear.

The 24-hour awake-sleep cycle owes primarily to rhythmicity generated by the suprachiasmatic nuclei of the hypothalamus. The natural human sleep-wake cycle defined by these nuclei is approximately 25 hours. These nuclei are "reset" on a daily basis by any of the host of "zeitgebers" in our daily lives—alarm clocks, hungry dogs pawing, family members prodding or shouting, but most importantly, by light via a direct retinal-suprachiasmatic pathway.

The importance of the various regions involved and of their tightly coordinated function becomes readily evident in sleep disorders. Cases 12-19 to 12-22 provide examples of dysfunction of specific components of the neural apparatus underlying sleep or of failure of coordination between these components (summarized in Table 12-4).

## Case 12-19

### Narcolepsy

*A 25-year-old man presents to clinic with a chief complaint of repeatedly falling asleep during the day. No matter how vigorous the activity he is engaged in, he will suddenly be seized with an overwhelming feeling of sleepiness, to which he must succumb. He will sleep for 5 to 15 minutes and then awake feeling refreshed. On further inquiry, he also relates periods, mainly when he is emotionally distraught, when he becomes so weak he must sit down lest he fall. He may awake from sleep at night and find himself completely unable to move for several minutes. When this first happened he was terrified but now he is quite used to it. He is also prone to very vivid dreams that tend to occur when he is about to awake.*

*Continued*

Higher Neural Functions

## Case 12-19—cont'd

**Comment:** *This patient has narcolepsy, a hereditary disorder of sleep function linked to certain allelic variants of genes on chromosome 6 at the HLA locus. He has the full narcolepsy tetrad: narcolepsy (tendency to fall asleep, regardless of the circumstances), cataplexy (weakness during emotional arousal), sleep paralysis, and hypnopompic hallucinations. Narcolepsy represents but one of a number of disorders in which one or more of the various components of REM sleep occur in the wrong context. Thus, normally we enter REM sleep only at night from stage III or IV sleep. Narcoleptics enter REM sleep directly from wakefulness. When the profound suppression of muscle tone produced by peri-locus ceruleus neurons during REM sleep occurs during wakefulness, it may produce sleep paralysis or cataplexy. Vivid dreams normally occur only during REM sleep, but in the context of the narcolepsy tetrad, they may occur during stage I sleep (hypnogogic [going to sleep] or hypnopompic [end of sleep] dreams). It is now apparent that narcolepsy is the result of a neurodegenerative and possibly autoimmune disease involving hypocretin/orexin secreting cells in the lateral hypothalamus. These cells have widespread projections that variously act to inhibit the hypnogenic neurons of the VLPO nucleus and excite neurons in the brainstem reticular formation responsible for arousal.*

## Case 12-20

### REM Sleep Behavior Disorder

*A 70-year-old man brings his wife to the clinic because she regularly flails about in her sleep, often striking him. She is studied overnight in the sleep laboratory. In the course of the night she is observed to be making coordinated movements of her arms that look like the movement of someone paddling a canoe. She is promptly awakened and asked if she was dreaming. She says yes—she was dreaming of paddling a canoe.*

**Comment:** *This patient has REM sleep behavior disorder. In this disorder, the peri-locus ceruleus neurons fail to suppress muscle tone during REM sleep. As a result, patients act out their dreams.*

## Case 12-21

### Night Terrors and Somnambulism

*A 7-year-old child is brought in by his alarmed parents because he frequently awakes at night screaming, at which times his heart is racing and he appears terrified but has no recall of any precipitating event or dream. Now and again, he also sleep walks.*

**Comment:** *Night terrors and somnambulism begin in stage IV sleep, probably occurring in relation to dreams which, because they do not occur during REM sleep, are not recalled. In sleep walking, there is no suppression of muscle tone so the dreams are enacted.*

## Case 12-22

### Insomnia

*There are two well-defined clinical disorders in which patients experience more or less permanent insomnia as a result of destruction of one of the hypnogenic centers. One is the rare syndrome of fatal familial insomnia, a rapidly progressive, inherited degenerative disorder, the etiology of which (prion disease) is similar to that of Creutzfeldt-Jakob disease and kuru in humans, scrapie in sheep, and mad cow disease. The disease affects a relatively circumscribed portion of the brain including the thalamus and the rostral hypnogenic center anterior to the hypothalamus.*

*Another more common cause of persistent hyposomnia or even insomnia is a stroke involving the caudal basis pontis, typically resulting from thrombotic occlusion of the basilar artery (see Fig. 8-38). These patients are usually "locked in" as they have substantially destroyed all corticobulbar fibers innervating cranial nerve nuclei together with descending motor systems, classically rendering them capable only of up and down eye movements which are produced by cranial nerve III and midbrain vertical gaze centers far rostral to the stroke. To the extent that the stroke extends beyond the basis pontis into the pontine tegmentum, it damages the pontine hypnogenic center, leading to insomnia. REM sleep is particularly severely affected.*

Sleep in general, but particularly REM sleep, may be associated with prominent autonomic activity. This activity may have an adverse impact on other organ systems, as exhibited in Case 12-23.

---

## Case 12-23

### Increased Autonomic Tone during REM Sleep

*A 60-year-old man with a history of high blood pressure, hypercholesterolemia, and heavy smoking develops exertion-related pressure-like precordial chest pain associated with shortness of breath and sometimes sweating and nausea. He is able to relieve his symptoms quite rapidly with sublingual nitroglycerin. Lately he has been fairly frequently awaking at 4 to 5 AM with chest pain.*

**Comment:** *This relatively common scenario can be related to the effect of lability in autonomic function during REM sleep, which as we have noted, predominates toward the latter part of the night. Increased sympathetic activity increases heart rate and contractility to the point that myocardial oxygen requirements exceed the capacity of stenotic coronary arteries to supply oxygen. Heart pain or angina results.*

---

The purpose of sleep remains mysterious. The idea that it has some restorative power is challenged by the existence of people who routinely sleep only an hour or two every 24 hours and feel perfectly fine. Prolonged sleep deprivation does not result in psychosis or other gross aberration of cognitive function. Rather, it results in what every one of us knows from personal experience, a feeling of exhaustion, sleepiness, inattentiveness, and difficulty maintaining concentration. REM sleep may be important in the consolidation of newly acquired declarative memories. Attempts to keep people awake for long periods of time eventually fail as they enter a sort of twilight zone in which, from moment to moment, they shift back and forth from sleep to wakefulness. There is some evidence that non-REM sleep deprivation is associated with deep aching muscle pain and abnormal sensitivity to pain, as Case 12-24 illustrates.

---

## Case 12-24

### Consequences of Deep Non-REM Sleep Deprivation

*A 45-year-old woman presents with chief complaint of constant total body pain. She admits to irritability and abnormal quickness to anger. She has memory difficulty characterized by a tendency to mislay things and to go places, only to forget the purpose of her journeys by the time she arrives. She complains of frequent stomach pains. She is often vaguely dizzy. She drops things and bumps into things. She worries that her feet swell. She sometimes gets short of breath. She is constantly fatigued. It takes her an hour to get to sleep, she typically awakes many times during the night, and rarely does she sleep past 4 AM.*

**Comment:** *This clinical scenario is very common. It often leads to extended diagnostic testing that ultimately serves only to convince the patient that she or he is seriously ill. Sleep deprivation in general, and possibly non-REM sleep deprivation in particular, are associated with muscle aching, preoccupation with vague physical complaints, fatigue, depressed mood, and irritability. The mechanisms for this are not understood. Absent-mindedness, dropping things, and bumping into things reflect impairment in attention and concentration due to sleep deprivation. In addition, these patients are often depressed, a factor that serves to amplify their attention to every bodily symptom, further increase their pain, and lead to worry. In two common sleep disorders, sleep apnea syndrome, and periodic limb movements of sleep, patients suffer from non-REM, slow wave sleep deprivation even though they appear to be getting a normal quantity of sleep. Because of repeated partial arousals (due either to transient inability to breath because of a collapsed airway, or because of repeated limb movements), they spend the entire night in stage I and II sleep.*

---

## ATTENTION: INTENTIONAL AND REACTIVE

At any one moment we are being bombarded by thousands of different sensory stimuli. *Attention* is the process whereby we focus on one single source of sensory stimuli, at the same time maintaining vigilance over other sensory input such that we can instantly shift our attention to a new stimulus source should the need arise. Attention may be *intentional* or *reactive*. You are presently deliberately focusing your attention on this written material, an example of intentional attention. However, if something bites your foot, you will promptly shift your attention in order to further investigate, an example of reactive attention. Frontal systems drive intentional attention. Simple stimuli, such as a painful bug bite, elicit reactive attention largely through brainstem and thalamic mechanisms. However, more complex stimuli, such as the passing of an old friend as you wander down the hall deep in thought, require sensory association, polymodal, and supramodal cortices in temporal and parietal lobe cortex to engage reactive attention. For any creature, survival demands a delicate and dynamic balance between intentional and reactive attention. For example, a rat engages intentional attention as it serially examines objects for their food value. However, it must maintain vigilance using its reactive attentional mechanisms as failure to detect a fast moving object (normally a potent stimulus to reactive attention) could rapidly result in the rat becoming someone's dinner.

The neural basis for attention is almost inseparable from the neural basis for the orienting response, in which the organism actually makes a movement, most often of the eyes but also of the head or even the whole body, in order to better assess the attended stimulus. The frontal eye fields (Brodmann's area 8) and the superior colliculus are the key structures involved in the orienting response (Fig. 12-31). The frontal eye fields receive input from dorsolateral prefrontal cortex relevant to intentional attention and input from area 7 and other posterior cortices relevant to reactive attention. The superior colliculi are primarily involved in reactive attention. In the context of brain damage, the dynamic balance between these neural systems may be disrupted and disorders of attention result.

Case 12-25 illustrates the consequences of disruption of attentional systems and the orienting response.

## Case 12-25

### Hemispatial Neglect

*A 65-year-old man experiences a large right hemisphere stroke. On examination he will not respond to any stimulus, visual or somatosensory, on his left side—he has a hemianopia and hemibody sensory loss. He appears unable to move his left side. He cannot be coaxed to look left or even to move his eyes beyond midline toward the left. He fails to eat the food on the left side of his plate or to wipe the left side of his mouth. As he talks, an unattended straw waggles precariously in the left side of his mouth. In order to better define the reasons for his deficits, his physician conducts some further tests. When vision is retested while the patient looks to the far right, the hemianopia disappears. When the patient's left arm is pulled across his midline into his right hemispace, the patient does detect some stimuli delivered to the hand and exhibits some capability for moving the hand. The patient is asked to bisect a long line drawn on a sheet of paper; his performance is shown in Figure 12-32. The patient is asked to cancel all the lines drawn on a sheet of paper; his performance is shown in Figure 12-33.*

*Three months later the patient has shown substantial recovery. He now readily responds to stimuli presented to his left side. He has spontaneous movement on the left side and nearly normal strength,* *although he does not use his left arm as readily as his right. That is, he exhibits a left hemiakinesia. Visual fields are retested: the patient is asked to look at the examiner's nose while the examiner raises one or two fingers in each of the visual quadrants. The patient is able to answer correctly in all four quadrants. However, he proves absolutely unable to avoid moving his eyes (saccading) to look directly at the examiner's hand whenever stimuli are presented on the left side: that is, he demonstrates a visual grasp on the left.*

**Comment:** *This patient exhibits the phenomenon of hemispatial neglect. It may be observed after lesions in a number of areas of the brain, all of which appear to make up part of arousal and attention systems. In humans it is most often seen with strokes involving the frontoparietal cortex, and it is typically far more severe after right hemisphere lesions, the reasons for which are only partially understood. Although the neglect syndrome is a complex phenomenon, the behavior described in this case vignette can be reasonably well understood, as Heilman, Watson, and Valenstein originally proposed, in terms of dysfunction of the arousal and attention systems discussed in this section. Acutely, he demonstrates severe impairment in both intentional and reactive attention and associated*

## Case 12-25—cont'd

defects in the orienting response due to the frontoparietal lesion (e.g., no stimulus will induce him to saccade over to the left to gather more visual information about that stimulus). His impairment in intentional attention is part of a more generalized disorder of intention toward the left hemispace related to right frontal dysfunction. Thus, he exhibits a left hemiakinesia, reflecting an inability to initiate any movement with the left body, not just orienting movements. When his left arm is brought into his right hemispace, where intentional aspects of behavior are driven by the left frontal lobe, the patient exhibits some ability to move the left arm, proving that he is not merely suffering from hemiparesis due to damage to motor systems. One might have surmised that his impaired vision in the left hemifield was due to damage to ascending visual pathways to occipital cortex. However, when both left and right retinotopic visual fields are brought into the attended (right) hemispatial field, the patient exhibits normal vision, proving that the "hemianopia" observed during straight ahead gaze was in fact due to inattention and not damage to visual pathways. Similarly, he is able to detect stimuli to the left hand when it is placed in right hemispace. The performance on the line bisection and line cancellation tasks demonstrates the effects of defects in both intentional and reactive attention: that is, to perform these tasks, we need to have a normal reactive attentional response to stimuli that appear in the left hemispace and we need to be able to actively direct both our attention and movement into the left hemispace.

One might ask why this patient's reactive attention was so severely disturbed given that his superior colliculi were intact. There is no good answer to this. We do know that in the course of acute injury, many parts of the nervous system exhibit severe, albeit transient, dysfunction even when they are not directly involved in the injury. This response is referred to as diaschisis. The best example of diaschisis is the syndrome of spinal shock that is observed after spinal cord trauma. Not only does the patient became paraplegic or quadriplegic with the injury, but he transiently loses all reflexes mediated by the uninjured but now disconnected lower spinal cord, reflexes which subsequently return, often in a hyperactive form because they are disconnected ("released") from higher inhibitory mechanisms. This phenomenon was discussed in motor systems. In the context of hemispatial neglect, it is common to transiently see severe disruption in all aspects of reactive attention, even those more primitive aspects mediated by the superior colliculus, perhaps because of a "shock" mechanism. As the patient recovers from his stroke, he provides good evidence of a disinhibited collicular reactive attentional mechanism: not only is he able now to detect visual stimuli presented in his left field of vision but he is unable to suppress an orienting response mediated by the right superior colliculus.

## SELECTIVE ENGAGEMENT

Attention is a process whereby we direct our senses at a specific, external stimulus. However, this process entails the recruitment of selected internal neural networks. For example, visual attention requires us to recruit networks in the ventral "what" visual pathway to further evaluate the form and color of the stimulus after networks in the dorsal "where" visual pathway have defined the location and movement of the object. It requires simultaneous disengagement of neural networks that were being used to attend to the previous stimulus we had focused upon. Attentional processes are but a special case of a more general process, selective engagement, that the brain uses to bring "on line" the networks needed to perform certain processes and to take "off line" networks that are no longer needed. In this way, the brain is able to keep order in its house of 100 billion member neurons.

There are undoubtedly many different selective engagement mechanisms. We will first discuss two mechanisms that seem to explicitly involve the process of bringing discrete neural networks on line, one involving corticocortical systems, the other corticothalamocortical systems. We will then review a number of systems involving biogenic amines (acetylcholine [ACh], dopamine [DA], norepinephrine [NE], serotonin [5-HT]) that, rather than bringing networks on line or off line, seem to influence the relative states of activity of different parallel network systems.

### Specific Network Recruitment

#### Corticocortical Systems

In 1985, Moran and Desimone performed a very revealing experiment in which they recorded from single red-light sensitive neurons in the inferior temporal cortex (a

*Higher Neural Functions*

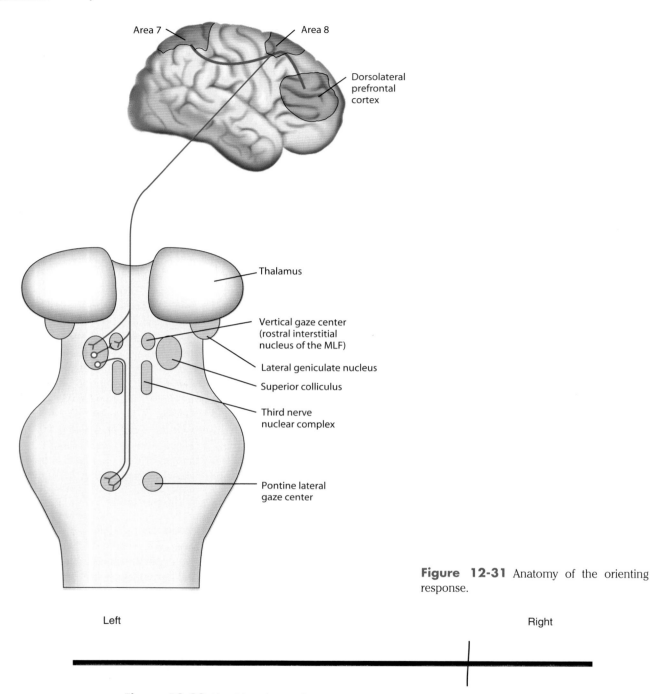

**Figure 12-31** Anatomy of the orienting response.

**Figure 12-32** Line bisection performance by a patient with hemispatial neglect.

visual association area in the "what" visual pathway) as a monkey looked at a red light and a green light. The monkey was intensively trained so that if the red light came on, it knew to move a lever quickly, thereby getting a reward of a squirt of apple juice. Under these circumstances, whenever the red light came on, the red-sensitive neuron would fire vigorously. However, if the monkey was trained to respond only to the green light (and was rewarded only for a response to the green light), the red-sensitive neuron ceased to respond, even when the red light came on. Thus, in order for the red-sensitive neuron to fire, it required simultaneous bottom-up input from the geniculocalcarine system conveying the light information and top-down input from higher neural systems, presumably the frontal lobes (see later discussion), that designated the behavioral significance of that light information. Thus, in order for the red light to fire the red-sensitive neuron, that neuron had to be selectively engaged by the frontal lobes. This selective engagement did not actually fire the red-sensitive neuron—it only biased that neuron such that it could be fired by the additional input of red light. When green-sensitive neurons were selectively engaged, red light no longer succeeded in firing the red-sensitive neuron. This ingenious experiment defines the neurophysiologic basis of attention as it is mediated by corticocortical (frontal-inferior temporal) systems, and exemplifies the process of selective engagement.

What is the evidence that prefrontal cortex is involved in bringing on line selected neural networks in sensory association cortices (as in the Moran and Desimone experiment), and possibly other, polymodal and supramodal association cortices? First, a host of well-documented and extensively studied connections between prefrontal cortex and posterior association cortices could provide the anatomic basis for selective

engagement processes. Beginning in the 1930s, a number of investigators began evaluating the behavioral effects of removal (ablation) of selected regions of the cerebral cortex in monkeys. One of the most robust findings from this research was that monkeys who had undergone bilateral ablation of dorsolateral prefrontal cortex were severely impaired on a particular task referred to as delayed response. In the delayed response task, the monkey watches as food is put into one of two food wells and the wells are covered. A screen then comes down for a period of time. When the screen is later lifted, the monkey can receive a reward by uncovering the baited food well. At first this seems like a simple memory task that would be solved by simply noting whether the left or the right well was baited and remembering "left" or "right." However, monkeys do not have the luxury of a language with this degree of specificity. Thus, they have to solve this problem in a different way, a way cleverly uncovered in research by Patricia Goldman-Rakic and Joaquín Fuster in the 1980s. During the delay period, neurons in the dorsolateral prefrontal cortex of monkeys continuously fire, selectively engaging the relevant neurons in the dorsal "where" visual pathway that are maintaining a representation of the location of the baited well. When these dorsolateral prefrontal neurons are unavailable because of the ablations, the monkey has no way of

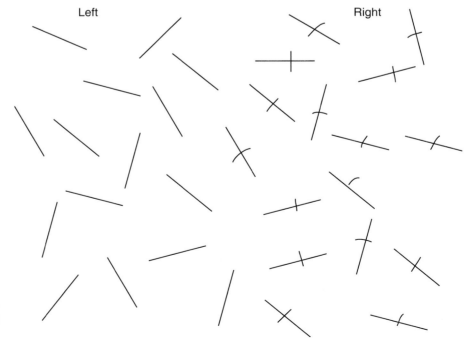

Left                Right

**Figure 12-33** Line cancellation performance by a patient with hemispatial neglect.

**Higher Neural Functions**

# FRONTAL CORTEX

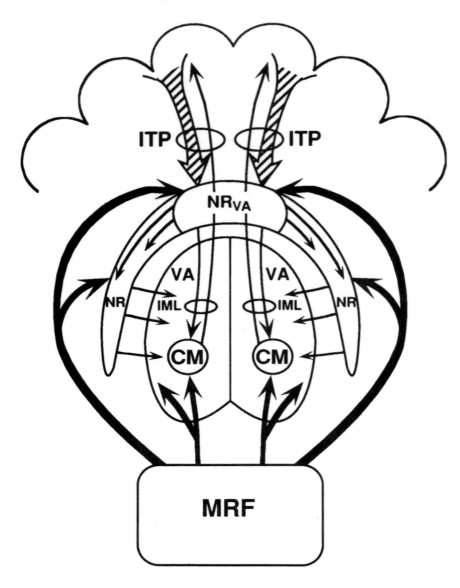

**Figure 12-34** Diagram of connections between the midbrain reticular formation (MRF), the thalamus, nucleus reticularis (NR), and prefrontal cortex that subserve arousal and one type of selective engagement (see text). ITP = inferior thalamic peduncle, the major white matter pathway connecting the prefrontal cortex with NR and the thalamus proper; VA = ventral anterior nucleus of the thalamus; $NR_{VA}$ = a portion of NR immediately anterior to VA that appears to be specialized for a role in mediating prefrontal control over selective engagement; CM = central median, one of the intralaminar nuclei that appears to be a major link in the prefrontal-NR system; IML = internal medullar lamina, the white matter sheet dividing the thalamus and enveloping CM that conveys prefrontal-CM connections. (From Nadeau SE, Crosson B. Subcortical aphasia. Brain Lang 58:355–402, 436–7–458, 1997.)

keeping the "where" pathway neural nets on line so that they can maintain a representation of the location of the baited well. Goldman-Rakic has referred to this process as maintenance of working memory, as the maintained representation represents a kind of temporary "chalkboard" memory trace. She and others have since provided evidence of a similar selective engagement mechanism at work in several other cognitive systems.

## Corticothalamocortical Systems

In the section on arousal, we noted that one mechanism by which the MRF maintains the brain state corresponding to arousal involves MRF projections to the thalamic reticular nucleus (NR). There are also projections from the prefrontal cortex to NR (Fig. 12-34). Whereas the connections between the MRF and NR serve to "open" the thalamic gate broadly, allowing free relay of information by all thalamic systems, it appears that the prefrontal-NR connections serve to selectively open specific regions of the NR gate, allowing information relay only by portions of selected thalamic systems. This potential attentional mechanism (and selective engagement mechanism) has received little study. Evidence suggests that, at least to some extent, it has been superseded by corticocortical systems (e.g., those defined by Moran and Desimone, Goldman-Rakic, Fuster, and others). For example, visual attention in monkeys does not appear to be influenced by this thalamic mechanism. However, the aphasia that can be seen in humans after certain thalamic lesions seems to reflect dysfunction of this particular selective engagement mechanism.

## Balance of Activity between Parallel Systems: Biogenic Amines

It is a great irony that although we have a host of drugs that we use to manipulate biogenic amine systems to treat serious neurologic and psychiatric disorders (see later discussion), and that most recreational drugs act by perturbing these systems, we have a very primitive understanding of their function. For this reason, much of the discussion in this section will be somewhat speculative, based on a mix of inference, neuroscientific data, and clinical experience.

Biogenic amines are supplied to the brain by dense concentrations of neurons in specific nuclei in the brainstem and basal forebrain. Biogenic amine systems have two properties that equip them for modulation of the balance of function between parallel systems: (1) A relatively small number of neurons, each with an enormous number of axonal endings (up to 2 million), project to a very large number of target neurons distributed in multiple systems; and (2) moment-to-moment fluctuations in the firing rate of biogenic amine neurons are relatively modest, suggesting that they are acting in a neurohormonal capacity, modifying the environment of target neurons, rather than sending target neurons specific information.

### Anatomy

There are two major concentrations of *acetylcholinergic neurons*. One makes up the core of the MRF, which subserves arousal. A second concentration is located in the basal forebrain and consists of a continuous band of cells extending from the nucleus basalis (of Meynert)

through a region called the diagonal band of Broca to the medial septal nuclei. It supplies projections to the entire cerebral cortex (mainly from the nucleus basalis) and the hippocampus (mainly from the medial septal nuclei) (Fig 12-35).

The major concentration of *dopaminergic neurons* is in the midbrain, within the substantia nigra just dorsal to the cerebral peduncles and in the space between the two substantia nigra, the ventral tegmental area. The substantia nigra projects mainly to the putamen, which is involved in motor function, and to the caudate nucleus, most of which is involved in prefrontal function (Fig. 12-35). The ventral tegmental area projects heavily to a ventral extension of the caudate nucleus, the nucleus accumbens (to be discussed further in Cycle 12-9). The nucleus accumbens is extensively interconnected with a number of structures in the limbic system, and there are direct dopaminergic projections from the ventral tegmental area to these same limbic structures. The ventral tegmental area also projects to the entire cerebral cortex.

The major concentration of *noradrenergic (norepinephrine) neurons* is in another pigmented nucleus, the locus ceruleus, located in the dorsolateral pons. The locus ceruleus projects to nearly all structures in the cerebrum.

The major concentration of serotonergic neurons is in a series of nuclei in the dorsal midline of the midbrain and pons known as the raphe nuclei. Like noradrenergic neurons, they project to nearly all structures in the cerebrum.

### Function

The extensive projections of each biogenic amine system from tiny nuclei to multiple disparate target structures suggests that each has but a single function that somehow applies to all targets. However, each system has a number of different receptors (see Chapter 4), and there is emerging evidence that the source nuclei, small as they are, do not operate in monolithic fashion.

The entire *acetylcholinergic system* in the basal forebrain appears to play a crucial role in the establishment of new memory (Table 12-5). Memory formation, both declarative (fact) and nondeclarative (the most important being procedural or skill memory), consists of alteration in the strengths of neural connections. We believe that much, perhaps most, of cerebral memory formation respects Hebbian principles, that is, interneuronal connection strengths are enhanced to the

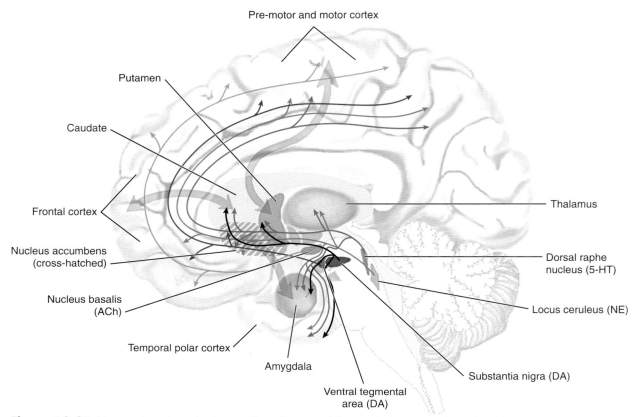

**Figure 12-35** Monoaminergic projections to the striatum and the cerebral cortex and relationships between components of the striatum and cortical systems. (5-HT = serotonin, NE = norepinephrine, DA = dopamine, ACh = acetylcholine)

extent that the connected neurons are simultaneously active. However, there is at least one other crucial ingredient to this process: there must be some signal that designates the activity represented by the mutually active neurons as important. This judgment originates primarily in the limbic system. It is communicated to the rostral cholinergic system, which then supplies a burst of cholinergic input to target cortices, communi-

cating to these cortices the "imprimatur" of the limbic system—the fact that the limbic system feels that this information is important and worth learning. Acetylcholine acts on target neurons in the cerebral cortex and the hippocampus to prolong the opening of NMDA glutamate-gated sodium/calcium channels (by delaying repolarization by interfering with the opening of potassium channels), thus gating into the cells more calcium,

**TABLE 12-5** Functions of Biogenic Amine Systems

| System | Function |
|---|---|
| Acetylcholine | Conveying limbic imprimatur to cortical neural networks in process of encoding new declarative and procedural memories |
| Dopamine | Basal ganglia: regulation of balance between direct and indirect pathways |
| | Nucleus accumbens: regulation of limbic tone |
| Norepinephrine | Promotion of arousal through excitation of nucleus reticularis and other mechanisms |
| | Regulation of balance between corticocortical and corticobulbar/corticospinal activity |
| | Regulation of balance between intentional and reactive attention |
| Serotonin | Regulation of balance between orbitofrontal-limbic and dorsolateral prefrontal systems |

which is necessary for production of the permanent changes in neural connectivity constituting memory. The limbic imprimatur regarding declarative memories is communicated via the medial septal nuclei to the hippocampus. The limbic imprimatur regarding both declarative and nondeclarative memories is communicated to the cerebral cortex via the nucleus basalis (see Cycle 10-6, Section C). To return to the main theme of this section, regulation of the balance between parallel systems: ACh appears to regulate the degree to which neurons in the cerebral cortex that are involved in information processing are simultaneously engaged in memory storage.

We will consider two major functions of the cerebral *dopaminergic system* (Table 12-5). First, DA appears to regulate the balance between the direct and indirect basal ganglia pathways (see Cycle 6-9). Thus, DA deficiency in the putamen in patients with Parkinson's disease results in excessive activity in the indirect pathway (which includes the subthalamic nucleus) with resultant insufficient thalamocortical transmission through the VL thalamic nucleus to SMA, premotor and motor cortex. Consequently, these patients exhibit akinesia and bradykinesia. Second, dopaminergic input to nucleus accumbens and limbic structures appears to influence the degree to which the limbic system participates in cognitive activity. When patients with schizophrenia experience positive symptoms (delusions and hallucinations), these experiences are so compelling that patients often become terrified and are prone to act on them, despite the fact that they are clearly contrary to perception, existing knowledge, and logical argument (see Cycle 12-9). That is, their limbic value judgment overwhelms all other potential influences on behavior. Dopamine receptor blocking agents, now in use for over 50 years, remain the single most effective treatment for acute psychotic breakdowns in schizophrenic patients.

Three potential *noradrenergic effects* on cerebral function will be cited here. First, there are well-established NE projections to the nucleus reticularis (NR). These projections exert an effect quite similar to that of ACh, promoting arousal by opening the thalamic gate. Norepinephrine must increase arousal by additional mechanisms, as noradrenergic drugs have a much greater impact on arousal than do cholinergic agents. Second, NE acts to regulate the signal-to-noise ratio in target neurons in the cerebral cortex. What does this mean? Most neurons maintain some level of background activity. This activity may be significantly increased by input from connected systems. The ratio of activity during input to activity without input is referred to as signal-to-noise ratio. Norepinephrine appears to have a different effect on signal-to-noise ratio in layer III cortical neurons than on layer V cortical neurons. Low NE levels increase signal-to-noise ratio in layer III neurons, whereas high NE levels increase signal-to-noise ratio in layer V neurons. Layer III neurons are the major source of corticocortical connectivity (intrahemispheric and transcallosal, interhemispheric). Layer V neurons are the major source of corticospinal and corticobulbar projections. Thus, low NE levels appear to promote the intracortical communication needed for cognitive activity, whereas high NE levels appear to promote the transmission from the cortex to the brainstem and spinal cord necessary to execute plans for action. Experiments in monkeys have shown that microstimulation of locus ceruleus during the cognitive component of tasks degrades task performance. However, just before the monkey initiates a response (having completed the necessary cognitive activity), neurons in locus ceruleus exhibit a burst of activity, which increases cortical NE concentrations, presumably setting the stage for layer V activity. Third, NE appears to regulate the balance between reactive attention and intentional attention. The best evidence of this is the success that has been achieved with drugs such as methylphenidate (Ritalin), which potentiate noradrenergic activity, in the treatment of attention deficit hyperactivity disorder (ADHD). Patients with this disorder, who are most often children, appear to be "bouncing off the walls" because they attend and orient to so many environmental stimuli. They have great difficulty deliberately focusing their attention on the task at hand, for example, school work. With Ritalin, they are able to achieve a better balance between reactive and intentional attention.

One possible function of 5-HT systems will be considered. To understand this, some historical perspective is needed. During the 1920s and 1930s, before the advent of pharmacologic treatments for depression, psychosis, and obsessive compulsive disorder, psychosurgery was developed to deal with the vast numbers of patients who languished in state mental hospitals, often in the most abject states. Although psychosurgery today is often viewed as a grotesque medical aberration, its impact was once considered to be so profound and so beneficial that one of its major developers, Egas Moníz, won the Nobel prize in medicine in 1939 for this work. Most psychosurgery is now considered unacceptable, but one operation, cutting of the white matter tracts projecting to and from posterior orbitofrontal cortex, remains a consideration in patients with refractory, ruminative depression and severe obsessive compulsive disorder. Alternatives to craniotomy, such as stereotactic radiosurgery of these pathways and electrical stimulation in the region of the ventral anterior limb of the internal capsule and the nucleus accumbens, are the subjects of active research. Patients with refractory, ruminative depression spend all their time going over and over their sources of guilt, their mistakes, and the expected negative consequences of any actions they might take. Patients with severe obsessive compulsive disorder spend their time doing their obsessive rituals, to the exclusion of everything else. Patients with either disorder are completely dysfunctional and suffer terribly. From a neural systems perspective, these patients appear to be "slaves" to their orbitofrontal-limbic systems. That is, all thoughts and plans for action are dictated exclusively by the orbitofrontal-limbic system, and the normal dynamic balance between this system and dorsolateral prefrontal cortex is lost. From this perspective, the salutary effect of orbitofrontal undercutting can be interpreted as redressing this imbalance by partially impairing the orbitofrontal-limbic system, thereby providing the opportunity for at least some thoughts and plans for action to be influenced by dorsolateral prefrontal systems. Although there continue to be sufficient patients with refractory ruminative depression and severe obsessive compulsive disorder to motivate research into nonpharmacologic approaches, in the present day, most such patients will respond, at least partly, to drugs that potentiate 5-HT systems, most notably the serotonin selective reuptake inhibitors (SSRIs) (e.g., fluoxetine [Prozac]). That is, SSRIs appear to alter the functional balance between dorsolateral and orbital prefrontal cortex such that the orbitofrontal-limbic system plays a relatively lesser role in defining thought and plans for action.

### Pharmacology

As we have noted, despite our primitive understanding of the functions of biogenic amine systems, a number of clinically important drugs act through these systems, and the effects of most drugs of abuse are mediated through these systems (Table 12-6).

## PRACTICE 12-7

**A.** A 75-year-old man with chronic atrial fibrillation embolizes a clot from the left atrium that ends up wedged at the rostral tip of the basilar artery. Predict his clinical symptoms.

**B.** A 65-year-old obese gentleman with a long history of loud snoring is observed by his wife to repeatedly stop breathing through the night. Each time, after 15 seconds or so, he makes some unsuccessful breathing efforts, obstructed by his transiently collapsed glottis, and ultimately exhibits a startle reaction accompanied by a deafening snore. He then continues to snore until the next episode. As a result, although he sleeps through the night, he never gets past stage II sleep. Predict the consequences of this disorder.

**C.** Visual fields are tested by confrontation in a 73-year-old woman with disseminated cortical pathology, worst in temporoparietal regions, due to Alzheimer's disease. She is asked to focus on the examiner's nose while he raises one or two fingers in each visual quadrant. The patient is absolutely unable to resist the urge to saccade to the examiner's moving hand. What is the mechanism of this *visual grasp*?

**D.** Relate the neglect syndrome to selective engagement mechanisms.

**E.** Refer back to the patient in Practice 12-4A. This patient's tumor was almost certainly benign—actually a histologic abnormality rather than a neoplasm. Would it be safe to remove it? Why or why not? (Hint: What impact might the surgery have on memory function and why?)

**F.** List some tasks requiring working memory.

**G.** A medical student develops a bad cold while preparing for an examination. Her friend recommends an over-the-counter cold remedy that contains an antihistamine, a drug with major anticholinergic effects. Knowing that neurons in the medial septal nuclei are cholinergic, do you think it would be a good idea for her to take this drug?

**H.** Patients with advanced Parkinson's disease uniformly develop hallucinations and many develop delusions. Levo-dopa and other dopamine agonists are the mainstay of treatment of Parkinson's disease. Predict their effect on hallucinations and delusions in these patients.

**TABLE 12-6** Functions of Biogenic Amine Systems

| System | Drug | Purpose | Effect |
|---|---|---|---|
| **Acetylcholine** (ACh) | *Agonists:* acetylcholinesterase inhibitors (donepezil, rivastigmine, galantamine) | Increase cortical ACh in patients with Alzheimer's disease, who experience degeneration of nucleus basalis | Slowing of rate of decline in cortical connectivity and attendant loss of knowledge |
| | *Antagonists* | Curb extrapyramidal effects of neuroleptics (e.g., trihexyphenidyl [Cogentin]); Treat bladder spasticity (e.g., oxybutynin); Hypnotics (e.g., diphenhydramine); Treat vertigo (e.g., scopolamine); Undesired side effects of various drugs (e.g., antihistamines, tricyclic antidepressants) | Impaired coding of declarative and possibly procedural memory; sedation through interference with neural transmission from midbrain reticular formation (MRF) |
| **Dopamine** (DA) | *Agonists:* (dopamine [given as levodopa], pramipexole, ropinirole) | Redress imbalance between direct and indirect basal ganglia pathways in Parkinson's disease | Improvement in akinesia, bradykinesia and rigidity |
| | *Antagonists:* (neuroleptics) | Reduce limbic influence on perception, recall and planning in psychosis | Reduction in agitation, hallucinations, delusions in schizophrenia |
| **Norepinephrine** (NE) | *Agonists:* therapeutic (e.g., methylphenidate, d-amphetamine) | Treat imbalance between attentional and intentional attention in ADHD | Improved ability to focus attention |
| | *Agonists:* (e.g., methamphetamine, cocaine) | Recreation: mechanisms uncertain | Increase arousal, sense of power and well-being, pleasure in ongoing activity; psychosis |
| | *Reuptake inhibitors:* (e.g., tricyclic antidepressants, venlafaxine) | Treat depression: mechanisms uncertain | Augment the effect of serotonergic agents |
| **Serotonin** (5-HT) | *Agonists:* (reuptake inhibitors) (antidepressants of all types) | Reduce impact of orbitofrontal limbic system on thinking, plans for action | Reduction in emotion evoked by events; improved functionality through improved recruitment of dorsolateral prefrontal systems in planning |
| | *Direct agonists:* lysergic acid diethylamide (LSD); methylene-dioxymethamphetamine (MDMA, Ecstasy) | Recreation: mechanisms uncertain | Altered consciousness, hallucinations |
| | *Antagonists:* Reserpine (depletes stores of 5-HT, DA, NE) | Treatment of hypertension | Depression in 20% of patients |

Higher Neural Functions

# Parallel Distributed Processing: The Relationship between Neural Microstructure and Higher Neural Functions

## Objectives

1. Be able to describe the essential features of parallel distributed processing (PDP).

2. Be able to describe how a PDP network can learn.

3. Be able to describe what is meant by a distributed representation at both the association cortex level and the neuronal level and give examples of each.

4. Be able to define the term inference in PDP and behavioral terms and provide examples of advantages and disadvantages of this facility.

5. Be able to define the term graceful degradation and explain the network basis for this phenomenon given either network damage or noisy input.

6. Be able to describe what is meant by bottom-up and top-down flow of activity and relate this to hallucinations and to interpretation of noisy input.

7. Be able to describe what is meant by parallel constraint satisfaction and give an example.

8. Be able to describe what is meant by a self-organizing system and indicate the ways in which the brain functions as such a system.

In this chapter we have attempted so far to provide a logical accounting for the higher neural functions most crucial to human behavior. Our approach has centered on the explication of fundamental neural systems. In the course of this, however, we have not answered perhaps the most fundamental question of all: how is it possible for individual neurons, whose currency is electrical impulses and squirts of neurotransmitter, to generate behaviors so wondrous and complex, that until quite recently, we dismissed the idea that they could be a product of mere biology, but instead had to reflect something mysterious and transcendent that we referred to as the mind? We are very far from a clear answer to this question, but in this section we will try to give you a flavor for a young discipline, *parallel distributed processing (PDP)*, often known as *connectionism*, that is rapidly providing major insights.

## PDP NETWORKS: BASIC OPERATING PRINCIPLES

The most fundamental insight of PDP, the one thing that literally defines the whole approach, is that *higher neural functions cannot be understood in terms of the behavior of single neurons, only as the joint interactive behavior of thousands or millions of neurons interconnected in neural networks*. In this section, we will try to give you a sense of how this is possible, and how the interactive behavior of large neural networks makes some strong predictions about brain functions, predictions that have been amply born out in studies of normal and brain-injured individuals. We are indebted

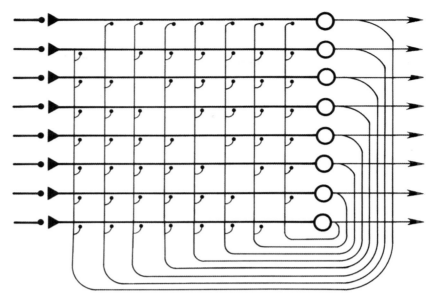

**Figure 12-36** An auto-associator network. (From McClelland JL, Rumelhart DE. A distributed model of human learning and memory. In McClelland JL, Rumelhart DE, PDP Research Group (eds). Parallel Distributed Processing, Vol. 2. Cambridge, MIT Press, 1986, pp. 170–215. © 1986 by The Massachusetts Institute of Technology.)

to James McClelland, David Rumelhart and their colleagues for much of what follows.

Figure 12-36 shows a very simple PDP network. It consists of a series of 8 units, each of which has an input (on the left) from outside the network and an output (to the right) to somewhere outside the network. Every unit is connected to every other unit, hence its name: auto-associator network. Networks like this one with up to thousands of units are programmed on computers, enabling simulations that test the ability of the networks and the assumptions engineered into them to emulate actual behavior (Box 12-1).

In a simulation, during each processing cycle, the computer calculates activation, input, and output values for every unit in the network. Input is calculated as the sum of the activation levels for all the units "synapsing" on a particular recipient unit, each activation level multiplied by the connection strength between the respective input unit and the recipient unit. Activation levels are often limited to a range, for example, between 0 and +1. Activation functions typically have a threshold value below which they are set to zero. Thus, low level activity is eliminated, something that helps to dampen noise in the system. Activation functions are also typically nonlinear, for example, resembling the sigmoid function of the hemoglobin-oxygen desaturation curve. This nonlinearity (coupled with the nonlinearity implicit in the threshold feature) provides the essential basis for the complexity of behavior of which PDP networks are capable (see further dis-

## BOX 12-1 Mathematics of PDP

The following is a formula frequently used to compute activation levels:

$$a_i(t) = \frac{1}{1 + e^{-net_i(t)}}$$

where $a_i(t)$ is the activation level of unit $i$ and $net_i(t)$ is the input to unit $i$ at a particular time $t$. This formula produces a sigmoid activation curve. The value of $a_i(t)$ in this case would range between 0 and +1. $Net_i(t)$ would be computed as follows:

$$net_i(t) = \sum_j a_j(t)w_{ji}$$

This says: take the activation level of each unit ($j$) connected to unit $i$, multiply it by the strength of the connection between that unit and unit $i$ ($w_{ji}$), then sum over all these units. An output is then computed for each unit. This typically takes the following form:

For $a_j(t) \leq \theta$,    $o_i(t) = 0$

For $a_j(t) > \theta$,    $o_i(t) = \frac{a_i(t) - \theta}{1 - \theta}$

This says that when the activation level of unit $i$ is greater than a threshold level $\theta$, the output of unit $i$, $o_i$, is a linear function of its activation level, ranging between 0 and 1.

**Higher Neural Functions**

cussion). These various properties also substantially mimic the behavior of neurons.

In this way, each unit functions as an individual microprocessor. Because the computer visits each unit every cycle, all the units end up acting essentially simultaneously and in parallel, hence the name *parallel* distributed processing.

Given their design, *PDP networks do not transfer information from one place to another. Rather, the information is stored in the connection weights. Activation flows from unit to unit throughout the network, eventually settling into a steady state that defines a representation.* The connection strengths constrain the flow of activation and define the steady states into which the network can settle.

## LEARNING BY PDP NETWORKS

In some PDP models, connection strengths between units ($w_{ij}$) are assigned (see Box 12-1). We will discuss an example of this later (the rooms-in-a-house network). However, more often, PDP networks are equipped to learn by themselves through their experience with the data by the incorporation of a learning subroutine. This type of training serves two purposes: (1) it is an efficient way (indeed the only practical way) of setting connection strengths in models that have hundreds of thousands of connections; and (2) it implicitly tests the capability of a neural-like model to learn from experience. Models are trained by supplying them, during each trial, with an input consisting of a pattern of activation levels across the input units. The model is then allowed to process that input until it settles into a steady state, which generates a stable pattern of activation levels across its output units. Now the learning subroutine is given the desired or target output pattern (the "correct answer"). It then mathematically compares the actual and correct output patterns and then makes a small adjustment to each of the connection strengths in the model (according to its relative contribution to the total error) such that the error generated during the next exposure to this input pattern is slightly smaller. Ultimately, through hundreds or thousands of exposures to the set of inputs, the learning subroutine succeeds in adjusting the connection strengths such that the model produces very close to the correct output for every input, that is, the error is reduced to close to zero. Models incorporating such learning devices have shown the capacity for learning astonishingly complex functions. In fact, neural net computers are now widely used to solve computational

problems in which there is a complex relationship between input and desired output that cannot be logically or systematically defined.

The human brain also exhibits enormous capability for learning to produce complex output that is optimal to the given circumstances. In the course of this, we implicitly learn rules, gaining implicit learning that may later be made explicit. For example, in learning to speak, we acquire a working vocabulary in the vicinity of 10,000 to 30,000 words and a facility for putting those words together in orderly sequences that implicitly obey rules of grammar, including word order, verb conjugation, using the proper person (she, you, they), and in many languages, the proper case (nominative, objective, etc.). One example provides particular insight into the complexity of this process: the formation of the English past tense. Many English verbs form the past tense simply by adding "-ed," for example, look-looked, need-needed, chase-chased. However, even here there is some irregularity: the past tense of look is pronounced "lookt," whereas the past tense of need is pronounced "needed." Many English past tenses involve substantially greater irregularities. Many verbs ending in t or d have an identical present and past tense: such as hit, cut, split, bid; or the past tense is formed by a switch in the final phoneme, such as spend-spent. Many verbs require one of a number of changes in their core: sing-sang, come-came, get-got, take-took, feel-felt, catch-caught. Some have completely different past tenses: go-went. Various books have codified these patterns of past-tense formation into "rules." However, we do not produce the past tense form of verbs by referring to the rules—we simply speak them, often with mistakes when we are young, ultimately with remarkable accuracy. McClelland and Rumelhart developed a 920-unit PDP model that learned to produce the past tense of English verbs when given the present tense. *Like humans, it learned strictly from experience (through its incorporated mathematical learning algorithm), but in the process it showed abundant evidence of having implicitly learned these rules. PDP networks equipped with learning algorithms demonstrate, like the brain, great power in detecting regularities in data and optimizing their response.*

## PDP: DISTRIBUTED REPRESENTATION AT THE LEVEL OF THE SINGLE NETWORK

The units in the models we have discussed have a neural-like character. As we shall see in a later example, the representation that a given network actually produces at any one instant is defined by the *pattern of activity* of all the units (or neurons) in the network. This is referred to as a *distributed representation*, hence the name parallel *distributed* processing. The term distributed representation means something slightly different here than it did earlier in the chapter because it refers to representation at the neuronal level. *Our actual perception of something consists of a grand representation distributed across various association cortices, each of which supports a component representation distributed across networks of neurons*. Thus, what we experience is defined by a hierarchy of distributed representations, the highest levels spanning different areas of the brain, the lowest levels spanning local networks of neurons. *Whereas the particular pattern of unit activity in a network at any one time defines a representation, the connection weights (synaptic strengths) define the capability of a network for generating particular representations. The information is in the connections*. In all the examples to be considered in this section, the units and the representations supported by them are defined in terms meaningful to us. However, units and representations in the brain need not be definable in terms that are meaningful to us, only in terms that make sense to brain systems that make use of these representations.

From this brief computational background, we will now consider two examples of PDP networks that will illustrate their behavior and power.

## ROOMS IN A HOUSE: AN AUTO-ASSOCIATOR NETWORK

This example involves a very simple auto-associator network that nevertheless captures the essential properties of information representation in the complex of association cortices that enable us to give meaning to the things we perceive.

The rooms of a house contain different items and have particular features that enable us to define each room in terms of its contents and features. Table 12-7 lists 40 room descriptors or features, each of which will correspond to a unit in this PDP model. In order to facilitate understanding (and computation!), we are employing a local representation in lieu of a distributed representation for these features, that is, each feature corresponds to a unit. Each unit is connected to every other unit in the network. The connection strengths or weights of each of these connections were determined by asking two raters to imagine an office and then say for each of the 40 descriptors whether it was appropriate for the office. This process was replicated for living room, kitchen, bathroom, and bedroom. This cycle was repeated 16 times, yielding a total of 16 judgments on each descriptor for each of 5 rooms. This provided the corpus of material that was "taught" to the network. In this particular instance, the weights of the connections in the network were set according to the probability that any two particular features would occur in conjunction, based upon the corpus of judgments rendered by the raters. Fig. 12-37 depicts the connection weight matrix that resulted.

In effect, we now have a miniature brain that operates on the basis of PDP. This brain can be operated by clamping one or more units at an activation level of 1 (in effect, stating that these features are present) and letting the system run until activation spreads from these units throughout the network and the network eventually reaches steady state. In principle, the network could reach any one of a very large number of binary steady states $(2^{40})$ (states in which every unit is either on or off), but in practice, it settles into one of only five different states. Figure 12-38 depicts that pattern of activation as it evolves and ultimately stabi-

Higher Neural Functions

### TABLE 12-7 The Forty Room Descriptors

| | | | | |
|---|---|---|---|---|
| ceiling | walls | door | windows | very-large |
| large | medium | small | very-small | desk |
| telephone | bed | typewriter | bookshelf | carpet |
| books | desk-chair | clock | picture | floor-lamp |
| sofa | easy-chair | coffee-cup | ashtray | fireplace |
| drapes | stove | coffeepot | refrigerator | toaster |
| cupboard | sink | dresser | television | bathtub |
| toilet | scale | oven | computer | clothes-hanger |

*Source:* From Rumelhart DE, Smolensky P, McClelland JL, Hinton GE. Schemata and sequential thought processes in PDP models. In McClelland JL, Rumelhart DE, PDP Research Group (eds). Parallel Distributed Processing, Vol. 2. Cambridge, MIT Press, 1986, pp 7–57.
© 1986 by The Massachusetts Institute of Technology.

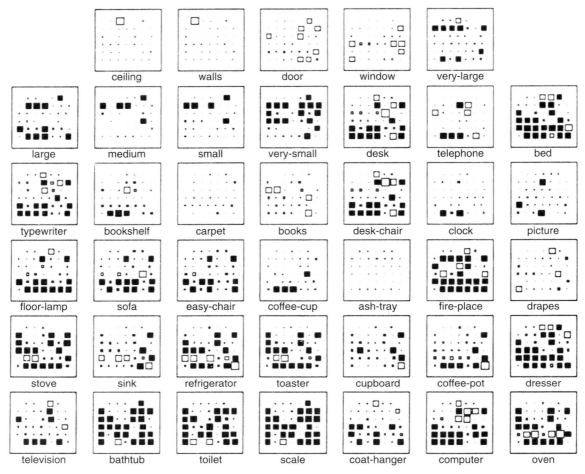

**Figure 12-37** Matrix of connection weights in the room-descriptor model. Small dark squares signify inhibitory connections, white squares excitatory connections. The size of a small square is proportional to the strength of the connection. The descriptor layout in each small square precisely replicates the descriptor layout in the entire figure. Referring to the large square in the bottom right corner, one can see that oven (bottom right location within this large square) has a strong negative connection to its neighbor immediately to the left, computer, but a strong positive connection to its diagonal neighbor, coffee-pot. (From Rumelhart DE, Smolensky P, McClelland JL, Hinton GE. Schemata and sequential thought processes in PDP models. In McClelland JL, Rumelhart DE, PDP Research Group (eds). Parallel Distributed Processing, Vol. 2. Cambridge, MIT Press, 1986, pp 7–57. © 1986 by The Massachusetts Institute of Technology.)

lizes when the features oven and ceiling are turned on. As can be seen, in the steady state that finally emerges, oven, coffee-pot, cupboard, toaster, refrigerator, sink, stove, drapes, coffee-cup, clock, telephone, small, window, walls, and ceiling are activated. This cluster of features implicitly defines a kitchen. Kitchen thus emerges as a particular pattern of activation of the network. The network contains in its connection weights the knowledge that enables us to elicit this representation. The kitchen representation is instantiated as a *distributed representation*. The capability for

eliciting this representation simply by activating one or more features produces *content addressable memory*. We do not have to know where the kitchen representation is stored, indeed, it is stored throughout this network; we simply have to evoke a feature of the representation and it comes to life, albeit in ephemeral form as a pattern of activation. By activating other features in this same network, we can elicit other schemata. For example, if we clamp ceiling and desk, a pattern of activation emerges that includes computer, ashtray, coffee-cup, picture, desk-chair, books, carpet,

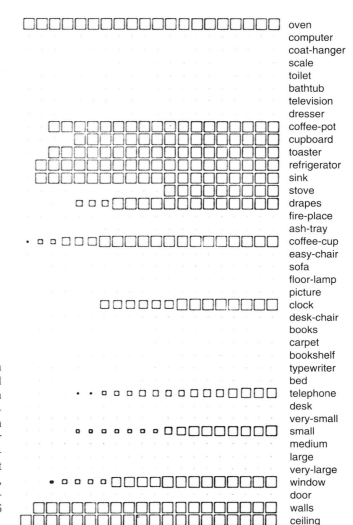

oven
computer
coat-hanger
scale
toilet
bathtub
television
dresser
coffee-pot
cupboard
toaster
refrigerator
sink
stove
drapes
fire-place
ash-tray
coffee-cup
easy-chair
sofa
floor-lamp
picture
clock
desk-chair
books
carpet
bookshelf
typewriter
bed
telephone
desk
very-small
small
medium
large
very-large
window
door
walls
ceiling

**Figure 12-38** Evolution of the pattern of activation in the room-descriptor network when the units ceiling and oven are clamped in the on position. Time elapses from left to right. The right-most column of squares corresponds to the final state of the network. The size of each square indicates the degree of activation of that particular feature unit. (From Rumelhart DE, Smolensky P, McClelland JL, Hinton GE. Schemata and sequential thought processes in PDP models. In McClelland JL, Rumelhart DE, PDP Research Group (eds). Parallel Distributed Processing, Vol. 2. Cambridge, MIT Press, 1986, pp. 7–57. © 1986 by The Massachusetts Institute of Technology.)

bookshelf, typewriter, telephone, desk, large, door, walls, and ceiling: unmistakably the representation of an office.

## Properties of the Network

This network exhibits several interesting properties. As we have seen, it is capable of supporting a number of completely different patterns of activity corresponding to completely different representations. Furthermore, representations can contain subrepresentations, reflecting the connectivity within the network; for example, easy-chair and floor-lamp nearly always go together, as do desk and desk-chair, window and drapes. Repre-

sentations can also blend: if we clamp both bed and sofa, we eventually activate television, dresser, drapes, fire-place, easy-chair, sofa, floor-lamp, picture, clock, books, carpet, bookshelf, bed, large, window, door, walls, and ceiling. This is in effect the representation for a large, fancy bedroom. The production of this representation provides an example of a modest bit of creativity. The raters whose judgments provided the basis for the connection weights were never asked what items were appropriate to a large fancy bedroom. Rather, the network *inferred* this representation from the knowledge it had been provided about the rooms of a house.

The capacity for inference underlies the ability of PDP models to *generalize*, to make an inference about a more general situation based upon knowledge of one or more specific aspects of the situation. Because living organisms are unlikely to encounter exactly the same situation more than once, the capacity for inference latent in the PDP nature of their brains both makes it possible to always generate some sort of response and maximizes the probability that that response will be appropriate. Presumably the same capacity underlies the human ability to generate rules and generalizations despite the fact that we actually experience a series of special instances. However, there are negative aspects to this capacity for inference and generalization. Thus, the room descriptor network may make errors of guilt by association: shown an easy-chair it will assume there is a floor-lamp nearby, even if in a particular instance there is none. More generally, it will *confabulate*; for example, if oven is clamped, it will tell you it "saw" a refrigerator, coffee-pot, toaster, etc., even though it actually "saw" only the oven. In fact, the room descriptor network, and indeed PDP networks in general, have no intrinsic way of distinguishing between elements they have seen and elements they have inferred. Humans also tend to make errors of guilt by association and to "remember" what they would have expected, even if it was not really there. This suggests that discriminating fact from inference requires, at least in part, transcendent cerebral mechanisms that are not intrinsic to the networks storing information. One such mechanism might be a form of value judgment rendered by the limbic system that serves to define a particular representation as factual. Another mechanism might be an appendage or elaboration of the network that links the representation to a particular time and place, that is, gives it the properties of episodic memory as opposed to mere semantic memory. Case 12-26 illustrates incorrect inference in the form of confabulation.

The room descriptor model provides us the basis for defining the mechanism of another key property of PDP models and of the brain itself: *graceful degradation*. A lesion of the brain does not produce fundamental reorganization or production of novel behavior. Rather, errors tend to be near misses. Network damage increases the probability of error rather than fundamentally altering function. As we shall see, the property of graceful degradation also means that PDP networks and the brain tend to work well in the face of ambiguity, incomplete data, or false information. How would the room descriptor network function if half of its units were randomly destroyed? Clamping oven now might lead to a pattern of

## Case 12-26

### Confabulation in Korsakoff's Syndrome

*A 65-year-old man with a lifelong history of alcoholism has developed the severe impairment of memory that characterizes Korsakoff's syndrome. He has lived in a nursing home for years. When asked if he has any family, he cheerfully answers affirmatively and tells you that in fact, they just visited him last week. The nurses shake their heads, indicating that this is not true—that the patient is confabulating. However, later you run into a nurse who has been employed at the nursing home for many years and she tells you that yes, the patient does have a delightful daughter and a couple of grandchildren, and that they did indeed visit—5 years ago.*

**Comment:** *Korsakoff's syndrome results from recurrent hemorrhagic necrosis of midline nuclei of the thalamus and the mammillary bodies, key links in the hippocampal system, as a result of thiamine deficiency. Consequently, these patients are impaired in their ability to establish new declarative memories and their ability to recall memories encoded over recent years. All declarative memory is affected but episodic memory is particularly impaired. Thus, this patient knows he has an adult daughter whom he loves, but he has no knowledge of exactly when he last saw her. It turns out he did actually see her at the nursing home but whether he actually recalled the place of the visit or simply provided a plausible answer is uncertain. Because the patient's recollection seemed to most of the nurses to be contrary to fact, it was labeled a confabulation. In fact, confabulations typically contain components of actual fact that seems fallacious only because these components are cast in an incorrect temporal or spatial context. This is a result of the particular impairment of episodic memory and perhaps the loss of ability to distinguish factual from plausible.*

activation that involves only oven, cupboard, toaster, refrigerator, sink, coffee-cup, and telephone. This distribution contains far fewer features than were activated in the intact network. Nevertheless, the distributed representation that is generated is still unmistakable: it is kitchen. Graceful degradation occurs because the information underlying "kitchen" is represented throughout the network and cannot be obliterated by damage to portions of the network.

It is helpful to view PDP networks as a form of hologram. Let us say we have a hologram that when projected yields a picture of a standing woman, elegantly dressed. If we project a fragment of that hologram, we may still be able to discern a standing woman but the state of her dress is no longer clear. If we take a still smaller fragment, we may be able to discern a human but the gender is no longer clear. If we take an even smaller fragment, we can discern in the projection only a slender vertical object: it could be a standing human, an obelisk, a fence post, or a tree stump. Thus, a hologram, like a PDP network, degrades gracefully.

## The Auto-Associator Network: Insights Into Thinking

The room descriptor network, humble as it is, provides some insight into cerebral processes that may underlie thinking. In the network, a representation of a concept is static, but because it represents a pattern of activation, it is intrinsically ephemeral. The replacement of one pattern by another, that is, one representation by another, instantiates a serial process. Successive "clamps" on units of the network, either by external stimuli (e.g., as the network "walks" from room to room), or by output from other connected networks (as the network "contemplates" moving about the house), may elicit successive representations. If the brain is viewed as a large collection of variously interconnected networks, then consciousness might correspond to the total complex of representations defined through selective engagement by the current pattern of activation in the cortex. In this view, successive stimuli in the environment serve to clamp the brain networks in different ways, leading to the instantiation of new representations. Our interpretation of a situation often leads to an action which in turn leads to an alteration in the constellation of representations, another action, etc. Therefore, the necessarily serial nature of motor activity entrains a serial change in representations.

Suppose we postulate the existence of two networks, one supporting a representation corresponding to the present situation, the other supporting a representation that is a model of the present situation. In the model, our own internal specification of some component (our internal clamp) allows us to see what representation would emerge, given that clamp, and compare it with the representation corresponding to the actual state of affairs. By such mental modeling, we can anticipate the consequences of our actions, constrained of course by the limits of our knowledge, which is stored in the connection strengths within the model network. We can also solve complex problems in our heads by serially altering a given representation in precise ways as if those changes were actually being effected in the environment. Thinking, in this conceptualization, corresponds to imagining we are doing the process externally by manipulating an internal network model of the external world. Our ability to solve problems depends in great part on the availability of model representations that we can then internalize. Models, it seems, are difficult to develop and are in good part culture-bound and evolve only gradually. A major aspect of schooling is teaching representational schemes. It may be that true creativity lies in developing internal model networks that implicitly support novel representations and in turn enable us to ask unprecedented "what if" questions about the external world.

## PATTERN ASSOCIATOR NETWORKS

Figure 12-39 depicts a simple pattern associator network. It transforms a pattern of activity across its input units into a pattern of activity across its output units. All the primary and association cortices that process input to the brain and produce output from the brain constitute collections of pattern associator networks that convert neural activity in one or more input patterns to neural activity in one or more different output patterns. For example, a group of parallel pattern associator networks translates activity in calcarine cortex into representations in "what" and "where" visual association cortices that define the meaning, location, and movement of the visualized object or scene. A pattern associator network transforms auditory phonologic representations into articulatory phonologic representations, providing the capacity for repetition, and instantiating knowledge about the characteristic phonemic sequences of a language.

Rather than develop a particular pattern associator network, we will focus on two related aspects of such networks: *top-down/bottom-up processing* and *noise tolerance*. In the brain, each primary sensory cortex and its association cortices can be viewed as a giant, multilevel pattern associator model in which input from the bottom end derives from the sensory organ itself, for example, the retina, and output from the top is to

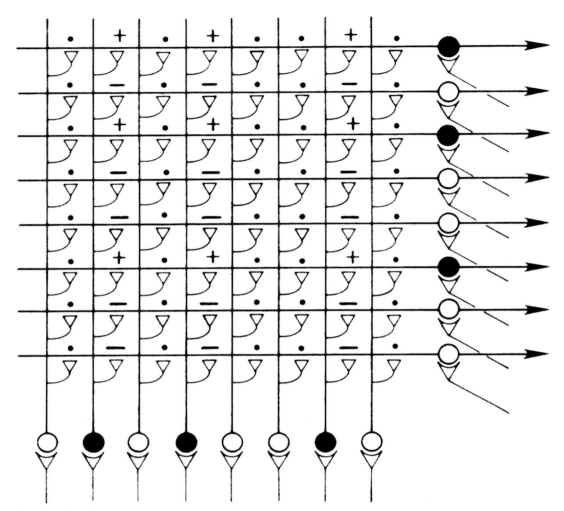

**Figure 12-39** A simple pattern associator network. The pattern of activity shown in the input units at the bottom elicits, via the system of input-output connections with their respective weights (denoted by + and – signs), the pattern of activity shown in the units at the right. (From Rumelhart DE, McClelland JL. On learning the past tenses of English verbs. In McClelland JL, Rumelhart DE, PDP Research Group (eds). Parallel Distributed Processing, Vol. 2. Cambridge: MIT Press, 1986, pp 216–271. © 1986 by The Massachusetts Institute of Technology.)

the ultimate auto-associator—the linked network of polymodal and supramodal association cortices that enables us to attach meaning to what we perceive. As it turns out, however, activation flow in the brain, as in many PDP networks, is two way, that is both from the bottom-up and the top-down. This has two particularly interesting consequences: a great tolerance for noisy input and a capacity for imagery, both of which we will explain in greater detail.

## Noisy Input

In our earlier discussion of graceful degradation, we cited relative preservation of function in the presence of damage as an important example. Tolerance for noisy input is another aspect of graceful degradation. Both reflect intrinsic properties of both PDP networks and the brain. Look at Figure 12-40.

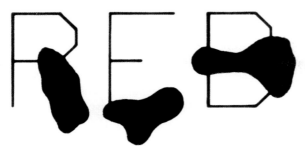

**Figure 12-40** Despite the obscured portions of letters, we read the word "red." (From McClelland JL, Rumelhart DE, Hinton GE. The appeal of parallel distributed processing. In Rumelhart DE, McClelland JL, PDP Research Group (eds). Parallel Distributed Processing, Vol. 1. Cambridge: MIT Press, 1986, pp 3–44. © 1986 by The Massachusetts Institute of Technology.)

If you look at each letter individually, you can make some guesses about what it might be, but you cannot tell unambiguously. Thus, the first letter might be "P" or "R," the second letter "E" or "F," and the third letter "B" or "D." However, when you look at the letters together, you are left with no doubt whatsoever that the word is "red" and that the letters are R, E, and D. In fact, you can arrive at this conclusion in an extraordinarily brief time and without conscious reflection. This capacity reflects bottom-up/top-down interactions within your brain networks supporting reading. The degraded letters generate bottom-up flow of activation from visual cortex that, unfortunately, is ambiguous: six different distributed letter representations will receive some activation, yielding a total of eight possible "words." However, when the bottom-up flow of activation spreads to polymodal and supramodal association cortices that provide the basis of meaning, only one of these eight words, "red," elicits meaning. This enables you to recognize it as a real word. Activation then spreads back down to the level of distributed letter representations (within unimodal visual association cortex—probably within the lingual and fusiform gyri in the medial inferior temporal lobes). This increases the activation levels of representations of R, E, and D, and reduces the activation levels of representations of P, F, and B, R, E, and D representations then have greater capability for inhibiting alternative letter interpretations through lateral flow of inhibitory activity (in much the same way that fireplace would inhibit sink in the room descriptor model). The result is that you develop a considerable sense of confidence that you are actually seeing the letters R, E, and D.

This capacity of hierarchical PDP networks to make sense of noisy input is of enormous value to us. Consider the experience of driving home on a rainy night. Despite the paucity of visual input, all moving, the host of false visual cues generated by reflections, and the visual noise generated by rain splattering on the windshield, we manage to extract a coherent perception that enables us to drive safely. Or consider the experience of carrying on a conversation in a loud party. Unfortunately, this mechanism for making the best of noisy input does not always work to our advantage. For example, it is the bane of our existence when it comes to correcting typographical errors because if a typed word sufficiently resembles its target to activate that target, top-down flow of activation will reinforce the component letters of the correct target, which in turn will reduce the activation of incorrect letters in visual perception of the typed word. The result is that we see what we intended to type, not what we actually typed.

## Imagery

Close your eyes and picture in your "mind's eye" what you would see if you opened them. The image you are generating is a faithful rendition, albeit a pallid one, of what you were actually seeing when your eyes were open. It is being generated by visual association cortices, but it is being generated from the top down. Consider for a moment how much your capacity for imagery, which resides in this capacity for top-down activation, enriches your life and enhances your cognitive capabilities. In the example just cited, the "mind's eye" image is a rather depleted rendition of the real thing. However, there are circumstances when the image may be far more vivid. We all experience this in dreams, which on occasion are so compelling we have at least momentary difficulty discriminating them from reality. In a more general sense, whenever we access a particular declarative memory, we are accessing distributed network representations from the top down.

Mind's eye images generated in sensory association cortices that cannot be discriminated from reality correspond to visual hallucinations. Analogous "images" generated in polymodal and supramodal association cortices correspond to delusions. Case 12-27 illustrates hallucinations and delusions in a patient with Parkinson's disease and mild dementia.

**Higher Neural Functions**

## Case 12-27

### Hallucinations in Parkinson's Disease

*A 70-year-old woman with a 20-year history of Parkinson's disease is seen in follow-up in a neurology clinic. Her husband reports that although she is generally doing pretty well on the medications she is taking, she has developed a serious problem with hallucinations and delusions. Her hallucinations usually consist of animals or strange people. She has a very persistent hallucination of gnarled, ragged little men she calls "trolls." Although at first she recognized the trolls as hallucinations, they have slowly evolved into a delusional system. She occasionally tries to strike trolls with a cooking implement when they appear on a kitchen counter. She insists that her husband drive the trolls out of the bathroom before she will use it. When they return from an evening engagement, she insists on remaining on the front porch until he clears the house of trolls.*

**Comment:** *The majority of patients with longstanding Parkinson's disease develop visual hallucinations. We believe that these derive from patterns of neural activity in visual association cortices that are generated from the top down from higher level, polymodal or supramodal cortices—rather than from the bottom up through visual input. Most of these patients recognize their hallucinations as unreal and are not bothered by them. Dysfunction in three systems appears to either potentiate hallucinations or lead from hallucinations to the generation of delusional systems: episodic memory, limbic valuation, and frontally mediated hypothesis testing. Poverty of perceptual input also appears to potentiate hallucinations. Each of these will be discussed at greater length below.*

### Episodic Memory

We noted earlier that PDP systems have no intrinsic mechanism for distinguishing fact from inference and that transcendent mechanisms are required to accomplish this distinction. Episodic memory links the representation generated by neural networks to a particular time, place, and circumstance. Being able to remember that she had had this particular strange experience before, to remember the various circumstances under which it occurred, the outcome of those occasions, and the assuring things that people said to her at those times would help her to identify the hallucinations as network inferences and not fact. Memory systems, most particularly episodic memory systems, are affected by common dementing processes, including those that occur in Parkinson's disease.

### Limbic Valuation

Second, patterns of neural activity generated in the limbic system may provide the sense of reality or unreality that helps us to distinguish fact from hallucinatory inference. On the other hand, it is possible that limbic representations actually lead, through limbic connections to sensory association cortices, to the top-down generation of hallucinatory patterns of activity. In demented patients, hallucinations are often linked to feelings of fear and lack of control resulting from cognitive deterioration that eventually evolve into paranoia. These limbic patterns of activity may render hallucinations sufficiently compelling that they are viewed as true perception, that is, they become delusions.

### Frontal Mediated Hypothesis Testing

Third, frontally mediated hypothesis testing normally leads us to check the reality of unusual sensory experiences. We perform "thought experiments," logically sorting through the details and circumstances of the sensory experiences. We may also plan actions to test the reality of these experiences. In dementia, there is often impairment in frontal systems, which may preclude coherent thought experiments and reality testing. Frontal systems may also have a perverse effect in certain disorders. If the limbic-derived sense of the reality of hallucinations is sufficiently strong, we may employ frontal systems to devise new and more elaborate delusional models of the external world that, in turn, support hallucinations as "logical" and "consistent" with reality. Such elaborate delusional systems are most often seen in schizophrenia (see later discussion).

### Poverty of Perceptual Input

Finally, rich sensory environments help us to distinguish hallucination from fact. Most of us have had the experience of lying awake at night and seeing a vague shape in the bedroom that we cannot recall or account for. On occasion, these perceptions may become sufficiently compelling to get us to stir and turn on a light briefly. Demented patients are far more likely to experience hallucinations and go through frightening delusional experiences at night than during the day. This has very practical implications: we can treat hallucinations and delusions in these patients by devices as simple as a night light and relatively benign drugs that aid sleep.

## PDP SYSTEMS IN A BROADER PERSPECTIVE

### Evidence of Parallel Distributed Processing in the Brain

This has been a very brief and in many ways fragmentary tour of PDP. However, we hope it has given you an intuitive sense of how complex behaviors can be generated by such humble microprocessors as neurons. One question many of you may have already asked is what is the evidence that PDP principles are actually instantiated in the brain? The answer is substantial and rapidly growing. For example, as your eyes saccade back to the beginning of each new line of text, the precise endpoint of that saccade is defined by a distributed representation in the superior colliculi—a pattern of activation involving all neurons in the superior colliculi. As you reach out to turn the page, the direction of your arm movement is defined by a distributed representation in motor cortex. As you are alerted by an unusual sound in the room, perhaps someone calling your name, the location of that sound is defined by a distributed representation in auditory cortices. The evolution of edge detectors, center-surround cells, motion detectors, and ocular dominance columns in visual cortex you read about in the vision chapter has been accounted for with remarkable cogency using PDP models. There is now a vast literature in this area, which is referred to as computational neuroscience.

### Chaos: The Science of Self-Organizing Systems

PDP probably strikes you as a somewhat strange and nonintuitive science. Actually, it represents a subfield of a fundamentally novel discipline that has burgeoned over the last 20 years—the science of self-organizing systems. Our basic intuitions about how things happen in nature originate in physics and chemistry, which are essentially deterministic disciplines. That is, they assume that one event leads to another in a way that can, at least in principle, be defined by an equation. The classical example is Newtonian mechanics. Unfortunately, this approach completely breaks down when it comes to describing the behavior of large numbers of entities governed by nonlinear functions over more than trivial periods of time—for example, turbulence. This science of self-organizing systems is referred to as chaos.[2] Although chaotic systems are not deterministic, they are not random either. They may display astonishing and intricate order: witness the regularity in certain cloud formations, dunes in a desert, leaves, flowers, snowflakes, and the persistence of the great red spot of Jupiter. In all these systems, the order we see emerges from the rule-bound behavior of very large numbers of simple units interacting with each other and their environment under certain conditions, for example, atmospheric water molecules contributing to cloud formation. The rules that ultimately provide the basis for the order govern only the individual units, not the entire system. Thus, rather than the system being organized by some superordinate principles, expressible mathematically (like Newtonian mechanics), the units within the system self-organize by virtue of the principles that govern only their own individual activity.

The brain is a chaotic system, both in its development and in its function. We begin life with a genetically determined array of neural connectivity. However, through the constant changes in the synaptic connection strengths of 100 billion neurons, each with over 1000 synaptic contacts, that original array is vastly transformed through our lifetimes and is constantly being altered from moment to moment. This evolution is guided by both genetic factors and experience. The effect of experience is achieved through Hebbian and other learning principles. The prolonged developmental period of humans allows great opportunity for experience to shape the rough neurodevelopmental processes set in motion and constrained by genetic factors. In this way, the modest brain-relevant information in the human genome can be parlayed into a structure that contains orders of magnitude of more

[2]For an outstanding introduction to this field, see Gleick J. *Chaos: Making a New Science.* New York, Viking, 1987.

Higher Neural Functions

information. The defining attribute of this developmental process is that it is completely unsupervised. Whatever order emerges derives from the various adaptive responses of 100 billion individual neurons and their synapses to their immediate neural environment, which in turn is heavily influenced by the sensory, autonomic, and hormonal environments. The remarkable degree of order achieved is strong testimony indeed to the power of the chaotic principles that define self-organizing systems.

The brain is chaotic in its function as well. Our instinctive recourse to deterministic and hierarchical principles leads us to view the frontal lobes as the supreme arbiters of behavior, everything else subserving the grand designs the frontal lobes elaborate. However, in many of the operations of daily life, we rely exclusively on other components of the nervous system and can be thankful that it is possible to keep the frontal lobes out of it. If we accidentally touch a hot stove, we certainly don't want our hand parked there long enough for the frontal lobes to formulate a plan—an agonizing, tissue-destroying 300+ ms. We rely on brainstem and spinal cord reflex mechanisms instead—a much speedier and more effective alternative. We rely on reactive attentional systems (temporoparietal and collicular) to warn us of potentially dangerous events or situations. The ultimate goal of the Olympic athlete is to leave his/her finely tuned sensorimotor systems to "do their thing" with minimal interference from cognitive and limbic systems—a feat only rarely achieved as anxiety takes its toll. These orderly responses emerge from completely undirected and unsupervised interactions of the entire cohort of neurons in the nervous system.

We are familiar with a host of other self-organizing systems, but are not very knowledgeable about this aspect of their behavior. The immune system is a self-organizing system in which interunit communication is mediated by chemical transmission at a distance and by fleeting ligand-membrane receptor interactions, rather than the more direct and considerably more sustained contact provided by electrochemical synapses in the brain. Cells within every organ system exhibit self-organizing behavior in organogenesis and repair. Evolution itself appears to exhibit self-organizing principles and is a prime example of chaos in action.[3]

---

[3]Richard Dawkins, in The Blind Watchmaker (New York, Norton, 1986), provides a particularly compelling and lucid account of Darwinian evolution from this perspective.

## PRACTICE 12-8

**A.** PDP networks are optimal for what is technically referred to as *parallel constraint satisfaction*—that is, arriving at a solution that optimally satisfies multiple demands or fits optimally with multiple different sources of information. Consider the sentence "The ball was thrown by the pitcher." The meaning of this sentence is instantly clear by the time you finish it. Now think about the nouns and the verb in this sentence. Do they have more than one potential meaning? How did you arrive at the correct meaning for each? What about the form of the sentence (the syntax)? Is the first noun in a sentence usually the perpetrator of the action (the "agent") or the recipient of the action (the "patient")? What are the clues to the slightly unusual syntax of this sentence?

We all process sentences sequentially, whether we hear them or read them. What do you think your brain was thinking?

**B.** Figure 12-41 shows a simple pattern associator network that converts the pattern on the top to the pattern on the right. In part *B* this same pattern associator is abbreviated using matrix notation. Just to update your faint recollections of matrix algebra, the top item in the output column is computed by multiplying each item in the input row at the top by the corresponding item in the first row of the matrix and adding. Thus, $(+1)(-0.25) + (-1)(+0.25) + (-1)(+0.25) + (+1)(-0.25) = -1$. Subsequent entries in the column on the right are computed in analogous fashion.

In part *C*, half the input to the pattern associator has been lost and in *D* one third of the pattern associator has been destroyed. Calculate the output patterns in *C* and *D*. What do you conclude regarding graceful degradation?

**C.** Cite some other examples of self-organizing systems.

**D.** Cite some common inferences encountered in daily life. Are these beneficial or harmful? Are humans the only creatures making use of inference?

**E.** All of us experience occasional slips of the tongue and word finding difficulty and all of us produce grammatical errors from time to time. Given your understanding of graceful degradation, predict the nature of errors made by aphasic patients.

**F.** Return to Case 12-8. How do you think this patient would do if actually given the correct tool? Why?

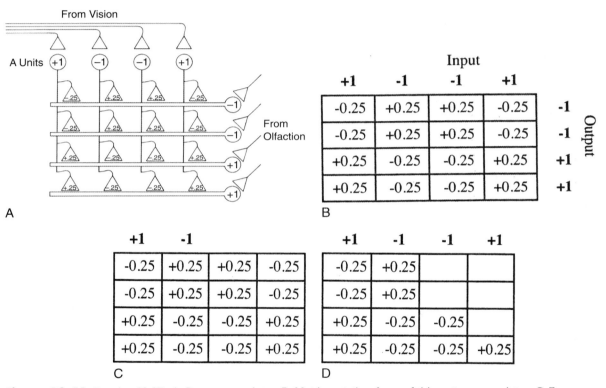

**Figure 12-41** Practice 12-8B. *A*, Pattern associator. *B*, Matrix notation form of this pattern associator. *C*, Fragmentary input. *D*, Damaged network. (*A* and *B* from McClelland JL, Rumelhart DE, Hinton GE. The appeal of parallel distributed processing. In Rumelhart DE, McClelland JL, the PDP Research Group (eds). Parallel Distributed Processing, Vol. 1. Cambridge: MIT Press, p 34. © 1986 by The Massachusetts Institute of Technology.)

# Cycle 12-9

# Integrated Brain Function

## Objectives

1. Be able to name the neural system whose dysfunction is most central to the state of depression and list other neural systems implicated in depression.

2. Be able to offer an explanation of depression in terms of a maladaptive state of reduced potential energy in PDP networks.

3. Be able to name the neural system for which dysfunction is most central to panic disorder and explain how this leads to more widespread alterations in neural systems supporting cognitive processing.

4. Be able to describe schizophrenia and list the major neural systems implicated in this disorder.

5. Be able to describe the development of schizophrenia in terms of the evolution of nonlinear dynamic systems.

6. Be able to describe briefly the neuroanatomy that accounts for the effectiveness of manipulations of biogenic amines (serotonin and norepinephrine in depression, dopamine in schizophrenia) in the treatment of these disorders.

The first seven cycles of this chapter detailed the neural systems responsible for the higher level functions of the brain. Daily living requires that these neural systems work together in an integrated fashion. The seemingly simple act of learning from this text requires the orbitofrontal-limbic assessment that it is a valuable endeavor, a dorsolateral frontal focus on the novelty of the material coupled with intentional attention to the words (lest the procedural memory of reading move you through several paragraphs without leaving a memory trace), dorsomedial frontal activity to initiate and sustain your reading, an intact visual association hierarchy, highly developed receptive language skills, plus intact recent and working memory systems that together accomplish the task of making this material a remote memory (in more ways than one).

Much of what we know about high level neural systems has developed from observing the effects of neurologic illnesses in humans (e.g., strokes, tumors, epilepsy, injuries) plus an ever-expanding array of anatomic, physiologic, and pharmacologic research in the laboratory. This cycle will examine integrated brain function through the lens of three common psychiatric disorders—major depression, schizophrenia, and panic disorder. These illnesses cannot be understood by focusing on single neural systems. Rather, they affect the activities and interactions of multiple higher level systems. Thus, an examination of these illnesses from the standpoint of functional neuroanatomy can inform us about the integrated operation of the human brain.

## Case 12-28

### Depression

*A 72-year-old widow was hospitalized for malnutrition and mutism. Prior to admission, she was living in her own home. Her family reported that for 3 months she gradually had become less interested in her usual social activities. For 6 weeks she had not ventured out of her house. They began taking food to her but she ate little. She took no interest in her personal appearance but cooperated when others washed and dressed her. She looked sad, developed insomnia, became forgetful, and talked about dying. She spoke only when others coaxed her into conversation, then eventually stopped talking completely. On admission, she weighed only 67 lb. A medical evaluation found malnutrition and dehydration. On neurologic examination, she did not respond to questions but passively allowed her cranial nerves, reflexes, and muscle tone to be tested. These findings were normal. A CT scan of the brain was normal. She was treated with a psychostimulant and an antidepressant. Within 3 days, she was eating on her own. One week later she was discharged home to live with her family, and within 2 months she resumed her usual activities in the community.*

**Comment:** *This patient suffered from major depressive disorder. Her symptoms of depression included her sad appearance, disturbances in sleep and appetite, memory deficits, anhedonia (loss of pleasure from usual activities), social withdrawal, profound lack of initiative, and recurrent thoughts of death. These symptoms reflect dysfunction in many brain regions, including frontal lobes, limbic areas, hypothalamus, hippocampus, and brainstem. Despite this, most episodes of major depression are not associated with anatomic central nervous system pathology. As in this case, the neurologic examination and neuroimaging studies typically are unremarkable.*

## MAJOR DEPRESSIVE DISORDER

Let us take a closer look at depressive symptoms (Case 12-28) from the standpoint of functional neuroanatomy. Patients with major depression experience a mix of persistent, negative emotional states such as sadness, anxiety, irritability, and anger. For poorly understood reasons, the emotional sense defined by the limbic system turns bleak. Depression is popularly thought to be triggered by an adverse event, but major depressive disorder often occurs without an identifiable precipitant. Even when associated with a loss or tragedy, depressive illness is more severe and longer lasting (months to years on average) than normal reactions to adversity. This suggests that the limbic definition of emotional sense is dysregulated in depressive disorders. That is, emotional sense becomes increasingly negative and does not return readily to a normal state.

However, major depression is not simply a disorder of negative emotions. Patients with depressive illness also have more pessimistic or catastrophic thoughts than normal individuals. They expect difficulties and poor outcomes, even in routine life circumstances. They undervalue formerly pleasurable activities and interpersonal interactions. In other words, as depressed patients' limbic systems signal sadness, anger, and irritability, limbic system links to other neural systems based in prefrontal and sensory association cortices lead to negative value judgments about the patient's memories, perceptions, activities, plans, and interactions with others. An effective form of psychotherapy for depression specifically targets the vicious circle of catastrophic thinking, perceptual bias, and negative emotions that are part of this disorder.

The symptoms of major depressive disorder also include disturbances of concentration, recent and working memory, sleep, appetite, energy level and sexual desire, as well as the development of suicidal thoughts. Concentration deficits point to dysfunction of the intentional attention system. Recent memory problems suggest abnormalities in hippocampal processing. Appetite changes and loss of libido are not surprising, given that the hypothalamus is the limbic system's primary effector structure. Disturbances of sleep and energy suggest that brainstem sleep and arousal centers function abnormally in major depression. Finally, the development of suicidality indicates that negative value judgments about oneself may overwhelm the usually strong, limbic-encoded instinct for self-preservation.

We do not have much knowledge about the circuitry that connects these higher neural systems. In fact, it is unlikely that one circuit links them all. This presents a challenge in understanding major depression as a single biologic entity. Any hypothesis must take into account the widespread symptomatology and reversible nature of the illness. The insidious onset of depressive symptoms suggests that a gradual degradation of function occurs in multiple brain systems. However, this dysfunction is reversible in almost all cases and does not leave an anatomic trace that can be detected with current technology. It is plausible that the neural dysregulation of depression begins in orbitofrontal-limbic circuitry. However, it is not clear what anatomic pathways allow this dysfunction to propagate throughout the brain.

Biogenic amine systems are clearly a crucial factor in depression. They provide a major avenue for treatment. Dysfunction in these systems may also be an important factor in the genesis of depression. Recall that biogenic amines affect general states of the brain such as sleep, arousal, and attentiveness. They also modify information processing in other neural systems (e.g., change signal-to-noise ratios). In other words, they set the background tone or stage on which higher neural systems operate. Biogenic amine systems project heavily to limbic structures such as the amygdala and to regions, such as nucleus accumbens, that are heavily interconnected with the limbic system (see Fig. 12-35). Furthermore, all effective treatments for depression enhance noradrenergic and/or serotonergic neurotransmission. Therefore, the leading biologic hypothesis about major depression states that dysregulation in biogenic amine systems negatively impacts the processing power of higher neural systems throughout the brain. Frontal lobes, hippocampus, hypothalamus, brainstem, and other areas do not sustain structural damage as they do in strokes or tumors. Rather, they may function poorly because the neurochemical environment in which they operate is suboptimal. Restoration of normal tone in the biogenic amine systems gradually reverses the dysfunction of these higher neural systems and relieves the constellation of symptoms that constitute major depression.

Our earlier discussion of PDP provides us an alternative way of viewing depression. In the rooms-in-a-house model, we noted that the network is theoretically capable of settling into $2^{40}$ different binary states (states in which some subset of the units is turned on—fully activated—and the remaining units are turned off). However, because of the mix of excitatory and inhibitory connections within the network, no matter which single room feature we clamp (turn on), activation levels in each of the 40 units increase or decrease until the network "settles" into one of five different patterns of activation, each corresponding to a room in the house. Each of these five different patterns can be usefully viewed as a deep valley in a "potential energy landscape" (in mathematical terms, optimal goodness of fit function). Just as a ball rolls downhill until it settles at the lowest point in the physical landscape (the point of lowest potential energy in the gravitational field), the rooms-in-a-house network moves downhill until it settles into a trough of minimal potential energy (or maximal goodness of fit). Which of the five troughs or valleys in the energy landscape the rooms-in-a-house network settles into is exclusively dependent on the input to the system.

Because the brain incorporates PDP principles, we think that brain function can usefully be viewed in terms of settling into various states of minimal "potential energy" or maximal goodness of fit. However, there are some important differences between the brain and the rooms-in-a-house model. Most obviously, the brain, or even subsystems within the brain, contains vastly more than 40 units (whether we conceive of the units as being neurons or columns of neurons). Furthermore, the relationships between units in the brain are considerably more complex than between those in the rooms-in-a-house model. The potential energy troughs into which a brain system settles are determined not just by the input, but also by the preexistent state of activation of the system. Finally, the energy landscape of a brain system can be changed to the degree that the connections between the units can be altered by experience.

Because of the vastly greater complexity of the brain, the energy landscape is marked not simply by high mountains and deep valleys—there are in addition small valleys, small hills within valleys, and ledges on the sides of hills and mountains. A neural system is potentially capable of settling into any minor concavity, even if it is only a ledge high on the side of an energy mountain. Furthermore, although every dip in the energy landscape represents, to one degree or another, a mathematical optimum, it may not correspond to a behaviorally adaptive state. For example, all of us are susceptible to developing a "tip of the tongue" state when we are speaking, in which we "know" exactly what we want to say, but cannot actually come up with the word. The frustrating persistence of this "tip of the tongue" state reflects a settling by language systems into a behaviorally maladaptive dip in the energy landscape. The state of the limbic energy landscape corresponding to clinical depression represents a vastly more dysfunctional and maladaptive situation, in which the affected person may barely be able to function, and suffers enormously.

It may take considerable "energy" to move from one valley in the energy landscape of a neural system to another valley. A simple metaphor may help understanding. Graphite and diamond are two stable forms of carbon. Diamond represents a vastly more stable state because the particular conformation of carbon atoms in diamond maximizes the strengths of the bonds between the atoms. However, despite the enormous energy advantages, graphite will not spontaneously transform into diamond. Rather, enormous heat and pressure must be brought to bear—the system must be transported over an extremely high peak in the energy landscape—before the carbon atoms of graphite will reorganize into a diamond configuration. This metaphor may be particularly apropos of states of the limbic system corresponding to depression. Whereas we usually move with great ease from state to state (word to word, concept to concept) in the energy landscape of language systems (except when we experience the "tip of the tongue" phenomenon), as yet undefined properties of the limbic system seem to make it extremely difficult to move out of a valley into which it has settled.

Manipulation of biogenic amine systems may represent a particularly effective means for providing the energy to lift the limbic system out of a deep, maladaptive valley corresponding to depression, thus allowing it to settle into a better valley. Psychological treatment, which leads to learning, changing connection strengths, provides a means for reshaping the energy landscape, in effect filling in the depression valley or building up the landscape around it so that the system is less likely to fall into this valley state.

## PANIC DISORDER

Anxiety is a universal experience that is usually adaptive and functional. It serves to alert us to events in our environment that require special attention. Anxiety can motivate us to prepare for an examination or become more vigilant when crossing a busy intersection during rush hour. However, when anxiety occurs without provocation or out of proportion to the event at hand (too intense or too long), it is considered pathologic (Case 12-29).

---

### Case 12-29

**Panic Disorder**

*A 32-year-old woman, while sitting on the couch watching television, rapidly develops overwhelming anxiety, a sensation that she cannot get enough air, chest pain, and tingling in her extremities. She is convinced at the time of the episode that she is going to die and has her husband call 911. Results of an emergency room evaluation are entirely normal and she returns home without an explanation for this terrifying event. Her second "spell" occurs at night and awakens her from sleep. Emergency evaluation again reveals no physical explanation for these episodes. In dread of the next attack, she begins to closely monitor any physiologic cues that her body may give her (changes in heart rate, skin temperature, breathing pattern) as early warnings of the next attack. Additionally, she begins to plan her day to avoid places where previous attacks have occurred and finds it more and more difficult to leave the "safety" of her house (agoraphobia).*

**Comment:** *This young woman has panic disorder. For poorly understood reasons and in seemingly unprovocative circumstances, she experiences the sudden generation of activity in her limbic system that corresponds to severe anxiety. Intense fear and distressing physical symptoms occur in the absence of any real threat to her. She makes catastrophic appraisals of these "false alarms" and develops a new, albeit inaccurate, notion of safety in her environment. Her remote memories of what is safe and what is not, laid down by her lifetime experiences, are updated to include her catastrophic appraisals. The frontal lobes bias sensory association cortex to respond to environmental stimuli such as reminders of previous attacks (refer again to selective engagement). Neurons in the amygdala and related limbic nuclei are conditioned to respond more intensely to somatic information, such as breathing and heart rate. The reciprocal connections from higher cortical areas to the amygdala and from the amygdala to brainstem areas offer neural circuitry that is sufficiently integrated to account for the subjective experience of fear, the physiologic arousal during a panic attack, and the cognitive appraisal of these episodes. Additionally, the intimate connections between the hippocampus and limbic structures account for the laying down of new memories of the experience that influence future appraisals of similar circumstances.*

Although neither the distributed representation of anxiety nor the precise mechanisms that generate it normally or pathologically are well understood, experimental data support the general concepts we have discussed. For example, a sense of anxiety has been evoked in humans undergoing neurosurgery by electrical stimulation in the amygdala, the anterior hypothalamus, and the periaqueductal gray. Measurement of regional cerebral blood flow, which is proportional to synaptic activity, using positron emission tomography (PET), has demonstrated increased blood flow in the anterior cingulate gyrus, the insula, and the amygdala during experimentally induced panic attacks.

Additional support for an interactive connectivity between these neural substrates is seen in the therapeutic interventions known to be effective in treating panic disorder. Medications can be used to block the actual episodes of panic. However, psychological treatment (cognitive-behavioral therapy) is often necessary for the patient to relearn how to make reasonable appraisals of internal cues (e.g., heart rate) and to once again experience benign settings (e.g., the mall) as nonthreatening.

## SCHIZOPHRENIA

Schizophrenia is an illness that involves deficits of multiple higher neural systems that substantially alter the inner thoughts of afflicted individuals and their interactions with the world (Case 12-30).

Patients with schizophrenia are challenged by deficits in several higher neural functions. The precise source of the positive symptoms is not known. Hallucinations are well-formed sensory phenomena (i.e., voices, not noises; fully developed visual images, not flashes of light) leading most researchers to conclude that they arise in higher level sensory association cortices. Delusions appear to be abnormal associations or faulty interpretations of perceptions and remote memories. Many delusions are related to the patient's life circumstances and historical era. Certain delusional themes, such as mind control, have been present throughout the ages, but specific false beliefs (e.g., the genetic engineering and computer chips in this case) use contemporary information. Therefore, patients with schizophrenia have the capacity to attain and retain memories, but for uncertain reasons, they either develop more faulty memory associations than the average person or fail to reject inaccurate associations as they arise.

### Case 12-30

#### Schizophrenia

*A 21-year-old man was brought into a hospital Emergency Department by his distraught parents. Seven months earlier, he had returned home from his junior year of college to work a summer job. During that time, his demeanor gradually changed. He quit the job because he felt he was being treated unfairly. He stopped socializing with his friends and began to spend long hours in his room playing computer games, searching the Internet, and writing a secret manuscript about mind control. He refused to return to college in the fall, saying that the purpose of his life had changed. For 6 weeks he had been "acting paranoid." He hung up the phone when other family members were using it. He watched reruns of Star Trek every day and seemed to talk silently to one of the characters. The patient reported that he had been hearing voices ever since a top secret society implanted "a genetically engineered, crystalline strontium computer chip" behind his left ear. His parents brought him to the hospital after they found him trying to "cut out the strontium" with a kitchen knife. The patient was admitted to the hospital and treated with risperidone, an antipsychotic medication that affects dopamine and serotonin in the brain. After 9 days, his auditory hallucinations and delusions about the strontium faded. He attempted to return to college the following semester, but withdrew because of increasing paranoid delusions. Back at home, he found a job in a warehouse. The risperidone kept most of his symptoms under control, though he occasionally talked about mind control and participated in few social activities other than work and church.*

**Comment:** *The cardinal features of schizophrenia include hallucinations (sensory experiences in the absence of external stimuli), delusions (unshakable, false beliefs), disorganization in thought processes (inability to put one idea after another in a logical order), avolition (reduced initiative), flattening of emotional expression, and alogia (diminution in spontaneous speech production). Hallucinations, delusions, and thought process abnormalities are termed "positive symptoms," while avolition, emotional restriction, and alogia are called "negative symptoms." Negative symptoms often lead to social isolation and withdrawal from friends and family.*

In the section on PDP, we discussed the fact that PDP networks cannot distinguish between representations generated from the top down and representations generated from the bottom up, a form of their intrinsic inability to distinguish fact from inference. From this standpoint, the positive symptoms of schizophrenia appear to be top-down processing gone awry. Hallucinations and delusions differ from the daydreams, fantasies, and remembrances that everyone experiences. These also are top-down phenomena (i.e., generated in widely distributed cortical association areas), but they can be identified readily as internally produced constructs, not responses to current environmental stimuli. Patients with schizophrenia cannot make this distinction regarding their hallucinations and delusions. This may be due to the strong links between sensory association cortices and the limbic system that lead to compelling emotional responses to these images (e.g., fear or paranoia). It may also be due to the inability of schizophrenics to use environmental stimuli to prove to themselves the falseness of their symptoms and to distinguish relevant from irrelevant stimuli, functions of dorsolateral prefrontal cortex and the intentional attention system, respectively.

The negative symptoms of schizophrenia appear to arise from altered activity of dorsolateral prefrontal and dorsomedial frontal lobe systems. Patients with prominent negative symptoms have difficulty forming strategies for dealing with novel situations and cannot shift well from one task to another. Compare these symptoms to the dorsolateral prefrontal syndrome discussed in Cycle 12-6. Patients with negative symptoms also appear to have little spontaneity or motivation in their behavior (avolition) and speech production (alogia). Initiation and maintenance of voluntary activities are dorsomedial frontal lobe functions.

The etiology of schizophrenia is not known, but the most prominent theory states that neural migration proceeds abnormally in utero. This migration defect is not widespread or severe enough to cause gross anatomic pathology. Rather, it is thought to be concentrated in neural networks that reciprocally connect the frontal lobes to the thalamus, ventral striatum, and limbic structures. These frontal-striatal-thalamic circuits may provide the neural substrate to continuously integrate sensory and motor functions with selective attention, value judgments, and motivation. All medications effective in treating schizophrenia block dopamine receptors in pathways that connect midbrain structures (e.g., ventral tegmental area) to the limbic system, a clear indication of the importance of the limbic system in the genesis of much schizophrenic symptomatology. However, recent data suggest more widespread pathology. For example, there may be abnormalities in neural circuits involving the thalamus (including sensory association and frontal systems) in schizophrenic patients. This might account for the prominent role that internally generated phenomena (e.g., hallucinations) play in schizophrenia and the relative lack of motivation that schizophrenics derive from external life events. It seems most accurate to view schizophrenia as a reflection of subtle defects in neural wiring that deform the integrated activity of higher neural systems. With the onset of schizophrenia, the parallel distributed systems that subserve normal processing of thoughts, sensory perception, and executive functions likely change state, settling into a condition that maintains the chronic illness. Treatments for schizophrenia can reduce symptoms but do not restore the affected neural systems to their premorbid state.

Our earlier view of the brain as a chaotic system (Cycle 12-8) may provide a useful way of analyzing the development of psychiatric disorders in general and schizophrenia in particular. In Cycle 12-8, we related both brain function and brain development to the properties of the brain as a chaotic system, but most of our discussion focused on brain function as we considered a particular type of chaotic system, parallel distributed processing. Here we will focus on brain development.

Chaotic systems are nonlinear dynamic systems. To understand what is meant by this term, and its implications, we will consider one simple nonlinear dynamic system. This system was described in 1963 by Edward Lorenz, a mathematician and a meteorologist at the Massachusetts Institute of Technology, in one of the most important scientific papers of the twentieth century. Lorenz's extraordinary insight, conveyed in this and two companion papers, constituted the birth of chaos theory. The system Lorenz described, involving three equations, was actually an oversimplified model of fluid convection. Here are the three equations:

$$\frac{dx}{dt} = 10(y - x)$$

$$\frac{dy}{dt} = -xz + 28x - y$$

$$\frac{dz}{dt} = xy - \frac{8}{3}z$$

You do not need to understand the details of these equations, or anything about fluid convection, to be

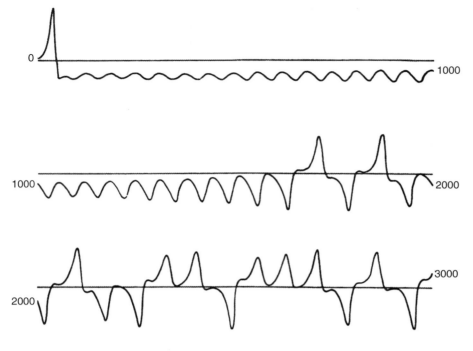

**Figure 12-42** Graph of the function of *y* for the first thousand iterations (top curve), the second thousand iterations (middle curve), and the third thousand iterations (bottom curve) for the Lorenz system. See text for details. (From Lorenz EN. Deterministic nonperiodic flow. J Atmospheric Sci 20:130–141, 1963. © American Meteorological Society.)

able to appreciate the remarkable behavior of the system these equations define. This is a nonlinear dynamic system, nonlinear because two of the equations involve multiplicative terms involving two of the variables ($xz$ and $xy$), and dynamic, because all three equations define the changes over time in $x$, $y$, and $z$. The equations describe continuous functions, but in order to simulate the system on a computer, a discrete time increment of 0.01 was used. Each time increment of 0.01 constitutes one iteration in the computation. Figure 12-42 shows the behavior of $y$ over the first 3000 iterations. The system has to be given an initial "nudge" (corresponding to the sharp peak at the beginning of the top curve of the figure, because, as you can see from the equations, if $x$, $y$, and $z$ are all zero, then $dx$, $dy$, and $dz$ will also be zero, and the system will sit forever at an unchanging steady state. After the brief nudge, $y$ settles down into mild oscillation about an average value of −8.4 (you actually do not need to worry about the literal values for any of the variables). If we watched this system for about 500, or even 1000 iterations, we might be inclined to say, enough is enough, yes, it oscillates a little, but it looks like a pretty well behaved, orderly system. However, at about iteration 1650, something dramatic happens, and the behavior of $y$ becomes disorderly and unpredictable—seemingly random.

Like hundreds of scientists before him, Lorenz could have thrown up his hands and left it there, con-

ceding that, yes, there are limits to our ability to define natural systems (the weather, in Lorenz's case) in precise mathematical terms over long periods of time, but some day. . . . However, Lorenz then plotted the evolving values of $x$, $y$, and $z$ over time in one three-dimensional coordinate system ("phase space") (Fig. 12-43). The graph plots the course of the system beginning at iteration 1400 ("14" in the figure). With each successive iteration after the 1400th, the successive values of $x$, $y$, and $z$ define a clockwise spiral tilted in one eighth of the cube of space defined along the $x$, $y$, and $z$ axes. In fact, from after the initial nudge to iteration 1650, the system continues in this relatively, but not absolutely predictable, spiral. However, after the 1650th iteration (as we saw in Fig. 12-42), a dramatic change occurs: the system begins to alternately spiral in two completely different regions, or domains, of space (forever as it turns out). However, Figure 12-43, unlike Figure 12-42, shows us that this behavior, heretofore seemingly random, is actually very orderly in a way we never could have imagined—it is chaotic. The temporal evolution of the system defines a butterfly wing–shaped object, a system-specific pattern commonly referred to in chaos theory as a "strange attractor." In short, "chaos" is by no means synonymous with random or unpredictable, but rather corresponds to a different type of order, the order evident in most natural systems, as we discussed at some length in the previous cycle.

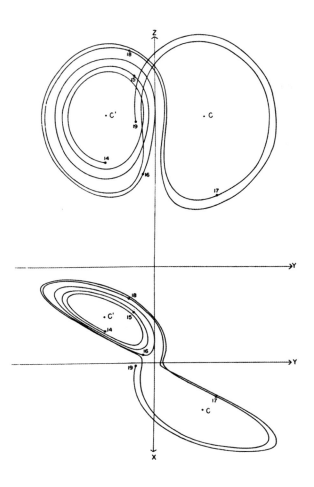

**Figure 12-43** Graph of the evolution of values of *x, y,* and *z* over time in the Lorenz system between iteration 1400 ("14") and iteration 1900 ("19"). The top graph plots the system in the *yz* plane and the bottom graph in the *xy* plane. C and C′ define the two major domains in which this chaotic system alternately resides. This type of graph, in which each point corresponds to a state of the system at a particular instant in time, is referred to as a phase space plot. See text for details. (From Lorenz EN. Deterministic nonperiodic flow. J Atmospheric Sci 20:130–141, 1963. © American Meteorological Society.)

How might this give us insight into the evolution of higher neural systems and of psychiatric disorders? What we have seen is that a very simple, nonlinear dynamic system, after a long period of minimally fluctuating and generally predictable behavior, suddenly starts bouncing back and forth between two completely different domains of mathematical space. This bouncing back and forth, when we see it in the light of a representation like that shown in Figure 12-43, is also orderly in its own way, and it clearly defines two very

different states of the system. Reconsider Case 12-30 in light of Figure 12-43. Suppose that the extraordinarily complex nonlinear dynamic system based upon orbitofrontal-limbic neural networks behaves substantially like the vastly simpler Lorenz system, and that 100 iterations corresponds to a year of life. For the first 16+ years of life, behavior, though fluctuating somewhat, appears to be relatively normal. Then between year 16 and year 17, behavior starts making detours into a fundamentally different, and as it turns out, extremely dysfunctional state. We might also be able to account for the oscillations in the behavior and experience of patients with bipolar affective ("manic-depressive") disorder as reflecting natural transitions between domains in a complex nonlinear dynamic system.

Why might some people remain in one, generally functional behavioral (and mathematical) domain all their lives, while others, like patients with schizophrenia and bipolar affective disorder, end up bouncing back and forth between different and, in some cases, highly dysfunctional domains? It turns out that the behavior of the system described by Lorenz's equations, and of nonlinear dynamic systems in general, is highly dependent on the initial conditions. In the case of Lorenz's equations, these are defined by the constants in the equations, which derive from thermodynamic science. In the brain, corresponding constants would logically derive from genetic and congenital factors, and to some degree, the accumulated experience of the individual. As we have noted, most schizophrenics have evidence of subtle neuroanatomic abnormalities, indicating that their brains were not perfectly normal to start with—that the initial conditions (reflected in the constants) were slightly altered. With very small adjustments in the constants, the time course of the chaotic behavior we observe can change dramatically, or the system can even end up spending its entire life oscillating in only one domain of mathematical space. In Lorenz's system, neither domain is "better" than the other one, but in the systems underlying human behavior, one domain may be adaptive and the other eminently maladaptive by virtue of its impact on experience and behavior (as in schizophrenia or bipolar affective disorder).

It is a very long reach indeed from Lorenz's very simple system to the neural systems defining emotional function. Many may think the reach is so long as to be simply incredible. Is there any more concrete evidence that the developmental evolution of any neural system can be understood in the terms we have been discussing? In fact, there is. We will briefly discuss one example. In Chapter 9, we noted that primary visual

*Higher Neural Functions*

cortex, V1, is organized, among other things, into ocular dominance columns: columns of neurons that respond almost exclusively to input from one eye. Columns at any given retinotopic location in V1 responding to input from the ipsilateral eye are located immediately adjacent to columns responding predominantly to input from the contralateral eye. In the newborn kitten, these ocular dominance columns are already in evidence, but they respond to input from both eyes, albeit somewhat more to input from the contralateral eye than from the ipsilateral eye. In a large number of experiments performed in the 1960s, Hubel and Wiesel and other investigators showed that if kittens are deprived of input to one eye, for example, by suturing the eyelid shut, that all columns in V1 ultimately show responsiveness only to input to the open eye. Even though retinal geniculocalcarine transmission from the sutured eye remained normal, when the suturing was removed, the kitten was effectively permanently blind in that eye. The same thing can happen in humans deprived of input from one eye (e.g., because of a congenital cataract [opacification of the lens]) and is referred to as amblyopia.

Amblyopia can be induced in kittens by lid suturing only during the first 3 weeks of life. Thereafter, even very sustained periods of monocular visual deprivation will have no effect. The mechanism underlying the existence of this "critical period" has been debated extensively. Some investigators have posited some kind of exogenous maturational factor. However, an early experiment by Hubel and Wiesel showed that temporary binocular blinding did not have nearly so disruptive an effect, suggesting that the changes produced by unilateral visual deprivation were due to a competitive interaction between the geniculocalcarine afferents serving the two eyes. Since then, Kenneth Miller and Michael Stryker have developed a simple PDP model of the geniculocalcarine system.[4] This model spontaneously develops ocular dominance columns as it is exposed to binocular visual input, and it develops amblyopia when deprived of input from one eye during the "critical period." The existence of the critical period reflects the fact that this model, and the visual system, are nonlinear dynamic systems. As such, they evolve over time and undergo extensive changes (in the case

of these particular systems, acquire extensive knowledge in the form of neural connections). As a result, only during a limited phase of their evolution are they dependent on binocular input for the development of normal patterns of connectivity, and therefore susceptible to interruptions in input from one eye. No exogenous "maturational factor" need be posited: the critical period is an intrinsic property of the evolution of these nonlinear dynamic systems.

In the case of schizophrenia, we surmised that the evolution of a nonlinear dynamic system, subserved by orbitofrontal-limbic cortex, eventuated in the appearance of spontaneous oscillations between two mathematical and behavioral domains, one highly dysfunctional. In the case of the visual system, far more concrete evidence and simulations using a specific and detailed neural network model (also a nonlinear dynamic system) provide evidence of a complex evolutionary pattern as well, one that eventuates not in oscillations between two domains, but one that demonstrates differential susceptibility to environmental influences in the course of its evolution. In both examples, the observed behavior can be explained entirely in terms of the evolutionary properties of a nonlinear dynamic system.

# PRACTICE 12-9

**A.** Explain, in terms of neural systems, why a depressed patient:
1. no longer enjoys normally pleasurable experiences in life (anhedonia);
2. declines to engage in projects or activities or pursue long-term goals;
3. has no appetite.

**B.** What biogenic amine projections are most likely to be important in the treatment of depression and why?

**C.** Explain why psychological treatment is often needed for patients with panic disorder even when the panic attacks are effectively treated pharmacologically. Can you relate this to energy landscapes in PDP networks?

**D.** Why might hallucinations be so compelling to schizophrenics?

**E.** What neural systems are implicated in the loss of spontaneity and initiative of schizophrenic patients and their difficulty in dealing with novel situations and shifting tasks?

---

[4]Miller KD, Stryker MP. The development of ocular dominance columns: Mechanisms and models. In Hanson SJ, Olson CR (eds). *Connectionist Modeling and Brain Function: The Developing Interface*. Cambridge, MIT Press, 1990, pp. 255–350.

**F.** Explain why dopamine blockers that target receptors in the limbic system are effective in treating only some of the symptoms of schizophrenia.

**G.** Explain in terms of nonlinear dynamic systems how genetic/congenital abnormalities in neural cytoarchitecture and major adverse experiences can have strong impact on the ultimate evolution of the brain. Explain why the timing of adverse experiences might be important.

## CYCLE 12-1

**A.** See Figure 12-1.

## CYCLE 12-2

**A.** Just as there are "what" and "where" visual systems, there is a "what" somatosensory system, represented by primary and secondary somatosensory neurons, and a "where" somatosensory system, represented in projections from postcentral gyrus to areas 5 and 7.

**B.** This patient has pure word deafness due to a stroke involving auditory cortex in the left hemisphere and connections from right auditory cortex to left hemisphere language cortex (Fig. 12-44). She is able to hear environmental sounds perfectly normally but is unable to decode the linguistic content of acoustic input. Thus, it becomes apparent that normal auditory processing consists of distributed processing of two rather differ-

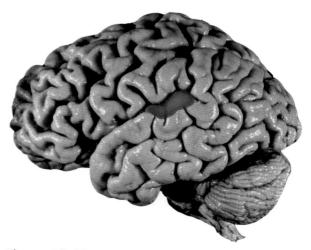

**Figure 12-44** Lesion in Practice 12-2B. Most of the infarct involves primary auditory cortex (Heschl's gyrus) and auditory association cortices on the superior surface of the temporal lobe, deep within the sylvian fissure.

ent acoustic attributes of auditory stimuli. Here the two hemispheres have different capabilities, the left decoding linguistic content and the right nonlinguistic content.

**C.** She has bilateral inferior quadrantanopias due to damage to superior medial occipital cortex bilaterally. Her ability to recognize, describe, and name objects is perfectly normal because the "what" visual pathway is completely spared. Her ability to point to and even to look at objects is also severely impaired because of destruction of the "where" visual pathway (referred to as optic ataxia and optic apraxia, respectively). She has Balint's syndrome (see also Case 9-6).

**D.** The patient is unable to read because left visual association cortex has been deprived of visual input due to the left calcarine infarct and the trajectory from right visual association cortex to left hemisphere cortex that supports reading has been destroyed by the lesion of the splenium of the corpus callosum. This is another example of disconnection of sensory association cortex from a supramodal cortex, as in Case 12-4. It was first described by Joseph Jules Dejerine in the 1880s. Because the right hemisphere can usually process single letters, these patients often read (very slowly) by spelling the words out aloud.

## CYCLE 12-3

**A.** This patient has Wernicke's aphasia due to a lesion of left area 22 (Wernicke's area) that damages the phonologic processor, connections to association cortices supporting meaning, and connections from dominant auditory association cortex to association cortices that would normally enable comprehension (Fig. 12-45). His aphasia corresponds to a combination of the aphasias described in Cases 12-6 and 12-7. He would not be expected to have a hemiparesis because Wernicke's area is quite distant from motor systems and is frequently damaged by stroke without involvement of motor pathways (Table 12-8).

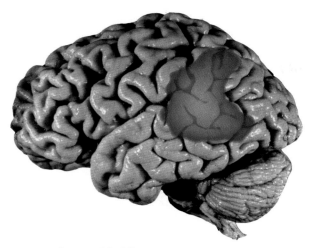

**Figure 12-45** Lesion in Practice 12-3A.

**B.** She would be severely impaired in the use of tools with her left hand because her right premotor cortex can no longer access the distributed representation of praxis in the left hemisphere. Graphesthesia in the left hand would also be severely impaired because even though her right hemisphere is capable of processing the sensory input, it cannot provide a verbal report or communicate its findings to the left hemisphere, which can provide a verbal report.

**C.** Getting lost reflects impairment in another aspect of visuospatial function and therefore localizes to the non-dominant hemisphere. Thus, this patient is unlikely to have a focal left hemispheric process, such as a tumor, and is far more likely to have a more diffuse, degenerative process. Most likely this is Alzheimer's disease. Getting lost is a classic symptom of Alzheimer's disease, in which the most severe cortical pathology is in the temporal and parietal lobes.

**D.** She would tell you that you sounded happy because the only information she can decode from your sentence is linguistic. Our understanding of spoken language is defined by a distributed representation, part linguistic (in the left hemisphere), part prosodic (in the right hemisphere).

**TABLE 12-8** Summary of Major Features of Disorders of Language Function

| Mechanisms Affected | Linguistic Features | Locus of Lesion | Common Term |
| --- | --- | --- | --- |
| Impaired verbal output due to damage to motor representations of phonemes | Labored, slurred speech | Frontal operculum (Broca's area) | Broca's aphasia |
| Disruption of phonologic processing in language production (loss of phonologic sequence knowledge) | Generation of phonemic paraphasias in spontaneous language and repetition | Posterior area 22 (Wernicke's area); area 40 | Conduction aphasia |
| Disruption of links between perisylvian language cortex and association cortices supporting meaning | Good repetition, no phonemic paraphasias, poor comprehension and empty, anomic spontaneous language | Temporoparietal cortex sparing the perisylvian region | Transcortical sensory aphasia |
| Disruption of links between perisylvian language cortex and association cortices supporting meaning plus damage to posterior portions of dominant perisylvian cortex supporting phonologic processing | Poor repetition, abundant phonemic paraphasias in spontaneous language and repetition (sometimes jargon), poor comprehension | Temporoparietal cortex including posterior perisylvian cortex | Wernicke's aphasia (in effect, transcortical sensory aphasia + conduction aphasia) |

Higher Neural Functions

## CYCLE 12-4

**A.** The man's lesion is in the vicinity of the left lateral septal nucleus. The story in this case, of sudden pronounced alterations in behavior, is highly characteristic of seizures in the limbic or frontal systems.

**B.** One would not expect the same results. Although the hypothalamus is the source of autonomic outflow that in a fundamental sense defines limbic function, behaviors elicited by hypothalamic stimulation are generated in the context of activity in the remainder of the limbic system. That context is usually very different in a caged laboratory animal than in a beloved pet.

**C.** This is a real phenomenon, mediated by limbic-autonomic connectivity. Even healthy laboratory animals placed in extremely stressful circumstances from which there is no escape can die (see Chapter 11).

## CYCLE 12-5

**A.** We would expect him to have Korsakoff's syndrome, which is characterized by both anterograde and retrograde deficits in declarative memory. The responsible lesions are in the mammillary bodies and the dorsomedial nuclei of the thalamus. If your answer included the anterior nuclear group of the thalamus, give yourself full credit, even though involvement of these nuclei has been inconsistent in pathologic studies. The periaqueductal lesions associated with Wernicke's encephalopathy account for the ophthalmoplegia (by virtue of destruction of nuclei and pathways involved in eye movement) and lethargy, stupor, and coma (by virtue of damage to the midbrain reticular activating system).

**B.** The effects of hippocampal lesions reflect the nature of the material processed by the hemispheres with which they are linked. Thus, left hippocampal lesions cause disproportionate impairment in verbal memory, whereas right hippocampal lesions cause disproportionate impairment in nonverbal memory. Prospective temporal lobectomy patients undergo a procedure call the Wada test in which one hemisphere of the brain is briefly anesthetized, allowing examiners to determine the verbal memory capability of the other hippocampus. In the ideal surgical candidate, damage to the temporal lobe in which the seizure focus lies is sufficiently severe and longstanding that declarative memory capability has already been largely subsumed by the opposite hemisphere.

**C.** Declarative memory acquisition would be affected because declarative memory formation depends on long white matter links within the hippocampal system and connections between the hippocampal system and the cerebral cortex.

**D.** Animals. Even though the representation of remote memories is widely distributed, the extent of this distribution reflects the fundamental modalities of the memory. Thus, our recall of animals is based disproportionately on visual representations in the inferior temporal lobes whereas our recall of tools depends to a relatively greater degree on "mind's hand" representations in frontal and parietal cortex.

**E.** One would expect procedural memory impairment due to premotor cortex disease.

**F.** This is but one of a variety of lines of converging evidence that tell us that there is far greater plasticity in the brain than we ever imagined, and that in fact sensorimotor systems undergo constant self-organizing adaptation to the demands that are being placed upon them. Thus, this tennis player allowed his sensorimotor systems to reshape themselves a little too much to the harsh demands of a life of leisure.

**G.** Even though smell is a minor sense in humans, olfactory stimuli can be extremely powerful evokers of prior memories, probably because olfactory connectivity with hippocampal structures assures that when present, a prominent olfactory stimulus leads to a major olfactory component in the distributed representation of that memory.

## CYCLE 12-6

**A.** Given the history, this patient is likely to have sustained fairly extensive damage to one of his frontal lobes from tumor, surgery, and radiation therapy, and some damage to the other from radiation. However, the behaviors described are largely localizable to the right dorsolateral frontal cortex. The tendency to produce constructions that only vaguely resemble the target, the perseverative retracing of lines, and the loss of capacity for critical judgment of one's own performance are typical. His echopraxia reflects an inability to resist the temptation to imitate the examiner's gesture. If you perform this test yourself with a

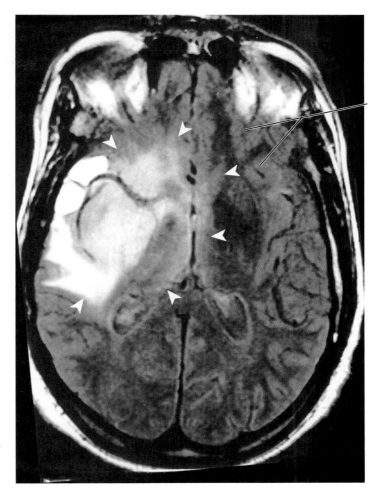

**Figure 12-46** Magnetic resonance image (MRI) of patient in Practice 12-6B. The borders of the tumor are indicated by arrowheads.

colleague, you will quickly appreciate that is it considerably easier to mimic than to produce the contrasting program.

**B.** This is a classic orbitofrontal syndrome, caused in this case by a primary brain tumor, a glioma (Fig. 12-46). The inappropriate humor, at times cruel, is referred to as witzelsucht.

**C.** This patient has Binswanger's disease, which is characterized by tiny strokes predominantly in the white matter adjacent to the bodies of the lateral ventricles and is caused by his longstanding high blood pressure (Fig. 12-47). Eventually these tiny lesions, which are more demyelinative than axonal, become nearly confluent. Frontal system function and declarative memory acquisition are most severely impaired because these systems are particularly dependent on the integrity of long white matter pathways. The periventricular location of these lesions causes particularly severe deficits in dorsomedial frontal function, hence the akinesia and loss of initiative, as well as gait apraxia and urinary incontinence. The clinical picture very much resembles that in communicating hydrocephalus.

## CYCLE 12-7

**A.** Cortical blindness due to bilateral occipital infarction caused by bilateral posterior cerebral artery occlusion, lethargy due to ischemia of the MRF and the thalamus, some combination of vertical gaze palsy and right or left CNIII palsy, and possibly hemiparesis or quadriparesis due to ischemia in one or both cerebral peduncles or caudal posterior limbs of the internal capsules.

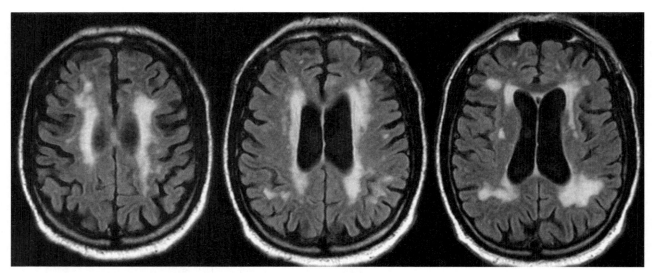

**Figure 12-47** Magnetic resonance image (MRI) of a patient with Binswanger's disease. The high signal (*white*) observed throughout the deep hemispheric white matter bilaterally indicates increased water content due to loss of myelination and, to a somewhat lesser extent, axons.

**B.** Even though total quantity of sleep is normal, this patient will be both REM and non-REM sleep deprived because he never got past stage II. Typically these patients function during the day much like you or I would had we stayed up all night. They have difficulty concentrating, tend to fall asleep all day long, at times under inappropriate circumstances such as at the dinner table or while in conversation, and may experience the pain associated with non-REM sleep deprivation. This is a common disorder.

**C.** The visual grasp is a reactive attentional orienting movement, most likely mediated in this case by the superior colliculi.

**D.** The neglect syndrome can usefully be viewed as a failure of selective engagement of much of the involved hemisphere, most often the right. Thus, not only are these patients typically inattentive to the left but they have problems engaging right frontal cortices to initiate behavior directed to the left and they typically have a very flat affect reflecting deficits in emotional expressive function. Some of these deficits might reflect direct damage to right hemisphere neural structures, such as premotor cortex, but as a rule, the lesion is not sufficiently extensive to account for the deficits in this direct way. This suggests that defective selective engagement is responsible.

**E.** No. Surgery would seriously risk damage to structures critical to declarative memory formation, includ-

ing the medial septal nuclei and the basal forebrain, which supply acetylcholine to the hippocampus and the cerebral cortex, respectively.

**F.** All tasks engaging the cerebrum require us to transiently bring on line selected neural networks—hence, working memory. Working memory is allocated as a by-product of other cerebral mechanisms engaged in task performance.

**G.** Not a good idea. The blockade of cholinergic input from the medial septal nuclei to the hippocampi, and from the nucleus basalis to the cerebral cortex, would adversely affect declarative memory acquisition, hardly the thing to do when preparing for a test.

**H.** Dopamine receptor blockers are the mainstay of treatment of patients with psychiatric disease associated with hallucinations and delusions, for example, schizophrenia. Therefore, quite predictably, dopaminergic agonists aggravate such symptoms in parkinsonian patients.

## CYCLE 12-8

**A.** A ball could be a spherical object or a dance. Threw could refer to propelling a ball or hosting a party, and for some might even briefly evoke the thought of throwing up. A pitcher could be a container or a baseball player. Thus, each major lexical item in this sentence is ambiguous. In English, the first noun in a sentence is overwhelmingly the agent or perpetrator. Not so in this sentence, which is in the passive voice. The most obvious clue to this is the "was . . . by" construction in the middle of the sentence, which indicates the passive voice. However, you were made aware that this sentence was probably in the passive voice earlier. Balls may fall or roll, but most often they are the object of an action.

There is good psychological evidence that the brain accesses to one degree or another many of the possible interpretations of a sentence as we process it and ultimately narrows the interpretations to one (if the sentence is not ambiguous). Americans are unlikely to think of anything other than a sport implement when they read the word "ball." If the sentence had been "The ball was thrown by the queen," most Americans would pause and possibly reread the sentence when they were suddenly confronted with the image of the queen on a baseball mound. People living in Great Britain might be expected to more equally activate the two major meanings of ball and thrown. Thus, parallel constraint satisfaction evolves over time.

**B.** See Figure 12-48. The amplitudes of the output are reduced relative to *A* and *B*, but the pattern of the output is identical—a clear demonstration of graceful degradation. In the brain, such reduced amplitudes generally translate into a reduced probability that the correct response will be generated. However, the likelihood of producing a completely novel response remains low.

**C.** Ant, bee, and termite colonies, social animals in general, coral. Bacterial colonization of mucous membranes might even be considered a crude self-organizing system. Ecosystems. The Gaia concept that the entirety of life on earth self-regulates to preserve a viable planet, if valid, would represent the grandest example of self-organization.

**D.** Our lives are predicated on a constant stream of inferences. All the myriad things that seem to remain constant from day to day lead us to infer that they will remain constant. Even our experience with things that are variable lead us to inferences about the expected range of variability. We thus readily detect rather modest alterations in the behavior of our friends and family members or in the movement of traffic on the way to work. Inferences enable us to proceed efficiently—we don't have to spend a lot of time thinking about what will change and what will stay the same. Inferences prepare us for important events. For example, we infer that crossing a major street will be dangerous and take due precautions. We infer that a final exam in medical school will be hard and important and study accordingly. Unfortunately, inferences are not always good. We often make simplistic or biased inferences about the quality of a particular person on the basis of a single encounter. Human beings in general appear to be extraordinarily susceptible to making invidious inferences about entire races or classes of people based on very fragmentary information. A significant part of what we "know" actually represents things we have inferred from very limited experience or as a logical extension of our conceptual framework. Frequently it turns out to be false. Although science is founded on hypothesis formation—in actuality, inferences—we tend to see what we expect to see (i.e., what we infer) and therefore often overlook important pieces of data. For the scientific clinician, making good inferences from the patient's chief complaint, formulating good hypotheses, will help in making the correct observations. Making multiple hypotheses (i.e., a differential diagnosis) that truly cover the disease possibilities in a given patient helps to assure that even though we tend to see what we expect to see, we have prepared ourselves with all relevant expectations. In other words, a good clinician simultaneously takes advantage of the intrinsic strengths of his/her neural net architecture and takes care to compensate for its intrinsic weaknesses.

Inferences are no less important to lower animals. Mosquitoes infer that objects with the appropriate

| +1 | −1 | | | |
|---|---|---|---|---|
| −0.25 | +0.25 | +0.25 | −0.25 | −0.5 |
| −0.25 | +0.25 | +0.25 | −0.25 | −0.5 |
| +0.25 | −0.25 | −0.25 | +0.25 | +0.5 |
| +0.25 | −0.25 | −0.25 | +0.25 | +0.5 |

| +1 | −1 | −1 | +1 | |
|---|---|---|---|---|
| −0.25 | +0.25 | | | −0.5 |
| −0.25 | +0.25 | | | −0.5 |
| +0.25 | −0.25 | −0.25 | | +0.75 |
| +0.25 | −0.25 | −0.25 | +0.25 | +1 |

**Figure 12-48** Pattern associator matrix calculations for Practice 12-8B: partial input (*left*) and damaged network (*right*).

Higher Neural Functions

olfactory signature are sources of nourishment. Unfortunately they are only too often correct. They also infer that a rapid change in the pattern of luminance warns of imminent disaster and are quick to take flight. This response probably leads to a lot of false alarms, as crude a sensory analysis as goes into it, but it has the critical outcome of helping to keep the mosquito alive.

**E.** To a very large extent, aphasic patients make the same types of language errors as normal people—they just make a lot more of them.

**F.** His performance would improve if not become entirely normal. In pantomiming, he must rely exclusively on the effect of top-down spread of degraded neural activity patterns. When given the tool to hold, he is provided a source of additional information which flows from the bottom up and serves to improve, if not completely correct, the tool use movement.

# CYCLE 12-9

**A. 1.** Perceptual input to sensory association systems no longer elicits patterns of activity in the limbic system that are "pleasurable."
**2.** Plans for projects, activities, and long-term goals developed through prefrontal cortices elicit patterns of activity in the limbic system that fail to validate and sustain those plans.
**3.** Pathologically altered patterns of neural activity in the limbic system are communicated to portions of the hypothalamus important to appetite and food intake.

**B.** Dorsal raphe (serotonin) and locus ceruleus (norepinephrine) projections to amygdala, limbic cortex, and nucleus accumbens. Nucleus accumbens has extensive interconnections with limbic cortices. Potentiation of the activity in these systems, by altering signal-to-noise ratio in the target structures, moves the limbic system out of the neural representations corresponding to the state of depression.

**C.** Patients with panic disorder utilize prefrontal and higher association cortices to generate logical explanations or hypotheses for their anxiety attacks. Frontally mediated intentional attention mechanisms lead them to attend to logically implicated environment cues. The expectation that these cues will lead to attacks causes anxiety, confirming the hypotheses and leading to repeated reenforcement of the pathologic theory. Psychological treatment may be necessary to break this vicious circle. In PDP energy landscape terms, psychological treatment alters the energy landscape.

**D.** Because the neural representations in sensory association cortices that correspond to hallucinations are linked to patterns of activity in the limbic system that correspond to an overwhelming sense of validity and urgency.

**E.** Prefrontal.

**F.** Although pathologic limbic states account for much of the core symptomatology of schizophrenia and are most amenable to alteration by dopamine receptor blockers, the neural abnormalities of schizophrenia are far more pervasive and involve other systems, particularly prefrontal, that are not susceptible to significant alteration by dopamine blockers.

**G.** Both genetic/congenital and major adverse experiences alter normal patterns of neural connectivity (neural connection strengths), and thus the initial conditions constraining the brain as a nonlinear dynamic system. Because of these alterations, the abrupt transitions to alternate states that may occur in such systems lead to alternative brain states that may be profoundly maladaptive. Unlike linear dynamic systems in which change is continuous and progressive, in nonlinear systems, the change may be inapparent for years and then occur suddenly in dramatic fashion.

The timing of adverse experiences may be crucial because only at certain states in the evolution of nonlinear dynamic systems are they susceptible to particular influences. Thus, occluding one eye in a newborn kitten will have a profound effect on the development of ocular dominance columns. However, occluding that eye 6 months later will have no effect because those columns are fully evolved by that time and cannot be "reversed" by blindfolding.

# List of Cases

# Index

Note: Page numbers followed by the letter f refer to figures; those followed by the letter t refer to tables; those followed by the letter c refer to cases; and those followed by the letter b refer to boxes.

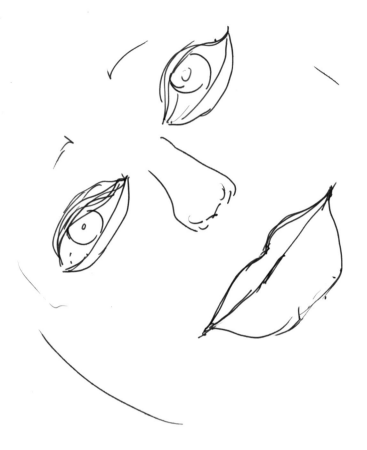